Critical Care Manual of Clinical Procedures and Competencies

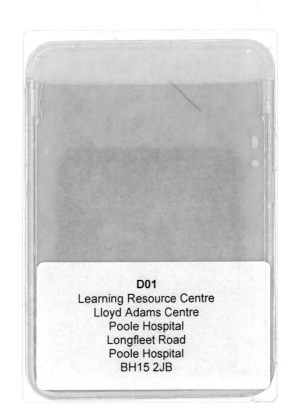

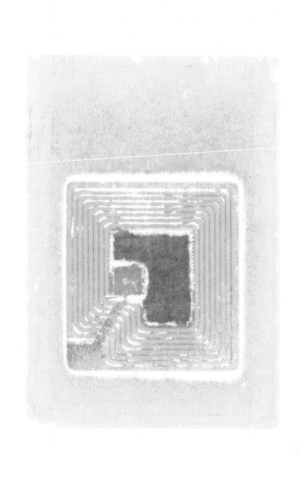

Critical Care Manual of Clinical Procedures and Competencies

Edited by

Jane Mallett
RN, BSc (Hons), MSc, PhD
Consultant in Health Care Development
Dorset, UK

John W. Albarran
RN, Dip N (Lon), BSc (Hons), PG Dip Ed, MSc, DPhil
Associate Professor in Cardiovascular Critical Care Nursing
Associate Head of Department for Research and Knowledge Exchange (Nursing & Midwifery)
Programme Manager for Doctorate in Health and Social Care
University of the West of England
Bristol, UK

Annette Richardson
RN, BSc (Hons), MBA
Nurse Consultant in Critical Care
Newcastle upon Tyne Hospitals NHS Foundation Trust
Newcastle upon Tyne, UK

Endorsed by

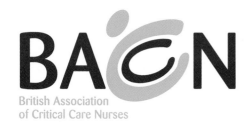

British Association
of Critical Care Nurses

WILEY Blackwell

This edition first published 2013
© 2013 by John Wiley & Sons, Ltd.

Registered office: John Wiley & Sons, Ltd, The Atrium, Southern Gate, Chichester, West Sussex, PO19 8SQ, UK

Editorial offices: 9600 Garsington Road, Oxford, OX4 2DQ, UK
The Atrium, Southern Gate, Chichester, West Sussex, PO19 8SQ, UK
2121 State Avenue, Ames, Iowa 50014-8300, USA

For details of our global editorial offices, for customer services and for information about how to apply for permission to reuse the copyright material in this book please see our website at www.wiley.com/wiley-blackwell.

Designations used by companies to distinguish their products are often claimed as trademarks. All brand names and product names used in this book are trade names, service marks, trademarks or registered trademarks of their respective owners. The publisher is not associated with any product or vendor mentioned in this book. It is sold on the understanding that the publisher is not engaged in rendering professional services. If professional advice or other expert assistance is required, the services of a competent professional should be sought.

The contents of this work are intended to further general scientific research, understanding, and discussion only and are not intended and should not be relied upon as recommending or promoting a specific method, diagnosis, or treatment by health science practitioners for any particular patient. The publisher and the author make no representations or warranties with respect to the accuracy or completeness of the contents of this work and specifically disclaim all warranties, including without limitation any implied warranties of fitness for a particular purpose. In view of ongoing research, equipment modifications, changes in governmental regulations, and the constant flow of information relating to the use of medicines, equipment, and devices, the reader is urged to review and evaluate the information provided in the package insert or instructions for each medicine, equipment, or device for, among other things, any changes in the instructions or indication of usage and for added warnings and precautions. Readers should consult with a specialist where appropriate. The fact that an organization or Website is referred to in this work as a citation and/or a potential source of further information does not mean that the author or the publisher endorses the information the organization or Website may provide or recommendations it may make. Further, readers should be aware that Internet Websites listed in this work may have changed or disappeared between when this work was written and when it is read. No warranty may be created or extended by any promotional statements for this work. Neither the publisher nor the author shall be liable for any damages arising herefrom.

Library of Congress Cataloging-in-Publication Data
Critical care manual of clinical procedures and competencies / edited by Jane Mallett, John W. Albarran, Annette Richardson.
    p. ; cm.
Includes bibliographical references and index.
ISBN 978-1-4051-2252-8 (pbk. : alk. paper)
I. Mallett, Jane, RGN. II. Albarran, John W. III. Richardson, Annette.
[DNLM: 1. Critical Care. 2. Critical Illness–therapy. 3. Monitoring, Physiologic. 4. Needs Assessment. WX 218]

616.02'8–dc23

2012044642

A catalogue record for this book is available from the British Library.

Wiley also publishes its books in a variety of electronic formats. Some content that appears in print may not be available in electronic books.

Cover image courtesy of the Editors
Cover design by Andy Meaden

Set in 9.5/11.5pt Sabon by Toppan Best-set Premedia Limited, Hong Kong
Printed in Singapore by Ho Printing Singapore Pte Ltd

1 2013

Contents

Chapter 1   Scope and delivery of evidence-based care   1

John W. Albarran and Annette Richardson

Chapter 2   Competency-based practice   11

Julie Scholes, Jo Richmond and Jane Mallett

Chapter 3   Recognizing and managing the critically ill and 'at risk' patient on a ward   27

Mandy Odell

Chapter 6   Monitoring of the cardiovascular system: insertion and assessment   173

Alan T. Platt, Sarah Conolly and Jonathan Round

Chapter 9   Continuous renal replacement therapies: assessment, monitoring and care   309

Annette Richardson and Jayne Whatmore

Chapter 10   Assessment and monitoring of analgesia, sedation, delirium and neuromuscular blockade levels and care   333

Phil Laws and Nicola Rudall

Chapter 11   Assessment and monitoring of neurological status   357

Margaret A. Douglas and Sarah E.C. Platt

Chapter 12   Assessment and care of tissue viability, and mouth and eye hygiene needs   381

Philip Woodrow, Judy Elliott and Pauline Beldon

Chapter 16   Rehabilitation from critical illness   489

Catherine I. Plowright and Christina Jones

Chapter 17   Withdrawal of treatment and end of life care for the critically ill patient   499

Natalie A. Pattison

Chapter 18   Cardiopulmonary resuscitation   531

Jackie S. Younker and Jasmeet Soar

List of contributors

John W. Albarran RN, DipN (Lon), BSc (Hons), PGDipEd, MSc, DPhil
Associate Professor in Cardiovascular Critical Care Nursing
Associate Head of Department for Research and Knowledge Exchange (Nursing and Midwifery)
Programme Manager for Doctorate in Health and Social Care
University of the West of England, Bristol

Micheala Allsop RN Dip, BSc (Hons)
Critical Care Research Nurse
Newcastle upon Tyne Hospitals NHS Foundation Trust

Andrew Baker MB, ChB, FRCA
Specialty Registrar, Anaesthesia and Critical Care
St James's University Hospital, Leeds

Pauline Beldon RN, PGDip
Tissue Viability Nurse Consultant
Epsom and St Helier University Hospitals NHS Trust

Elaine Coghill BSc (Hons), PGDipEd, MSc
Quality and Effectiveness Lead
Newcastle upon Tyne Hospitals NHS Foundation Trust

Sarah Conolly MB, BS, FRCA
Consultant in Anaesthesia and Intensive Care Medicine
James Cook University Hospital, Middlesbrough

Maureen Coombs RN, PhD, MBE
Professor of Clinical Nursing (Critical Care)
Graduate School of Nursing Midwifery and Health
Victoria University Wellington and Capital and Coast District Health Board, Wellington, New Zealand

Margaret A. Douglas RN, BSc (Hons), PGDip, MEd
Senior Lecturer
Northumbria University, Newcastle upon Tyne

Judy Dyos RN, PGDip, MSc
Lead Nurse Critical Care Education
University Hospital Southampton NHS Foundation Trust

Judy Elliott RN, BSc (Hons), MSc
Tissue Viability Nurse
East Kent Hospitals University NHS Foundation Trust

Vanessa Gibson RN, RNT, CertEd, PGDip, AdDip, MSc
Teaching Fellow and Principal Lecturer Critical Care
Northumbria University, Newcastle upon Tyne
Professional Advisor, National Board British Association of Critical Care Nurses

Karen Hill RN, BSc (Hons), MSc
Acuity Practice Development Matron
University Hospital Southampton NHS Foundation Trust
Lecturer in Critical Care Nursing
Southampton University
National Secretary, British Association of Critical Care Nurses

Christina Jones MPhil, PhD, CSci, MBACP, DHip
Nurse Consultant Critical Care Rehabilitation and Honorary Reader
Whiston Hospital, Liverpool
Institute of Ageing and Chronic Disease, University of Liverpool

Phil Laws MA, MRCP, FRCA, DipICM, EDIC, DipClinEd, FFICM
Consultant in Intensive Care Medicine and Anaesthesia
Newcastle upon Tyne Hospitals NHS Foundation Trust

Jane Mallett RN, BSc (Hons), MSc, PhD
Consultant in Health Care Development
Dorset

D.J. McWilliams BSc (Hons)
Clinical Specialist Physiotherapist – Critical Care
University Hospitals Birmingham NHS Foundation Trust

Ian Nesbitt MBBS, FRCA, DICM, FFICM
Consultant in Anaesthesia and Critical Care
Freeman Hospital, Newcastle upon Tyne

Mandy Odell RN, PGDip, MA, PhD
Nurse Consultant, Critical Care
The Royal Berkshire NHS Foundation Trust, Reading

Natalie A. Pattison RN, BSc (Hons), MSc, DNSc
Senior Clinical Nursing Research Fellow
The Royal Marsden NHS Foundation Trust

Alan T. Platt RN, BSc (Hons), PGDipEd, MSc
Senior Lecturer
Northumbria University, Newcastle upon Tyne

Sarah E.C. Platt MBBS, FRCA, DICM, FFICM
Consultant in Anaesthesia and Intensive Care
Royal Victoria Infirmary, Newcastle upon Tyne

Catherine I. Plowright RN, BSc, MSc, MA
Consultant Nurse Critical Care
Medway NHS Foundation Trust
Honorary Lecturer
Canterbury Christ Church University

Annette Richardson RN, BSc (Hons), MBA
Nurse Consultant Critical Care
Newcastle upon Tyne Hospitals NHS Foundation Trust

Jo Richmond RN, BSc
Corporate Nurse
Heart of England Foundation Trust

Jonathan Round MB, BS, FRCA
Specialty Registrar in Anaesthetics
Northern Deanery

Nicola Rudall BPharm (Hons), MSc, MRPharmS
Senior Lead Clinical Pharmacist, Perioperative and
Critical Care
Newcastle upon Tyne Hospitals NHS Foundation Trust

Kirsty Rutledge RN, BSc (Hons)
Sister, Critical Care
Newcastle upon Tyne Hospitals NHS Foundation Trust

Julie Scholes RN, DipN, DANS, MSc, DPhil
Professor of Nursing, Director of Post Graduate Studies,
Brighton Doctoral College
University of Brighton

Jasmeet Soar MA, MB, BChir, FRCA, FFICM
Consultant in Anaesthesia and Intensive Care
Medicine
Southmead Hospital, Bristol

Amanda Thomas BAppSc(Phy), MAppSc(Ex&SpSc),
MCSP, MACPRC
Clinical Specialist Physiotherapist
The Royal London Hospital

David Waters RN, PGDip, BA (Hons)
Senior Lecturer in Critical Care
Buckinghamshire New University, Uxbridge

Jayne Whatmore RN, Dip Health Studies
Sister, Critical Care
Newcastle upon Tyne Hospitals NHS Foundation Trust

Simon M. Whiteley MA, FRCA, FFICM
Consultant in Anaesthesia and Intensive Care
Leeds Teaching Hospitals NHS Trust

Philip Woodrow MA, RN, DipN, PGCE, MA
Practice Development Nurse, Critical Care
East Kent Hospitals University NHS Foundation Trust

Jackie S. Younker RN, PGCertEd, MSN
Senior Lecturer in Nursing
University of the West of England, Bristol

Foreword

In the last 15 years the majority of medical disciplines have adopted competency-based training as the standard approach to education. Nursing programmes were well in advance of doctors in this respect, having recognised for a long time the need to define professional practice (and hence the practitioners) in terms of knowledge, skills, attitudes and behaviours. This approach has been a powerful tool for creating a 'product specification' for clinicians whose abilities can so profoundly alter their patients' lives. Moreover, competencies make clear those elements which are unique to a particular discipline, and those which are shared between disciplines. There are few specialties in which shared and complementary competencies are more important for teamworking than intensive care medicine, and this has been given visible expression through the European CoBaTrICE competencies which have been adopted by both the ICM physician programme and Advanced Critical Care practitioners in the UK.

Critical Care Manual of Clinical Procedures and Competencies takes this work forward by linking competencies to their underlying rationale and to the evidence required to demonstrate their acquisition, contained within the framework of an accessible textbook. This is a valuable method of linking knowledge acquisition to reflective learning in the workplace.

Competence alone is not enough however, particularly in the complex and fast-changing world of critical care. New scientific knowledge converted into best practice guidelines may stand the test of time or may be found to be wrong as further research evidence accumulates. The competent practitioner must therefore also be a critical and questioning professional. The first two chapters of this Manual very properly discuss the nature of evidence in practice, and how research evidence and practice experience should be integrated. If this Manual succeeds in fostering both competence and critical capacity it will have done much to improve patient care.

Julian Bion
Professor of Intensive Care Medicine
University of Birmingham
Birmingham, UK

Foreword

'See one, do one, teach one' as a means of passing on clinical skills and abilities from one generation to the next may sound fine in principle and indeed served the professions well for many centuries. However, in our modern world such simple concepts in the learning process have, by necessity, become much more complex.

Critically ill patients (and their families) expect and deserve competent, skilled and professional care, anything less can and will kill them. It has been unacceptable for some decades now to allow anything but skilled and qualified nurses care for critically ill patients in health facilities even in the poorest of countries.

In the UK, there are 60 million people, of whom 1% are nurses (600,000), and of this number approximately 5% are critical care nurses (30,000) caring for about 6000 critically ill patients at any given time. If we assume that the chances of a clinician failing to follow a standardized clinical procedure resulted in serious harm or death had a probability of one in a thousand cases on any given day, then six critically ill patients will be seriously harmed or killed by such failings today in the UK! The risk of error, harm and death for critically ill patients is very real and very present and the potential for such harm to occur on any given day will be escalated when staff are poorly skilled and do not follow standardized, evidence based clinical procedures and care. We have a profound and humbling duty as nurses and clinicians to ensure only correct protocols and procedures of care and treatment are followed.

Critical Care Manual of Clinical Procedures and Competencies is a detailed, thoughtful and necessary resource to inform nurses and clinicians of the correct procedure to follow when caring for the critically ill patient and their family. Evidence based, practical procedures and competencies are described in sufficient detail to assist the practising clinician to understand and apply their skills safely.

Edited by critical care nursing and practice development leaders, and informed by dozens of respected experts in their respective specialties, *Critical Care Manual of Clinical Procedures and Competencies* sets a necessary standard for the delivery of safe and effective care in the field of critical care. It is an essential reference for all who lead, teach and practise in critical care.

Ged Williams
Executive Director of Nursing & Midwifery,
Gold Coast Hospitals & Health Service
Professor of Nursing, Griffith University, Gold Coast
Founding Chair/Past President,
World Federation of Critical Care Nurses
Former Director, World Federation of Societies
of Intensive Care and Critical Care Medicine
Founding President, Australian College
of Critical Care Nurses

Preface

Background

The inspiration for the *Critical Care Manual of Clinical Procedures and Competencies* goes back many years. I edited three editions of The Royal Marsden Hospital Manual for Clinical Nursing Procedures (RMH Manual) (1992, 1996 and 2000) and was overwhelmed by the response of professionals to a text that brought together a set of evidence-based procedures concerning cancer care. The RMH Manual was (and still is) viewed as an essential text and a 'bible' for nursing. The *Critical Care Manual of Clinical Procedures and Competencies* (*Critical Care Manual*) has developed from this tradition.

Vision and purpose

The *Critical Care Manual* aims to support optimum treatment and care for patients who are critically ill. In order to develop evidence-based procedures and the elements of competency required for each area, an open-minded approach has been utilised to consider whether there is enough evidence to support new specific clinical interventions and to challenge, as appropriate, current methods. This has involved rigorous examination of research findings, expert clinical consensus and existing practice by international experts. Hopefully, the result is a *Critical Care Manual* that will prove to be a useful resource to underpin the advancement of critical care practice and education. The next few years will reveal readers' views.

Scope

The *Critical Care Manual* differs from the RMH Manual in several ways. First, the focus is patients who are critically ill (levels 1 to 3, based on the classification devised in England [DH 2000]). The text, therefore, is aimed at a wide range of practitioners caring for critically ill patients, or those who are undertaking education in this area. Second, the patient and their requirements are seen as central to the management of critical illness. This necessitates a multidisciplinary team approach rather than individual profession-based procedures and competencies (although it is understood that

a specific group of professionals is more likely to undertake some of the procedures than others). Third, to assist further with integrated governance and education, fundamental and specific competencies have been developed and incorporated into the chapters.

The emphasis of the *Critical Care Manual* is 'general' critical care. Specialist critical care, such as that provided for patients with severe burns and/or large wounds, was felt to be beyond the scope of this particular version. This has enabled the first edition of the *Critical Care Manual* to be detailed, in depth and to include some specific management of patients. However, the editors would welcome practitioners' opinions on areas that it would be appropriate to include in the next edition. Organ donation may be one such topic.

Organisation and content

The *Critical Care Manual* has been broadly organised to guide practitioners from the tenets of critical care and the imperative for practitioner competency, through recognition of clinical deterioration, immediate critical care and care of those with multi-organ failure.

More specifically, the text first elucidates the development of the most recent concepts of critical care and its classification. The nature of evidence-based practice and, importantly, the principle of patient-centred practice is also debated (Chapter 1). In relation, Chapter 2 covers the relevance of competency-based practice to healthcare delivery and puts forward a framework for fundamental and procedure-related competencies (Fundamental Competency Statements and Specific Procedure Competency Statements respectively). The former are based on the fundamental patient needs highlighted within the Essence of Care 2010 (DH 2010) and include essential concerns such as communication, respect and dignity, pain management and safety, etc. When demonstrating competency to conduct a procedure it is important that both Fundamental and Specific Procedure competencies are met. This is because the inclusion of assessment of fundamental care facilitates a shift from evidence-based practice towards a more patient-centred approach. Every chapter includes Specific Procedure Competency Statements associated with each procedure.

However, for brevity the Fundamental Competency Statements are not repeated in each chapter. The competency statements have been designed to be able to be easily used in differing organisations' documentation.

The subsequent chapters cover the management of critical illness through a patient's potential journey, including inter alia:

- timely recognition of a deteriorating and critically ill patient on the ward (Chapter 3 provides an immediate perspective of assessment and interventions which are expanded in depth in later chapters)
- admission to a critical care unit (Chapter 4)
- clinical assessment and monitoring specific systems, such as the respiratory and cardiovascular systems, and neurological status
- clinical management of particular aspects of critical illness, for instance hydration and nutrition (via oral, enteral and parental routes); tissue viability; mouth and eye hygiene
- clinical interventions, for example titration of inotropic and vasopressor medication; continuous renal replacement therapy; analgesia and neuromuscular blockade; sleep promotion; physical mobility and exercise interventions (Chapters 5 to 14)
- physiological effects of the transfer of critically ill patients (such as horizontal and vertical gravitational forces) (Chapter 15)
- rehabilitation from critical illness (Chapter 16)
- withdrawal of treatment and end of life care (Chapter 17)
- cardiopulmonary resuscitation using the latest guidance from the Resuscitation Council (Chapter 18).

It is hoped that the *Critical Care Manual* will be of use to practitioners outside Europe, although it has been written from a UK perspective.

Acknowledgements

The *Critical Care Manual* would never have come to fruition without the expertise, understanding and guidance of my fellow editors, John Albarran and Annette Richardson, both of whom are eminent in the critical care arena. They have shown great patience as I have attempted to deconstruct the rationales for 'this is the way it is done'.

I would also like to thank all the authors for their diligence, thoroughness and professionalism in producing an excellent and readable final manuscript – sometimes to a very short deadline. I hope they are pleased with the outcome.

In addition, I would like wholeheartedly to thank the staff at Wiley-Blackwell for their support and dedication. In particular, and throughout the whole process, Beth Knight has been an exceptional and kind guide. Also, Catriona Cooper, for her hard work, clarity and support; and Rachel Coombs and James Benefield, who provided help at the beginning of the process.

Finally I would like to thank Ruth Swan, for her serenity and unfailing assistance in the closing stages of 'proofing'.

Jane Mallett
Consultant in Health Care Development

References

Department of Health (2000) *Comprehensive Critical Care: a review of adult critical care services*. London: DH.

Department of Health (2010) *Essence of Care 2010*. London: DH.

List of abbreviations

2,3-DPG	2,3-diphosphoglycerate	BIA	bio-electrical impedance analysis
5-FU	5-fluorouracil	BiPAP	bi-level positive airway pressure ventilation
AAC	augmentive or alternative communication	BIPAP	bi-level ventilation
AACCN	American Association of Critical Care Nurses	BLS	basic life support
ABCDE	airway, breathing, circulation, disability, exposure	BMA	British Medical Association
		BME	black and minority ethnic
A&E	Accident and Emergency	BMI	Body Mass Index
ABG	arterial blood gas	BNF	British National Formulary
ABPI	Ankle to Brachial Pressure Index	BOC	British Oxygen Company
ADH	antidiuretic hormone	B/P Sphyg	sphygmomanometer
ADL	activities of daily living	BPI	Brief Pain Inventory
ADR	adverse drug reaction	BSE	bovine spongiform encephalopathy
AED	automated external defibrillator	CAD	coronary artery disease
AFO	ankle foot orthosis	CARES	Cancer Rehabilitation Evaluation System
AHP	allied health professional	CAUTI	catheter-associated urinary tract infections
AIDS	acquired immune deficiency syndrome	CBT	cognitive behaviour therapy
AKI	acute kidney injury	CCA	critical care assistant
ALARP	as low as reasonably practicable	CCU	critical care unit
ALI	acute lung injury	CD	controlled drug
ALS	advanced life support	cfu	colony-forming units
ALT	alanine aminotransferase	CIPNM	critical illness polyneuromyopathy
ANH	acute normovolaemic haemodilution	CJD	Creutzfeldt–Jakob disease
ANP	atrial natriuretic peptide	CML	chronic myeloid leukaemia
ANS	autonomic nervous system	CMV	cytomegalovirus
ANTT	aseptic non-touch technique	CNS	central nervous system
AORN	Association of Perioperative Registered Nurses	CO	cardiac output
		COAD	chronic obstructive airways disease
AP	anteroposterior	COMA	Committee on Medical Aspects of Food Policy
APTR	activated partial thromboplastin ratio		
ARDS	acute respiratory distress syndrome	COPD	chronic obstructive pulmonary disease
ARSAC	Administration of Radioactive Substances Advisory Committee	COSHH	Control of Substances Hazardous to Health
		CPAP	continuous positive airway pressure
AST	aspartate aminotransferase	CPET	cardiopulmonary exercise testing
AT	anaerobic threshold	CPP	cerebral perfusion pressure
ATC	around the clock	CPR	cardiopulmonary resuscitation
AV	atrioventricular	CRRT	continuous renal replacement therapy
BACCN	British Association of Critical Care Nurses	CRP	C-reactive protein
BAL	bronchoalveolar lavage	CSAS	Chemotherapy Symptom Assessment Scale
BCG	bacille Calmette-Guérin	CSF	cerebrospinal fluid/colony-stimulating factor
BCSH	British Committee for Standards in Haematology		
		CSS	Central Sterile Services
BE	base excess	CSU	catheter specimen of urine

CT	computed tomography
CVAD	central venous access device
CVC	central venous catheter
CVP	central venous pressure
CVVH	continuous veno-venous haemofiltration
CVVHD	continuous veno-venous haemodialysis
CVVHDF	continuous veno-venous haemodiafiltration
CXR	chest X-ray
DBE	deep breathing exercises
DF	dorsiflexion
DFLST	decision to forego life-sustaining treatment
DH	Department of Health
DIC	disseminated intravascular coagulation
DM	diabetes mellitus
DMSO	dimethyl sulphoxide
DNA	deoxyribonucleic acid
DNACPR	do not attempt cardiopulmonary resuscitation
DNMBD	depolarizing neuromuscular blocking drug
DO_2	oxygen delivery
DPI	dry powder inhaler
DRE	digital rectal examination
DVLA	Driver and Vehicle Licensing Agency
DVT	deep vein thrombosis
EAPC	European Association of Palliative Care
EBM	evidence-based medicine
EBN	evidence-based nursing
EBP	evidence-based practice
EBRT	external beam radiotherapy
EBV	Epstein–Barr virus
ECF	extracellular fluid
ECG	electrocardiogram
ECM	extracellular matrix
ECMO	extracorporeal membrane oxygenation
EDTA	ethylenediaminetetra-acetic acid
EEG	electroencephalogram
EGFR	epidermal growth factor receptor
EIA	Equality Impact Assessment
ELISA	enzyme-linked immunosorbent assay
EMG	electromyogram
EMLA	eutectic mixture of local anaesthetics
EMS	electrical muscle stimulation
ENT	ears, nose and throat
EOG	electro-oculogram
EOLC	end of life care
EPO	erythropoietin
EPUAP	European Pressure Ulcer Advisory Panel
ERV	expiratory reserve volume
$ETCO_2$	end tidal CO_2
ETT	endotracheal tube
EUPAP	European Pressure Ulcer Advisory Panel
F(Fr)	French (gauge)
FBC	full blood count
FCS	fundamental competency statement
FEES	fibreoptic endoscopic evaluation of swallowing
FFI	fatal familial insomnia
FFP	fresh frozen plasma
FiO_2	fractional inspired oxygen
FRC	functional residual capacity
FTSG	full-thickness skin graft
FVC	forced vital capacity
GABA	gamma-aminobutyric acid
GCS	Glasgow Coma Scale
G-CSF	granulocyte-colony stimulating factor
GEDV	global end diastolic volume
GEF	global ejection fraction
GFR	glomerular filtration rate
GGT	gamma-glutamyl transferase
GI	gastrointestinal
GMC	General Medical Council
GM-CSF	granulocyte macrophage-colony stimulating factor
GP	general practitioner
GSL	general sales list
GTN	glyceryl trinitrate
HADS	Hospital Anxiety and Depression Scale
HBsAg	hepatitis B surface antigen
HBV	hepatitis B virus
HCA	healthcare assistant
HCAI	healthcare-acquired/associated infection
HCV	hepatitis C virus
HDN	haemolytic disease of the newborn
HDR	high dose rate
HDU	high-dependency unit
HEPA	high-efficiency particulate air
HFOV	high-frequency oscillation ventilation
HIV	human immunodeficiency virus
HLA	human leucocyte antigen
HME	heat and moisture exchange(r)
HOOF	home oxygen ordering form
HPA	Health Protection Agency
HR	heart rate
HSC	Health Service Circular/Health and Safety Commission
HSE	Health and Safety Executive
IASP	International Association for the Study of Pain
IBCT	incorrect blood component transfused
IC	inspiratory capacity
ICD	implantable cardioverter defibrillator
ICF	intracellular fluid
ICP	intracranial pressure
ICRP	International Commission on Radiological Protection
ICS	intraoperative cell salvage
ICSI	intracytoplasmic sperm injection
ICU	intensive care unit
IgM	immunoglobulin M
IJV	internal jugular vein
ILCOR	International Liaison Committee on Resuscitation
IMV	intermittent mandatory ventilation
INR	international normalized ratio

IPCT	infection prevention and control team
IPEM	Institute of Physics and Engineering in Medicine
IPPB	intermittent positive pressure breathing
IRMER	Ionizing Radiation (Medical Exposure) Regulations
IRR	infra-red radiation
IRV	inspiratory reserve volume
ISC	intermittent self-catheterization
ITBV	intrathoracic blood volume
IV	intravenous
IVC	inferior vena cava
IVF	in vitro fertilization
IUI	intrauterine insemination
JPAC	Joint UKBTS/NIBSC Professional Advisory Committee
KGF	keratinocyte growth factor
KVO	keep vein open
LANSS	Leeds Assessment of Neuropathic Symptoms and Signs
LBC	liquid-based cytology
LCP-ICU	Liverpool Care Pathway for Intensive Care Units
LCT	long-chain triglyceride
LDR	low dose rate
LMA	laryngeal mask airway
LMN	lower motor neurone
LMWH	low molecular weight heparin
LP	lumbar puncture
LPA	Lasting Power of Attorney
LVEDP	left ventricle end diastolic pressure
MAC	*Mycobacterium avium intracellulare*
MAOI	monoamine oxidase inhibitor
MAP	mean arterial pressure
MBP	mean blood pressure
MC&S	microscopy, culture and sensitivity
MCT	medium-chain triglyceride
MDA	Medical Devices Agency
MDI	metered dose inhaler
MDT	multidisciplinary team
ME	medical examiner
MET	medical emergency team
MEWS	Modified Early Warning System
MHRA	Medicines and Healthcare Products Regulatory Agency
MI	myocardial infarction
MIC	minimum inhibitory concentration
MLD	manual lymphatic drainage
MPQ	McGill Pain Questionnaire
MRI	magnetic resonance imaging
MRSA	meticillin-resistant *Staphylococcus aureus*
MSAS	Memorial Symptom Assessment Scale
MSCC	metastatic spinal cord compression
MSU	midstream specimen of urine
NANDA	North American Nursing Diagnosis Association

NAVA	neurally adjusted ventilatory assist
NBTC	National Blood Transfusion Committee
NCEPOD	National Confidential Enquiry into Patient Outcome and Death
NEWS	National Early Warning System
NDNMBD	non-depolarizing neuromuscular blocking drug
NG	nasogastric
NHS	National Health Service
NHSCSP	NHS Cervical Screening Programme
NHSE	National Health Service Executive
NICE	National Institute for (Health and) Clinical Excellence
NIV	non-invasive ventilation
NMC	Nursing and Midwifery Council
NMDA	N-methyl-d-aspartate
NMDS	neuromuscular blocking drug
NPA	nasopharyngeal airway
NPSA	National Patient Safety Agency
NPUAP	National Pressure Ulcer Advisory Panel
NPWT	negative pressure wound therapy
NRS	numerical rating scales
NRT	nicotine replacement therapy
NSAID	non-steroidal anti-inflammatory drug
NSAT	Newcastle Sleep Assessment Tool
NSF	National Service Framework
ODP	operating department practitioner
OGD	oesophagogastroduodenoscopy
ONS	Oncology Nursing Society
OPA	oropharyngeal airway
OSCE	objective structured clinical examination
OT	occupational therapist
OTC	over the counter
OTFC	oral transmucosal fentanyl citrate
P	pharmacy medicines
PA	posterior anterior
$PaCO_2$	partial pressure of carbon dioxide
PACU	peri-anaesthesia care unit
PAD	preoperative autologous donation
PAO_2	partial pressure of alveolar oxygen
PAP	pulmonary artery pressure
PART	patient-at-risk team
PAWP	pulmonary artery wedge pressure
PC	*Pneumocystis carinii*
PCA	patient-controlled analgesia
PCEA	patient-controlled epidural analgesia
PCS	postoperative cell salvage
PCV-VG	pressure control ventilation-volume guarantee
PDPH	postdural puncture headache
PDT	percutaneous dilatational tracheostomy
PE	pulmonary embolism/pulmonary embolus
PEA	pulseless electrical activity
PEEP	positive end-expiratory pressure
PEF(R)	peak expiratory flow (rate)
PEG	percutaneous endoscopically placed gastrostomy

PEP	postexposure prophylaxis	SCI	spinal cord injury
PET	positron emission tomography	SCNS	Supportive Care Needs Survey
PF	plantar flexion	SCUF	slow continuous ultrafiltration
PGD	patient group direction	SDF	stromal cell-derived factor
PGSGA	patient-generated subjective global assessment	SGA	subjective global assessment
PHCT	primary healthcare team	SHOT	Serious Hazards of Transfusion
PICC	peripherally inserted central catheter (long line)	SI	Système International
		SIMV	simulated intermittent mandatory ventilation
PN	parenteral nutrition	SIMV-PC	synchronized intermittent mandatory ventilation pressure control
PNS	peripheral nervous system		
POA	preoperative assessment	SIMV-VC	synchronized intermittent mandatory ventilation volume control
POCT	point-of-care testing		
POM	prescription-only medicine	SIRS	systemic inflammatory response syndrome
PPE	personal protective equipment		
PPV	pulse pressure variation	SL	semi-lunar
PrP	prion protein	SLD	simple lymphatic drainage
PSAR	Pain and Assessment Records	SLE	systemic lupus erythematosus
PSCC	primary/benign spinal cord compression	SLEDD	sustained low-efficiency daily diafiltration
PSD	patient-specific direction	SLT	speech and language therapist
psi	pounds per square inch	SNRI	serotonin-norepinephrine reuptake inhibitor
PT	physiotherapist	SOP	standard operating procedure
PTFE	polytetrafluoroethylene	SPCS	specific procedure competency statement
PTHrp	parathormone-related polypeptide	SPI	Social Problems Inventory
PTSD	post traumatic stress disorder	SPN	Safer Practice Notice
PTSS-14	Post Traumatic Syndrome 14 Question Inventory	SpO_2	saturation of haemoglobin by oxygen
		SRHH	Self-Report Health History
PUO	pyrexia of unknown origin	SSG	split-thickness or split skin graft
PVC	polyvinylchloride	SSI	surgical site infection
PVD	peripheral vascular disease	SSRI	selective serotonin reuptake inhibitor
PVR	pulmonary vascular resistance	SUI	serious untoward incident
PWO	partial withdrawal occlusion	SV	stroke volume
RA	right atrium	SVC	superior vena cava
RAP	right atrial pressure	SvO_2	mixed venous oxygen saturation
RAS	reticular activating system	SVR	systemic vascular resistance
RASS	Richmond Agitation and Sedation Scale	swg	standard wire gauge
RBC	red blood cell	TACO	transfusion-associated circulatory overload
RCA	root cause analysis	TA-GVHD	transfusion-associated graft-versus-host disease
RCN	Royal College of Nursing		
RCS	Royal College of Surgeons of England	TB	tuberculosis
RCUK	Resuscitation Council UK	TCA	tricyclic antidepressant
REM	rapid eye movement	TCI	target-controlled infusion
RIG	radiologically inserted gastrostomy	TED	thromboembolic deterrent
RNI	reference nutrient intake	TENS	transcutaneous electrical nerve stimulation
ROSC	return of spontaneous circulation	TIVA	total intravenous anaesthesia
RSV	respiratory syncytial virus	TLC	total lung capacity
RSVP	reason, story, vital signs, plan	TLD	thermoluminescent
RTO	Resuscitation Training Officer	TNP	topical negative pressure therapy
RTOG	Radiation Therapy Oncology Group	TPI	*Treponema pallidum* immobilization
RV	residual volume	TPN	total parenteral nutrition
SA	sinoatrial	TRALI	transfusion-related acute lung injury
SABRE	Serious Adverse Blood Reactions and Events	TRSC	Therapy Related Symptom Checklist
SARS	severe acute respiratory syndrome	TSE	transmissible spongiform encephalopathy
SaO_2	arterial oxygen saturation	TSS	toxic shock syndrome
SBAR	Situation-Background-Assessment-Recommendation	TT	tracheostomy tube
		TTO	to take out
SBO	small bowel obstruction	TURP	transurethral resection of prostate
SCC	spinal cord compression	TV	tidal volume
		UH	unfractionated heparin

UMN	upper motor neurone	VF	ventricular fibrillation
UTI	urinary tract infection	VPF	vascular permeability factor
V/Q	ventilation/perfusion	V/Q ratio	ventilation/perfusion ratio
VAD	vascular access device	Vt	tidal volume
VAP	ventilator-associated pneumonia	VT	ventricular tachycardia
VAT	venous assessment tool	VTE	venous thromboembolism
VC	vital capacity	VTM	viral transport medium
vCJD	variant Creutzfeldt–Jakob disease	WBC	white blood cell
VCV	volume control ventilation	WBP	wound bed preparation
VDRL	Venereal Disease Research Laboratory	WHO	World Health Organization
VDS	verbal descriptor scales	WOB	work of breathing
VEGF	vascular endothelial growth factor	WR	Wassermann reaction

Chapter 1

Scope and delivery of evidence-based care

John W. Albarran[1] and Annette Richardson[2]

[1]University of the West of England, Bristol, UK
[2]Newcastle upon Tyne Hospitals NHS Foundation Trust, Newcastle upon Tyne, UK

Critical Care Manual of Clinical Procedures and Competencies, First Edition.
Edited by Jane Mallett, John W. Albarran, and Annette Richardson.
© 2013 John Wiley & Sons, Ltd. Published 2013 by John Wiley & Sons, Ltd.

Importance of critical care

Healthcare around the world, to a greater or lesser degree, encompasses the treatment and care of people with a wide range of conditions. Some will be critically ill and clinical decisions and interventions will have immediate and fundamental impact on whether they live and/or their degree of recovery. It is, therefore, imperative that treatment and care of critically ill patients is the best that can be provided. Excellence, however, requires appropriate interventions with a strong evidence base and practitioners[1] who are competent to deliver treatment and care. The aim of *Critical Care Manual of Clinical Procedures and Competencies* is to support optimum treatment and care for patients who are critically ill by detailing the latest research and rationales for evidence-based procedures and competencies in each specific area. As such, the manual is ideally placed to be used as a reference and resource for advancing critical care practice and education.

Background and classification of critically ill patients

Critical care[2] has developed considerably over many years, with a number a key policies and initiatives emphasizing and escalating the pace of change. A significant transformation took place following the publication of the critical care modernisation policy document entitled 'Comprehensive Critical Care' (DH 2000a). This strategy document led to a restructure of the organization of critical care services by advocating that provision of care should extend beyond the walls of intensive care units and be comprehensive in meeting patients' needs. It highlighted the provision of care within a continuum of primary, secondary and tertiary care, with the greater part of services in the secondary care setting. It set out the vision for how critical care should be delivered, replacing the division of intensive care beds and high dependency beds with a classification system focused on levels of care (Table 1.1). 'Critical care' is a global definition, and is used as an umbrella term for intensive and high dependency care and includes the care of critically ill patients on the ward (DH 2000a: 7).

The classification system provides a blueprint for delivering critical care services along a continuum which spans from managing the healthcare needs of patients with multi-organ failure patient (level 3) to those at risk of their condition deteriorating (level 1). Individuals whose needs can be met on general hospital wards without support from the critical care outreach teams are not considered critically ill (level 0).

Table 1.1 Classification of critically ill patients (DH 2000a, © Crown copyright 2011)

Classification	Definition
Level 0	Patients whose needs can be met through routine ward care in an acute hospital
Level 1	Patients at risk of their condition deteriorating, or recently relocated from higher levels of care, whose needs can be met on an acute ward with additional advice and support from a critical care team
Level 2	Patients requiring more detailed observation or intervention, including support for a single failing organ system or postoperative care, and those 'stepping down' from higher levels of care
Level 3	Patients requiring advanced respiratory support alone or basic respiratory support together with support of at least two organ systems. This level includes all complex patients requiring support for multi-organ failure

The organization of care for different categories of patient varies according to patient requirements and also how this is accommodated by the local service. At present, patients with level 3 needs are generally cared for in a clinical area that is designated primarily for this category of patient and is often referred to as an intensive care unit. This is because this group need high levels of monitoring, intervention and organ support that requires specialist expertise and equipment. Sometimes the level 3 care facility is also a 'specialty only' unit (such as patients with neurological problems or burns).

Patients with level 2 and 1 needs are cared for in a variety of settings. These include a designated level 2 and/or 1 unit (which may or may not include specialist-only beds); specific area/beds within a level 3 facility (which may or may not include specialist-only beds); and specific area/beds within a level 0 care facility (which may or may not include specialist-only beds). Patients requiring level 2 and 1 care on a level 0 care facility are often there on a temporary basis with the support of the multidisciplinary critical care outreach team.

While the levels of critical care (1 to 3) are clearly defined (DH 2000a) and therefore allow for a joint understanding of the needs of patients and the required level of care, a variety of service organizations' designations and terms have been used to describe critical care facilities; these include intensive care unit (ITU or ICU), critical care unit (CCU), high dependency unit (HDU), special care unit (SCU) and post-anaesthetic care unit (PACU). It is important, therefore, that the patient's needs and the care facility are clearly and accurately identified and that all involved in service planning and provision and delivery of care have a shared understanding in order to effectively and efficiently meet the patient's requirements. For the purposes of this manual the term 'critical care' follows that of more recent documentation and developments and refers to patients requiring care at levels 1 to 3.

---

[1] In this text the term practitioner is used to refer to all staff who deliver care. This includes, for example, doctors, therapists, dieticians, nurses, etc. It also extends to healthcare assistants involved in delivery of care.

[2] The term 'critical care' is generally intended to include care and treatment.

It is worth noting that as well as the varying levels of critical care requirement and the locations where this care can be delivered, the characteristics of the patient population are important in determining the level of care required. The considerable heterogeneity of the patients is a challenge, as differences in age and sex; type, trajectory and duration of disease; co-morbidities and complications all cause difficulties in defining a patient requiring critical care (Vincent and Singer 2010).

The varying patient characteristics and the complexity of caring for the critically ill has resulted in the requirement for teams of multidisciplinary specialist critical care practitioners to deliver the care, including: doctors, nurses, advanced critical care practitioners, physiotherapists, dieticians and healthcare assistants engaged in patient care. Although at times specific individuals within the team are involved in the delivery of particular aspects of the care, the overall delivery of critical care is highly reliant on teamwork and the ability of a number of varied types of practitioner to deliver the care over time. Therefore throughout this manual the term critical care practitioner (or practitioner) will be used to represent the various specialist critical care roles.

National guidance

Over the past few years NHS strategies have focused on improving quality, patient care safety, patient outcomes and cost effectiveness of treatment and care (DH 2007a, 2009, 2010a; Richardson 2011). To achieve this, the critical care modernisation strategy recommended that guidelines, standards and protocols for critical care be developed by multiprofessional staff (DH 2000a)[3] (*see also* Table 1.2). In 1999, the National Institute for Clinical Excellence was introduced to act as a politically independent body aimed at improving the quality of care by setting national standards, developing evidence-based guidelines for a variety of conditions and issuing guidance on patient safety (Sibson 2011). It was high-profile examples (such as the Bristol Royal Inquiry [BRI 2001] into children's heart surgery) that have in part served to precipitate key developments and changes in how healthcare professionals' competence is monitored (Sibson 2011). In an attempt to regain public confidence and control the spiralling economy, the NHS engaged in implementing a series of wide-reaching measures. These were devised to reduce risks by ensuring that clinical interventions were informed by an evidence base, regular auditing of practice, and by the maintenance of staff performance and competency. Alongside these NHS initiatives were the rising public expectations for more explicit justification and rationale for interventions used in patient care and for increased engagement with service users in the evaluation of healthcare services (Williams 2006; NICE 2007, 2009).

[3] Although the use of guidelines is not unique to critical care, it is central objective of the NHS strategy.

In summary, the policies and changes to the NHS and critical care have collectively spearheaded improvements in the delivery and management of critical care services, resulting in greater inter-professional collaboration serving to enhance patient outcomes. Stemming from these changes has been the establishment of patient care pathways, a more coherent and systematic approach to the early identification of patient at risk of deterioration, more effective use of critical care beds, and improvements in length of critical care unit stay, discharge rates and mortality rates (Williams 2006).

Evidence-based practice

Concomitantly with major organizational changes and reforms, a new evangelical movement in the form of evidence-based medicine (which was subsequently a term applied to other professions in the form of evidence-based practice/healthcare, nursing) became embedded within the NHS and radically transformed the overall culture, clinical management of patients and research activity (Davies and Nutley 1999; Trinder and Reynolds 2000; Craig and Smyth 2002). Universal acceptance and adoption of this phenomenon was unparalleled within healthcare and led to the establishment of international networks of evidence-based practice communities and support as exemplified by the Cochrane Collaboration. According to Trinder and Reynolds (2000: 12), factors such as economic constraints and concerns by health practitioners and the public over standards of clinical practice made evidence-based practice intellectually and intuitively appealing and a natural way forward, quite simply 'a product of its time'. Prior to this point, many interventions and practices for patients had been based on rituals, traditions and the individual preferences of clinicians. In many instances, practices and interventions lacked a scientific basis and were potentially detrimental to patients' wellbeing and recovery (Swinkels et al. 2002). This approach to care and treatment was expensive, did not provide a standardized approach to management, even for patients with the same conditions and in turn led to inconsistency in outcomes. For the purposes of this chapter, the term 'evidence-based practice' is used, as it can be considered a more generic term for the wider healthcare professions.

Definitions

Evidence-based medicine/practice (EBP) has been defined as:

> the conscientious, explicit and judicious use of current best evidence in making decisions about the care of individual patients, based on skills which allow the doctor to evaluate both personal experience and external evidence in a systematic and objective manner.
> (Sackett et al. 1997: 71)

In the above definition it is implied that the expertise of clinicians and patient choice should be integrated with best

Table 1.2 Differences between protocols, procedures and guidelines

Protocols	Procedures	Guidelines
A protocol should be developed by a multidisciplinary team with the aim of providing a complete account of the steps required to deliver care or treatment to a patient Typically they are either developed locally to implement national standards (such as National Service frameworks or guidelines produced by NICE; see below) or to establish care provision drawing from the best available evidence in the absence of nationally agreed benchmarks (Institute for Innovation and Improvement 2011)	Procedures are operational elements that arise from local protocols. They are applicable to individual patients with each detailing the order of activities to be performed It is not uncommon for these to be developed prior to writing a protocol and they should also be underpinned by the best evidence	Clinical guidelines are systematically developed statements that seek to support healthcare professionals and patients' decision making under specific circumstances (Thomas and Hotchkiss 2002) Guidelines can cover conditions (asthma), symptoms (chest pain), clinical procedures (endotracheal suctioning) and responses (resuscitation of unresponsive and unconscious people). Again, guidelines are intended to reduce variations in practice, to optimize care and treatment, and provide the means of increasing the accountability of healthcare professionals. The effectiveness of guidelines is based on a systematic appraisal of research and meeting a series of key criteria that include reliability and validity of data, cost-effectiveness and clinical applicability (Thomas and Hotchkiss 2002). The development of clinical guidelines is a labour-intensive process that demands skill in critical appraisal, time to systematically evaluate the quality of research, consultation with experts, and therefore may take two years to complete (Snowball 1999)

evidence, derived from specific sources of empirical data, to inform decisions about the care of individual patients (Gray 2009). In practical terms, EBP is the systematic evaluation of published evidence to assess the effectiveness of current practices, and novel or established interventions (Hewitt-Taylor 2003). Best research evidence in this context is described as:

> clinically relevant research, often from the basic sciences of medicine, but especially from patient centred clinical research.
>
> (Sackett et al. 2000: 1)

The above statements specify the direction of what should happen and describe practical techniques to address the chasm between research and clinical care (Trinder and Reynolds 2000). In particular, research that has direct application to patient care is differentiated from clinical studies without immediate and practical relevance. The focus on clinical relevance is intended to help healthcare practitioners concentrate their attentions on research that benefits patients and improves the delivery of high-quality care provision. The inclusion of structured methods for systematically evaluating research is pivotal in supporting healthcare practitioners to assess the merits and contributions of research to their field. Finally, EBP offers a platform to enable practitioners to make decisions that reflect research findings and to apply empirical data to the care and management of individual patients (Trinder and Reynolds 2000).

In contrast, clinical expertise applies to:

> the ability to use our clinical skills and past experience to rapidly identify each patient's unique health state and diagnosis, their individual risks and benefits of potential interventions, and their personal values and expectations.
>
> (Sackett et al. 2000: 1)

Integrating patient values is about addressing:

> the unique preferences, concerns and expectations each patient brings to the clinical encounter and which must be integrated into clinical decisions if they are to serve the patient.
>
> (Sackett et al. 2000: 1)

Overall, EBP is about developing vision whereby the quality of care can be advanced not only through the application of patient-centred clinical research but by incorporating systematically generated research-based knowledge, the expertise derived from practice, and the preferences and perspectives of those under the care of healthcare providers (Pearson and Craig 2002). According to Trinder and Reynolds (2000), a key element of EBP, aside from providing directions about what should happen, is the provision of practical approaches and guidance for resolving the gaps between research and patient care. The evidence-based practice ideology also incorporates a framework for making clinical decisions drawn from clinical studies for applying these to individual patients.

Delivering care that is based on evidence of effectiveness can standardize service delivery, improve diagnostic techniques, optimize health outcomes and maximize the use of healthcare resources (Bick and Graham 2010). EBP can also enable clinical staff to respond to the needs and demands of changing patient demography (Cook et al. 1996). Similarly, evidence-based clinical effectiveness can be defined as a set of specific clinical interventions which, when used for a particular patient or population, achieves its purposes. The intention is to maintain and improve health and secure the greatest possible health gain from available and limited resources (DH 2007b). The ideology has also served to overcome the gap between research and clinical practice by encouraging enquiry directed at improving patient outcomes.

The ultimate aims of evidence-based practice can be summarised as being to:

1   provide appropriate and effective care
2   standardize treatments
3   make best use of available resources
4   improve outcomes
5   promote safety and reduce harm.

Youngblut and Brooten (2001) provide a useful distinction between practice supported by evidence and practice based on evidence. In the former, for example, articles, but not necessarily research, may be retrieved to support and continue a practice or protocol. In the case of the latter, the evidence from well-designed research studies is systematically reviewed, the recommendations are identified and the practice/protocol is amended accordingly. While the benefits of evidence-based practice have been well documented in terms of standardizing care, cost effectiveness, improving the quality of care, and mortality and morbidity outcomes, there are studies reporting that many critical care practitioners do not appreciate the value of research to their role and are unfamiliar with methods of accessing and systematically evaluating data from published work (Bucknall et al. 2001; Pravikoff et al. 2005). It has been acknowledged that the development of the EBP movement requires that healthcare practitioners are trained in interpreting and using research data, and that research findings are widely disseminated to facilitate their accessibility (Cook et al. 1996; Trinder and Reynolds 2000; Newman and Roberts 2002).

Debates on the nature of 'evidence'

There are many areas of contention and confusion regarding evidence-based practice, many of which concern definitions of 'what counts as evidence' and how it differs from 'science,' 'research' and 'clinical effectiveness' (Swinkels et al. 2002; Murray et al. 2008). Key challenges have also related to the meaning that patients, family members, healthcare professionals and other stakeholders attribute to the concept of EBP. In broad terms, 'evidence' may comprise findings generated from research, understandings from basic sciences, clinical expertise and expert opinion (Youngblut and Brooten 2001). It may also encompass knowledge from expert patients; indeed, those with chronic conditions are well informed about their conditions and current treatments. This reflects the current consensus that evidence in delivering patient care can come from a number of sources (Bick and Graham 2010).

This view is in stark contrast with the EBP dogma, where data from experimental, quasi-experimental trials and case control studies (which embrace 'quantitative research' designs) are accorded higher status than other forms and sources of evidence. This is due to the perception that data from these study types is associated with a more scientific (positivist), bias-free, (so-called) objective and rigorous traditions (Murray et al. 2008) (see Table 1.3). Consequently, it is believed that the results of such studies can be replicated and applied to wider populations. Importantly, these studies are instrumental in establishing the safety and effectiveness of clinical interventions and in confidently predicting responses to therapeutic measures (Hewitt-Taylor 2003). Within the hierarchy of evidence, large, properly designed randomized controlled trials (RCTs) are considered by some as the 'gold standard' for determining cause-and-effect relationships and as such have greater potential to influence clinical decision making. However, the results of a single study are usually not sufficient to support a wholesale adoption of either a treatment or clinical intervention. Nevertheless, evidence analysed as part of a systematic review of RCTs may produce findings to either recommend the cessation of accepted treatments and diagnostic tests or the implementation of more accurate, reliable and effective substitutes. Consequently, data produced from RCTs have dominated debates on what counts as evidence, causing confusion for many healthcare practitioners and other healthcare stakeholders (Swinkels et al. 2002).

Table 1.3 Hierarchy of evidence levels

Level	Descriptor
I	Evidence obtained from at least one systematic review of multiple well-designed randomized controlled trials
II	Evidence obtained from a least one properly designed randomized controlled trial of appropriate size
III	Evidence from well-designed trials without randomization; cohort, time series or matched case-controlled studies
IV	Evidence from well-designed non-experimental studies from more than one centre or research group
V	Opinions of respected authorities, based on clinical evidence, descriptive studies and reports of expert committees

Proponents of the hierarchy of evidence are critical about data from qualitative studies due to the lack of control, objectivity, rigour and because of their inability to generalize the findings to a wider population (Swinkels et al. 2002). 'Qualitative studies' are typically concerned with understanding human behaviour, experiences and reactions to events, and as such often rely on semi-structured interviews, observations and interpreting data sources such as photographs, biographies, diaries, historical archives and other textual material. However, in developing clinical practice it is not always methodologically or ethically appropriate to use RCTs to study particular aspects of care. In addition, not all practice aspects important to patients can be studied through clinical trials for ethical, cultural and political reasons (Youngblut and Brooten 2001). Studying the experiences and perceptions of patients can provide useful insights and understandings, unveiling the challenges and difficulties they encounter during critical care unit admission that cannot be captured through quantitative data. Qualitative data and subsequent analysis can also provide insights into whether some treatments are acceptable to patients and highlight directions for possible interventions (MRC 2000, 2008). Critics of the EBP argue that an over-reliance on experimental studies displaces the role of intuitive judgements, unsystematic clinical experience and pathophysiological rationale in guiding decisions about the care of patients (Goding and Edwards 2002; Swinkels et al. 2002).

Viewing evidence through a single lens offers a distorted perspective of knowledge and evidence, and in the case of quantitative outlook, the approach reduces and objectifies patients into numerical values. Adopting a purely quantitative approach will obscure the opportunity to capture the multidimensional nature of a patient's experiences and perceptions of their illness. Hek (2000) and Mckenna (1999) advocate including the perspectives of patients, family members or carers and the expertise of clinicians, and combining these with data from rigorous and robust studies to produce a more individualized and informed approach to decision making. This perspective is aligned with notions of patient centeredness and holistic care delivery (Hek 2000). Increasingly, research councils now advocate the inclusion of exploratory qualitative studies involving patients to inform the development of complex interventions trials in helping to assess acceptability, compliance, issues of sample recruitment, retention and delivery of intervention (MRC 2000, 2008).

Two further areas of debate revolve around the commissioning and funding of research and on the outcomes of RCTs. Increasingly, many large international RCTs are funded by industry, often with little input from patient groups or other key stakeholders, the outcomes of which may be primarily driven by commercial interests. While public and patient engagement in the UK is contributing to health service development (DH 2004; NICE 2010), this involvement needs to expand to developing the research agenda that reflects the health needs and priorities of society. The introduction of Academic Health Science Networks

(2012) seeks to encourage greater collaboration between a number of stakeholders, including industry partners, to drive forward the dissemination of innovations, the translation and promotion of research, and to support education and training to enhance the delivery of high-quality care provision which is responsive to the needs of the population and which benefits the economy (DH 2012).

Turning to the results of RCTs, the outcomes are primarily focused on implementing treatments that apply to the average patient, rather than the individual. This distinction is of importance to service users. However, despite the above debates there has been growing recognition, within critical care and beyond, that qualitative data and analysis can complement quantitative findings and contribute to the effectiveness of care measures and improve professional practice and the overall quality of the research (Nordgren et al. 2008; Rusinová et al. 2009). A qualitative approach to research can also illuminate contextual features, as well as the success or failure of interventions by understanding patients and healthcare practitioners' acceptance and/or rejection of treatments and EBP respectively (Britten 2010).

To counter and challenge the traditional evidence-based hierarchy, Rycroft-Malone et al. (2004) have proposed an alternative for a broader evidence base that emphasises and places patients centre stage. It is further argued that effective practice is determined through practitioner interactions and relationships with patients and this can be assessed by drawing up several sources of evidence (see Figure 1.1).

The integration of these elements allows for scientific and empirical sources to meld together with practitioner expertise and patient preferences in a more holistic approach. Importantly, knowledge gained from practice and personal knowledge associated with life experiences of dealing with different contexts and patient situations accords a wealth of expertise that practitioners (and some patients and carers) contribute to the decision-making process. This proposed

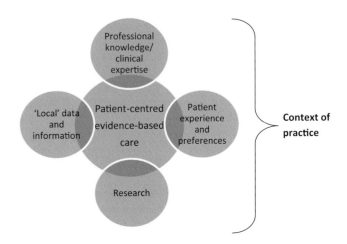

Figure 1.1 Four sources of evidence base for patient-centred practice. (From Rycroft-Malone et al. 2004. Reproduced with permission from Wiley.)

framework recognizes that integrating evidence from research is vital, but care must also reflect the individual's experiences, values and preferences, and the practitioner has a key role in mediating interventions to ensure compliance and improved patient outcomes (Rycroft-Malone et al. 2004). Local context can provide a wealth of sources that can shape and improve practice; this can include local and national policies, audits of practice, patient stories and population demographics. All these should be incorporated to inform the evidence base that guides the delivery of patient-centred healthcare. An example of how patient, carer and practitioners' expertise and research can be brought together is the development of benchmarks for fundamental care (DH 2010b). This document (*Essence of Care 2010*) was designed to reflect patients' and carers' views of their health and social care needs and preferences. It can be used with other sources of evidence to improve patient-centred care (*see also* Chapter 2). In summary, the Rycroft-Malone model offers an alternative approach in understanding evidence-based practice, it acknowledges that scientific knowledge is key to informing decisions, but it equally acknowledges that practitioners draw on a variety of important sources to guide and shape patient care.

Another related concept emanating from North America is the best 'patient-focused practice' model (McCauley and Irwin 2006), which likewise challenges approaches to delivering individualized patient care (Kjörnsberg et al. 2010). The values behind patient-focused practice aim to promote a holistic patient-centred approach and increase practitioner–patient interactions, where communication, continuity of care and congruence are central concepts (McCauley and Irwin 2006; Kjörnsberg et al 2010). There is also an emphasis on multidisciplinary collaboration, patient and public involvement in decisions affecting care giving with more open consideration to including multiple sources of evidence and perspectives.

Supporting evidence-based practice

In practical terms, there are many activities within healthcare that can support evidence-based practice and clinical effectiveness, and these can be split into three main components. The inclusion of service users is important and part of an overall NHS strategy (Thomas and Hotchkiss 2002). The following should be in place nationally and locally within organizations.

- First, setting evidence-based standards through the development of local and national evidence based guidelines, protocols and procedures (Thomas and Hotchkiss 2002). Guidelines, procedures and protocols are a mainstay for improving standards of care, reducing patient risk and enhancing the quality of service provision. They all aim to achieve the same outcomes, but have distinctive functions (*see* Table 1.2). Another development includes the introduction of 'care bundles' that are a collection of guidance developed from a strong research base. They are another example of how patient outcomes can be systematically improved and complications reduced by standardizing practice (Fulbrook and Mooney 2003; McClelland 2007; Tolentino-Delos Reyes et al. 2007; Wip and Napolitano 2009; Robb et al. 2010).

- Second, activities supporting delivery of evidence-based standards/effective care such as providing staff with knowledge and skills, clinical decision support systems and assessment of competencies (Dawes et al. 2000). Developing and maintaining generic and specialist competencies through ongoing assessment are the cornerstones for guaranteeing that standards are high and that patient risk is minimized (these issues are explored further in Chapter 2).

- Third, a quality process of improving patient care and outcomes through the systematic review of practice and measuring performance change against recognized standards (DH 2007b). Clinical audit is a mechanism that enables healthcare professionals to regularly monitor and review their practice against agreed national benchmarks. Where practice is below standard or where there is need to assess the impact of new service on patient outcomes, measures before and after the implementation of the change/innovation are compared to determine whether improvements have occurred. Inter-professional and cross-institutional working is regarded as pivotal in improving patient outcomes through developing critical care pathways and in translating research findings into practice (DH 2012).

Integrated governance

Evidence-based practice is an integral part of the Clinical Governance framework and was developed in response to escalating costs of healthcare, quality and standards of patient care, increased public interest in safety and effectiveness of clinical interventions (DH 1998; NHSE 1999). The Clinical Governance framework and subsequently Integrated Governance (DH 2006) framework are part of a wider strategy to improve quality of patient services and the effectiveness of decision making by emphasizing greater accountability among NHS organizations and staff for:

- continuous quality improvement
- safeguarding high standards of care
- promoting patient safety
- creating an environment for excellence to flourish.

Critical to the successful implementation of the Integrated Governance agenda is the promotion of the increased use of evidence-based guidelines and the development of systems, processes and a national infrastructure of support and performance monitoring (McSherry and Pearce 2007). To assist these processes, new bodies such as the National Institute for Clinical Excellence, the Commission for Health Improvements and National Service Frameworks were established (Thompson and Learmonth 2002). The subsequent development of national and local standards in the form of specialty-based guidance and protocols were ways of engaging with and developing a culture of quality enhancement, thereby meeting clinical governance objectives. Integrated Governance seeks to continue strengthening organizational and professionals' obligation in improving the quality of care (DH 2006). This can be achieved through raising the standards of care, promoting patient safety, minimizing variations in care outcomes and improving access to healthcare services while underpinning decisions on the most current evidence known to be effective for the target population (NHSE 1999; DH 2006, 2012).

Keeping updated, expanding the knowledge base and maintaining professional competency are seen as integral expectations of healthcare practitioners and core strands of the governance strategies. A commitment to lifelong learning by practitioners (DH 2000b) is recognized as vital to maintaining standards and advancing the quality of patient care. In many ways this manual supports and moves forward this agenda by providing a robust framework for developing skills, knowledge and competency of healthcare professionals within the discipline of critical care practice.

Another key component to clinical and integrated governance (DH 2006) is risk management. Risk management can be defined as practising safely, aiming to develop good practice and avoiding or reducing the occurrence of harm to patients (McSherry and Pearce 2007). Adverse events in relation to healthcare practice are often preventable and may happen due to the following.

- Failure to strictly follow procedures in the care of patients.
- Technical failure/inappropriate and incorrect use of medical equipment.
- Poor records, documentation and intra-professional communication.
- Healthcare practitioners performing tasks for which they have not been trained or deemed to be competent.
- Failure to act and respond appropriately.

In 2000, the National Patient Safety Agency was set up to address many of these issues and create an NHS culture that would aim to improve patient safety. It sought to systematically learn from and analyse organizations' experiences, and to share these with others through the production of alerts, guidance and strategies to reduce harm.

A further national development supporting evidence-based practice was the establishment of the National Institute of Clinical Effectiveness (NICE). NICE (2008) bases decisions on published evidence, expert panels and evidence developed from real-life experiences. NICE attempts to ensure the evidence is of good quality and is relevant, and includes specialists who are invited to share their experience and advice on how guidance might be put into practice. Patient and carer involvement is equally vital to providing an understanding of what matters most to them and their families. In this way, NICE makes recommendations in the form of guidance for care based on best evidence of clinical and cost-effectiveness (Bick and Graham 2010).

Despite concerns regarding the nature of evidence, there is consensus that to improve patient outcomes, clinical treatments and care should be delivered in a standardized manner, be cost-effective, low risk, and informed by the findings of rigorous and robust research. The preferences of patients must be considered and respected, and decisions should embrace the expertise of frontline healthcare professionals. Delivering high-quality care that reflects national standards is the remit of all healthcare practitioners regardless of grade or organizational status. In this manual, we aim to guide critical care practitioners to develop skills, knowledge and clinical competence, to promote their confidence and comprehensively advance their practice within the field of critical care and beyond. To achieve these aims and objectives the chapters have been structured to facilitate depth of learning, skills and competence in a range of patient situations.

Using this book

The aim of book is to help practitioners make informed decisions about care of the critically ill based on appraisal of the best evidence available. Following Chapter 2, which introduces the competency framework, each subsequent chapter has been formatted with the following subheadings.

- Definition of the practice area – an operational definition reflecting the aspects of care and/or treatments to be addressed.
- Aims and indications – an overall aim that outlines what healthcare professionals should achieve in delivering care. The indications reflect the conditions under which the care is required to be implemented.
- Background
  - Anatomy and physiology – to support applied understanding of treatments/interventions and their relevance in improving patient outcomes, it is essential that clinicians have a sound grasp of related anatomy, physiology and pathophysiology. This in-depth awareness will also facilitate recognition of potential adverse side effects associated with individual treatments.
  - Evidence and current debates – although there is strong evidence for many interventions used in everyday clinical practice, there are areas and activities where there is little empirical data and guidance is based on consensus views of leading experts. In these sections, debates and controversies regarding novel therapies and the abandonment of certain interventions is reviewed.
  - Review of detailed components of practice area.
- Guidelines, trouble shooting and competency tools – the competency framework is outlined in Chapter 2 and principles applied thereafter.
- References, background reading, websites.

References

Bick D and Graham ID (2010) The importance of addressing outcomes of evidence-based practice. In: Bick D and Graham ID (eds) *Evaluating the Impact of Implementing Evidence-based Practice*. Oxford: Wiley-Blackwell.

Bristol Royal Infirmary inquiry (2001) Kennedy I (chairman) *Learning from Bristol: the report of the public inquiry into children's heart surgery at the Bristol Royal Infirmary 1994-1995*. Bristol: Bristol Royal Infirmary.

Britten N (2010) Qualitative research and the take-up of evidence based practice. *Journal of Research in Nursing* 15(6): 537–544.

Bucknall T, Copnell B, Shannon K and McKinley D (2001) Evidence based practices are critical care nurses ready for it? *Australian Critical Care* 14(3): 92–98.

Cook DJ, Sibbald WJ, Vincent J-L and Cerra F for the evidence based medicine critical care group (1996) Evidence based critical care medicine: what is it and what can it do for us? *Critical Care Medicine* 24(2): 334–337.

Craig JV and Smyth L (eds) (2002) *The Evidence-based Practice Manual for Nurses*. Edinburgh: Churchill Livingstone.

Davies HTO and Nutley SM (1999) The role of evidence in public sector policy and practice: the rise and rise of evidence in health care. *Public Money and Management* 19: 9–15.

Dawes M, Davies P, Gray A et al. (2000) *Evidence-based Practice: a primer for health professionals*. Edinburgh: Churchill Livingstone.

Department of Health (1998) *A First Class Service: quality in the New NHS*. London: HMSO.

Department of Health (2000a) *Comprehensive Critical Care: a review of adult critical care services*. London: DH.

Department of Health (2000b) *The NHS Plan: a plan for investment, a plan for reform*. London: DH.

Department of Health (2004) *Patient and Public Involvement in Health: the evidence for policy Implementation*. London: DH. http://www.dh.gov.uk/en/Publicationsandstatistics/Publications/PublicationsPolicyAndGuidance/DH_4082332 [accessed 24 July 2012].

Department of Health (2006) *The Integrated Governance Handbook (2006)*. http://www.dh.gov.uk/en/Publicationsandstatistics/Publications/PublicationsPolicyAndGuidance/DH_4128739 [accessed 18 December 2011]

Department of Health (2007a) *The NHS Plan*. London: DH.

Department of Health (2007b) *Report of the High Level Group on Clinical Effectiveness*. London: DH.

Department of Health (2009) *NHS 2010–2015: from good to great. Preventative, people focussed, productive*. London: DH.

Department of Health (2010a) *Equity and Excellence: liberating the NHS*. London: DH.

Department of Health (2010b) *Essence of Care 2010*. London: The Stationery Office.

Department of Health (2012) *Academic Health Science Networks*. London: DH.

Fulbrook P and Mooney S (2003) Care bundles in critical care: a practical approach to evidence-based practice. *Nursing in Critical Care* 8(6): 249–255.

Goding L and Edwards K (2002) Evidence-based practice. *Nurse Researcher* 9(4): 45–57.

Gray M (2009) *Evidence-based Healthcare and Public Health (3e)*. Edinburgh: Churchill Livingstone.

Hek G (2000) Evidence-based practice: finding the evidence. *Journal of Community Nursing* 14: 19–22.

Hewitt-Taylor J (2003) Reviewing evidence. *Intensive and Critical Care Nursing* 19: 43–49.

Institute for Innovation and Improvement (2011) *Quality and Service Improvement Tools*. http://www.institute.nhs.uk/quality_and_service_improvement_tools/quality_and_service_improvement_tools/protocol_based_care.html [accessed 18 November 2011].

Kjörnsberg A, Karlsson N, Babra A and Wadensten B (2010) Registered nurses' opinions about focused- patient care. *Australian Journal of Advanced Nursing* 28(1): 35–44.

McCauley K and Irwin RS (2006) Changing the work environment in intensive care units to achieve patient-focused care. The time has come. *American Journal of Critical Care* 15: 541–548.

McClelland H (2007) Can care bundles improve the quality in emergency care? *Accident and Emergency Nursing* 15: 119–120.

McKenna H, Cutliffe J and McKenna P (1999) Evidence-based practice: demolishing some myths. *Nursing Standard* 11: 39–42.

McSherry R and Pearce P (2007) A guide to Clinical Governance. In: *Clinical Governance: a guide to implementation for healthcare professionals* (Chapter 3) Oxford: Blackwell Publishing.

Medical Research Council (2000) *MRC Guidelines for Good Practice in Clinical Trials*. London: MRC.

Medical Research Council (2008) *Developing and Evaluating Complex Interventions: new guidance*. London: MRC.

Murray S, Holmes D and Rail G (2008) On the constitution and status of 'evidence' in the health sciences. *Journal of Research in Nursing* 13(4): 272–280.

NHSE (1999) *Clinical Governance: quality in the new NHS*. London: DH.

National Institute for Health and Clinical Excellence (2007) *Acutely Ill Patients in Hospital: recognition and response to acute illness in adult patients in hospital*. http://www.nice.org.uk/CG50 [accessed 24 July 2012].

National Institute for Health and Clinical Excellence (2008) *NICE: our guidance sets the standard for good healthcare*. http://www.nice.org.uk/aboutnice/whatwedo/what_we_do.jsp?domedia=1&mid=EE5AA72F-19B9-E0B5-D4215C860E77FD2E [accessed 8 August 2011].

National Institute for Health and Clinical Excellence (2009) *Rehabilitation After Critical Illness (NICE Guideline NG83)*. http://www.guidance.nice.org.uk/cg83 [accessed 24 July 2012].

National Institute for Health and Clinical Excellence (2010) *Patient and Public Involvement*. http://www.nice.org.uk/getinvolved/patientandpublicinvolvement/patient_and_public_involvement.jsp [accessed 24 July].

Newman M, and Roberts T (2002) Critical appraisal I: is the quality of the study good enough for you to use the findings? In: Craig JV and Smyth L (eds) *The Evidence-based Practice Manual for Nurses*. Edinburgh: Churchill Livingstone.

Nordgren L, Asp M and Fagerberg I (2008) The use of qualitative evidence in clinical care. *Evidence Based Nursing* 11: 4–5.

Pearson M and Craig JV (2002) The context of evidence-based practice. In: Craig JV and Smyth L (eds) *The Evidence-based Practice Manual for Nurses*. Edinburgh: Churchill Livingstone.

Pravikoff DS, Tanner AB and Pierce ST (2005) Readiness of US nurses for evidence-based practice. *American Journal of Nursing* 105(9): 40–51.

Richardson A (2011) 'The big three': quality safety and cost. *Nursing in Critical Care* 16(5): 220–221.

Robb E, Jarman B, Suntharalingam G et al. (2010) Using care bundles to reduce in-hospital mortality: quantitative survey. *British Medical Journal* 340: 861–863.

Rusinová K, Pochard F, Kentish-Barnes N et al. (2009) Qualitative research: adding drive and dimension to clinical research. *Critical Care Medicine* 37(Suppl): S140–S146.

Rycroft-Malone J, Seers K, Tichen A et al. (2004) What counts as evidence based practice? *Journal of Advanced Nursing* 47(1): 81–90.

Sackett DI, Richardson WS, Rosenberg W and Haynes RB (1997) *Evidence Based Medicine: how to practice and teach EBM.* London: Churchill Livingstone.

Sackett DL, Strauss SE, Richardson WS et al. (2000) *Evidence Based Medicine: how to practice and teach EBM (2e).* London: Churchill Livingstone.

Sibson L (2011) *Urgent Care Handbook: professional practice.* London: Quay Books.

Snowball R (1999) Critical appraisal of clinical guidelines. In: Dawes M, Davies P, Gray A et al. (eds) *Evidence-based Practice: a primer for healthcare professionals.* Edinburgh: Churchill Livingstone.

Swinkels A, Albarran JW, Means R et al. (2002) Evidence-based practice in health and social care: where are we now? *Journal of interprofessional Care* **16**(4): 335–347.

Thomas L and Hotchkiss R (2002) Evidence-based guidelines. In: Craig JV and Smyth RL (eds) *The Evidence-based Practice Manual for Nurses.* Edinburgh: Churchill Livingstone.

Thompson L and Learmonth M (2002) How can we develop an evidence based culture? In: Craig JV and Smyth RL (eds) *The Evidence-based Practice Manual for Nurses.* Edinburgh: Church-ill Livingstone.

Tolentino-Delos Reyes A, Ruppert S and Shiao S-Y (2007) Evidence-based practice: use of the ventilator bundle to prevent ventilator-associated pneumonia. *American Journal of Critical Care* **16**: 20–27.

Trinder L with Reynolds L (2000) *Evidence-based Practice: a critical appraisal.* Oxford: Blackwell Science.

Vincent JL and Singer M (2010) Critical care: advances and future perspectives. *Lancet* **376**: 1354–1361.

Williams C (2006) The dynamic context of critical care provision. In: Scholes J (ed.) *Developing Expertise in Critical Care Nursing.* Oxford: Blackwell Publishing.

Wip C and Napolitano L (2009) Bundles to prevent ventilator associated pneumonia: how valuable are they? *Current Opinions in Infectious Diseases* **22**: 159–166.

Youngblut JM and Brooten D (2001) Evidence-based nursing practice: why is it important? *AACN Clinical Issues* **12**(4): 468–476.

Chapter 2

Competency-based practice

Julie Scholes,[1] Jo Richmond[2] and Jane Mallett[3]

[1]University of Brighton, Brighton, UK
[2]Heart of England Foundation Trust, West Midlands, UK
[3]Dorset, UK

Critical Care Manual of Clinical Procedures and Competencies, First Edition.
Edited by Jane Mallett, John W. Albarran, and Annette Richardson.
© 2013 John Wiley & Sons, Ltd. Published 2013 by John Wiley & Sons, Ltd.

Introduction

The critical care environment has a rapid work flow, with a patient case-mix requiring highly technical and complex interventions delivered by a workforce that is constantly changing (Laporta et al. 2005). An ageing population means the burden of acute and chronic illness will increase and this will have a direct impact on the demand for critical care services internationally. There is a 'persistent shortage' of intensive care practitioners, notably nurses with specialist skills (DH 2010b: 8). These factors are indicative of increased risk to patient safety and clinical error (Pedreira 2011). In the UK (Hutchings et al. 2009) and the USA,[1] it is predicted that there will be a shortfall in critical care physicians, pharmacists and nurses. Shortfalls in specialist staff have a direct correlation to adverse patient outcomes (Kelley et al. 2004). The problem is international and therefore hospitals cannot rely on recruiting staff from abroad to meet the demand (DH 2010b). Innovative strategies for staff development, education and training are required that meet the needs not only of professional staff but also of support workers (DH 2010b).

Competence-based training programmes provide a framework to facilitate staff in learning new skills and consolidating existing skills (Skills for Health 2010). Providing such programmes attracts new staff to the critical care unit (CCU) and contributes to staff retention (Morris et al. 2009). In times of staff shortage, hospital-based practice facilitation, education preparation and training needs assessment prevail so staff can be facilitated without leaving the workplace (RCN 2003). Frequently this provision is constructed around competence-based delivery. Competence implies a performance irrespective of role. That is, the capability of an individual to perform a task is of more significance than their professional background or position. However, that is not to deny that professional background and role might well advantage an individual towards competence or indeed excellent performance as a consequence of their clinical experience (Scholes 2006). Politically, a position whereby a competent individual can perform irrespective of role enables services to 'evolve and adapt to the unpredictable health care environment' in the context of 'tighter financial' pressures (DH 2010b: 13). The philosophical and political issues that surround competency in critical care practice and the implications for patient safety and quality of care will be critically explored below.

Defining competence

Competence is when a person has sufficient skill, knowledge and capability to be suitable or sufficient for purpose, and qualified to provide a service (*Oxford English Dictionary*). Personal competence is the capacity to function and perform, based upon level of attainment, level of knowledge to underpin the competency, and interpersonal abilities to be adaptive and to respond (Kedge and Appleby 2010). When these definitions are transposed into professional competence, performance becomes more specific.

The first element of professional competence is to recognize one's limitations: the recognition of the care that can be provided safely and independently and the actions that require co-dependence on other healthcare professionals (NMC 2010). Clinical decisions about when to act, when to wait, when to accrue more clinical information and/or evidence, and when to refer to others are all part of competent performance (Fero et al. 2009). This implies knowledge, skills, appropriate attitudes, and the ability to perform safely and correctly (Axley 2008). Professional competence is the application of knowledge to inform decision making that initiates the physical performance of activities associated with that domain of practice for which the individual can be held to account by virtue of their professional role. As such, professional competence implies compliance with professional codes of practice and a standard of performance that is monitored by professional bodies. Entry to the profession is determined when a threshold of competence has been assessed, and removal from the professional register is the ultimate sanction should performance drop below the standard. Professional competence in critical care practice implies additional specialist knowledge and skill to effectively care for patients with complex and dynamic conditions requiring respiratory support and support of at least two other organ systems, as well as meeting the needs of the patient's family (Endacott and Scholes 2010).

Competence acquisition

Competence is dependent on context and circumstances in which people operate, and yet competent practitioners are expected to be able to apply *basic competencies* in any environment.[2] The degree of skilled performance might

---

[1] In the USA, critical care provision is estimated to cost 1% of the Gross Domestic Product (Kelley et al. 2004). In the UK, costs for intensive care were estimated on cost per patient day (Audit Commission 1999) and was estimated to cost between £675 and £725 million, inflating by 5% per annum. However, considerable variation is evident in these estimated costs because there is no standardized costing methodology (Seidel et al. 2006). Recently, payment by results (Pbr) has attempted to implement a national tariff for critical care services based on the number of 'organs supported'. This approach has also been subject to criticism because no consistent methodology or robust whole system assessment of data has been scrutinized (Flynn 2010). What seems to be fairly consistently supported is that nurses are the single most expensive cost component in the support of the critical ill patient (Audit Commission 1999).

[2] For example, a practitioner would be expected to apply basic competencies of managing a cardiac arrest both in an intensive care unit and in a different environment, such as a lift. There should be a baseline recognition, intervention, ventilation of the patient, etc., possibly use of a defibrillator (if deemed competent to perform this task and the equipment was available), and calling for assistance. Failure to recognize, or act to provide basic life support, in both circumstances would be considered grossly incompetent. Furthermore, competence would imply a risk assessment when transferring an unstable patient who might suffer a cardiac arrest in the lift. In this instance, failure to provide adequate expertise (appropriately trained personnel) and emergency resuscitation equipment on that transfer could be deemed an incompetent judgement.

decrease when functioning in a novel environment (Benner et al. 1996), but there is an expectation of a minimal standard for core professional competencies. For example, performing mouth care might be considered a fundamental skill acquired on a course. When applied to the unconscious intubated patient, competent mouth care requires situated clinical know-how (for example, additional assessment, considerations and care), dexterity and skilled performance. Prior to staff being allowed to perform any skill they should be deemed safe to practice, and the assessor should have been deemed competent to assess another's competence. There are tiers of competence and any assessment of performance is inextricably linked with both the quality of care and patient safety (Axley 2008; Pedreira 2011).

To acquire competence is deliberative, that is, it is intentional; one seeks to learn and to ensure evaluation on performance to confirm competence has been achieved (Levett-Jones and Lathlean 2009). Employers should provide access to education, training and facilitation to ensure the workforce is competent (Department of Health Emergency Care 2005), and the employee should seek to learn all that is required to become competent. How someone has acquired the competence often informs the assessor's decision on the competent performance. Therefore, a student's systematic and thorough approach to learning and indeed their motivation to learn, might provide the assessor with greater confidence in confirming competent performance than a summative review or snapshot of one activity.

The assessment of competence is subjective (Eraut 1994). The personal traits of the individual being assessed influence any decision about performance (Duffy 2003). For example, a positive attitude, being interested in the task, preparedness to develop further and good communication skills are considered factors to strengthen competence (Nikula et al. 2009). The business of positively acquiring competence and being assessed as competent are iterative, developmental and transformative (Scholes 2006).

Defining the specialty

To work in critical care requires specialist skills. These skills are often in short supply (DH 2010b). In part this has been due to the traditional way in which the critical care specialist has been prepared. For example, when making reference to a competent specialist in critical care nursing,[3] the World Health Organization (WHO) defines the practitioner as someone who has undertaken a post-registration programme that enables them to demonstrate:

- a well-developed knowledge base that enables them to meet the complex needs of the critically ill patient
- specialist skills in both technological and caring dimensions

- expertise to make sound and rapid clinical judgements
- ability to recognize and manage the ethical issues inherent within the critical care environment (WHO 2003).

Access to critical care specialist nursing education has changed. In the early 1990s, the provision of intensive care training courses had shifted from 'front loading' education (secondment to centres that provided a full-time programme of intensive care nurse training [Ellis 1994]) to work-based learning (undertaking the course after having worked in CCU and continuing to practise in that unit one day as a supernumerary student, the next as a member of staff [Endacott et al. 2003]). At the same time, shortfalls in critical care nurses meant that units were often recruiting students at the point of qualification and qualified nurses without any prior knowledge or experience of critical care. These practitioners struggled to adapt to the demands of critical care and staff turnover was high, with considerable cost to the organization (O'Sullivan 2002). In response to this, junior practitioners who awaited specialist training needed baseline critical care competencies to help them adapt to the environment and function safely (RCN 2003). These competency programmes ensured a 'quality-assured' performance before a practitioner was allowed to practise unsupervised (Durston and Rance 1995).

These induction programmes sometimes had an element of rotation to different critical care localities to broaden the practitioner's scope of experience. Invariably the focus of learning on these rotational pathways was sharpened by competency statements and supported by training packages delivered within the practice setting. However, the scope of these competencies became extensive, overambitious and, in some circumstances, they became a substitute for the old ENB 100[4] (a 24-week preparation programme in intensive care nursing) but without the theory. The supernumerary period in which these competencies were to be acquired varied considerably by unit and region (Scholes and Endacott 2002). Newly qualified nurses sometimes demonstrated a knowledge deficit in basic anatomy, physiology and pharmacology, and therefore the competency programmes had to address this alongside the clinical performance of the neophyte practitioner. This demonstrated that the use of competency frameworks can illuminate requirements for remedial theoretical intervention as well as structures by which to assess skilled performance.

Competency-based curriculum

Since the 1980s the movement towards competency-based education has affected most practice-based and/or public

---

[3] The vast majority of the examples in the literature are focused on nursing.

[4] The Joint Board in Nursing Certificate 100 Intensive and Critical Care Nursing certificate (a six-month clinical programme in 'centres of excellence') had been considered the gold standard of post-registration clinical nursing qualifications. It was replaced in the mid-1990s by the English National Board ENB 100, a part-time course that could be completed within one or two years (Scholes and Endacott 2002).

services (Eraut 1994). The factors bringing about this shift were multifactorial, but for the purposes of this review the focus is on four phenomena: flexibility, public expectation, the expanding curriculum and the reduction in time spent in training.

1 Flexibility of staff

Competent performance can be constructed as the capacity and capability of the practitioner to perform irrespective of their qualification. This approach allows managers to redeploy staff in response to:

- surge events or crises (e.g. response to mass casualties related to terrorist attacks or surges in need related to pandemics)
- staff shortage or cost efficiency drives to provide support workers to substitute for more expensive staff (Scholes and Vaughan 2002).

The cost-effectiveness of substitution roles is in question for nursing and medicine. For example, a nurse practitioner substituting for a GP may receive lower remuneration but spend more time on patient assessment and interventions than the doctor (Venning et al. 2000), demonstrating no clear evidence in cost saving at the point of care delivery (Laurant et al. 2005). Although the literature has advocated the contribution of advanced practitioners and physician assistants[5] in the intensive care setting, there is scant evidence to determine the impact they have on patient outcomes and any cost saving these roles provide (Kleinpell et al. 2008). This requires further robust research and health economic evaluation to determine the cost-effectiveness of these roles. The same applies to practitioners who substitute for nurses. There is little evidence that where support workers provide services otherwise delivered by qualified nurses this saves money, but there is evidence that critical care assistants (CCAs) make a significant contribution to ease workload pressures on qualified nurses, enabling them to care for sicker patients. Reluctance to delegate specific nursing tasks to CCAs can result in them being underused (McGuire et al. 2007) and extra demands being placed on qualified nurses who have to supervise their work (McLeod 2001), and retention of the trainees is variable (Hind et al. 2000). Where these initiatives have been undertaken cost saving is rendered neutral by the expense of additional patient complications (Buchan and Dal Poz 2002), although

more recent studies have found no adverse impact on care (McGuire et al. 2007).

2 Public expectation

In response to widening public expectation to participate in care decisions and critical consumerism that extended into evaluations of care provided by the public sector, greater attention is paid by the provider (NHS indemnity[6]) to delivering skilled and competent performance. Demand from an ageing population and an increase in the management of chronic diseases has led to greater emphasis on those who receive the service having a say or being consulted on how that service is delivered. Competency frameworks help to make explicit what the consumer can expect and realistically what the provider can deliver.

3 The expanding curriculum

The expanding curriculum and diversity of subject domains taught in preparatory and post-registration programmes to meet generic competency (e.g. sociology, computer literacy, equality and diversity) meant less time was spent focusing on traditional subjects (e.g. anatomy and physiology). There was criticism about how this widening body of knowledge might not be considered 'essential' and did not provide for core skills to underpin transferable clinical competencies on qualification (e.g. UKCC 1999; Scholes et al. 1999). In recognition of this, competency frameworks were created to remedy shortfalls and focus the attention of the learners on essential clinical skills (UKCC 2001; Scholes et al. 2004; DH 2008), alongside the generic skills of lifelong learning and critical appraisal of research to ensure the practitioner could be self-directing.

4 Reduction in time for clinical apprenticeships

The reduction in time spent on clinical apprenticeships and/or the proportion of the training programme spent in clinical practice has reduced significantly over the past 20 years (Girbes et al. 2010). This has meant less time for students to acquire clinical competence in their preparation programmes and resulted in a political call for this to be rectified (UKCC 1999; DH 2008; Girbes et al. 2010). Several strategies were adopted to remedy this. The first aimed to provide remedial competency frameworks to ensure newly qualified staff could function effectively in practice. Second, there was also a demand for educational institutions to reframe their curriculum for the preparatory programmes to ensure alumni were fit for practice and purpose (ibid). Third, there was a determination by hospital managers that

---

[5] A seminal study by Rudy et al, 1998) compared the contribution of advanced practitioners (APs) and physician's assistants (PAs) with resident physicians in critical care. They found that performance was similar but the APs and PAs were directed to the care of less sick and younger patients. Further PAs and APs were more likely to spend longer with nurses talking about patient care and interacting with the patient's families and taking account of the patient's social history, and spent more time on research and administration. Patient outcomes were similar for both the APs and PAs and resident physicians (Ruby et al, 1998).

[6] NHS bodies are legally liable for the negligent acts and omissions of their employees (the principle of vicarious liability), and should have arrangements for meeting this liability. This is known as NHS indemnity. This insurance covers the actions of staff in the course of their NHS employment and also the people who are contracted by the NHS to work in their organization (including voluntary and charitable volunteers) (DH 2007a and b).

any time spent in practice was to be directed and productive. Competency frameworks provided the structure to direct learning as well as demonstrate outputs or outcomes of that learning transformed into competent performance.

Competency and the relationship with integrated governance

Integrated governance is a term used to describe different types of activity related to the improvement of the quality of care (Smith 2005). These organixation-wide activities include:

- continuing professional education
- clinical effectiveness and clinical audit
- risk management
- research and development
- fostering a climate of openness and accountability set within good management systems.

The philosophical shift from clinical governance to integrated governance is exemplified by a learning organization that brings together discrete areas of quality management activity under one umbrella oriented by the theoretical compass of self-organizing systems (Department of Health 2006a). A learning organization learns from excellent performance but also from the analysis of mistakes. Self-assessment and unit-based (e.g. intensive care unit/department of specialist provision) audit of clinical practice and patient outcome help to monitor activity with a direct purpose to enhance quality. Critically, integrative governance relies on individual integrity, accountability and responsible behaviour (Smith 2005).

Competency frameworks help individuals understand the threshold standard of performance, either as an assessor or when being assessed: they increase the performance level (Fero et al. 2009). Through competency frameworks practitioners can be co-managers of quality within the integrated system. Leadership and vision are necessary within the system to forward plan and determine roles in varying circumstances. Competency frameworks help to determine the performance of an individual that might not be linked to the professional qualification they hold. Therefore, competency frameworks offer hospitals some organizational resilience when coping with significant external change, be that financial expediency or surge capacity to respond to excess demand and staff redeployment (Christian et al. 2006).

As demand for health and social care increases, reconfiguring who does what and when demands an integration, and in some situations a reconfiguration of services. Increasingly, cross-boundary and cross-sector working (e.g. the blurring of health/social care provision) is likely to become the norm (Jackson et al. 2008). This creates new challenges for integrated governance that includes delivery from health, social care and third sector (such as charity providers) partnerships. Competency frameworks are essential because they define what the practitioner can do irrespective of the title of their role. However, functionality is not the only issue when considering competence. Performance is contingent on

salient decision making, even if that relates to referral to others. Traditionally, the theory underpinning certain competencies might reside more within one profession's domain than another. Knowledge can be reconfigured to underpin certain activities, but disaggregation of too many theoretical principles can lead to fragmentation that is counterproductive. Therefore, this needs to be considered when generating competencies for a new specialty within a specialist service. For example, when developing competency for an ethics consultant for CCU, the preferred model may remain a medic with ethics training (Chwang et al. 2007) because that individual has the prerequisite theoretical knowledge and clinical know-how.

The reconfiguration of services demands a more radical approach and challenges practitioners to consider undertaking competencies outside their usual sphere of practice and beyond their theoretical foundations. This idea is made possible by the availability of a computerized evidence base. However, the computerized evidence requires there to be an accurate diagnosis on which to base the evidence in the first instance. Therefore, when considering competence, particularly for those for whom the field of practice is novel, there is a need to provide sufficient knowledge to help orientate the practitioner to context. In addition, in the UK there is a shift from time-based to competency-based training for practitioners (Girbes et al. 2010). Therefore someone can demonstrate competence at their own pace, be that accelerated or deferred, rather than wait for the course of a programme. However, Girbes et al. (2010) caution, within this approach it is important to define a minimum time frame for the *acquisition of experience* prior to assessment of competence, to ensure performance can accommodate complexity and not just functional capacity.

With integrated governance, a pivotal condition is reliance on an individual's responsibility and accountability for their practice. When considering competence for someone who is well rehearsed in the field of practice, it is essential to provide an 'amnesty' in which a declaration can be made for the need for refresher skills. For example, it cannot be assumed that people under the age of 30 have information technology literacy skills and those over the age of 30 have not (Kingsley and Kingsley 2009). 'Skill fade' (that is, the loss of performance without regular rehearsal) may require remedial intervention to bring performance back to the required standard and to keep competencies fresh, for example resuscitation skills (Gemke et al. 2007). Learning something new may generate a contradiction that renders past understanding of a foundational theoretical or practice principle faulty. The learner will need time to reframe their thinking and reconstruct their practice and this might cause a decrease in performance until the new practice is well rehearsed and the practitioner is ready to be assessed as competent. Importantly, this phase requires appropriate supervision and support to ensure patient safety. Collaborative team working can help to accommodate different levels of individual performance and allow for constant and dynamic learning transformations wherein the individual demonstrates significant change and development in their practice and professional identity.

Competency frameworks are never static but require regular revision in response to the changing healthcare environment and to new technologies. For example, with increasing emphasis on the tightened financial climate, it has been suggested that cost assessment of clinical procedures may become a core competency (Chandawarkar et al. 2007).

Assessing competence: when and how

Assessing competence is normally confined to sufficient performance to merit competence. Qualitative distinctions or degrees of competence create a level of ambiguity inconsistent with either being competent and correct or incompetent and in error. Gatekeepers (such as the Nursing and Midwifery Council, General Medical Council and the Healthcare Professions Council) of the professions can determine threshold standards that have to be achieved to gain registration and/or licence. The novice practitioner either meets them or does not. However, strategies to enhance the competence of professionals in post are generally reframed as aspirational goals to enable individuals to strive to meet a desired standard through lifelong learning and continuing professional development (Buckley et al. 2009). The potential damage created by imposing post hoc professional competencies and auditing whether practitioners have met this standard on a given date could potentially create tension with employment laws (EFTA Surveillance Authority 2010). It has been suggested that this type of clinical audit can form part of monitoring and supervision arrangements within integrated governance (Jackson et al. 2008), but with the express purpose of learning from mistakes rather than using this strategy to be punitive. The outcome of an error investigation might conclude that a practitioner exhibited below-threshold performance and recommendations are made for remedial intervention to redress the shortfall. However, performance below that which might be expected for entry to the profession could result in referral to the registering authority and potential loss of licence to practice.

Competence is observable and assessable (Manley and Garnett 2000) and can be measured. It is assumed that it is possible to recognize competence and easily identify incompetent performance. What is perhaps more challenging is recognizing and acting on performance that is weak but not obviously faulty, but gives sufficient grounds to raise concern about independent, unsupervised practice in a diverse array of circumstances. Herein lies the difficulty for those who are to determine whether or not a practitioner is competent and how to assess that.

Competency statements define the specialty, but determining what competencies make up a specialty requires considerable deliberation and debate before final consensus can be reached. The following should be considered when developing competencies.

1   The features of the competence which can be indentified need to be achievable, realistic and relevant.

2   How the competencies are to be measured and the threshold or minimum standard above which performance is deemed to be competent.

3   The conditions of performance. The competence is realistic to achieve in the context of assessment (i.e. that anxiety relating to performance be taken into account but the degree to which performance is moderated by the stress of assessment is relative to the real-world situation or stressful circumstance in which that competence might be called upon).

4   That the performance is likely to be sustained beyond the event of assessment.

5   The validity of the competence (it assesses what it is intended to assess).

6   The reliability of the competence (the same outcome would be achieved when assessing a comparable student or the same outcome if the competence was observed by a different assessor).

7   Whether to provide opportunity to remediate poor performance, for the student to be reassessed and the reasonable timescale in which this might be repeated.

In addition, the aim of enabling learning through assessment and determining qualitative criteria to distinguish and reward different levels of performance (above the basic minimum) might be considered. However, given the complexity in disentangling all the issues listed from 1 to 7, qualitative criteria to reward above-average performance might be considered desirable rather than essential.

The risk in writing competencies is to dissect and detail relevant behaviours, knowledge and performance that overcomplicates the range of competencies to be assessed and the burden for the assessor and the individual being assessed. For example, Buckley's team identified 327 competencies for critical care (medicine) and 276 for pulmonary medicine, and categorized these as essential or relevant (Buckley et al. 2009). When attempting to define threshold standards for national or international competencies, the diversity of contexts has to be considered and assimilated to take account of culture, disparate provision of services, feasibility of technical competencies and accessibility to provide certain practices. In these circumstances, competence is more likely to be described at a level of abstraction that ensures more generic application, thus reducing the overall number of competencies but also the specificity of each one (Eraut 1994). In contrast to Buckley et al. (2009), The European Society of Intensive Care Medicine undertook a project to define the minimum standard of competence to be expected of a doctor who wanted to practise as an intensive care specialist. The CoBaTrICE (Competency Based Training in Intensive Care Medicine in Europe and other world regions) project generated 102 competence statements grouped into 12 domains[7] (CoBaTrICE 2009). Here we can see two shifts,

[7] The 12 domains are: resuscitation; diagnosis; disease management; interventions; procedures; peri-operative care; comfort and recovery; end of life care; paediatric care; transport; safety and management; professionalism.

first CoBaTrICE have addressed the more generic label of intensive care specialist from the specialists within the specialism described by Buckley et al. (2009), but also how the level of abstraction reduced the overall number of competency statements to accommodate local differences in practice across Europe and other world regions.

The same situation arose when attempting to determine national competencies for critical care nursing practice (Scholes and Endacott 2002). Similar to CoBaTrICE, the initiative was generated in response to workforce mobility and the professional disquiet at the difference in performance and capability demonstrated by practitioners when they moved from one locality to another. For the intensive care nurses this was even more problematic because they might have held the same respected qualification (the ENB 100 certificate), but practitioners were judged on where they had completed the ITU programme rather than certificate (ibid). The distinctions came about because some students were based in district general hospitals and were gaining a very different experience to those who might be based at a 'centre of excellence' or tertiary specialist unit. These data were gathered before the widespread introduction of high dependency units and the assessment of levels of patient dependency to befit the criteria for admission to CCU. Therefore, some students were educated in units that had patients who had one organ failure and were not ventilated and therefore fell outside the DH guidelines for the admission to CCU (Audit Commission 1999). However, this meant that although some nurses in district general hospital CCUs might have had less experience in managing complex patients, they benefited from being able to practise more autonomously. The concern was the difference, and a desire to generate a minimum standard, especially as the English National Board for Nursing, Midwifery and Health Visiting were to be disbanded and local universities were to provide the courses (i.e. what was to be taught in college could become highly variable). The disparity in patient dependency and service provision meant that staff in different localities required different competencies to ensure local relevance. This led to the term 'practice-competency gap' – whereby a set of competencies are determined to be desirable by service commissioners, but the practitioner has no opportunity to gain that type of clinical experience to either rehearse or consolidate those skills in the ITU in which they were employed (Scholes and Endacott 2003). At the time (2001–03), particular concern was directed towards caring for a patient undergoing haemofiltration and renal replacement therapy. Advances in technology and investment in robust training programmes now mean that such support is standard practice in many critical care units. But the practice-competence gap remains a contemporary phenomenon, and a comparable situation in 2011 would be lack of experience in managing a patient undergoing extracorporeal membrane oxygenation (ECMO). This treatment may only be used infrequently and be required in response to, for example, a flu pandemic (a surge demand) (Boschert 2009). Therefore, the requisite skills might quickly become redundant outside peak demand unless rehearsed in clinical simulation laboratories. Clinical simulation, using a framework such as 'First to Act' (Kinsman et al. 2012) enables practitioners to focus on responding to emergencies and can consolidate competencies that might rarely be experienced in everyday practice, but require a robust response when they do arise.

Objective Structured Clinical Evaluation (OSCE) and simulation

Clinical competence can be assessed using Objective Structure Clinical Evaluation (OSCE). This technique enables relative control over environmental variables and also assists in reducing the subjective element of assessment (Walsh et al. 2009). Critics argue that the OSCE reduces competence to tasks, which are reviewed out of context, and that specific attention to the minutiae of performance overrides the holistic interaction. To redress this, the assessment of competent performance and decision making in response to a changing scenario is undertaken in high-fidelity simulation environments that reflect as closely as possible the real world of practice.

OSCEs and learning in simulation laboratories can confront the learner with the limits of their performance. There is no place to attribute or hide error. This can create performance anxiety and stress for some practitioners. However, exposure to this type of experience can create an opportunity for contradiction (being made aware that what they thought they knew was in fact faulty or inadequate) that can trigger powerful and meaningful learning to redress shortfalls in performance. This approach to assessing competence is useful especially when assessing the performance of a new skill. Capturing performance on video and then replaying this to students for them to self-evaluate their actions and give an account of their decision making provides rich research data, but also serves as an invaluable educational opportunity (Endacott et al. 2010). The use of video and self-evaluation of their performance gives back control to the learner and helps them to identify learning needs and further skill development to enhance their competence. It is critical that learners are facilitated to make a constructive critical analysis of their performance. The sequence in which the facilitator asks questions is just as important as the higher-order questions (questions of increasing complexity that require problem solving rather than memorised responses) that are asked (Barnum 2008). The learner should be sensitively debriefed to maximize learning from the experience. Simulation can also improve competence and confidence (Cooke et al. 2008). This approach could prove very useful when attempting to up-skill staff undertaking substitution roles in times of peak demand.

Linking the technical with humanistic care

Competence is informed by theory and practice. When referring to competent performance of a critical care practitioner, skilled performance of a task cannot be separated from situated, salient decision making and empathic engagement with the patient (Nikula et al. 2009). Therefore, a competent critical care practitioner would practise using an evidence base, but that needs to be blended with situated ethical decision making and recognition of the individual patient's needs. Patient needs include technical curative dimensions as well as fundamental care needs (Box 2.1), indeed there are particular challenges in the environment of critical care units to provide care for people who are critically ill (Table 2.1). In view of this, the person-centred outcomes within Essence of Care 2010 (DH 2010a) have been used to devise a set of fundamental competency statements (FCS) (Table 2.2) to represent the needs of all patients, not only those being cared for within a critical care environment. They also relate to all practitioners and support care workers. The FCS should always be considered, whatever the critical care competency. The specific competencies for critical care practice are set out in the following chapters in this manual. A generic format has been devised for FCS and specific procedure competency statements (SPCS) (*see* Table 2.2), which can be developed for competency (for example, Table 2.3 includes the specific procedure competency statements for transpulmonary cardiac output monitoring using thermodilution (example PiCCO®)). It is important to realize that both FCS and SPCS are considered within each competency.

However, there are specific challenges created by the critical care environment that need to be considered when practising any competence, including meeting fundamental care needs. The specific nuances and particulars of any one moment are defined by the circumstances of the patient's condition, the unit and the parties engaged in care provision (*see* Table 2.1 for examples of the challenges that may present when demonstrating the competence of meeting fundamental care needs within the critical care environment).

The challenges (Table 2.1) demonstrate that when delivering a technical skill in critical care so much more needs to be considered than the procedure. The critical care context often enhances the complexity of performance and the needs of the patient at any given moment in time. To perform competently also requires due regard to the needs of colleagues, the patient's family and other staff and visitors on the unit. The novice will approach their practice attending

---

Box 2.1 Fundamental needs

People's need for:

- effective communication
- respect and dignity
- a care environment that meets needs and preferences
- safety
- food and drink
- prevention and management of pain
- personal hygiene to meet needs and preferences
- maintenance of skin and underlying tissues
- bladder, bowel and continence care
- control over their care
- health and wellbeing
- record keeping that promotes high-quality care

Essence of Care (DH 2010a)

Table 2.1 Challenges in critical care of meeting fundamental competencies

Examples of challenges that may occur within critical care when meeting fundamental care needs	
Communication	Requirement to: - communicate with semi-conscious, sedated, paralysed or unconscious people - communicate with people who are unable to speak. For example, patients with a tracheostomy - communicate with people who have altered levels of perception induced by drugs, trauma and an alien environment - recognize that the critical care environment is highly technical and will be confusing or frightening for patients, relatives and carers - make complex and technical information understandable to a layperson - ensure that the patient's best interests have been taken into account when participating in a decision for treatment - recognize that significant others may have compromised capacity to make decisions in times of shock, emotional distress and exhaustion - gain the trust and understanding of the patient, relatives and carers to add to the therapeutic success of interventions - share complex information accurately with members of the multidisciplinary team to ensure continuity of care
Respect and dignity	Requirement to: - preserve modesty while meeting the need to expose the patient for therapeutic interventions and personal care - consider the need for a chaperone during intimate procedures - provide privacy when performing clinical care - recognize individual needs and beliefs

Table 2.1 (*Continued*)

Examples of challenges that may occur within critical care when meeting fundamental care needs

Care environment	Requirement to: ■ maintain patient comfort while safely handling and positioning equipment ■ maintain and comply with specific health and safety standards during a procedure ■ provide a therapeutic environment by balancing the need for alarms, noise, light, etc., with the need for the patient to have sleep and periods of calm
Safety	Requirement to: ■ risk assess an intervention and implement safety measures. For example, exposure to X-rays or the administration of medication
Food and drink	Requirement to: ■ balance nutritional and hydration needs within the complexity of deranged physiology and altered states and/or conditions sometimes therapeutically induced
Prevention and management of pain	Requirement to: ■ anticipate pain management requirements in the unconscious patient ■ provide alternative methods of pain control such as PCA (patient-controlled analgesia) ■ balance methods of pain control that do not compromise function and capacity to progress ■ recognize pain signs and symptoms in a semi-conscious patient ■ distinguish between pain and anguish
Personal hygiene	Requirement to: ■ meet the individual's need for oral care when intubated ■ recognize the individual personal hygiene needs in spite of altered body image ■ anticipate that some procedures will alter a patient's personal hygiene needs. For example, insertion of a urinary catheter will require additional meatal cleansing ■ provide assistance for personal hygiene following the procedure if required, for example due to perspiration, leakage of blood, etc.
Prevention and management of pressure ulcers	Requirement to: ■ anticipate the risk of pressure damage and reduce that risk. For example, by supporting tubes, administration sets, masks, etc. ■ recognize that altered physiology and nutrition can compromise skin integrity ■ inspect the skin for early signs of tissue damage
Bladder, bowel and continence care	Requirement to: ■ anticipate that interventions such as enteral and parenteral feeding may affect bowel action ■ provide ongoing care for urinary catheters, stomas, etc.
Self-care	Requirement to: ■ recognize the limited capacity to perform self-care and maximize any opportunity to promote independence and control over care ■ understand the concept of living wills, advanced directives, etc. ■ support and supervise significant others to undertake care
Health and wellbeing	Requirement to: ■ assist family and carers to make choices about time away from the patient in order to eat regular meals and to rest
Record keeping	Requirement to ■ maintain detailed contemporaneous records of specific care interventions and medicines management ■ implement documented plan for continuing care following a specific procedure
Prevention and management of infection control	Requirement to: ■ conduct procedures, where relevant, in an aseptic manner ■ take appropriate infection prevention and control precautions according to the situation
Valid consent	Requirement to: ■ ensure the patient's best interests have been taken into account when participating in decision making ■ recognize relatives' compromised capacity to make decisions in times of shock, emotional distress and exhaustion

Table 2.2 Generic format for fundamental competency statements and specific procedure competency statements

Fundamental competency statements	Examples of evidence of competence that may be assessed by, for instance, observation or written reflection of practice (for example assessor's, people's and/or carer's feedback)
Effective communication Demonstrate effective communication in terms of interpersonal skills, assessment of communication needs, information sharing and empowering people to communicate. Identify any issues relating to communication with people, including: ■ people who do not speak English ■ people who have mental and physical needs ■ children Demonstrate effective communication skills with carers, colleagues and members of the multidisciplinary health or social care team	*May be demonstrated by:* ■ providing an explanation of the procedure in an understandable manner and checking of the person's (parental or guardian's) understanding ■ reducing the person's anxiety ■ organizing the time and place of the procedure with the multidisciplinary team ■ acting to reduce risks with the multidisciplinary team ■ organizing valid consent ■ providing alternative means of communication for people unable to speak due to intubation/tracheostomy for example
Respect and dignity Demonstrate care that is focused on respect for the individual in terms of attitude and behaviour, confidentiality, privacy, dignity and modesty	*May be demonstrated by:* ■ appropriate screening of the person during the procedure to ensure privacy and dignity ■ maintaining the person's modesty while the procedure is undertaken ■ using attitude and behaviour to inspire confidence showing compassion ■ ensuring cultural needs are met wherever possible
Care environment Demonstrate how to meet people's environment needs and preferences in terms of safety, access, comfort, cleanliness, tidiness, maintenance, storing of equipment and infection control in relation to all aspects of fundamental care	*May be demonstrated by:* ■ ensuring relevant infection control guidance is followed ■ ensuring correct preparation and disposal of equipment ■ putting the bed at the right height with brakes on, etc. ■ using the correct personal protective equipment (PPE) ■ disposing of clinical waste appropriately following the procedure ■ clearing space for procedure
Safety Demonstrate how to make people, their carers, visitors and staff feel and be safe, secure and supported	*May be demonstrated by:* ■ ensuring the immediate area is safe, for example free from clutter, and clean ■ ensuring that resuscitation equipment is available and working correctly
Food and drink Demonstrate how to meet people's nutrition and hydration needs and preferences	*May be demonstrated by:* ■ ensuring the person has access to food and drink if appropriate, for example by moving a bed table into position and placing a drink where the person can reach it
Prevention and management of pain Demonstrate how to meet people's and carers' pain management needs that optimize function and quality of life	*May be demonstrated by:* ■ ensuring the person has adequate analgesia before, during and following the procedure ■ ensuring appropriate assessment and management of pain ■ considering positioning of cushions and or pillows as a way of reducing discomfort ■ explaining the person's analgesia regimen
Personal hygiene Demonstrate how to meet people's personal hygiene needs and preferences according to individual and clinical needs	*May be demonstrated by:* ■ providing assistance for personal hygiene following the procedure if required. This may be necessary, for example, due to perspiration, leakage of blood, etc.
Prevention and management of pressure ulcers Demonstrate how to maintain or improve the condition of people's skin and underlying tissues	*May be demonstrated by:* ■ advising the person how to reduce the risk of tissue damage due to pressure ■ assessing a person's wound site as per management plan ■ providing support for tubing to reduce pressure
Bladder, bowel care and continence care Demonstrate how to meet people's bladder and bowel needs	*May be demonstrated by:* ■ providing an opportunity before a procedure for the person to pass urine ■ ensuring continence and/or assisting person to manage incontinence

Table 2.2 (*Continued*)

Fundamental competency statements	Examples of evidence of competence that may be assessed by, for instance, observation or written reflection of practice (for example assessor's, people's and/or carer's feedback)
Self-care Demonstrate how to enable people to have control over their care	*May be demonstrated by:* ■ educating the person on how best to mobilize ■ ensuring the person understands the future plan of care and their agreed contribution
Health and wellbeing Demonstrate how to support people to make healthier choices for themselves and others	*May be demonstrated by:* ■ teaching breathing exercises ■ providing literature about procedure
Record keeping Demonstrate how people benefit from records that promote communication and high-quality care	*May be demonstrated by:* ■ ensuring that accurate documentation of the procedure takes place ■ commencing and reviewing the wound management plan, drainage chart, etc.
Prevention and control of infection Demonstrate how to prevent and control the spread of infection	*May be demonstrated by:* ■ ensuring relevant infection control guidance is followed
Valid consent Demonstrate how to: ■ explain and discuss the procedure with the *person* ■ ensure the *person's* understanding ■ gain the *person's* consent Demonstrate an understanding of: ■ reasons for obtaining valid consent ■ issues concerning mental capacity	*May be demonstrated by:* ■ people's understanding and agreement of the procedure

Specific procedure competency statements	Evidence
Complete assessment against relevant fundamental competency statements	
Demonstrate ability to: ■ teach and assess or ■ learn from assessment	Examples of evidence of teaching, assessing and learning
Identify risks, potential problems and complications for (subject of competency) and how to prevent or manage them	Examples of evidence of competency for specific procedures may include: ■ direct observation of procedure
Demonstrate knowledge and understanding of local and national policies, guidance and procedures in relation to (subject of competency)	■ testimonial from people, carer and/or staff members ■ teaching session for peers ■ completion of a reflective text, workbook, or educational package
Demonstrate knowledge and understanding of evidence base in relation to (subject of competency)	■ examination ■ test
Demonstrate skills that are required in relation to (subject of competency)	■ discussion with supervisor/mentor in relation to (subject of competency)
Prepare equipment required in relation to (subject of competency)	
Demonstrate the correct technique for the procedure in relation to (subject of competency)	

to rudimentary or single components (Benner 1984). They might well be slow, reading small chunks of information and responding to their assessment through the performance of elemental tasks. The expert can perform technically competent tasks with exquisite attention to fundamental care needs that the practitioner might not have deliberately considered: they are simply a component of their artistic performance of expert critical care practice. The majority will sit mid way between these two polar extremes. It is important to note, that competence is not achieved if all that is demonstrated is technical competence without attention to the fundamental care needs of the patient. Equally, competence is not conferred if a procedure is performed inadequately however expert the delivery of fundamental care needs.

The fundamental competency statements (Table 2.2) are designed to be used with specific competency statements to

Table 2.3 Example of how specific procedure competency statements can be used to assess a procedure

Complete assessment against relevant fundamental competency statements (*see* Chapter 2, pp. 20, 21)	Evidence
Specific procedure competency statements for transpulmonary cardiac output monitoring using thermodilution (e.g. PiCCO®)	**Evidence of competency for transpulmonary cardiac output monitoring using thermodilution (e.g. PiCCO)**
Demonstrate ability to: ■ teach and assess or ■ learn from assessment.	Examples of evidence of teaching, assessing and learning.
Identify indications for monitoring using the transpulmonary cardiac output monitoring using a thermodilution system, including: ■ haemodynamic instability ■ shock ■ sepsis ■ lung injury ■ pulmonary oedema ■ organ failure ■ high-risk surgical patients.	*May be demonstrated by:* ■ discussion with supervisor/mentor, providing an explanation of the indications for monitoring using the transpulmonary cardiac output monitoring using a thermodilution system.

Demonstrate skills that are required in relation to caring for a patient with a thermodilution transpulmonary cardiac output monitoring system.
■ Safe and correct set up of the system components in line with manufacturer's guidelines, including:
  1. collection of correct components
  2. correct connection to the monitoring device and patient monitor
  3. correct input of patient data.
■ Correct calibration/zeroing of catheter and arterial waveform in accordance with manufacturer's guidelines.
■ Correct configuration and calibration of system in line with manufacturer's guidelines, including:
  ■ correct set-up of calibration components
  ■ correct administration of the thermodilution indicator solution in line with manufacturer's guidelines and following local and national policies for medicine management.
■ Re-calibration in line with local and manufacturer's guidelines
■ Correct securing of catheter, transducers and cables following local policy and manufacturer's guidelines.
■ Ensure that waveforms and parameters are displayed at all times and alarms appropriately set.
	May be demonstrated by:
	■ direct observation and discussion with supervisor/mentor of correct procedure for set up of:
	  ○ relevant components
	  ○ calibration/zeroing
	  ○ securing
	  ○ monitor display
	  ○ alarms
	■ discussion with supervisor/mentor of relevant manufacturer, local and national guidelines and policies
	■ discussion with supervisor/mentor of the rationale for the agreed haemodynamic parameter settings.

Demonstrate an understanding of: ■ the rationale for the haemodynamic parameters agreed and set by the multidisciplinary team.	
Demonstrate skills that are required in relation to preventing potential catheter infection. ■ Observe dressing for signs of infection, use visual infusion phlebitis (VIP) chart or local equivalent. ■ Change dressing as required – follow local policy.	*May be demonstrated by:* ■ discussion with supervisor/mentor ■ direct observation of the procedure ■ acting to reduce risk with the multidisciplinary team.

Table 2.3 (*Continued*)

Complete assessment against relevant fundamental competency statements (*see* Chapter 2, pp. 20, 21)	Evidence
Specific procedure competency statements for transpulmonary cardiac output monitoring using thermodilution (e.g. PiCCO®)	**Evidence of competency for transpulmonary cardiac output monitoring using thermodilution (e.g. PiCCO)**

Demonstrate knowledge and understanding of local and national policies, guidance, in relation to infection control.

Identify the contraindications, risks, potential problems and complications of the thermodilution transpulmonary cardiac output monitoring system, and how to prevent or manage them, including:

Contraindications:
- peripheral arterial vasoconstriction
- damped arterial trace
- CVP in femoral vein (over estimate)
- intra-aortic balloon pumps
- inaccurate readings:
  - aortic aneurysm
  - pneumonectomy
  - aortic stenosis.

Complications:
- venous/arterial access
- bleeding at site
- pneumo+/- haemothorax
- air embolism
- arterial puncture
- nerve injury
- venous thrombosis.

In use:
- incorrect calibration
- erroneous data
- misinterpretation of data.

May be demonstrated by:
- acting to reduce risk with the multidisciplinary team
- correctly assessing haemodynamic status following local guidelines
- communicating in a timely and appropriate manner any changes or concerns regarding haemodynamic observations with the multidisciplinary team
- able to deliver clinical care while limiting adverse affects of the thermodilution transpulmonary cardiac output monitoring system
- direct observation of the procedure.

Demonstrate knowledge and understanding of evidence base in relation to the impact of clinical interventions upon haemodynamic status.

Demonstrate knowledge and understanding of evidence base in relation to the transpulmonary cardiac output monitoring technique using a thermodilution system.
- Waveforms
- Parameters:
  1. arterial pressure (AP)
  2. mean arterial blood pressure (MAP)
  3. heart rate (HR)
  4. stroke volume (SV) and index (SVI)
  5. cardiac output (CO)
  6. cardiac index (CI)
  7. systemic vascular resistance (SVR) and index (SVRI)
  8. global end-diastolic volume (GEDV) or index (GEDI)
  9. intra-thoracic blood volume (ITBV) or index (ITBI)
  10. stroke volume variation (SVV%)
  11. pulse pressure variation (PPV%)
  12. extravascular lung water (EVLW) or index (ELWI)
  13. pulmonary vascular permeability index (PVPI)
  14. global ejection fraction (GEF%)
  15. cardiac function index (CFI)
  16. left ventricular contractility (dP/mx).

May be demonstrated by:
- discussion with supervisor/mentor
- direct observation of the procedure
- correctly assessing haemodynamic status following local guidelines
- communicating in a timely and appropriate manner any changes or concerns regarding the validity of observations with the multidisciplinary team.

(*Continued*)

Table 2.3 (*Continued*)

Complete assessment against relevant fundamental competency statements (*see* Chapter 2, pp. 20, 21)	Evidence
Specific procedure competency statements for transpulmonary cardiac output monitoring using thermodilution (e.g. PiCCO®)	**Evidence of competency for transpulmonary cardiac output monitoring using thermodilution (e.g. PiCCO)**
Demonstrate knowledge and understanding of the potential problems that can occur during monitoring with the system and how to troubleshoot these, including: ■ calibration problems ■ inappropriate measurements.	*May be demonstrated by:* ■ direct observation and discussion with supervisor/mentor of correct procedure for troubleshooting: 　○ calibration problems 　○ inappropriate measurements ■ discussion with supervisor/mentor of relevant manufacturer, local and national guidelines and policies.

enable staff to achieve competence in fundamental care *and* specific clinical procedures. It is intended that the FCS are used to educate and assess staff in carrying out *any* procedure at *any* competency level. As such, the FCS can be included as part of any national or local organization's relevant education package or framework. The FCS can, therefore, be used with the Knowledge and Skills Framework,[8] Skills for Health Common Core Competencies (for example, Common/Core Competencies for Advanced Practitioners).[9]

Using the FCS, fundamental care is not assessed in isolation from other clinical activities. Staff cannot be deemed competent unless they can demonstrate that they meet people's relevant fundamental care needs *as well as* adequately conducting the procedure. It is important to note that it is the competence of staff in delivering the relevant fundamental aspects of care *when conducting a clinical procedure* that is being assessed using the FCS. In view of this the FCS should be considered each time a procedure is carried out and assessed concurrently.

The fundamental competency statements and specific procedure competency statements may be developed for any procedure or intervention. In this way the patient's fundamental needs are considered at the same time as competently performing complex clinical skills. The following chapters in this manual will focus on individual critical care procedures and competencies. While reading, the practitioner should always consider how their practice can be extended

to enhance the care and opportunities of recovery for their patient.

References and further reading

Audit Commission (1999) *Critical to Success. The place of efficient and effective critical care services within the acute hospital.* London: Audit Commission.

Axley L (2008) Competency: a concept analysis. *Nursing Forum* **43**(4): 214–222.

Babl FE and Sharwood LN (2008) Research governance: current knowledge among clinical researchers. *Medical Journal of Australia* **188**(11): 649–652.

Barnum MG (2008) Questioning skills demonstrated by approved clinical instructors during clinical field experiences. *Journal of Athletic Training* **43**(3): 284–292.

Benner P (1984) *From Novice to Expert: excellence and power in clinical nursing practice.* Menlo Park: Addison-Wesley, pp. 13–34.

Benner P, Tanner C and Chesla C (1996) *Expertise in Nursing Practice: caring, clinical judgement and ethics.* New York: Springer Publishing Company.

Boschert S (2009) Flu pandemic pushing demand for ECMO. Optimal use of ECMO debated. *CHEST Physician.* http://www.chestnet.org/accp/article/flu-pandemic-pushing-demand-ecmo [accessed 22 December 2010].

Buchan J and Dal Poz M (2002) Skill mix in the health care workforce: reviewing the evidence. *Bulletin of the World Health Organization* **80**(7): 575–580. http://www.scielosp.org/scielo.php?pid=S0042-96862002000700010&script=sci_arttext&tlng=en [accessed 21 December 2010].

Buckley JD, Addrizzo-Harris DJ, Clay AS et al. (2009) Multisociety task force recommendations of competencies in pulmonary and critical care medicine. *American Journal of Respiratory and Critical Care Medicine* **180**(4): 290–295.

Chandawarkar RY, Taylor S, Abrams P et al. (2007) Cost-aware care: critical core competency. *Archives of Surgery* **142**(3): 222–226.

Christian MD, Hawryluck L, Wax RS et al. (2006) Development of a triage protocol for critical care during an influenza pandemic. *Canadian Medical Association Journal* **175**(11): 1377–1381.

Chwang E, Landy DC and Sharp RR (2007) Views regarding the training of ethics consultants: a survey of physicians caring for patients in ICU. *Journal of Medical Ethics* **33**(6): 320–324.

[8] Department of Health (2004) *The NHS Knowledge and Skills Framework* (NHS KSF and the Development Review Process. London: DH. http://www.dh.gov.uk/prod_consum_dh/groups/dh_digitalassets/@dh/@en/documents/digitalasset/dh_4090861.pdf (accessed 13 June 2010).

[9] Skills for Health. *Nationally Transferable Roles Template. Advanced Practitioner Roles.* http://www.skillsforhealth.org.uk/Search-Results.aspx?searchQuery=common+core (accessed 13 June 2010).

CoBaTrICE (2009) The CoBaTrICE Web page. http://www.cobatrice. org/Data/ModuleGestionDeContenu/PagesGenerees/en/02-competencies/7.asp [accessed 15 December 2010].

Cooke JM, Larsen J, Hamstra SJ and Andreatta PB (2008) Simulation enhances resident confidence in critical care and procedural skills. *Fam Med* **40**(3): 165–167.

Department of Health (1997) *Report on the Review of Patient-Identifiable Information.* http://www.dh.gov.uk/prod_consum_dh/groups/dh_digitalassets/@dh/@en/documents/digitalasset/dh_4068404.pdf [accessed 9 February 2012]

Department of Health Emergency Care (2005) Quality Critical Care. Beyond Comprehensive Critical Care. A report by the Critical Care Stakeholder Forum http://www.dh.gov.uk/prod_consum_dh/groups/dh_digitalassets/@dh/@en/documents/digita-lasset/dh_4121050.pdf [accessed 16 January 2013].

Department of Health (2006a) Integrated Governance Handbook. A handbook for executives and non-executives in health care organisations http://www.dh.gov.uk/prod_consum_dh/groups/dh_digitalassets/@dh/@en/documents/digitalasset/dh_4129615.pdf [accessed 16 January 2013].

Department of Health (2006b) *Records Management: NHS Code of Practice part one.* http://www.dh.gov.uk/prod_consum_dh/groups/dh_digitalassets/@dh/@en/documents/digitalasset/dh_4133196.pdf [accessed 9 February 2012].

Department of Health (2007a) *NHS Information Governance – Guidance on Legal and Professional Obligations.* http://www.dh.gov.uk/prod_consum_dh/groups/dh_digitalassets/@dh/@en/documents/digitalasset/dh_079619.pdf [accessed 9 February 2012].

Department of Health (2007b) Powers to Extend Membership of NHS Indemnity Schemes. http://www.dh.gov.uk/en/Publicationsandstatistics/Legislation/Actsandbills/HealthandSocialCareBill/DH_080451 [accessed 28 July 2011].

Department of Health (2008) *Modernising Allied Health Professions (AHP) Careers: a competence-based career framework.* http://www.dh.gov.uk/en/Publicationsandstatistics/Publications/PublicationsPolicyAndGuidance/DH_086264 [accessed 28 July 2011].

Department of Health (2009) *Records Management: NHS Code of Practice part two.* http://www.dh.gov.uk/prod_consum_dh/groups/dh_digitalassets/documents/digitalasset/dh_093024.pdf [accessed 9 February 2012].

Department of Health (2010a) *Essence of Care 2010.* http://www.dh.gov.uk/prod_consum_dh/groups/dh_digitalassets/@dh/@en/@ps/documents/digitalasset/dh_119978.pdf [accessed 31 July 2011].

Department of Health (2010b) *Liberating the NHS: developing the health care workforce.* A consultation on proposals. DH 20.12.10. London: DH.

Department of Health (2010c) *Social Care Information Governance.* http://www.dh.gov.uk/en/Managingyourorganisation/Informationpolicy/Informationforsocialcare/DH_4075306 [accessed 9 February 2012].

Department of Health (2011) *The Care Record Guarantee. Our Guarantee for NHS Care Records in England.* http://www.nigb.nhs.uk/pubs/nhscrg.pdf [accessed 9 February 2012].

Duffy K (2003) *Failing Students: a qualitative study of factors that influence the decisions regarding assessment of students' competence in practice.* www.nmc-uk.org/documents/. . ./Kathleen_Duffy_Failing_Students2003.pdf [accessed 24 June 2011].

Dullenkopf A, Rothen HU, Swiss CoBaTrICE group (2009) What patients and relatives expect from an intensivist–the Swiss side of a European survey. *Swiss Medical Weekly* **139**(3–4): 47–51.

Durston M and Rance A (1995) Bringing the theory-practice gap in the ITU with in-service education. *Intensive and Critical Care Nursing* **11**: 233–236.

EFTA Surveillance Authority (2010) *Recognition of Professional Qualifications.* http://www.eftasurv.int/internal-market-affairs/areas-of-competence/persons/professional-qualifications/ [accessed 26 November 2010].

Ellis H (1994) Education for critical care nurses. In: Millar B and Burnard P (eds) *Critical Care Nursing Caring for the Critically Ill Adult.* London: Ballière Tindall.

Endacott R and Scholes J (2010) Minimal training requirements for ICU nurses. In: Flaatten H, Moreno R, Putensen C and Rhodes A (eds) *European Intensive Care Society Medicine Organisation and Management of Intensive Care.* Berlin: Medizinisch Wissenschaftliche Verlagsgesellschaft.

Endacott R, Scholes J, Freeman M and Cooper S (2003) The reality of clinical learning in critical care settings: a practitioner: student gap? *Journal of Clinical Nursing* **12**: 778–785.

Endacott R, Scholes J, Buykx P et al. (2010) Final year nursing students' ability to assess, detect and act on clinical cues of deterioration in a simulated environment. *Journal of Advanced Nursing* **66**(12): 2722–2731.

Eraut M (1994) *Developing Professional Knowledge and Competence.* London: Falmer Press.

Fero LJ, Witsberger CM, Wesmiller SW et al. (2009) Critical thinking ability of new graduate and experienced nurses. *Journal of Advanced Nursing* **65**(1): 139–148.

Flynn M (2010) Critical Care Network Briefing Regarding the Department of Health Update of Payment by Results for Critical Care. www.scnetworks.nhs.uk/index.php [accessed 24 June 2011].

Gaiser RR (2009) The teaching of professionalism during residency: why it is failing and a suggestion to improve its success. *Anesthesia and Analgesia* **108**(3): 948–954.

Gemke RJ, Weeteling B and van Elburg RM (2007) Resuscitation competencies in paediatric specialist registrars. *Postgraduate Medical Journal* **83**(978): 265–267.

Girbes A, Beishuizen A and Zijlstra J (2010) Minimal Training requirements for ICU physicians. In: Flaatten H, Moreno R, Putensen C and Rhodes A (eds) *European Intensive Care Society Medicine Organisation and Management of Intensive Care.* Berlin: Medizinisch Wissenschaftliche Verlagsgesellschaft.

Hind M, Jackson D, Andrewes C et al. (2000) Health care support workers in the critical care setting. *Nursing in Critical Care* **5**: 31–39.

Hutchings A, Durnard M, Grieve et al. (2009) *Evaluation of the Modernization of Adult Critical Care Services.* London: NIHR. www.sdo.nihr.ac.uk/files/project/133-final-report.pdf [accessed 24 June 2011].

Jackson C, Nicholdson C, Doust J et al. (2008) Seriously working together: integrated governance models to achieve sustainable partnerships between health care organisations. *Medical Journal of Australia* **188**(8 Suppl): S57–S60. http://www.nja.com.au/public/issues/188_08_210408/jac11093_fm.html

Johnson M, Ormandy P, Long A and Hulme C (2004) The role and accountability of senior health care support workers in intensive care units. *Intensive & Critical Care Nursing* **20**: 123–132.

Kedge S and Appleby (2010) Promoting curiosity through the enhancement of competence. *British Journal of Nursing* **19**(9): 584–587.

Kelley M, Chalfin D, Crandall E et al. (2004) The Critical Care Crisis in the United States. A Report From the Profession *CHEST* **125**(4): 1514–1517. http://chestjournal.chestpubs.org/content/125/4/1514.full [accessed 22 December 2010].

Kingsley KV and Kingsley K (2009) A case study for teaching information literacy skills. *Brirish Medical Council Medical Education* **29**(9): 7.

Kinsman L, Buykx P, Cahmpion R et al. (2012) The FIRST(2)ACT simulation program improves nursing practice in a rural Australian hospital. *Australian Journal of Rural Health* **20**(5): 270–4. doi:10.1111/j.1440-1584.2012.01296.x.

Kleinpell R, Wesley Ely E and Grabenkort R (2008) Nurse practitioners and physician assistants in the intensive care unit: an evidence based review. *Critical Care Medicine* **36**(10): 2888–2897.

Laporta DP, Burns J and Doig CJ (2005) Bench-to-bedside review: dealing with increased intensive care unit staff turnover: a leadership challenge. http://ccforum.com/impress/cc3543 [accessed 15 December 2010].

Laurant M, Reeves D, Hermens R et al. (2005) Substitution of doctors by nurses in primary care. *Cochrane Database Syst Rev* **18**(2): CD001271.

Levett-Jones T and Lathlean J (2009) The Ascent to Competence conceptual framework: an outcome of a study of belongingness. *Journal of Clinical Nursing* **18**: 2870–2879.

Manley K and Garbett R (2000) Playing Peter and Paul: reconciling concepts of expertise with competency for a clinical career structure. *Journal of Clinical Nursing* **9**: 347–359.

McGuire A, Richardson A, Coghill E et al. (2007) Implementation and evaluation of critical care assistant role. *Nursing in Critical Care* **12**(5): 242–249.

McLeod A (2001) Critical care assistants: from concept to reality. *Nursing in Critical Care* **6**: 175–181.

Mental Capacity Act (2005) http://www.legislation.gov.uk/ukpga/2005/9/pdfs/ukpga_20050009_en.pdf [accessed 09 February 2012].

Morris LL, Pfeifer P, Catalano R et al. (2009) Outcome evaluation of a new model of critical care orientation. *American Journal of Critical Care* **18**(3): 252–259.

Nikula AE, Rapola SPT, Hupli MI and Leino-Kilpi HT (2009) Factors strengthening and weakening vaccination competence *International Journal of Nursing Practice* **15**: 444–454.

Nursing and Midwifery Council (2010) *The Code of Professional Conduct*. London: NMC. http://www.nmc-uk.org/Nurses-and-midwives/The-code/The-code-in-full/ [accessed 26 November 2010].

O'Sullivan R (2002) Developing an intensive care unit induction programme. *Nursing Times.Net* **98**(3): 42.

Pedreira M (2011) The art of nursing: crossing the quality chasm and promoting patient safety in critical care. *Nursing in Critical Care* **16**(4): 161–163.

Royal College of Nursing (2003) *Guidance for Nurse Staffing in Critical Care*. London: RCN. http://www.rcn.org.uk/__data/assets/pdf_file/0008/78560/001976.pdf [accessed 21 December 2010].

Rubulotta F, Gullo A, Iapichino G et al. (2009) The Competency-Based Training in Intensive Care Medicine in Europe (CoBa-TrICE) Italian collaborative: national results from the Picker survey. *Minerva Anestesiologica* **75**(3): 117–124.

Rudy E, Davidson L, Daly B et al. (1998) Care activities and outcomes of patients cared for by acute care nurse practitioners, physician assistants, and resident physicians: a comparison. *American Journal of Critical Care* **7**(4): 267–281.

Scholes J (2006) *Developing Expertise in Critical Care Nursing*. Oxford: Blackwell.

Scholes J and Endacott R (2002) *Evaluation of the Effectiveness of Educational Preparation for Critical Care Nursing*. London: English National Board for Nursing, Midwifery and Health Visiting. Available via the NMC website.

Scholes J and Endacott R (2003) The practice competency gap: challenges that impede the introduction of national core competencies. *Nursing in Critical Care* **8**(2): 68–77.

Scholes J and Vaughan B (2002) Cross-boundary working: implications for the multiprofessional team. *Journal of Clinical Nursing* **11**(3): 399–408.

Scholes J, Endacott R and Chellel A (1999) *Diversity and Complexity: a documentary analysis and literature review of critical care nursing*. Researching Professional Education Series No13. London: ENB.

Scholes J, Freeman M, Gray M et al. (2004) *Evaluation of Nurse Education Partnership*. Final report. www.brighton.ac.uk/inam/research/projects/partnerships_report.pdf

Seidel J, Whiting P and Edbrooke D (2006) The cost of intensive care. *Continuing Education in Anaesthesia, Critical Care & Pain* **6**(4): 160–163.

Skills for Health (2010) *Skills and Labour Market Intelligence Report for England 2010*. http://www.skillsforhealth.org.uk/workforce-planning/research-and-labour-market-intelligence-services/ [accessed 22 December 2010).

Smith J (2005) Sixth Shipman Inquiry. In: *Integrated Governance Handbook 2006*. http://www.dh.gov.uk/en/Publicationsandstatistics/Publications/PublicationsPolicyAndGuidance/DH_4128739 16.72012.

Taylor CA, Taylor JC and Stoller JK (2008) Exploring leadership competencies in established and aspiring physician leaders: an interview-based study. *Journal of General Internal Medicine* **23**(6): 748–754.

Tetzlaff JE (2007) Assessment of competency in anesthesiology. *Anesthesiology* **106**(4): 812–825.

United Kingdom Central Council for Nursing, Midwifery and Health Visiting (1999) *Fitness for Practice*. London: UKCC.

United Kingdom Central Council for Nursing, Midwifery and Health Visiting (2001) *Fitness for Practice and Purpose*. The report of the UKCC's Post Commission Development Group. London: UKCC.

Venning P, Roland M, Roberts C and Leese B (2000) Randomised controlled trial comparing cost effectiveness of general practitioners and nurse practitioners in primary care. *British Medical Journal* **320**(7241): 1048–1053.

Walsh M, Hill-Bailey P and Koren I (2009) Objective structured clinical evaluation of clinical performance an integrative review. *Journal of Advanced Nursing* **65**(8): 1584–1595.

World Health Organization (2003) *WHO Europe Critical Care Nursing Curriculum*. www.euro.who.int/document/e81552.pdf [accessed 23 December 2010].

Chapter 3

Recognizing and managing the critically ill and 'at risk' patient on a ward

Mandy Odell

The Royal Berkshire NHS Foundation Trust, Reading, UK

Critical Care Manual of Clinical Procedures and Competencies, First Edition.
Edited by Jane Mallett, John W. Albarran, and Annette Richardson.
© 2013 John Wiley & Sons, Ltd. Published 2013 by John Wiley & Sons, Ltd.

Definition

Critical illness is an illness where a patient is suffering from a severe failure of one or more of their organs such as the heart, lung or kidneys (Intensive Care Society 2011). This can be caused by conditions such as myocardial infarction, cerebrovascular accident, poisoning, pneumonia, surgical complications, major trauma as a result of road traffic accidents, a fall, burns, an industrial accident or violence.

Aims and indications

The aim of recognizing and managing the critically ill or 'at risk' ward patient is to detect the deteriorating patient as quickly as possible so that appropriate plans can be made about the ongoing care of the patient.

Timely detection of patients' deterioration and appropriate clinical interventions can minimize the likelihood of serious adverse events, including cardiac arrest and death (NICE 2007). However, there are indications that for some patients, deterioration is not recognized or not acted on in a timely manner (NPSA 2007).

Background

Signs and symptoms of patients 'at risk' of deterioration or who are critically ill

A deteriorating patient is identified by worsening physiological signs and symptoms. However, recognizing physiological deterioration can be complex and is influenced by many factors, such as:

- individual physiological response that may vary widely
- age
- functional capacity
- gender
- culture
- past medical history.

It may be possible to predict where there is a risk of deterioration. This can occur when patients in hospital are relatively stable, but have the potential to develop critical illness, such as while waiting to undergo major surgery, or following surgery that carries a high risk of complications. The patient can have a period of physiological deterioration before they become critically ill, or the patient may suddenly become critically unwell (as in a severe myocardial infarction).

Recognizing and judging the degree of patient deterioration is complicated by the fact that it is a process that can result in complete recovery or death, with or without clinical intervention. In addition, the patient's past medical history and current diagnosis can affect the context within which physiological deterioration is viewed. In some patients it is an inevitable precursor to death following a life-limiting illness, while in other patients it is an undesirable complication that needs prompt and effective management to prevent further deterioration.

The pathophysiological course of deterioration is common to most patients regardless of their specific underlying clinical condition (Smith 2003), and the signs and symptoms can be observed as the body responds to poor organ perfusion. These signs and symptoms arise through the activation of the autonomic nervous system that is a physiological response to hypoxia, hypotension and stress. This 'flight-or-fight' response is the body's attempt to maintain adequate circulation to oxygenate vital organs and results in increased heart rate and respiratory rate, dilation of airways, dilation of the blood vessels supplying vital organs such as the heart, and constriction of blood vessels to non-essential organs (Tortora and Derrickson 2011). Where this physiological compensation is failing, the common signs may be confusion due to decreased oxygen to the brain, a decrease in blood pressure and/or poor urine output due to the body's attempt to preserve a circulating volume of fluid. The deteriorating patient can therefore be identified by changes in their vital signs that can include temperature (Silva et al. 2006; Prytherch et al. 2010), heart rate (Goldhill et al. 1999; Goldhill and McNarry 2004; Cuthbertson et al. 2007), respiration rate (Hillman et al. 2001; Hodgetts et al. 2002; Kause et al. 2004; Cuthbertson et al. 2007), blood pressure (Hillman et al. 2001) and oxygen saturation (Jacques et al. 2006; Cuthbertson et al. 2007). Other symptoms, such as new confusion or reduced conscious level (Schein et al. 1990), changes in skin colour (mottled, grey or blue) and skin temperature (very hot, cool or cold) can give additional clues to the severity of the patient's deteriorating physical condition.

The adverse signs and symptoms exhibited by deteriorating patients can be detected using the assessment system of Airway, Breathing, Circulation, Disability and Exposure (ABCDE) (Smith 2003). The ABCDE assessment process is a comprehensive approach that enables identification of the major signs and symptoms of the deteriorating patient, so that appropriate clinical interventions can be instigated that may prevent further deterioration (Smith 2003). The ABCDE approach will be fully explored later in this chapter.

The complexity of detecting and managing the deteriorating ward patient requires skill and experience, and there is evidence that ward practitioners have had problems with responding appropriately (McQuillan et al. 1998; McGloin et al. 1999). NICE (2007) and NPSA (2007) reported that the signs of deteriorating patients were frequently not acted on by practitioners.

Ward patients can suffer physiological deterioration for many different reasons and which may be as a result of:

- an individual response to an illness
- an injury
- a response to a noxious intervention (such as chemotherapy)
- an adverse incident (such as a medication error)
- a natural end of life event.

Care of patients whose condition is deteriorating

In the worst cases, the patient may require admission to the level 3 care facility, suffer a cardiac arrest and/or die. Patients who suffer an in-hospital cardiac arrest have a very poor chance of survival (Weil and Fries 2005). In spite of efforts to improve the resuscitation process (resus.org.uk), survival following cardiac arrest remains at approximately 14% (Weil and Fries 2005). To try and address these poor outcomes, attention has been focused on how to prevent cardiac arrest (Schein et al. 1990; Bedell et al. 1991; Franklin and Mathew 1994). These studies highlighted the presence of detectable physiological signs and symptoms in a large number of patients who went on to suffer a cardiac arrest. The signs and symptoms could be used to provide information on which to base an early intervention; however, in many cases they had been missed, neglected or poorly managed.

'Suboptimal' care was highlighted by McQuillan et al. (1998), who identified that patients being admitted to 'intensive care' from the general wards often had their deterioration missed, misinterpreted and/or mismanaged. The main factors that contributed to suboptimal care were thought to be as a result of a:

- failure of the organization
- lack of knowledge
- failure to appreciate clinical urgency
- lack of supervision
- failure to seek advice.

(McQuillan et al. 1998)

Other studies reported both poor monitoring of vital signs in acutely ill patients and a failure to report these abnormal changes to more senior practitioners (Smith and Wood 1998; McGloin et al. 1999; Hodgetts et al. 2002).

Concerns about the concept of the poorly managed, acutely ill ward patient were reflected in a report on critical care published by the Audit Commission in 1999. The publication reported that:

> Critical care units may become the backstop for a poorly performing hospital. Poor general care can result in patients needing critical care. This inflates the number of critical care beds required. Poor care may happen in A&E, the admissions unit, the operating theatre or on the wards. It can happen due to organisational failures, communication breakdowns, failure to seek consultant or specialist advice, failure to spot or act on danger signs, and failures in supervision and on-call response (Audit Commission 1999: 48).

A number of recommendations that came out of the report were to:

- improve the skills of ward nurses and doctors in the detection of critical illness

- agree 'danger signs' of the deteriorating patient
- develop critical care outreach (CCO) services to support ward staff in managing patients at risk of deterioration and critical illness.

(Audit Commission 1999)

In 2000, the Department of Health published a review of adult critical care services (DH 2000), supporting the Audit Commission's (1999) recommendations in the implementation of rapid response systems across England and Wales. This consisted of the introduction of critical care outreach (CCO) teams and early warning scoring (EWS) systems. Both CCO and EWS initiatives were intended:

- **to avert admissions** by identifying patients who are deteriorating and either helping to prevent admission or ensuring that admission to a critical care bed happens in a timely manner to ensure best outcome
- **to enable discharges** by supporting the continuing recovery of discharged patients on wards and post discharge from hospital, and their relatives and friends
- **to share critical care skills** with staff in wards and the community ensuring enhancement of training opportunities and skills practice and to use information gathered from the ward and community to improve critical care services for patients and relatives.

(DH 2000: 14–15) (*See also* Chapter 1)

Rapid response systems

'Rapid response' systems have been implemented and developed in order to assist the detection of deterioration and support clinical decision making (Audit Commission 1999; DH 2000). 'Rapid response' is a universal term that describes the processes involved in these systems from a worldwide perspective (DeVita et al. 2006). The systems tend to consist of two phases. The initial phase of deterioration detection commonly involves monitoring and recording vital signs. Once deterioration is recognized the patient is referred to a more expert clinical team. The second phase is where the expert team assesses and clinically manages the patient (DeVita et al. 2006).

Monitoring and recording vital signs can be supported by an early warning scoring system that consists of scoring pre-set physiological parameters, such as respiratory rate and heart rate. The scores for each parameter are then aggregated to give a final score that denotes how deranged the patient's vital signs are from normal. The development and refining of these early warning systems may provide a more robust method in which to identify and define the deteriorating patient (see below and Table 3.1).

Rapid response systems, consisting of early warning systems and critical care outreach teams, have evolved in response to the recognition of suboptimal care of deteriorating patients on general wards (Audit Commission 1999; DH

Table 3.1 National Early Warning Score (NEWS)* (adapted from Royal College of Physicians 2012)

Physiological parameters	3	2	1	0	1	2	3
Respiration rate	less than or equal to 8		9–11	12–20		21–24	greater than or equal to 25
Oxygen saturations	less than or equal to 91	92–93	94–95	greater than or equal to 96			
Any supplemental oxygen		Yes		No			
Temperature	less than or equal to 35.0		35.1–36.0	36.1–38.0	38.1–39.0	greater than or equal to 39.1	
Systolic BP	less than or equal to 90	91–100	101–110	111–219			greater than or equal to 220
Heart rate	less than or equal to 40		41–50	51–90	91–110	111–130	greater than or equal to 131
Level of consciousness				A			V, P, or U

*The NEWS initiative flowed from the Royal College of Physicians' NEWSDIC, and was jointly developed and funded in collaboration with the Royal College of Physicians, Royal College of Nursing, National Outreach Forum and NHS Training for Innovation.

2000; NICE 2007; NPSA 2007). The concept of early warning systems originated in Australia with the development of the medical emergency team (MET) – an experienced critical care team who are alerted by ward practitioners when the patient displays signs of pre-determined abnormal physiological signs and symptoms (Lee et al. 1995). The MET plays a similar role to cardiac arrest teams, but the aim is that they attend the patient before they deteriorate to a cardiac arrest. The MET assesses the patient's condition and implements appropriate clinical interventions and treatment plans. Similar rapid response teams and early warning systems have been developed in England and Wales (Morgan et al. 1997; Goldhill et al. 1999).

The most common CCO team model in the UK consists of experienced critical care nurses responding to referrals from the wards, and working with ward practitioners in the detection and management of deteriorating patients (DH 2003). In a survey of 71 hospitals using EWS, 62 reported that they used an aggregated type of score similar to that first published by Morgan et al. (1997) (DH 2003). However, the physiological parameters used and their weighted ranges may vary where they have been locally developed and implemented. While these locally adapted early warning systems may work well within the individual organizations, the differences in the systems mean that it is difficult to compare data, undertake large-scale research, or compare research findings between different hospitals.

In 2005, the National Confidential Enquiry into Patient Outcome and Death (NCEPOD 2005) published a study on the care of medical patients admitted to all intensive care units in the UK (excluding Scotland). This highlighted the continued problems with the recognition of deteriorating patients and the poor level of senior medical input. Out of 1235 patient records it was found that 22% had incomplete early warning scores, and 42% of 439 cases had inappropri-

ate or delayed therapy. In 162 cases there were considerable time delays between the first gross physiological abnormality recorded and subsequent 'ICU' referral, and of these 66% had delays of greater than 12 hours. As a consequence the National Institute for Health and Clinical Excellence (NICE) published guidance on the recognition and response to acute illness in adults in hospital (NICE 2007). This aimed to establish best practice in the observation of patients, care planning, staff competencies and organization of care. The recommendations included the use of physiological early warning systems for all adults in acute hospital settings (NICE 2007).

In partnership with NICE, the National Patient Safety Agency (NPSA) published its fifth report, *Safer Care for the Acutely Ill Patient* (NPSA 2007). This document details the nation wide analysis of reported patient safety incidents. These data are submitted voluntarily so can be incomplete and subject to bias; however, the incidents contributed to an overall picture that highlighted system weaknesses and helped guide practice change. The report concentrated on 107 cases out of 1804 reported incidents that had resulted in the death of a patient during 2005. Of the 107 cases, 64 were deemed by expert reviewers to be as a result of deterioration not being recognized or acted upon and 43 as a result of problems with resuscitation after a cardiorespiratory arrest (NPSA 2007). There was insufficient detail in the information provided in three cases to understand the contributing factors, but in the remaining 104 incidents, it was found that the following themes contributed to the suboptimal care of the patient:

- no observations were made on the patient for a prolonged period of time, meaning changes in vital signs were not detected (14 cases)
- abnormal vital signs were not recognized and so action was not taken (30 cases)

- deterioration was recognized and reported, but there was a delay in the patient receiving medical attention (17 cases)
- lack of in-depth knowledge and skill of practitioners resulting in a delay in starting resuscitation, failing to call resuscitation team or failing to attempt resuscitation (43 cases).

(NPSA 2007: 10)

As a result of these findings the NPSA recommended a number of key actions:

- improving the recognition of patients who are at risk, or who have clinically deteriorated
- appropriate monitoring of vital signs
- accurate interpretation of clinical findings
- calling for help early enough and ensuring that help is forthcoming
- training and skills development
- ensuring that appropriate equipment and drugs are available.

(NPSA 2007: 23)

Ongoing problems with poor use of early warning systems and utilization of rapid response teams have been complicated by a lack of a universally accepted early warning system that has been sufficiently empirically tested (Gao et al. 2007). Prytherch et al. (2010) have developed a seven-point early warning score that has been evaluated using 198 755 sets of observations of acute medical admission patients. Using in-hospital mortality, the VitalPac Early Warning Score (ViEWS) had been shown to be the best-validated early warning score to date. The new National Early Warning Score (NEWS) was built on the ViEWS criteria and improves discrimination of the risk of acute mortality (Royal College of Physicians 2012) (see Table 3.1).

Assessing and managing the deteriorating patient

The assessment and management of the deteriorating patient needs to be undertaken within a framework of safe practice that minimizes the risk and optimizes the outcome for the patient (Institute of Medicine 1999). No assessment or clinical intervention should be undertaken without the clinician being deemed competent and feeling confident about undertaking the practice (NMC 2008) (see also Chapter 2). If there is any doubt, then help from a more expert clinician should be sought as soon as possible. Response to the deteriorating patient and critical illness should be locally agreed within each hospital (NICE 2007), but if there is any concern that the patient is critically ill and deteriorating to a possible cardiac arrest, then a cardiac arrest call should be put out immediately (Resuscitation Council 2011).

Knowing the patient's history and diagnosis is useful in helping to make informed decisions about the individual's ongoing care, and medical records and recent laboratory results and investigations should be reviewed (Smith 2003), but neither are essential (Cooper and Cramp 2003). The main aim in managing the deteriorating, acutely ill patient is rapid assessment and resuscitation in order to make the patient safe, rather than making a definitive diagnosis (Smith 2003). Using a systematic assessment like the ABCDE approach (Smith 2003) ensures that the things that will rapidly kill the patient are treated first (Cooper and Cramp 2003). An obstructed airway will cause irreversible brain damage and/or death within 3–4 minutes (Adam et al. 2010) and so is the first priority in the ABCDE assessment process. Breathing is the next priority as poor respiratory function will kill the patient faster than cardiac problems or bleeding (Smith 2003). A comprehensive approach to the assessment is necessary in order that any unexplained signs and symptoms can be satisfactorily explored. This may require input from others with different areas of expertise, such as cardiologists or renal physicians if specific cardiac or renal problems are identified.

Information about the patient's normal state can be helpful. This will include their vital signs, such as normal oxygen saturations if they have chronic respiratory problems. If the patient normally has a low saturation and is on home oxygen it will help guide practitioners on targeting optimal oxygen saturations for that patient. Also knowing the patient's functional abilities, such as independence and mobility, will help with ongoing clinical decision making, such as appropriateness of escalating care or making decisions on limitations of treatment and Do Not Attempt Cardio-Pulmonary Resuscitation (DNACPR) decisions. This additional vital information can be gained from talking to the patient and their family. No one knows the patient better than themselves or those closest to them. Patients and relatives also need to be involved in decisions about ongoing care, especially if their condition is critical and there are concerns about the benefits of complex interventions such as ventilation and renal dialysis. It is as important to carefully assess and manage the dying patient, as well as those who may go on to receive intensive care (see also Chapter 17).

The following section presents the ABCDE approach, covering basic anatomy and physiology as well as the assessment and initial management of the acutely ill, deteriorating patient. Further details of how to manage patients requiring specific level 3 care is detailed in subsequent chapters.

ABCDE assessment process

The ABCDE assessment process is intended as a rapid bedside assessment of the patient. The main points, brief synopsis of some of the basic assessment methods that can be used and some of the simple immediate interventions are outlined in Table 3.2. These will be discussed more fully in the following section.

A – Airway

The aim of the airway assessment is to establish the patency of the airway and assess the risk of deterioration in the

Table 3.2 The ABCDE assessment process*

		Assessment method	Clinical interventions
A	Airway	**Look** to identify: ■ whether chest movement is 'see-saw' or absent ■ whether skin colour is blue or mottled **Feel**: ■ whether breath is exhaled from mouth or nose **Listen** for: ■ whether there is air entry and exit ■ whether the patient can talk to you	If patient is showing signs of obstructed airway then carry out the following: ■ head tilt and chin lift ■ jaw thrust ■ use airway adjuncts ■ administer high-flow oxygen
B	Breathing	**Look** for: ■ symmetrical chest movement ■ effort needed to breathe **Measure**: ■ respiratory rate ■ oxygen saturation ■ arterial blood gases **Listen** for: ■ breath sounds and added sounds	Position the patient to optimize respiratory function. Consider providing: ■ high-flow oxygen (10–15 L/min) ■ humidification ■ nebulizers ■ assisted breathing using a mask and reservoir bag
C	Circulation	**Look** at: ■ the skin colour **Feel** and **measure** a pulse for: ■ rate ■ volume ■ regularity **Feel** the: ■ peripheral skin temperature **Measure** the: ■ central temperature ■ blood pressure ■ capillary refill time ■ urine output **Monitor** the: ■ heart rhythm	Ensure venous access is available Consider giving fluid for hypovolaemia and low urine output Insert indwelling urethral catheter
D	Disability	**Look** for: ■ decerebrate or decorticate (abnormal) posturing **Measure**: ■ level of consciousness ■ pupil reaction ■ blood glucose levels ■ pain levels	Protect airway Assist breathing using a mask and reservoir bag Replace low levels of glucose Reverse noxious medications Give analgesia and anti-emetic
E	Exposure	**Look** at: ■ the exposed body and the abdomen and legs for abnormalities **Look** at: ■ the medical notes, drug charts and observation charts for further information	Maintain a safe environment, and privacy and dignity

*Consider seeking help from more senior practitioners if there are concerns that: the patient is continuing to deteriorate; a cardiac arrest is imminent; or if more advanced or specialist skills are required. Reproduced with the kind permission of the Resuscitation Council (UK).

patient's ability to protect their airway with an effective cough and gag reflex. The patient's airway can be clear, partially obstructed or completely obstructed. Obstruction of the airway is a medical emergency and can rapidly lead to cardiac arrest (Resuscitation Council 2011). Airway obstruction can be caused by the following:

- blockage by foreign body, blood, vomit, secretions, local swelling, or the patient's tongue
- central nervous system depression that causes a loss of airway protection reflexes.

Assessing the airway

The patient should be **observed** for chest movement and the airway assessed for patency by **listening** for abnormal noisy breath sounds. Normally, the patient should be breathing quietly, with a simultaneous rise and fall of the abdomen. Normal breathing does not fully recruit the intercostal muscles, but mostly utilizes the diaphragmatic muscle. When the diaphragm contracts it moves down effectively increasing the thoracic space and producing a negative pressure, which induces air entry. The increase in thoracic volume causes a concomitant decrease in abdominal volume, which causes the abdomen to slightly expand. The patient will work harder to breathe if the airway is partially blocked and this will involve recruitment of the intercostal and accessory muscles. If the airway is completely blocked then paroxysmal breathing may be observed where the chest and abdomen rise and fall alternatively and in a vigorous manner to attempt to overcome the obstruction. This will only be observed in the first few minutes of a complete airway obstruction, as the patient will quickly become hypoxic, leading to a respiratory and cardiac arrest. In a partially obstructed airway, the patient may be sitting up and leaning forward (if the patient is able) to optimize their breathing; this is because the upright position enables fuller expansion of the lungs, increased perfusion to the lower lung fields and helps in the use of accessory muscles (Mangione 2000). There may also be an accompanying stridor (an inspiratory wheeze caused by narrowing of the upper airways). Other sounds of a partially obstructed airway are snoring, expiratory wheezing, or gurgling (Resuscitation Council 2011). In some conditions affecting the airway, such as in epiglotitis, the patient may also be drooling.

If the breath sounds are quiet, then air entry should be confirmed by **observing** chest or abdomen for symmetrical chest expansion, by **listening** and **feeling** for air flow at the mouth and nose, or by **listening** for breath sounds with a stethoscope (*see also* Chapter 5). It may be necessary to lift the patient's chin and tilt their head to ensure a patent airway while listening and feeling for breathing (Resuscitation Council 2011).

If the patient is awake and responding, the airway patency should be established by getting the patient to talk. The patient should be asked to cough, as this enables a rapid assessment of conscious level and whether their responses are appropriate.

Treating a compromised airway

An obstructed airway is a medical emergency and a cardiac arrest call should be made if there is any doubt about resolving the obstruction immediately. The patient should be laid flat, the head tilted back and the chin lifted. This will help clear the airway obstruction caused by the relaxation of the soft tissues (Moule and Albarran 2009). High-flow oxygen (15L/minute via a non-rebreathe mask) should be applied. If the patient is not breathing, then basic life support should be commenced (Resuscitation Council 2011). Airway adjuncts may be needed to assist maintenance of the airway.

Airway adjuncts

If the patient is unable to maintain their own airway, adjuncts may be required such as:

- nasopharyngeal airway (NPA)
- oropharyngeal airway (OPA)
- laryngeal mask airway (LMA)
- endotracheal tube (ETT) (*see also* Chapter 5).

If the airway is compromised with secretions then suction of the airway may be required.

Airway suction

Suction apparatus should be available for all patients in hospital. If there are suspicions, or signs, that the patient may have aspirated, such as gurgling or seeing food or fluid in the airway, it may be necessary to clear the patient's oropharynx using a rigid oropharyngeal suction catheter, for example a Yankauer catheter. Suction can induce a gag response that may result in the patient vomiting and aspirating, so the suction device should be gently inserted into the oropharynx only as far as can be visibly seen so as not to elicit a gag reflex and cause the patient to vomit.

Any airway problems must be relieved before progressing to assessing and managing breathing.

B – Breathing

Respiratory function is driven centrally by the medulla oblongata and pons in the brain. The role of the respiratory system is to maintain optimal levels of carbon dioxide (CO_2) and oxygen (O_2). Central chemoreceptors in the medulla and cerebrospinal fluid, and peripheral receptors in the walls of arteries monitor levels of CO_2, O_2 and hydrogen concentration (acidity). If the concentration of CO_2 rises (hypercapnia) or acidity is increased (lowering of the pH), the respiratory centre is stimulated to increase the rate and depth of breathing. Conversely, the respiratory centre is not stimulated to increase the rate and depth of breathing if CO_2 drops or the pH rises. If O_2 levels drop (hypoxia) the peripheral chemoreceptors are stimulated, also resulting in an increased respiratory rate and depth (Tortora and Derrickson 2011).

Table 3.3 Normal arterial blood gas values

	Normal range
Partial pressure of oxygen in arterial blood (PaO_2)	10.0–13.0 kPa
Partial pressure of carbon dioxide in arterial blood ($PaCO_2$)	4.7–6.0 kPa
pH of arterial blood	7.35–7.45

Reproduced with the kind permission of the Resuscitation Council (UK).

An indication of the amount of gas dissolved in the blood can be obtained using its partial pressure (Pa), which is measured in kPa or mmHg (Tortora and Derrickson 2011). In addition, pH (a measure of hydrogen ion concentration on a logarithmic scale from 1 to 14, where pH changes inversely with hydrogen ion concentration) can be used to measure the acidity or alkalinity of arterial blood. Normal arterial blood gas values are highlighted in Table 3.3, but are more fully explained in Chapter 5.

Assessing breathing

Breathing function should only be assessed after the airway has been judged as adequate, although some information about respiration function can be gathered during the initial airway assessment, such as how fast the patient is breathing and the effort that the patient is using.

How the patient is positioned and how they respond, as well as their colour and breathing pattern, give valuable signs about the effectiveness of their respiratory function. A patient who is struggling to breathe will be evident. If conscious, they will look very uncomfortable, and will be stressed and panicking. The patient will also tend to position themselves upright or slightly leaning forward in an attempt to maximize the effectiveness of their breathing. The patient's skin colour might be grey or blue, denoting hypoxia, and they may be unable to talk in full sentences before taking another breath.

Respiratory rate

Normal respiratory rate is between 12 and 20 breaths/minute (Prytherch et al. 2010). The chest should expand equally with each breath. A high respiratory rate is an early compensatory mechanism to optimize organ perfusion, and it may be a symptom of a number of conditions that include lung disease, cardiac disease, drug intoxication, endocrine disorders, or anxiety. A low respiratory rate may be indicative of a metabolic disorder, drug intoxication, neurological dysfunction, or exhaustion. Neurological conditions and brain injury can impede the respiratory centre in the brain and cause respiratory abnormalities or respiratory arrest (Iggulden 2006).

The respiratory rate should be measured by counting the number of breaths that a patient takes over one minute. The breath can be determined through observing the rise and fall of the chest. The patient may inadvertently alter their respiratory rate if they are aware of being observed, so it may be necessary to distract the patient by holding their pulse while counting the breaths. Doing this will also tend to prevent the patient talking (and so making it difficult to count respirations), as they will be reluctant to disturb you if they think you are counting.

Oxygen saturation

Oxygen saturation is a measure of the amount of oxygen attached to haemoglobin molecules as a percentage of the maximum that can be carried in the erythrocytes. It is assessed using an oxygen saturation probe, commonly applied to the end of the finger. Optimum oxygen saturation should be 96% and above (Prytherch et al. 2010). The British Thoracic Society (2008) recommends a target oxygen saturation of between 94 and 98%, with a minimum level of 88%. In patients who are peripherally vasoconstricted, the saturation probe may not adequately detect the underlying circulation and give a low or no reading. While this may not be a true reflection of the patient's saturation, it is indicative of a poor circulation. An assessment of breathing and circulation will give an indication of whether the problem is more likely to be respiratory or circulatory, or both. Where a saturation probe cannot pick up a reading, or there are concerns about the patient's breathing, then an arterial blood gas (ABG) analysis should be undertaken. More detail regarding respiratory assessment and pulse oximetry can be found in Chapter 5.

Blood gas analysis

The ABG is a test that provides information about the levels of oxygen and carbon dioxide in the blood and the blood pH. Other useful measures from an ABG are bicarbonate and lactate levels, which can give further information about potential metabolic disorders. The results of an ABG give more in-depth information about the effectiveness of respiratory function than pulse oximetry.

More information about arterial blood gas sampling can be found in Chapter 5.

Chest auscultation

The chest should be auscultated with a stethoscope to confirm whether air is entering the lungs, whether both lungs have equal air entry and whether there are any additional abnormal sounds such as wheezing and crackles.

Treating abnormalities of breathing

The assessment of breathing will detect any abnormalities such as rapid or slow respiration rate, unequal lung expansion, abnormal patterns of breathing and low oxygen saturations. Abnormalities of breathing can be due to a primary problem with the respiratory system itself, such as asthma, pneumonia, or chronic obstructive pulmonary disease (COPD), or as a response to other conditions such as diabetic ketoacidosis, neurological malfunction, or sepsis. It is important to find the cause of the respiratory problem, but initial treatment to support respiration should not be delayed waiting for a definitive diagnosis (Cooper and Cramp 2003).

Treatment should begin with simple measures before progressing to more complex interventions if the patient's condition does not improve. The following steps can be taken to assist the patient who has breathing difficulties.

Oxygen

High-concentration oxygen should be given to all critically ill patients (British Thoracic Society 2008). In the majority of patients who are acutely unwell and deteriorating, 10–15L of oxygen per minute should be given via a non-rebreathe mask (Smith 2003) (Figure 3.1). A small percentage of patients with COPD will develop respiratory depression if given high-flow oxygen. This is due to their chronic physiological adaptation to abnormal high $PaCO_2$ levels and low PaO_2 levels. Raising the concentration of O_2 in the blood will reduce their stimulus to breathe (Smith 2003). In this situation, additional oxygen should be carefully controlled by using an oxygen mask through which the inspiratory oxygen concentration can be controlled (for example a Venturi mask). The patient should be closely observed for respiratory depression, seen by a reduction in respiratory rate and/or tidal volume.

Positioning

The patient should be positioned appropriately. A patient having breathing difficulties might find great relief in sitting upright or sitting leaning forward on to a bed table. This recruits a greater area of lung for gas exchange and can markedly improve respiratory function. Conversely, a patient who is profoundly hypovolaemic may not be able to tolerate an upright position. It is only through assessment, comparing risks and what is most comfortable for the patient that these decisions can be taken.

Nebulizers

A nebulizer is a medical device used to provide a suspension of droplets in a gas for inhaling drugs, or for humidification (Yentis et al. 2000). A short-acting beta$_2$ agonist, such as nebulized salbutamol, will produce bronchodilation and relieve a wheeze (British National Formulary 2011). A 0.9% sodium chloride nebulizer will act as a humidifier and help loosen tenacious secretions. Nebulizers given on the wards can be driven by oxygen or air (flow rate set as per manufacturer's instructions) depending on the needs of the patient.

Humidification

Inspired air is normally humidified in the naso/oropharynx before it reaches the trachea (Yentis et al. 2000). Patients with rapid respiratory rates or who are receiving cold, dry oxygen are likely to have excess drying of their airways and secretions. This causes increased thickness of secretions and mucous plugging. Humidifying inspired oxygen can greatly relieve these symptoms (see also Chapter 5).

C – Circulation

The aim of assessing the circulatory system is to determine the effectiveness of the cardiac output, which is essential for the adequate oxygenation of the vital organs. Cardiac output is the volume of blood ejected from the heart each minute and is equal to the stroke volume (the volume of blood ejected after each contraction) multiplied by the heart rate:

Cardiac output = stroke volume × heart rate.

Stroke volume is regulated by three factors:

- preload
- afterload
- contractility.

(Tortora and Derrickson 2011)

Preload is the effect of stretching the right ventricle prior to contraction and is determined by the volume of blood that fills ventricles at the end of diastole (Tortora and Derrickson 2011). If there is inadequate filling of the heart due to hypovolaemia, the cardiac output (and blood pressure) will fall (Smith 2003).

Afterload is the arterial pressure against which the heart has to contract and is determined by the tone of the blood vessels. An increase in afterload, or vascular resistance, such as in hypertension, can cause the cardiac output to decrease (Tortora and Derrickson 2011). A reduced vascular resistance can be caused by a reduction in the activity of the sympathetic nervous supply, such as in sepsis, drug toxicity, spinal cord damage and epidural anaesthesia (Smith 2003).

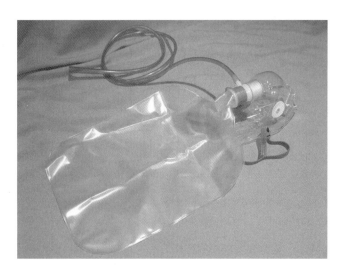

Figure 3.1 Non-rebreathable mask (from Moule and Albarran 2009, reproduced with permission from Wiley).

Contractility is the force of the contraction of the heart muscle. A reduction in contractility will cause the cardiac output to fall. Common causes of reduced cardiac contractility are: myocardial infarction, cardiac valve dysfunction, fluid loss, sepsis and pulmonary embolism (Smith 2003).

Assessing circulation

Circulation is third phase of the ABCDE assessment and is assessed once the airway and breathing have been assessed and appropriately treated.

Blood pressure

Blood pressure (BP) measurement is an indication of the effectiveness of the cardiac output. Normal BP ranges from 100/60 mmHg to 140/90 mmHg (Dougherty and Lister 2011). Mean arterial pressure (MAP) is the average blood pressure throughout the cardiac cycle and is calculated as follows:

$$MAP = \text{diastolic BP} + (\text{systolic BP} - \text{diastolic BP})/3.$$

(Smith 2003) (*see also* Chapter 5 for other calculations methods of MAP)

Adequate organ perfusion is dependent on an adequate MAP. Most organs require a MAP of 70 mmHg or above to function adequately (Smith 2003). Low blood pressure is often a late sign in the deteriorating patient as it represents a failure of the body's compensatory mechanisms, such as an increase in the peripheral vascular resistance and a decrease in urine output. Pulse pressure is the difference between the systolic and diastolic pressures. A low pulse pressure (less than 25% of the systolic pressure) can be an indication of shock. The commonest physiological abnormality prior to death is hypotension (systolic BP less than 90 mmHg) (Hillman et al. 2001). The NEWS system (Royal College of Physicians 2012) scores the systolic BP as abnormal at less than 111 mmHg.

Blood pressure can be measured manually or automatically using a blood pressure cuff on the patient's upper arm (on rare occasions it is sometimes necessary to use the lower arm or leg if access is difficult). BP can also be monitored via an indwelling arterial catheter (this is usually only undertaken in a critical care area). Blood pressure is often measured automatically using an oscillometric device on the ward. However, if there is no confidence about the reading, or the machine indicates an error in recording, a manual auscultatory sphygmomanometer should be used. This will allow a decision to be made as to whether the electronic machine is not functioning, or is insufficiently sensitive to ascertain an accurate blood pressure reading.

Heart rate

Heart rate is detected by palpating the pulse from an artery that lies near the surface of the skin, which is most commonly the radial artery in the wrist, but the carotid, brachial, and femoral arteries can also be used (Dougherty and Lister 2011). Normal heart rate is between 60 and 100 beats per minute (bpm). A rate below 60 bpm is considered bradycardic and a rate above 100 bpm is considered tachycardic (Mangione 2000).

The heart rate needs to be assessed relative to the patient's normal physiological condition. For example, a young fit individual with a normal heart rate of 65 bpm may be acutely unwell with a heart rate of 95 bpm, whereas a patient who has atrial fibrillation may normally have a heart rate of 105 bpm.

A tachycardia can be a normal response to increased exercise, but it may be a compensatory effect of poor cardiac output. If the stroke volume is diminished the body will react by increasing the heart rate in an attempt to maintain cardiac output.

As well as the rate, the pulse should also be felt for quality and regularity; a thready pulse is a sign of poor cardiac output, while there may be a bounding pulse in sepsis (Smith 2003). If there are any abnormalities detected with the pulse then a 12-lead electrocardiogram (ECG) should be undertaken.

Temperature

Normal temperature ranges from 36.8°C to 37.9°C, and can be influenced by age, gender, exercise and the time of day (Medicines and Healthcare Products Regulation Agency 2005). There are a number of thermometer devices available that can be used to measure temperature:

- Mercury in glass: the mercury contained in the glass vial expands when it is heated and can be read according to the corresponding markings (MHRA 2005).
- Chemical (phase change): a piece of plastic with small cavities containing a chemical mixture (which differs according to the manufacturer), each of which have a different melting point. The temperature change is symbolized by changing colour beneath a clear polymeric film (MHRA 2005).
- Electronic contact: a thermistor changes resistance in a metal wire according to increasing temperature (MHRA 2005).
- Infrared sensing: an optical sensor, usually a thermopile, can detect infrared emissions from a hot object (MHRA 2005).

There are also different body sites where the temperature can be measured:

- oral
- rectal
- axilla
- ear
- forehead.

The combination of the devices and sites used will influence the temperature measurement result (MHRA 2005).

A number of factors should be taken into consideration when choosing devices and sites to measure the patient's temperature, including degree of accuracy, comfort, dignity, invasiveness, complexity and expense. The hazardous nature of mercury has discouraged its general use (European Council Directive 2007/51/EC). Evidence regarding the poor reliability of tympanic measurement (Giuliano et al. 1999; Farnell et al. 2005) and the limitations in the range of temperature measurement of chemical devices (www.mhra.gov.uk [accessed December 2011]) has meant that the electronic contact device should be the one of choice for patients who are acutely ill.

A fever is an abnormally raised temperature caused when the anterior hypothalamus sets the core temperature to a level higher than the individual's normal temperature. This is most commonly caused by viral or bacterial infections and bacterial toxins (Tortora and Derrickson 2011). Hyperthermia occurs when the temperature regulator is set at the normal level but there is an elevated temperature. For example, due to status epilepticus or adverse reaction to medication (Dougherty and Lister 2011). There are grades of pyrexia ranging from 38°C (low grade). Hyperpyrexia is 40.0°C and above and is considered life threatening. It can be caused by, for instance, damage to the hypothalamus or bacteraemia (Dougherty and Lister 2011). It is important to understand the reason for the rise in a patient's temperature as the care will vary depending on causation. A core temperature below 35°C is termed hypothermia (Kumar and Clark 2006), and depending on the degree of hypothermia, the patient can have a number of clinical features including confusion, drowsiness, muscle stiffness and ECG changes. It is usually due to exposure to low temperatures and can be exacerbated by alcohol. Complications of hypothermia include pancreatitis, oliguria, cardiac arrhythmias and aspiration pneumonia (Kumar and Clark 2006).

Capillary refill time

Capillary refill time (CRT) is a useful simple measure of peripheral circulation. The patient's hand should be at the level of their heart and the top of the patient's finger pressed for 5 seconds to blanch the skin, and then released (Mangione 2000). Normal circulation should return to the fingertip within 3 seconds. If the colour of the patient's finger returns to normal within 1 second, it is a sign of a hyperdynamic state, such as in sepsis. If the CRT is longer than 3 seconds it could indicate hypovolaemia or poor circulation. CRT can also be tested by pressing for 5 seconds on the skin of the sternum in the centre of the chest.

Urine output

In health, urine output is 0.5–1 mL/kg/h. A group called the Kidney Disease Improving Global Outcomes (KDIGO) recently produced a consensus definition for acute kidney injury (AKI) and classified it by varying degrees of rising creatinine levels and deteriorating urine output (Kellum and Lameire 2012) (*see* Chapter 9).

A reduction in urine output is a normal initial physiological response to hypovolaemia. This autonomic nervous system response is activated by renal and hormonal autoregulation, which is a compensatory reaction to a decrease in blood pressure. Along with vasoconstriction of the arterioles and veins of the skin and abdominal viscera, the renal arterioles are also constricted, reducing blood flow to the kidneys. This has two effects: it conserves blood volume by reducing urine output, and it permits greater blood flow to other body tissues (Tortora and Derrickson 2011). If hypovolaemia and low blood pressure are left untreated, the reduced blood supply to the kidneys will result in acute kidney injury (NCEPOD 2009). Poor urine output (less than 200 mL over 24 hours) has been significantly associated with death (Jacques et al. 2006). Keeping the patient adequately perfused and maintaining optimal urine output helps in preventing renal problems.

Treating problems with circulation

The main immediate treatment for hypovolaemia and hypotension is the establishment of intravenous access and giving fluids.

Fluids

It is vital to establish intravenous access for any critically ill patient (Smith 2003) so that emergency fluids and drugs can be given more effectively. The most common gauge sizes of intravenous devices are 18, 20 and 22 (although it should be noted that needles are gauged in odd numbers). The gauge measurement relates to the inverse of the external diameter of the device (Phillips et al. 2011). Larger gauge numbers indicate a smaller diameter (Dougherty and Lister 2011).

The choice of intravenous access size will depend on the flow rate required and the size of the patient's vein. In the deteriorating patient the veins may have collapsed due to hypovolaemia, and so a larger gauge needle (that is, a needle with a smaller bore) will have to be used until the patient has been adequately fluid resuscitated.

Each gauge needle has a maximum flow rate and these may vary slightly between manufacturers, but are generally as follows:

18 gauge	103 mL/min	6.18 L/h
20 gauge	67 mL/min	4.02 L/h
22 gauge	42 mL/min	2.52 L/h

These flow rates can be found on the label of the device used.

Hypovolaemia should ideally be treated with the type of fluid that the patient has lost, such as blood. However, for immediate fluid resuscitation 250–500 mL aliquots of Hartmanns soution or other balanced electrolyte, calcium-free crystalloid solutions should be used to prevent hyperchloremic acidosis (Perel and Roberts 2011; Shaw et al. 2012).

Aliquots of fluid should be titrated against the patient's responses detected by their vital signs and physical assessment. The aim is a reduction in heart rate, increased urine output, peripheral warming and rise in blood pressure, with a systolic blood pressure of at least 100 mmHg. By continuously reassessing the patient, the effect of the intravenous fluid can be evaluated. If the patient still has signs of hypovolaemia after 2 L of fluid then more expert help should be sought, from more senior practitioners or the critical care team (*see also* Chapters 6 and 8).

D – Disability

Disability involves the review of the patient's neurological status and its assessment should only be undertaken once A, B and C have been optimized, as these parameters can all affect the patient's neurological status.

Assessing disability

The rapid bedside monitoring of the patient's neurological function involves three areas: the assessment of conscious level using the 'AVPU' system (see below); pupil reaction; and blood glucose levels.

The AVPU system

A rapid assessment of conscious level can be conducted at the bedside by using the 'Awake, responding to Voice, responding to Pain, or Unresponsive' (AVPU) system (Smith 2003). The patient should be approached and observed to see if they have their eyes open and are taking an interest and responding normally to their environment. This would be assessed as 'Awake'.

If the patient has their eyes closed, but opens them when they are spoken to, then they are assessed as 'responding to Voice'. However, a judgement needs to be made when a patient is naturally asleep, as physiologically this is not considered an altered level of consciousness.

The patient who doesn't respond to voice should be shaken gently to try to elicit a response. If there is still no response then painful stimuli should be applied. If the patient responds to painful stimuli, then the level of consciousness is 'responds to Pain'. The most common methods of applying painful stimuli to test the patient's response are:

- nail bed compression
- supraorbital pressure
- sternal rub
- trapezius squeeze
- earlobe pressure.

The most appropriate method is the trapezius squeeze as it does not effect a spinal reflex, and causes the least trauma to the patient (Adam et al. 2010).

The patient can respond to painful stimuli in a number of ways, which can give information about the level of any cerebral impairment, ranging from higher to lower then absent neurological responses:

- localize to pain by trying to push away the painful stimulus
- withdrawal from the source of pain
- limb flexion
- limb extension
- no response.

A patient not responding to pain is 'Unresponsive'.

If there are any concerns about the patient's level of consciousness, then a more in-depth assessment using the Glasgow Coma Scale (GCS) should be undertaken and further help should be sought. A patient with a level of consciousness at **P** or **U**, equivalent to a GCS of 8 or less, needs to be managed by a practitioner who is competent at airway management, as the as patient's airway may be at risk (*see also* Chapter 11 for GCS).

Pupil reaction

Pupil reaction is also tested to assess for any abnormalities. Pupils should be assessed for size, shape and symmetry. The pupils should be between 2 and 6 mm in width (depending on the amount of light in the environment), round and of equal symmetry. The pupils should briskly constrict to light. Abnormalities in pupil response can be due to congenital defects, previous ocular injuries, the effects of certain drugs, or brain injury (*see* Chapter 11 for more detail).

Blood glucose level

Blood glucose levels should be assessed to rule out hypoglycaemia, which is a common cause of reduced consciousness level in hospital patients. Hypoglycaemia is a blood glucose level less than 3 mmol/L. Blood glucose levels may be abnormally raised as a result of the stress of critical illness (Tortora and Derrickson 2011).

Treating disorders of consciousness level

The main aims in managing patients on the general ward with disordered consciousness level is to treat simple problems (such as hypoglycaemia), and also to maintain the patient's safety. This should take place prior to accessing higher levels of care and undertaking more complex investigations.

Maintaining a safe airway

Ongoing low levels of consciousness are a risk to the patient and the attending practitioner needs to be skilled in airway management. This may involve using manual airway manoeuvres and adjuncts (see above and Chapter 5). Placing the patient in the recovery position may minimize airway obstruction from the tongue and aspiration of stomach contents, but it does not prevent these complications, so a

Table 3.4 Treatment of hypoglycaemia

Consciousness level of patient	Unconscious	Conscious and able to swallow
Treatment	1 mg of glucagon can be given subcutaneously, intramuscularly, or intravenously or 50 mL of 20% glucose can be given intravenously into a large vein via a large-bore needle	Give a sugary drink such as Lucozade, Coca-Cola, or Ribena or 10 g or 20 g dextrose gel (for example, 1–2 GlucoGel tubes) can be squeezed between the teeth and gums
If the patient is on an insulin infusion it should be stopped immediately		

(BNF 2011)

patient with a low level of consciousness should always be closely observed. The patient may require further investigations and transfer to higher levels of care, so the wider healthcare team should be consulted and further action taken to preserve the airway.

Hypoglycaemia

The treatment for hypoglycaemia is outlined in Table 3.4.

Opiate reversal

If opiates might have caused a reduced level of consciousness then 0.4–2 mg naloxone (an opiate antagonist) can be given intravenously every 2–3 minutes as required to a maximum of 10 mg. Naloxone has a short half-life (45–70 minutes) and the effects may wear off before the effects of the opioid so the patient needs to be closely monitored in case their conscious level falls again (Resuscitation Council 2011). Reversing the effects of the opioid for central nervous system depression will also reverse its analgesic effects so the patient will need alternative pain relief.

E – Exposure

By the time the assessment reaches 'E' (Exposure) there should be a good understanding of the patient's problems, initial clinical interventions should be under way and the patient should be showing signs of improvement. The patient can be fully assessed by removing any clothing and bedding. The patient's abdomen and skin should be assessed for the presence of rashes, swelling, haemorrhage, or any excessive losses from drains or bowels. This information all helps to complete the assessment and provide information about their condition. It is essential to keep the patient informed about what is happening and to maintain the patient's dignity at all times. Observation charts, clinical notes and results from investigations can also all be reviewed for any additional information that can inform the assessment and ongoing plan of care for the patient.

If the patient is not improving or is critically unwell, then help should be obtained immediately from senior practitioners caring for the patient, rapid response teams, or the emergency cardiac arrest team (depending on local infrastructure).

Table 3.5 SBAR communication tool

SBAR	Suggested information
Situation	State: ■ your name ■ which ward/area you are on Identify: ■ the patient you are calling about ■ the current situation that prompted the call (including raised EWS if indicated)
Background	State: ■ when the patient was admitted and their diagnosis ■ any significant medical history ■ any prior procedures, interventions, or relevant results
Assessment	Detail: ■ your current assessment of the patient's condition NB Your ABCDE assessment can be used for this
Recommendation or referral	State: ■ what you have already implemented ■ what you need (be clear about your expectations) ■ what you recommend

Calling for help

Whenever calling for help or handing over patient details to another practitioner, effective communication is vital to save time and ensure all the relevant information has been given. A recommended system for improving the clarity of communication between practitioners is the Situation, Background, Assessment, Recommendation (SBAR) model (www.institute.nhs.uk). A guide to SBAR is given in Table 3.5.

A systematic approach to communication can promote more effective and efficient communication between practitioners, resulting in improved care and outcome for the patient. If there is any major concern about the patient then the cardiac arrest team should be called immediately.

Summary

This chapter has reviewed the factors relating to the recognition and immediate management of the deteriorating ward patient. The background to the phenomenon of patient deterioration has been explored, and the national and international development of strategies, such as rapid response systems, have been explained. Recognition and management of the deteriorating ward patient can be enhanced by using an initial rapid bedside assessment system. The ABCDE assessment system has been described, demonstrating simple bedside assessment skills, utilizing look, listen and feel techniques. Initial management of the deteriorating patient has been highlighted by the use of simple manoeuvres and interventions. The following chapters will explore these issues more fully.

A competency framework is outlined below that encompasses the skills for the early recognition and initial management of the deteriorating ward patient.

Procedure guideline 3.1: **Blood pressure measurement (manual) for a patient in bed (adapted with permission from the Royal Marsden Hospital Manual of Clinical Nursing Procedures)**

Essential equipment

- A range of cuffs
- Sphygmomanometer, working and calibrated
- Stethoscope
- Documentation
- Alcohol handrub
- Detergent wipes

Optional equipment

- Pillow if required to provide extra arm support.

Action	Rationale
1 Where possible, explain and discuss the procedure with the patient. If the patient lacks the capacity to make decisions the practitioner must act in the patient's best interests.	To ensure that the patient understands the procedure and gives their valid consent. To ensure the patient's best interests are maintained (Mental Capacity Act 2005).
2 Wash hands using bactericidal soap and water or bactericidal alcohol handrub, and dry.	To minimize the risk of infection.
3 Establish whether the patient has any of the following conditions: ■ lymphoedema or are at risk ■ an arteriovenous fistula ■ trauma to their arm ■ brachial artery surgery.	To ensure there are no contraindications to using a particular arm.
4 Provide a standardized environment which should be relaxed and temperate. The patient needs to be as comfortable as possible in bed.	To enable comparisons to be drawn with prior blood pressure results. Variations in temperature and emotions can alter blood pressure readings.
5 Ensure the manometer is no more than 1 metre away, vertical and at eye level.	If using a mercury manometer, the meniscus should be close to eye level or the angle of vision will mean an inaccurate result will be taken. With an aneroid scale, the eye level should be equal with the centre of the gauge.
6 Ensure the cuff is the correct size for the arm. The cuff bladder length should be 80% of the arm circumference and its width 40%.	Small cuffs give falsely high readings and large cuffs give falsely low readings.

7 Check the patient's arm is: (a) placed at heart level (midsternal level) (b) supported and free from clothing (c) ensure the patient's legs are not crossed.	(a) If the arm is lower than heart level it can lead to falsely high readings, and vice versa. (b) Diastolic pressure can increase by up to 10% if the arm is unsupported. (c) Blood pressure results can be falsely high if the patient has their legs crossed.
8 Wrap the cuff of the sphygmomanometer around the arm. (a) Have the bladder centred over the artery and superior to the elbow. The lower edge of the cuff should be 2–3 cm above the brachial artery pulsation. (b) Ensure the cuff bladder is not twisted. (c) Do not apply the cuff too tightly.	(a) To obtain an accurate reading, and so that the artery can easily be palpated. (b) So the cuff can be inflated properly. (c) Too tight a cuff may cause discolouration and ischaemia of the extremities.
9 Connect the tubing on the cuff to the manometer.	To ensure a pneumatic connection between the cuff and the machine.
10 Ask the patient to stop talking, eating and so on, during the procedure.	Activity can cause the manometer to record a falsely high blood pressure.
11 Palpate the brachial artery while pumping air into the cuff using the bulb. Once the pulse can no longer be felt rapidly inflate the cuff for further 20–30 mmHg.	Inflating the cuff to only 20/30 mmHg above the predicted systolic level prevents undue discomfort. The brachial pulse is advocated rather than the radial pulse and doing this locates the correct position for stethoscope placement.
12 Deflate the cuff and the point at which the pulse reappears approximates the systolic blood pressure.	This provides an indication of systolic pressure and can ensure accurate results in those who have an auscultatory gap.
13 Deflate the cuff completely and wait 15–30 seconds.	To allow venous congestion to resolve.
14 The stethoscope should be firmly, but without too much pressure, placed on bare skin over the brachial artery where the pulse is palpable. The bell of the stethoscope may hear the tone of the Korotkoff sounds better. However, the diaphragm has a larger surface area and is easier to hold in place.	If the stethoscope is in contact with material it may distort the Korotkoff sounds. Applying pressure with the stethoscope may partially occlude the artery.
15 Inflate the cuff again to 20–30 mmHg above the predicted systolic blood pressure.	To ensure an accurate measurement.
16 Release the air in the cuff slowly (at an approximate rate of 2–3 mmHg per pulsation) until the first tapping sounds are heard (first Korotkoff sound). This is the systolic blood pressure.	The cuff should not be deflated too quickly as this may result in inaccurate readings being taken.
17 Continue to slowly release the air, listening to the Korotkoff sounds; the point at which the sounds disappear is the best representation of the diastolic blood pressure (fifth Korofkoff sound). Continue to deflate the cuff slowly until you are sure the sounds have disappeared (after another 10–20 mmHg).	To ensure an accurate diastolic blood pressure and that you note any irregularities, such as if the sounds never disappear or disappear significantly below the fourth Korotkoff sound.
18 Once no further sounds can be heard, the cuff should be rapidly deflated.	To prevent venous congestion to the arm.

(Continued)

Procedure guideline 3.1: (Continued)

19 If you need to recheck the blood pressure wait 1–2 min before proceeding.	Venous congestion may make the Korotkoff sounds less audible.
20 Inform patient that the procedure is now finished.	To reassure the patient.
21 Wash hands using bactericidal soap and water or bactericidal alcohol handrub, and dry. Clean bell of stethoscope and cuff with detergent wipe (no alcohol).	To minimize the risk of infection.
22 Document fully as soon as the measurement has been taken and compare with previous results.	To: ■ provide an accurate record ■ monitor effectiveness of procedure ■ reduce the risk of duplication of treatment ■ provide a point of reference or comparison in the event of later questions ■ acknowledge accountability for actions ■ facilitate communication and continuity of care. (NMC 2008; GMC 2013; HCPC 2012)

Procedure guideline 3.2: Automated blood pressure measurement (adapted from Philips 2008)

Essential equipment

- A range of cuffs
- Non-invasive blood pressure monitor, working and calibrated
- Documentation
- Alcohol handrub
- Detergent wipes

Optional equipment

- Pillow if required to provide extra arm support.

Action	Rationale
1 Where possible, explain and discuss the procedure with the patient. If the patient lacks the capacity to make decisions the practitioner must act in the patient's best interests.	To ensure that the patient understands the procedure and gives their valid consent. To ensure the patient's best interests are maintained (Mental Capacity Act 2005).
2 Wash hands using bactericidal soap and water or bactericidal alcohol handrub, and dry.	To minimize the risk of infection.
3 Establish whether the patient has any of the following conditions: ■ lymphoedema or are at risk ■ an arteriovenous fistula ■ trauma to their arm ■ brachial artery surgery.	To ensure there are no contraindications to using a particular arm.
4 Provide a standardized environment which should be relaxed and temperate. The patient needs to be as comfortable as possible in bed.	To enable comparisons to be drawn with prior blood pressure results. Variations in temperature and emotions can alter blood pressure readings.
5 Ensure the cuff is approved for the specific blood pressure monitor.	To ensure compatibility of equipment and an accurate reading

6 Ensure the cuff is the correct size for the arm. The cuff bladder length should be 80% of the arm circumference and its width 40%.	Small cuffs give falsely high readings and large cuffs give falsely low readings.
7 Check the patient's arm is: (a) placed at heart level (midsternal level) (b) supported and free from clothing (c) ensure the patient's legs are not crossed.	(a) If the arm is lower than heart level it can lead to falsely high readings, and vice versa. (b) Diastolic pressure can increase by up to 10% if the arm is unsupported. (c) Blood pressure results can be falsely high if the patient has their legs crossed.
8 Apply the cuff: (a) to the arm at the same level as the patient's heart, with the marking on the cuff matching the brachial artery location. (b) Ensure the cuff bladder is not twisted. (c) Do not apply the cuff too tightly.	(a) To ensure an accurate reading. If the arm is lower than heart level it can lead to falsely high readings, and vice versa. (b) So the cuff can be inflated properly. (c) Too tight a cuff may cause discolouration and ischaemia of the extremities.
9 Regularly check the patient's skin quality and extremity of cuffed limb for colour and warmth.	If skin quality changes, or extremity circulation is being affected (for example, the limb is white, blue and cool), then the cuff site should be changed.
10 Connect the cuff to the tubing and plug the tubing into the blood pressure connector on the monitor. Ensure air tubing is not compressed or restricted.	To ensure a clear pneumatic connection between the cuff and the monitor. To ensure accurate blood pressure reading.
11 Ask the patient to stop talking, eating and so on, during the procedure.	Activity can cause the monitor to record a falsely high blood pressure.
12 Ensure the monitor is configured to the blood pressure readings required (systolic, diastolic, mean pressure).	To ensure that the correct reading is taken. The required information is displayed on the monitor.
13 Check and configure the required alarm limits.	To ensure the monitor alarms are set appropriate for the patient.
14 Using the 'set up' menu select measurement type (manual or automatic) and frequency.	The type and frequency of blood pressure monitoring will depend on the patient's condition.
15 Regularly check the patient's extremity (action 9) and adjust the frequency according to the patient's condition.	To minimize patient discomfort and complications from frequent blood pressure readings.
16 Inform the patient about the process and frequency for recording the blood pressure.	To reassure the patient.
17 Wash hands using bactericidal soap and water or bactericidal alcohol handrub, and dry.	To minimize the risk of infection.
18 Document as soon as the measurement has been taken and compare with previous results.	To: ■ provide an accurate record ■ monitor effectiveness of procedure ■ reduce the risk of duplication of treatment ■ provide a point of reference or comparison in the event of later questions ■ acknowledge accountability for actions ■ facilitate communication and continuity of care. (NMC 2008; GMC 2013; HCPC 2012) To ascertain the trend of the patient's blood pressure in order to determine care required.
19 Between patients or when required, clean the cuff with detergent wipe (no alcohol).	To minimize the risk of infection.

Procedure guideline 3.3: Pulse measurement (adapted with permission from the Royal Marsden Hospital Manual of Clinical Nursing Procedures)

Essential equipment

- A watch with a second hand
- Alcohol handrub
- Observations chart
- Black pen

- A stethoscope (if counting the apical beat)
- Electronic pulse measurement device, for example pulse oximeter, blood pressure measuring device, or cardiac monitor

Action	Rationale
1 Wash and dry hands.	To prevent cross-infection.
2 Where possible, explain and discuss the procedure with the patient. If the patient lacks the capacity to make decisions the practitioner must act in the patient's best interests.	To ensure that the patient understands the procedure and gives their valid consent. To ensure the patient's best interests are maintained (Mental Capacity Act 2005).
3 Where possible, measure the pulse under the same conditions each time.	To ensure continuity and consistency in recording.
4 Ensure that the patient is comfortable and relaxed. Ideally the patient should refrain from physical activity for 20 minutes.	To ensure that the patient is comfortable. Strenuous activity will result in falsely elevated readings.
5 Place the first and second, or in addition the third, finger along the appropriate artery and apply light pressure until the pulse is felt.	The fingertips are sensitive to touch. Practitioners should be aware that the thumb and forefinger have pulses of their own and therefore these may be mistaken for the patient's pulse.
6 Press gently against the peripheral artery being used to record the pulse.	The radial artery is usually used as it is often the most readily accessible.
7 The pulse should be counted for 60 seconds.	Sufficient time is required to detect irregularities in rhythm or volume. If the pulse is regular and of good volume subsequent readings may be taken for 30 seconds and then doubled to give beats per minute. If the rhythm or volume changes on subsequent readings then pulse must be taken for 60 seconds.
8 Record the pulse rate on appropriate documentation. Additional factors such as the rhythm, volume and skin condition (dry, sweaty or clammy) may be described in the patient's clinical notes.	To: ■ provide an accurate record ■ monitor effectiveness of procedure ■ reduce the risk of duplication of treatment ■ provide a point of reference or comparison in the event of later questions ■ acknowledge accountability for actions ■ facilitate communication and continuity of care. (NMC 2008; GMC 2013; HCPC 2012) To monitor differences and detect trends; any irregularities should be brought to the attention of the appropriate senior practitioners. Additional qualitative characteristics of the pulse may aid diagnosis of the patient's condition.
9 Where possible, discuss result and any further action with the patient.	To involve the patient in their care and provide assurance of a normal result or explain the actions to be undertaking in the event of an abnormal result.
10 Wash and dry hands or decontaminate with alcohol handrub.	To prevent the risk of cross-infection.

Procedure guideline 3.4: Temperature measurement (adapted with permission from the Royal Marsden Hospital Manual of Clinical Nursing Procedures)

Essential equipment

- Electric contact thermometer device
- Disposable probe covers
- Alcohol handrub

Action	Rationale
1 Where possible, explain and discuss the procedure with the patient. If the patient lacks the capacity to make decisions the practitioner must act in the patient's best interests.	To ensure that the patient understands the procedure and gives their valid consent. To ensure the patient's best interests are maintained (Mental Capacity Act 2005).
2 Wash and dry hands.	To minimize the risks of cross-infection and contamination.
3 Remove thermometer from the base unit and ensure the lens is clean and not cracked. Use a dry wipe to clean if required.	A dirty or damaged lens may affect the accuracy of the reading. Alcohol-based wipes should not be used as this can lead to a false low temperature measurement.
4 Place disposable probe cover on the probe tip, ensuring the manufacturer's instructions are followed.	The probe cover protects the tip of the probe and is necessary for the functioning of the instrument.
5 Gently place the probe tip with cover into the axilla with direct skin contact.	The axillary site is more comfortable and safer to use than oral site in the deteriorating patient.
6 Ask the patient, or help them, to clamp their arm close to their body.	To ensure skin contact and prevent air around the probe, causing a false low temperature measurement.
7 Activate the measurement device according to the manufacturer's instructions.	To commence the temperature measurement.
8 Remove probe tip from the axilla as soon as the thermometer display indicates it is complete.	To ensure procedure is carried out for allocated time.
9 Read the temperature display and document in the patient's records and compare with previous results.	To: - provide an accurate record - monitor effectiveness of procedure - reduce the risk of duplication of treatment - provide a point of reference or comparison in the event of later questions - acknowledge accountability for actions - facilitate communication and continuity of care. (NMC 2008; GMC 2013; HCPC 2012) Deviations from normal temperature ranges may require urgent clinical attention.
10 Release the probe cover according to the manufacturer's instructions and discard probe cover into domestic waste bin.	Probe covers are for single use only.
11 Wipe thermometer clean and replace in base unit.	To reduce the risk of cross-infection.

Competency statement 3.1: Specific procedure competency statements for recognizing and managing the deteriorating patient

Complete assessment against relevant fundamental competency statements	Evidence
Specific procedure competency statements for recognizing and managing the deteriorating patient	**Evidence of competency for recognizing and managing the deteriorating patient**
Demonstrate ability to: ■ teach and assess or ■ learn from assessment.	Examples of evidence of teaching, assessing and learning.
Demonstrate an understanding of which patients may be at risk of deterioration, including: ■ response to an illness ■ following an injury ■ following surgery ■ following discharge from critical care ■ a response to a noxious intervention (such as chemotherapy) ■ an adverse incident (such as a medication error) ■ a natural end of life event.	By discussion with senior practitioners/mentor/tutor. By prioritization demonstrated in observation frequency. Through teaching/delegation of more junior staff.
Have an understanding of the evidence regarding patient deterioration including: ■ NICE and NPSA reports.	By discussion with senior practitioners/mentor/tutor. Teaching session with peers.
Understand the significance of the early warning scoring system (particularly NEWS [Royal College of Practitioners 2012]) and critical care outreach (CCO) team.	By discussion with senior practitioners/mentor/tutor. Through evidence of observation charts recordings and utilization of CCO team. Through teaching session for peers.
Have an understanding of local policies and procedures with regard to patient observation practice.	By discussion with senior practitioners mentor/tutor. Be able to access and recall the main points of the policy.
Demonstrate appropriate frequency and completeness of patient observations and recording of vital signs, including: ■ heart rate ■ blood pressure ■ temperature ■ respiration rate ■ oxygen saturation ■ urine output ■ level of consciousness.	Through evidence of observation records. Through teaching sessions for peers.
Be able to carry out an ABCDE assessment.	Through observation by more senior practitioner or CCO team member.
Demonstrate proper documentation of ABCDE assessment.	Evidence in clinical records.
Identify which interventions may benefit the patient following the ABCDE assessment.	By discussion with senior practitioners/mentor/tutor. Evidence in clinical records.
Identify possible complications for deteriorating patients, including: ■ increasing levels of care requirements ■ consequence of poor organ perfusion (kidney, brain, gastrointestinal, skin and limb) ■ increasing need for respiratory support ■ increasing need for cardiovascular support ■ transferring to higher levels of care ■ long-term outcome and morbidity ■ impact on relatives/carers ■ end of life issues.	By discussion with senior practitioners/mentor/tutor. Through teaching sessions for peers. Reviewing case studies.

References and further reading

Adam S, Odell M and Welch J (2010) *Rapid Assessment of the Acutely Ill Patient.* Oxford: Wiley-Blackwell.

Audit Commission (1999) *Critical to Success.* London: Audit Commission.

Bedell SE, Deitz DC, Leeman C and Delbanco TL (1991) Incidence and characteristics of preventable iatrogenic cardiac arrests. *Journal of the American Medical Association* **265**(21): 2815–2820.

British National Formulary (2011) *British National Formulary 62.* London: British Medical Association and Royal Pharmaceutical Society.

British Thoracic Society (2008) Guideline for emergency oxygen use in adult patients. *Thorax* 63(Supp VI): vi1–vi68.

Cooper N and Cramp P (2003) *Essential Guide to Acute Care.* London: BMJ Books.

Cuthbertson BH, Boroujerdi M, McKie L et al. (2007)Can physiological variables and early warning scoring systems allow early recognition of the deteriorating surgical patient? *Critical Care Medicine* 35(2): 402–409.

Department of Health (2000) *Comprehensive Critical Care. A review of adult critical care services.* London: The Sationery Office.

Department of Health (2003) *The National Outreach Report, The NHS Modernisation Agency.* London: DH.

DeVita MA, Bellomo R, Hillman K et al. (2006) Findings of the first consensus conference on medical emergency teams. *Critical Care Medicine* 34(9): 2463–2478.

Dougherty L and Lister S (eds) (2011) *The Royal Marsden Hospital Manual of Clinical Nursing Procedures* (8e). Oxford: Wiley.

Farnell S, Maxwell L, Tan S et al. (2005) Temperature measurement: comparison of non-invasive methods used in adult critical care. *Journal of Clinical Nursing* 14(5): 632–639.

Franklin C and Mathew J (1994) Developing strategies to prevent in-hospital cardiac arrest: analysing responses of physicians and nurses in the hours before the event. *Critical Care Medicine* 22(2): 244–247.

Gao H, McDonnell A, Harrison DA et al. (2007) Systematic review and evaluation of physiological track and trigger warning systems for identifying at-risk patient on the ward. *Intensive Care Medicine* 33: 667–679.

General Medical Council (2013) *Good Medical Practice.* London: GMC. http://www.gmc-uk.org/gmp2013 [accessed 25 March 2013].

Giuliano KK, Scott SS, Eliot S and Giuliano AJ (1999) Temperature measurement in critically ill orally intubated adults: a comparison of pulmonary artery core, tympanic, and oral methods. *Critical Care Medicine* 27(10): 2188–2193.

Goldhill DR and MacNarry AF (2004) Physiological abnormalities in early warning scores are related to mortality in adult inpatients. *British Journal of Anaesthesia* 92(6): 882–884.

Goldhill DR, White SA and Sumner A (1999) Physiological values and procedures in the 24h before ICU admission from the ward. *Anaesthesia* 54: 529–534.

Health and Care Professions Council (2012) *Standard of Conduct, Performance and Ethics.* London: HCPC. http://www.hpc-uk.org/assets/documents/10003B6EStandardsofconduct,performance andethics.pdf [accessed 16 November 2012].

Hillman KM, Bristow PJ and Chey T et al. (2001) Antecedents to hospital deaths. *Internal Medicine Journal* 31: 343–348.

Hodgetts TJ, Kenward G, Vlachonikolis IG et al. (2002) The identification of risk factors for cardiac arrest and formulation of activation criteria to alert a medical emergency team. *Resuscitation* 54(2): 125131.

Iggulden H (2006) *Care of the Neurological Patient.* Oxford: Blackwell Publishing.

Institute of Medicine (1999) *To Err is Human. Building a Safer Health System.* Washington, DC: National Academy Press.

Intensive Care Society http://www.ics.ac.uk/patients___relatives/what_is_intensive_care_ [accessed 2 August 2011].

Jacques T, Harrison GA, McClaws ML and Kilborn G (2006) Signs of critical conditions and emergency responses (SOCCER): a model for predicting adverse events in the inpatient setting. *Resuscitation* 69(2): 175–183.

Kause J, Smith G, Prytherch D et al. (2004) A comparison of antecedents to cardiac arrests, deaths and emergency intensive care admissions in Australia and New Zealand, and the United Kingdom-the ACADEMIA study. *Resuscitation* 62: 275–282.

Kellum JA and Lameire N (2012) KDIGO clinical practice guidelines for acute kidney injury. *Kidney International Supplements* 2(1). http://www.kidney-international.org

Kumar P and Clark M (eds) (2006) *Clinical Medicine* (6e). Edinburgh: Elsevier.

Lee A, Bishop G, Hillman KM and Daffurn K (1995) The medical emergency team. *Anaesthesia and Intensive Care* 23(2): 183–186.

Mangione S (2000) *Physical Diagnosis Secrets.* Philadelphia: Hanley and Belfus Inc.

McGloin H, Adam S and Singer M (1999) Unexpected deaths and referrals to intensive care of patients on general wards. Are some cases potentially avoidable? *Journal of the Royal College of Physicians of London* 33(3): 253–259.

McQuillan P, Pilkington S, Allan A et al. (1998) Confidential inquiry into quality of care before admission to intensive care. *British Medical Journal* 316(7148): 1853–1858.

Medicines and Healthcare Products Regulation Agency (2005) *Thermometer Review: UK market survey* (MHRA 04144). London: Department of Health.

Mental Capacity Act (2005) http://www.legislation.gov.uk/ukpga/2005/9/pdfs/ukpga_20050009_en.pdf [accessed 9 February 2012].

Morgan RJM, Williams F and Wright MM (1997) An early warning system for detecting developing critical illness. *Clinical Intensive Care* 8(2): 100.

Moule P and Albarran JW (eds) (2009) *Practical Resuscitation for Healthcare Professionals.* Oxford: Wiley-Blackwell.

National Confidential Enquiry into Patient Outcome and Death (2005) *An Acute Problem?* London: NCEPOD.

National Confidential Enquiry into Patient Outcome and Death (2009) *Adding Insult to Injury.* London: NCEPOD.

National Institute for Health and Clinical Excellence (2007) *Acutely Ill Patients in Hospital.* London: Centre for Clinical Practice.

National Patient Safety Agency (2007) *Safer Care for the Acutely Ill Patient: learning from serious incidents.* London: NPSA.

Nursing and Midwifery Council (2008) *The Code: standards of conduct, performance and ethics for nurses and midwives.* London: NMC.

Perel P and Roberts I (2011) *Colloids vs Crystalloids.* The Cochrane Collaboration. John Wiley and Sons.

Philips (2008) *Intellivue Patient Monitor Instructions for Use.* Chapter 10. Germany: Philips.

Phillips S, Collins M and Dougherty L (2011) *Venepuncture and Cannulation.* Oxford: Wiley-Blackwell.

Prytherch DR, Smith GB, Schmidt P and Featherstone PI (2010) ViEWS – towards a national early warning score for detecting adult inpatient deterioration. *Resuscitation* 81: 932–937.

Resuscitation Council UK (2011) *Advanced Life Support* (6e). London: Resuscitation Council UK.

Royal College of Physicians (2012) *National Early Warning Score (NEWS) Standardising the assessment of acute-illness severity in the NHS.* Report of a Working Party. London: RCP. http://www.

rcplondon.ac.uk/sites/default/files/documents/national-early-warning-score-standardising-assessment-acute-illness-severity-nhs.pdf [accessed 27 January 2013].

Schein RM, Hazday N, Pena M et al. (1990) Clinical antecedents to in-hospital cardiopulmonary arrest. *Chest* **98**(6): 1388–1392.

Shaw AD, Bagshaw SM, Goldstein SL et al. (2012) Major complications, mortality and resource utilisation after open abdominal surgery: 0.9% saline compared to Plasma-Lyte. *Annals of Surgery* **255**(5): 821–829

Silva E, Akamine N, Salomao R et al. (2006) Surviving sepsis campaign: a project to change sepsis trajectory. *Endocrinology Metabolic Immune Disorder Drug Targets* **6**(2): 217–222.

Smith AF and Wood J (1998) Can some in-hospital cardio-respiratory arrests be prevented? *Resuscitation* **37**: 133–137.

Smith G (2003) *ALERT. Acute Life Threatening Events Recognition and Treatment.* University of Portsmouth.

Tortora GJ and Derrickson B (2011) *Principles of Anatomy and Physiology* (13e). New Jersey: John Wiley & Sons.

Weil M and Fries M (2005) In-hospital cardiac arrest. *Critical Care Medicine* **33**(12): 2825–2830.

Yentis SM, Hirsch NP and Smith GB (2000) *Anaesthesia and Intensive Care A to Z.* Oxford: Butterworth Heinemann.

Chapter 4

Admitting a critically ill patient

Vanessa Gibson[1] and Karen Hill[2]

[1]Northumbria University, Newcastle upon Tyne, UK
[2]University Hospital Southampton NHS Foundation Trust and Southampton University, Southampton, UK

Critical Care Manual of Clinical Procedures and Competencies, First Edition.
Edited by Jane Mallett, John W. Albarran, and Annette Richardson.
© 2013 John Wiley & Sons, Ltd. Published 2013 by John Wiley & Sons, Ltd.

Definition

Admitting a critically ill patient is the (recognition of their degree of illness and) transfer of the patient to a clinical area where practitioners with specialist expertise and competence, and the necessary equipment, are available to care appropriately for the patient.

Aims and indications

The aims of a critical care unit (which here is taken to include level 1, 2 and 3 patients; *see* Chapter 1 for definitions of levels) include:

- to ensure an appropriate level of critical care
- to ensure appropriate equipment is available
- to be cost effective.

Indications for admission to a critical care facility include the need for:

- additional and/or invasive monitoring
- single, double, or triple organ system monitoring and support
- respiratory and/or ventilator support
- amelioration of major uncorrected physiological abnormalities

- extended postoperative care
- preoperative physiological optimization
- additional clinical advice for practitioners caring for the patient
- appropriately trained and skilled critical care practitioners from a range of disciplines.

Background

This chapter has been written to give a broad overview of the immediate preparation and care of a patient being admitted to a critical care facility. The following chapters provide more depth into specific aspects of critical care and, therefore, include the relevant detailed anatomy and physiology.

Critical care services have developed largely as a result of innovations in medicine and surgery. In 2000, the Department of Health recommended that the existing labels, and organization of services, of 'high dependency' and 'intensive care' be replaced by a classification and service remodelling that focuses on the level of care that individual patients need (DH 2000) (*see* Chapter 1). This classification was expanded in 2002 and again in 2009 by the Intensive Care Society (ICS 2002a, 2009) (*see* Table 4.1).

Level 3 is the highest, most specialized level of continuing patient care and treatment, the primary objective of which

Table 4.1 Examples of care activities requiring different levels of care (ICS 2009) (*see also* Chapter 1)

Level of care and broad categories of care activities required by patient	Examples of specific care activities required by patient
Level 0	
Patients requiring hospitalization: ■ needs can be met through general ward care	Oral medication Bolus intravenous medication Patient-controlled analgesia Observations less frequently than 4 hourly
Level 1	
Patients recently discharged from a higher level of care	
Patients in need of additional monitoring, clinical input or advice	Observations at least 4 hourly Physiotherapy or airway suctioning at least 6 hourly, but not more than 2 hourly
Patients requiring 'critical care outreach' service support	Abnormal vital signs monitoring – but not a higher level of care
Patients requiring staff with special expertise and/or additional facilities for at least one aspect of critical care delivered in a general ward environment	Renal replacement therapy (stable chronic renal failure) Epidural analgesia Tracheostomy care
Level 2	
Patients needing single organ system monitoring and support	*Respiratory* More than 50% inspired oxygen Within 24 hours of tracheostomy insertion Non-invasive ventilation or CPAP Physiotherapy or suctioning at least every 2 hours *Cardiovascular* Continuous ECG and invasive pressure monitoring – unstable Care for haemodynamic instability due to hypovolaemia/haemorrhage/sepsis Single infusion of vasoactive drug with appropriate monitoring

Table 4.1 (*Continued*)

Level of care and broad categories of care activities required by patient	Examples of specific care activities required by patient
Patients needing preoperative optimization: ■ requiring invasive monitoring and treatment to improve organ function	Haemodynamic/respiratory resuscitation or optimization Insertion of invasive monitoring
Patients needing extended postoperative care: ■ extended postoperative observation is required either because of the nature of the procedure and/or the patient's condition. Included in this group would be patients needing short-term, i.e. less than 24 hours, routine postoperative ventilation who are otherwise well with no other organ dysfunction, e.g. fast-track cardiac surgery patients	*Procedure* Major elective surgery Emergency surgery in unstable or high-risk patient Care for increased risk of postoperative complications/interventions/ monitoring *Patient* Intermediate surgery in patient above 70 years or American Association of Anesthesiology III or IV (severe system disease with functional limitation or worse)
Patients needing a greater degree of observation and monitoring	Observation and monitoring that cannot be safely provided at level 1 or below, judged on the basis of clinical circumstances and ward resources
Patients moving to 'step down' care (that is a lower level of care than currently received)	Care above level 1 or 0 but no longer need level 3
Patients with major uncorrected physiological abnormalities: ■ these physiological abnormalities if uncorrected are likely to indicate a patient requiring at least level 2 care. Patients with lesser degree of abnormality may also require level 2 or 3 care	Care required for: ■ respiratory rate above 40 breaths/min ■ respiratory rate above 30 breaths/min for greater than 6 hours ■ heart rate greater than 120 beats/min ■ temperature less than 35°C for more than 1 hour ■ hypotension, e.g. systolic BP less than 80 mmHg for more than 1 hour ■ Glasgow Coma Score (GCS) less than 10 and at risk of acute deterioration
Level 3	
Patients needing advanced respiratory monitoring and support: ■ excluded from this group would be patients needing short-term, i.e. less than 24 hours, routine postoperative ventilation who are otherwise well with no other organ dysfunction, e.g. fast-track cardiac surgery patients. If ventilatory support exceeds 24 hours or other significant organ dysfunction develops these patients require level 3 care	Care required for: ■ respiratory failure from any cause that requires invasive, positive pressure mechanical ventilatory support ■ bi-level positive airway pressure (BiPAP) via any form of tracheal tube ■ extracorporeal respiratory support
Patients needing monitoring and support for two or more organ systems, one of which may be basic or advanced respiratory support	Syncronized intermittent mandatory ventilation (SIMV) or continuous mandatory ventilation (CMV) and continuous intravenous vasoactive drugs SIMV or CMV and haemofiltration Care for high-risk patients undergoing major surgery who are likely to require advanced respiratory support and monitoring/support of other organ systems Continuous intravenous medication to control seizures and supplementary oxygen/airway monitoring
Patients with chronic impairment of one or more organ systems sufficient to restrict daily activities (co-morbidity) and who require support for an acute reversible failure of another organ system	Care for: ■ severe ischaemic heart disease and major perioperative haemorrhage ■ COPD requiring home oxygen presenting with sepsis related to immunosuppression ■ angina on mild exercise and bronchopneumonia requiring CPAP

is the recovery of the patient to leaving hospital. (The return of a patient to a level 2 or 1 care facility is only the first step in this progression.) It is distinguished from the care and treatment pertaining to a specialty procedure of limited duration (such as a surgical operation, plasma exchange, or haemodialysis), although level 3 care may include these procedures.

Level 2 and 1 care is for 'Patients requiring more detailed observation or intervention including support for a single failing organ system or post-operative care and those "stepping down" from higher levels of care' (DH 2000: 10). Level 1 and 2 facilities, therefore, are for patients who require less specialized care and may include (but are not limited to):

- patients with invasive arterial monitoring, central venous pressure monitoring
- patients requiring epidural analgesia
- patients requiring opioid intravenous infusions for pain control
- patients no longer requiring level 3 care but who are not yet well enough to be returned to a general ward.

A level 1 or 2 care facility can act as a 'step up' or 'step down' facility and be either single specialty or multispecialty. This will influence the mix of cases and the skills required to care for patients (*see* Chapter 1).

In 2009, the Intensive Care Society published a framework of the levels of care provision for patients to assist in the decision-making process of appropriate admission to critical care units (see Table 4.1). The purpose of this framework was to support efficient and effective utilization of critical care facilities. Level 2 and level 3 patients are usually managed in designated critical care areas. However, there are many level 1 patients on the wards at risk of deterioration, or who are transferred out of level 2 or 3 areas, whose condition can change. These will require the support of critical care teams such as critical care outreach or medical emergency teams (ICS 2002b). In this context it is important that practitioners on the wards are able to recognize a patient who is deteriorating, respond appropriately and escalate care concerns in a timely manner (NICE 2007) (*see* Chapter 3).

Calling for appropriate assistance

The deteriorating patient needs to receive expert support and early intervention, thus minimizing further deterioration, in a timely manner (Rivers et al. 2001). To manage a deteriorating patient and facilitate timely admission to a level 2 or 3 care facility (that is, a critical care facility) there should be internal mechanisms for calling for help from the patient's clinical teams or critical care outreach teams. Delays in admission to critical care facilities can be attributed to lack of transfer equipment, bed capacity issues, or

availability of appropriately trained staff and, conversely, can lead to reduced outcomes (Young et al. 2003).

Calling for assistance has been shown to be most effective when the correct information and language is used when referring a patient to medical staff (Adam et al. 2010). Hospitals should support a healthcare-associated communication framework for referring acutely ill and deteriorating patients to other practitioners, for example a Situation, Background, Assessment and Recommendation (SBAR) system (Wacogne and Diwaker 2010). There is further evidence that the use of early warning scoring systems assists nurses to make more convincing referrals to more senior practitioners or critical care outreach teams (Andrews and Waterman 2005) and helps the receiving practitioner prioritize the calls that they have received. An effective referral can influence the timeliness of response and treatment to the patient (*see* Chapter 3 for details).

The decision to admit a patient to critical care facility is usually made consultant to consultant (NICE 2007). National guidelines are in place in the UK regarding recognition and response to acute illness (NICE 2007). It is imperative that admission to a critical care facility is not delayed, as there is a significant association between time to admission (or delayed admission) and survival rates in terms of a negative outcome for the patient (Cardoso et al. 2011; McQuillan et al. 1998; Young et al. 2003). In addition, NICE (2007) stresses that delay in recognition of acute illness may result in subsequent inappropriate management. Use of 'early warning' or 'track and trigger' systems is also recommended to monitor all adult patients in acute hospital settings (NICE 2007). These early warning systems are designed to alert staff to a deteriorating patient and facilitate timely admission into a critical care facility. Such tools score physiological parameters such as respiratory rate, heart rate, blood pressure, oxygen saturation and temperature (NICE 2007), which when abnormal should trigger a response to seek advice from a critical care outreach team or the patient's clinical team (*see* Chapter 3 for more detail). Further assessment by practitioners may result in a transfer to a critical care facility.

Admission of a patient to a level 2 or 3 care facility

Admissions to level 2 or level 3 facilities can be categorized into:

- planned (or elective) admissions
- emergency admissions.

Planned admissions

The term 'planned admissions' includes those who are awaiting major/high-risk elective surgery (However, patients requiring repatriation to the critical care facility from which they were initially transferred may also have their admissions planned as the transfer would be discussed and agreed between the current and initial critical care facility.) This is because recovery, outcome and mortality are more favourable when care is planned and managed in a level 2 or level 3 facility immediately after surgery. Lack of access to critical care facilities has been associated with increased post-surgical mortality (Jhanji et al. 2008). The decision to plan a patient's admission may be influenced by the duration of surgery, technicality of surgery, previous medical history, or the potential for perioperative complications. In such situations critical care can provide a period of intense observation, monitoring, or treatment that would not be feasible in a general ward. Patients undergoing elective, high-risk surgery should be booked into a critical care facility with as much notice as possible. Good practice requires that, wherever possible, the surgeon or anaesthetist should ensure the availability of a critical care bed prior to commencement of the surgery.

It is important that theatre practitioners communicate with critical care practitioners throughout the surgery in relation to the progress and condition of the patient. This is in order to liaise with the family, and also to ensure that the correct facilities to care for the patient are available following the operation. Towards the end of surgery critical care practitioners should also be informed of:

- the patient's stability
- any adverse events while in theatre
- the patients physiological status (cardiovascular [*see* Chapter 6], respiratory [*see* Chapter 5] etc.)
- specific treatment and care required.

Details on admission should include all of the above as well as more detailed instructions or information concerning:

- medication
- fluids required
- positioning
- pain management
- wound management, etc.

(NICE 2007, 2009; ICS 2011)

Some hospitals now have additional locations for patients following planned uncomplicated operations, called extended recovery areas, post-anaesthetic care units, 'fast-track' systems, or specialist observation areas on wards. These facilities, which may provide level 1, 2 and/or 3 care, have been developed to increase critical care capacity for some postoperative patients and as a result reduce the number of cancelled operations that rely on such resources. This development is an attempt to minimize the cancellation of planned surgery and enable emergency admissions to critical care facilities in a timely fashion due to reduction in competition for the same bed resources (ICS 2002a).

Emergency admissions

Critically ill patients who are admitted to hospital are usually assessed by one of the general medical, surgical, or specialist teams who have responsibility for admitting patients. If the patient requires a higher level of monitoring, ventilatory support, initiation of inotropic support (*see* Chapter 7), or haemofiltration therapy (*see* Chapter 9), further clinical review should be sought from senior critical care practitioners who will make a decision on the appropriateness of admission to a critical care facility. Where appropriate, the patient's and/or family's and GP's opinions should be taken into account as to where the care is provided. While the patient is waiting for transfer they should be receiving treatment from critical care practitioners. The period of time from decision to admission may be protracted when a unit is full and other patients need to be discharged from a critical care unit to facilitate the admission of the new patient. Liaison between the critical care unit and emergency department is important to assist in the updating of information and to provide progress reports on the timeline for admission. During this period it is judicious to ascertain information that may influence the location of the patient within the critical care unit to which they will be transferred, e.g. the need for infection prevention precautions which may necessitate the need for a cubicled bed space.

On admission to a critical care facility all necessary equipment and required practitioners should be available. The bed and surrounding space should be prepared for general requirements and the specific needs of the patient. This should include equipment to:

- support the patient's airway (for example airway adjuncts)
- support breathing (for example correct type of ventilator, tubing, attachments, etc.)
- support circulation (fluids, blood, medication, syringe pumps, etc.)
- assess neurological status and manage any disability
- meet the specific requirements of the patient (such as pressure area care, wound management).

Recording status on admission

Prior to and following admission to the critical care facility many activities are required to set up monitoring equipment, and initiate necessary interventions and physiological tests to direct the management of the patient. However, it is vital for immediate and future management of the patient to record status on admission.

The following should be assessed on admission:

- Airway (patency)
- Breathing (rate, rhythm etc)
- Circulation (haemodynamic status)
- Disability (neurological status)
- Exposure/Everything else (for example, rashes, swelling, etc.).

Other assessments may be required on admission but it is essential to record the above as a matter of priority to ensure rapid assessment and treatment, and to maintain patient safety. The patient may require a number of other assessments (*see* Procedure guideline 4.2) that should be undertaken as soon as possible after admission. These might include:

- nutritional assessment and presence of nasogastric tube
- height and weight, and calculation of Body Mass Index (BMI)
- assessment for risk for venous thromboembolic disease (VTE)
- pain assessment
- risk of falls
- sleep assessment
- infection risk
- rehabilitation assessment.

Establishing a rapport with the patient

Whether admission to a critical care facility is planned or an emergency it is a very stressful time for patients (Wikehult et al. 2008). Therefore it is important that staff establish a rapport with patients immediately. Some patients will be unconscious or semi-conscious on admission, while others may be awake. Communication with these patients requires competent communication skills. First, and prior to admission, specific practitioners should be allocated to the patient. They will be responsible for the preparations described above, but also and, equally important, the psychological wellbeing of the patient being admitted. Care should start with simple introductions by practitioners, for example their name and status, and this should apply to all patients whether conscious or not. If possible, it should be established how the patient would like to be addressed. A simple explanation of reasons for admission to the critical care facility should also be given and followed by explanations of any procedures. Patients will be frightened and possibly confused, therefore information should be repeated (Adam and Osbourne 2005). However, it has been reported that actions and remarks within critical care units are not only remembered by patients and relatives but may continue to affect patients 6 months after their discharge (Russell 1999). Practitioners should minimize moments of fear and pay extra attention to verbal and non-verbal cues of fear (Wikehult et al. 2008). Therefore it is important to remember fundamental elements of care, such as providing information and seeing the patient as a human being in the drama of admitting a patient to a critical care facility (Hofhuis et al. 2008).

Establishing a rapport with family and carers

The patient's admission to a critical care facility is a very stressful time for family members and friends. Supporting relatives is a vital part of the role of all critical care practitioners. Damboise and Cardin (2003) note that it is a multidisciplinary task to understand the needs of relatives. If the admission is planned the patient and relatives may have had an opportunity to visit the critical care unit preoperatively or practitioners may visit the patient on the ward prior to the operation to introduce themselves and discuss admission to the critical care unit (Adams and Osbourne 2005).

While the patient is receiving initial treatment relatives should be shown to an area where they can sit. This may be a general waiting area or private room, depending on the facilities available in the critical care unit. A member of staff (often a receptionist) should be allocated to greet and care for relatives, prior to them seeing the patient. It must be remembered that first impressions count and that this initial contact will be vital in future relationships with relatives. It is also important to establish who is accompanying the patient to facilitate appropriate communication. The role of a receptionist in the critical care unit waiting room has been identified as key to facilitating communication between critical care practitioners and families (Deitrick et al. 2005). In addition, staff should be mindful of the need for confidentiality. Relatives will be frightened and will need to be reassured that the patient is being treated, and information will need to be repeated. It is important to foster an environment that protects the physical and emotional health of severely stressed relatives (Lederer et al. 2005). Staff should complete any necessary documentation and ensure they have obtained relevant details of relatives and the main person to contact.

Relatives should not just be shown to a waiting area and left alone. Bournes and Mitchell (2002; 58) describe waiting as 'an agonising doubt and uncertainty that is isolating, distressing and frustrating'. Relatives should be given a realistic time frame for how long they may be expected to wait before seeing the patient. If the waiting time is prolonged the relatives should receive regular updates. Relatives have highlighted the importance of constantly knowing what is happening (Karlsson et al. 2011). At the earliest opportunity practitioners responsible for caring for the patient should meet with the relatives. They should introduce themselves and establish to whom they are talking. Woodrow (2012) makes reference to duty of care and the duty to maintain confidentiality. If patients are unable to express their wishes about what information can be shared, practitioners must be very cautious about giving out information (NMC 2008). If it is appropriate to do so practitioners should discuss what has been happening to the patient. The relatives should then be prepared for entering the critical care area and what the patient may be like, for example unconscious, presence of a breathing tube, unable to speak, etc.

It is possible that relatives may wish to be present throughout the admission process. Practitioners must judge if this is appropriate, for instance in the case of a vulnerable adult. If relatives are present a practitioner should be allocated to support and provide ongoing explanation to the relatives as to what is happening to the patient. Much debate exists around witnessed resuscitation (cardiovascular and other types of resuscitation) (*see* Chapter 17).

Once admission is established information should be given to relatives regarding how to contact the critical care unit, visiting, etc. This should be provided both verbally and in writing.

Procedure guideline 4.1: Admitting a patient to the critical care unit

Preparation of the critical care unit and bed space for admission

Equipment

Equipment will vary according to the needs of the patient but usually includes items in the following categories:
- personal protective equipment
- appropriate bed/mattress/pillows and linen
- emergency equipment (for example bag and valve mask)
- oxygen and air supply
- airway adjuncts
- suction system/equipment
- ventilation system/equipment
- monitoring equipment
- infusion devices and systems
- ways for maintaining privacy and dignity

Procedure Action	Rationale
1 Identify the level of care required by the patient.	To ensure the patient receives the most appropriate level of care.
2 Identify the most suitable bed space for the patient being admitted, i.e. open bay or cubicle.	To ensure the safety and comfort of the patient and to avoid moving the patient following admission. To reduce the risk of cross-infection. To reduce the risk of acquiring infection.
3 Check that the bed space is stocked with personal protective equipment required by staff as per local protocol.	To ensure the safety of both patients and staff. To reduce the risk of cross-infection. To reduce the risk of acquiring infection.
4 Identify the most suitable type of bed/mattress available for the patient and ensure bed is made up with clean linen. This will depend on prior knowledge of skin condition, weight, etc.	To ensure the patient is cared for on the most appropriate bed. For example, in relation to pressure area care, fractures, weight, chest problems. To avoid the risk of transferring or moving the patient following admission.
5 Ensure the bed and space around the bed have been cleaned and disinfected prior to admission and in accordance with local policy.	To minimize the risk of cross-infection.
6 Ascertain if emergency equipment is available and has been checked. This will include bag and valve mask, oxygen, airway adjuncts in a range of sizes, suctioning equipment, intubation equipment, emergency drugs and defibrillator.	To ensure equipment is working and is available if required in case of sudden deterioration of the patient on admission or if ventilator malfunction occurs, or if the patient requires intubation or re-intubation.
7 Check that the bed space is stocked with any equipment required for patient care and sufficient numbers of disposable items are available.	To ensure availability of equipment required for patient timely care. To minimize the risk to the patient of equipment not being available or time away from the patient area for practitioners to retrieve equipment.
8 Set up and test ventilator or other respiratory equipment as per manufacturer's instructions (*see* Chapter 5).	To ensure equipment is working and to minimize risk to the patient.

(Continued)

Procedure guideline 4.1: *(Continued)*

9 Set up and test monitoring equipment. Ensure monitoring equipment has been zeroed to atmospheric pressure and calibrated as per manufacturer's instructions. To include alarm limits appropriately set according to unit protocols.	To ensure equipment is working and to minimize risk to the patient. Failure to zero and calibrate monitoring equipment will lead to inaccurate readings and therefore possible mismanagement of the patient.
10 Ensure all suctioning equipment is set up and connected to correct wall vacuum unit. Check that the suction gauge records an increase in negative pressure on occlusion to the suction tube and suction is felt on the finger on occluding the open end of the suction tube. Test the system to ensure that it is working.	To ensure equipment is working and to clear the patient's airway or clear vomit as required.
11 Ensure emergency oxygen supply is available. Check cylinder is full and flow meter is attached and functioning.	To provide an alternative source of oxygen from the piped oxygen. To ensure equipment is working and to minimize risk to the patient should there be a fault with piped oxygen supply (NPSA 2009).
12 Ensure all documentation required by the patient is available in the bed space.	To ensure documents are available for timely recording the patient's status on admission and thereafter.

Procedure guideline 4.2: Recording status on admission

Equipment will vary according to the needs of the patient but will need to encompass that used for appropriate assessment, for example an 'ABCDE' assessment (*see* Chapter 3) including, inter alia:

- stethoscope
- monitoring equipment, such as that to measure arterial blood gases, blood pressure, central venous pressure, or to assess cardiac rhythms
- ventilator equipment, such as tidal volume, minute volume, ventilator pressures and respiratory rate
- glucometer
- pulse oximeter
- thermometer
- endotracheal cuff pressure monitor
- charts and/or personal computer and patient's clinical notes to guide assessment and record information, including those for assessing (where appropriate):

   – vital signs
   – fluid input, output and balance
   – neurological status
   – pressure ulcer risk
   – venous thromboembolism risk
   – nutritional status
   – falls risk
   – pain
   – sleep
   – blood gases
   – blood biochemistry and haematology.

Procedure Action	Rationale
1 Where possible, explain and discuss the need to undertake an assessment, take observations on admission with the patient and/or relatives if appropriate. If the patient lacks the capacity to make decisions the practitioner must act in the patient's best interests.	To ensure that the patient understands the procedure and gives their valid consent. To ensure the patient's best interests are maintained (Mental Capacity Act 2005).
2 Refer to any local procedures for documenting status of patient on admission.	To ensure practitioners comply with local hospital guidelines and governance.

3 Use recognized assessment framework to assess patient status, e.g. ABCDE approach.	To ensure a systematic approach is taken to assessment (Smith et al. 2002).
4 Determine if the patient is conscious and able to speak. Assess the patient's ability to speak in full sentences, whether they are alert and orientated and note the presence of any noisy breathing such as stridor (see also Chapters 5 and 11). Note the presence of any type of airway and document in records.	If the patient is able to speak this indicates a patent airway. The type of airway adjunct should be documented for future records to provide accurate medical notes and reduce time delays in future.
5 Assess airway patency by feeling for movement of expired air, and listening for inspiration and expiration.	To ensure airway patency.
6 If there are any concerns about airway obstruction lift the patient's chin and tilt back the head while protecting the cervical spine. Perform endotracheal suction.	To clear airway and preserve life. Suctioning assists in the removal of any foreign body or mucus obstructing the airway.
7 Assess breathing status, which should include: rate, rhythm, depth, symmetry, colour, use of accessory muscles and oxygen saturation. Document oxygen delivery device and percentage of oxygen being delivered.	To ascertain the patient's actual respiratory status on admission and assess potential for deterioration and any immediate intervention. To ensure accurate records are kept in case of any future questions or discrepancy (O'Driscoll et al. 2008).
8 Assess the patient's circulation including: capillary refill time, limb temperature, peripheral pulses, central pulses, blood pressure, heart rate, cardiac rhythm, central venous pressure (if being measured), 12 lead ECG and dosages of any vasopressor drugs being administered (*see* Chapters 3 and 6). For patients who are cold, peripherally shut down, or are receiving vasoconstrictor drugs, assessing capillary refill by pressing on the sternum with the thumb may be more appropriate.	To detect the patient's actual or potential risk of haemodynmic instability on admission and the need for any immediate intervention (Smith et al. 2002). To obtain admission data for later comparison.
9 Check the patient's temperature.	To determine if the patient is normothermic or requires any immediate action to either reduce or raise temperature.
10 Check fluid status, document any IV fluids being administered and check urine output.	To assess the patient's fluid balance on admission and the need for any immediate intervention. To ensure fluids are being administered as per prescription and records are being kept accurately.
11 Check any vasopressor or other drugs being administered on admission and cross-check with prescription and document.	To ensure safety of patient and that drugs are being administered as per prescription and records are being accurately recorded.
12 Check all vascular access for patency and signs of infection/inflammation at site of insertion. Document as appropriate for local policy.	To ensure that the vascular access is patent and functional in an emergency situation. To detect infection early (DH 2007).

(Continued)

Procedure guideline 4.2: (*Continued*)

13 Assess neurological status using either GCS or 'Alert, Voice, Pain, Unresponsive' (AVPU) system as per local policy. Record findings accurately, recording the best response, what stimulation was applied, where stimulus was applied and how much pressure was required to elicit a response. Check pupil reaction to light.	To assess the patient's neurological status and determine the need for any immediate intervention or further investigation or referral to specialist teams (Iankova 2006). Documentation of precise findings is necessary to ensure continuity of assessment and avoid future misinterpretations (NMC 2008). To assess the size, shape and equality of the pupils as an indication of brain injury/impairment.
14 Check blood glucose using locally agreed protocol.	To assess the patient's blood glucose for hypoglycaemia or hyperglycaemia and determine the need for any immediate intervention.
15 Undertake a pressure ulcer risk assessment using the local protocol/tools/scales. Check the status of the patient's skin and document any abnormalities, redness, wounds and drains. If appropriate to move the patient, roll to check their back, sacrum, heels and head.	To determine the pressure ulcer risk. To determine the appropriate turning regime. To determine the appropriate bed surface for the patient (Waterlow 2005; DH 2009) (*see also* Chapter 12). To ensure the condition of wounds and drains are documented on admission.
16 Undertake an infection risk assessment. Obtain relevant baseline specimens as per local septic screening protocol.	To ensure the patient receives prompt and correct treatment if any infections are present on admission. To ensure the patient receives appropriate isolation facilities and to determine infection risk to other patients and staff.
17 Obtain patient history from the patient if appropriate.	To determine the patient's view of illness and gather additional information for full assessment of the patient (Robertson et al. 2009).
18 Review notes and charts.	To gather additional information for full assessment of the patient (Smith et al. 2002).
19 Perform systematic examination of the patient once all immediate life-saving interventions have been carried out.	To provide a full and detailed assessment of the patient to determine any abnormalities and to direct further management of the patient. To ensure that nothing was missed on initial assessment on admission (Robertson et al. 2009).
20 Review results of any investigations performed.	To provide a full assessment of the patient's status. To confirm any abnormalities or deterioration from previous tests. To aid future management of the patient (Robertson et al. 2009).
21 Undertake a VTE risk assessment using local assessment tool. Complete documentation. Apply any necessary aids or administer any prescribed anticoagulants.	To determine the risk of development of VTE. To prevent development of VTE (ICS 2008; NICE 2010a).
22 Undertake a nutritional assessment and assessment of the patient's BMI using local assessment tool. Complete documentation. Refer patient to dietician as per local protocol. Administer any prescribed nutrition.	To ensure early nutrition is commenced and to avoid malnutrition (NICE 2006).

23 Undertake a pain assessment using local assessment tool suitable for critically ill patients. Complete documentation and administer any prescribed analgesia.	To ensure patient comfort. To avoid complications of pain (Carroll et al. 1999).
24 Undertake a sleep assessment using local assessment tool suitable for critically ill patients. Complete documentation and implement appropriate strategies to promote sleep.	To ensure the patient gets adequate sleep. To avoid sleep deprivation and potential delirium (Borthwick et al. 2006; NICE 2010b). *See also* Chapter 13.
25 Undertake a falls assessment where appropriate. Utilize a local falls assessment tool.	To ensure risk of falls is identified and strategies are implemented to prevent falls (Halm and Quigley 2011).
26 When the patient's clinical condition allows undertake assessment to determine risk of long-term physical and psychological problems.	To ensure that the patient receives early referral for a comprehensive physical and/or psychological assessment by staff with expertise in critical care rehabilitation (*see* Chapter 16).
27 Document assessment, treatment and care.	To: ■ provide an accurate record ■ monitor effectiveness of procedure ■ reduce the risk of duplication of treatment ■ provide a point of reference or comparison in the event of later questions ■ acknowledge accountability for actions ■ facilitate communication and continuity of care. (NMC 2008; GMC 2013; HCPC 2012)

Competency statement 4.1: **Specific procedure competency statements for admission to the critical care unit**

Complete assessment against relevant fundamental competency statements	Evidence
Specific procedure competency statements for admission to the critical care unit	**Evidence of competency for admission to the critical care unit**
Demonstrate ability to: ■ teach and assess or ■ learn from assessment.	Examples of evidence of teaching, assessing and learning.
Demonstrate knowledge of local and national guidelines and protocols for admission of patients to the critical care unit. Demonstrate knowledge of own responsibilities and role and responsibilities of other team members.	*May be demonstrated by:* ■ ability to locate protocols and guidelines ■ discussion with supervisor/mentor.
Established details of patient being admitted, including: ■ name ■ date of birth (if known) ■ rationale for transfer ■ preliminary diagnosis ■ admitting consultant/team ■ source of admission, e.g. A&E, theatres, ward, etc. ■ expected time of admission.	*May be demonstrated by:* ■ observation and discussion with supervisor/mentor.

(Continued)

Competency statement 4.1: *(Continued)*

Prepare critical care team for admission by allocating appropriate practitioner to the following tasks: ■ practitioner with primary responsibility for initial assessment and management of patient ■ completion of initial documentation/handover ■ care/support for relatives.	*May be demonstrated by:* ■ observation by supervisor/mentor.
Demonstrate ability to set up bed area and prepare any other equipment: ■ bed area is cleaned and prepared in line with local infection control policy ■ ventilator is set up and tested ■ resuscitation equipment is present and checked ■ airway/intubation and suction equipment is present and checked ■ monitors are switched on and checked ■ fluids and administration sets are made ready ■ bed area is stocked with associated equipment as per local protocols ■ availability and stocks of drugs are checked ■ need for protective clothing.	*May be demonstrated by:* ■ ability to locate infection control policy ■ discussion with supervisor/mentor ■ observation of correct preparation and assembly of equipment by supervisor/mentor ■ teaching session for peers.
Demonstrate knowledge of relevant infection control policies associated with admission to the critical care unit: ■ MRSA etc. status of patient ■ samples/tests required ■ need for protective clothing.	*May be demonstrated by:* ■ ability to locate infection control policy ■ discussion with supervisor/mentor ■ teaching session for peers.
Demonstrate understanding of holistic care of patients: ■ establish rapport with patient ■ introduce self ■ explain status and role ■ establish how patient wishes to be addressed.	*May be demonstrated by:* ■ discussion with supervisor/mentor ■ observation by supervisor/mentor.
Demonstrate knowledge of local and national guidelines on moving and handling patients and back care: ■ choose appropriate device for transfer of patient ■ demonstrate knowledge and skills in using hoist, etc. ■ check equipment is ready ■ prepare and coordinate team ■ explain procedure to patient ■ transfer patient to critical care facility ■ position patient appropriately (*see also* Chapter 14).	*May be demonstrated by:* ■ ability to locate moving and handling policy ■ discussion with supervisor/mentor ■ observation of correct choice, preparation and assembly of equipment by supervisor/mentor ■ observation of procedure by supervisor/mentor ■ teaching session for peers.
Demonstrate knowledge and skills for the correct connection of patient to monitoring and ventilator equipment.	*May be demonstrated by:* ■ discussion with supervisor/mentor ■ observation of correct preparation and assembly of equipment by supervisor/mentor ■ observation of procedure by supervisor/mentor ■ teaching session for peers.

Demonstrate knowledge and understanding of initial assessment of patient: ■ patent airway ■ respiratory rate ■ heart rate ■ systolic blood pressure ■ level of consciousness ■ GCS/AVPU ■ oxygen saturation ■ temperature ■ presence of IV access and other tubing ■ presence of drugs and infusions ■ presence of drains, etc.	*May be demonstrated by:* ■ discussion with supervisor/mentor of importance of initial assessment ■ teaching session for peers.
Demonstrate ability to identify priorities of care/treatment: ■ interpret findings from initial assessment ■ decide on immediate management plan ■ delegate urgent tasks.	*May be demonstrated by:* ■ discussion with supervisor/mentor of priorities of care ■ formulation of patient management plan ■ teaching session for peers.
Demonstrate knowledge of the importance of patient hand over from primary team.	*May be demonstrated by:* ■ discussion with supervisor/mentor ■ teaching session for peers.
Demonstrate knowledge of importance of completion of documentation using an agreed, standardized local format.	*May be demonstrated by:* ■ discussion with supervisor/mentor ■ observation of completion of documentation.
Demonstrate knowledge of the importance of communicating with anyone accompanying the patient: ■ establish rapport with accompanying relatives/friends/carers ■ introduce self ■ explain status and role ■ establish relationship to patient ■ provide initial information as appropriate ■ ensure confidentiality ■ document relatives' details, including contact details, next of kin, main person to be point of contact between relatives ■ provide relatives with information about the critical care unit both verbally and in writing.	*May be demonstrated by:* ■ discussion with supervisor/mentor ■ observation of discussion/interview with relatives by supervisor/mentor ■ observation of completion of documentation by supervisor/mentor ■ location of written materials ■ teaching session for peers.

References and further reading

Adam S, Odell M and Welch J (2010) *Rapid Assessment of the Acutely Ill Patient*. Oxford: Wiley-Blackwell.

Adam SK and Osbourne S (2005) *Critical Care Nursing. Science and Practice* (2e). Oxford: Oxford University Press.

Andrews T and Waterman H (2005) Packaging: a grounded theory of how to report physiological deterioration effectively. *Journal of Advanced Nursing* 52: 473–481.

Borthwick M, Bourne R, Craig M et al. (2006) *Detection, Prevention and Treatment of Delirium in Critical Care Patients*. United Kingdom Clinical Pharmacy Association.

Bournes DA and Mitchell CJ (2002) Waiting: the experience of persons in a critical care waiting room. *Research in Nursing and Health* 25(1): 58–67.

Cardoso LTQ, Grion CMC, Matsuo T et al. (2011) Impact of delayed admission to intensive care units on mortality of critically ill patients: a cohort study. *Critical Care* 15: R28. http://ccforum.com/content/15/1/R28

Carroll KC, Atkins PJ, Herold GR et al. (1999) Pain assessment and management of critically ill post-operative and trauma patient: a multisite study. *American Journal of Critical Care* 2(8): 105–117.

Considine J, Thomas S and Potter R (2009) Predictors of critical care admission in emergency department patients triaged as low to moderate urgency. *Journal of Advanced Nursing* **65**(4): 818–827.

Damboise C and Cardin S (2003) Family-centered critical care: how one unit implemented a plan. *American Journal of Nursing* **103**(6): 56AA–56EE.

Deitrick L, Ray D, Stern G et al. (2005) Evaluation and recommendations from a study of a critical care waiting room. *Journal for Healthcare Quality* **27**(4): 17–25.

Department of Health (1996) *Guidelines on Admission to and Discharge from Intensive Care and High Dependency Units*. London: Department of Health NHS Executive.

Department of Health (2000) *Comprehensive Critical Care: a review of adult critical care services*. London: DH.

Department of Health (2007) *High Impact intervention No 1: central venous catheter care bundle*. London: DH.

Department of Health (2009) *NHS 2010–2015: from good to great. Preventative, people centred, productive*. London: DH.

General Medical Council (2013) *Good Medical Practice*. London: GMC. http://www.gmc-uk.org/gmp2013 [accessed 25 March 2013].

Halm MA and Quigley PA (2011) Reducing falls and fall related injuries in acutely and critically ill patients. *American Journal of Critical Care* **6**(20): 480–484.

Health and Care Professions Council (2012) *Standard of Conduct, Performance and Ethics*. London: HCPC. http://www.hcpc-uk.org/assets/documents/10003B6EStandardsofconduct,performanceandethics.pdf [accessed January 2013].

Hofhuis JG, Spronk PE, van Stel HF et al. (2008) Experiences of critically ill patients in the ICU. *Intensive and Critical Care Nursing* **24**: 300–313.

Iankova A (2006) The Glasgow Coma Scale clinical application in Emergency Departments. *Emergency Nurse* **14**(8): 30–35.

Intensive Care Society (1997) *Standards for Intensive Care Units*. London: ICS.

Intensive Care Society (2002a) *Levels of Critical Care for Adult Patients*. London: ICS Standards.

Intensive Care Society (2002b) *Guidelines for the Introduction of Outreach Services*. London: ICS.

Intensive Care Society (2008) *Venous Thromboprophylaxis in Critical Care. Standards and Guidelines*. London: ICS.

Intensive Care Society (2009) *Levels of Critical Care for Adult Patients*. London: ICS Standards.

Intensive Care Society (2011) *Guidelines for the Transport of the Critically Ill Adult* (3e). London: ICS Standards.

Jhanji S, Thomas B, Ely A et al. (2008) Mortality and utilization of critical care resources amongst high-risk surgical patients in a large NHS trust. *Anaesthesia* **63**: 695–700.

Karlsson C, Tisell A, Engstrom A and Andershed B (2011) Family members' satisfaction with critical care: a pilot study. *Nursing in Critical Care* **16**(1): 11–18.

Lederer MA, Goode T and Dowling J (2005) Origins and development: the critical care family assistance program *Chest* **128**(3): 65S–75S.

McQuillan P, Pilkington S, Allan A et al. (1998) Confidential enquiry into quality of care before admission to intensive care. *British Medical Journal* **316**(7148): 1853–1858.

Mental Capacity Act (2005) http://www.legislation.gov.uk/ukpga/2005/9/pdfs/ukpga_20050009_en.pdf [accessed 9 February 2012].

National Institute of Health and Clinical Excellence (2006) *Nutrition Support in Adults*. London: NICE.

National Institute of Health and Clinical Excellence (2007) *NICE Clinical Guideline 50. Acutely ill patients in hospital. Recognition of and response to acute illness in adults in hospital*. London: NICE.

National Institute of Health and Clinical Excellence (2009) *Critical Illness Rehabilitation*. London: NICE.

National Institute of Health and Clinical Excellence (2010a) *NICE Clinical Guideline 92. Reducing the risk of VTE (deep vein thrombosis and pulmonary embolism) in patients admitted to hospital*. London: NICE.

National Institute of Health and Clinical Excellence (2010b) *NICE Clinical Guideline 103. Delirium: diagnosis prevention and management*. London: NICE.

National Patient Safety Agency (2009) *Rapid Response Report NPSA/2009/RRR006: Oxygen Safety in Hospitals*. London: NPSA. www.nrls.npsa.uk/alerts [accessed 22 December 2011]

Nursing and Midwifery Council (2008) *The Code: standards of conduct, performance and ethics for nurses and midwives*. London: NMC. http://www.nmc-uk.org/Documents/Standards/The-code-A4-20100406.pd [accessed 15 February 2012].

O'Driscoll BR, Howard LS, Davison AG et al. (2008) Guideline for emergency oxygen use in adult patients. British Thoracic Society Emergency Oxygen Guideline Group. Thorax 63 Supplement VI. www.brit-thoracic.org.uk

Rivers E, Nguyen B and Havstad S (2001) Early goal-directed therapy in the treatment of severe sepsis and septic shock. *New England Journal of Medicine* **345**: 1368–1377.

Robertson CE, Nicol EF, Douglas G and Macleod J (2009) *Macleod's Clinical Examination* (12e). Edinburgh: Elsevier Churchill Livingstone.

Russell S (1999) An exploratory study of patients' perceptions, memories and experiences of an intensive care unit. *Journal of Advanced Nursing* **29**(4): 783–791.

Smith GB, Osgood VM, Cranes S and ALERT Course Development Group (2002) ALERT – a multi-professional training course in the care of the acutely ill adult. *Resuscitation* **53**(3): 281–283.

Waterlow J (2005) *Pressure Sore Prevention Manual*. Taunton: Waterlow.

Wacogne I and Diwakar V (2010) Handover and note taking: the SBAR approach. *Clinical Risk* **16**(5): 173–175.

Wikehult B, Hedland M, Marsenic M et al. (2008) Evaluation of negative emotional care experiences in burn care. *Journal of Clinical Nursing* **17**: 1923–1929.

Woodrow (2012) *Intensive Care Nursing. A framework for practice* (3e). London: Routledge.

Young MP, Gooder VJ, McBride K et al. (2003) Inpatient transfers to the intensive care unit: delays are associated with increased mortality and morbidity. *Journal of General Internal Medicine* **18**: 77–83.

62

Chapter 5

Assessment, monitoring and interventions for the respiratory system

Maureen Coombs,[1] Judy Dyos,[2] David Waters[3] and Ian Nesbitt[4]

[1]*Victoria University Wellington and Capital and Coast District Health Board, Wellington, New Zealand*
[2]*University Hospital Southampton NHS Foundation Trust, Southampton, UK*
[3]*Buckinghamshire New University, Uxbridge, UK*
[4]*Freeman Hospital, Newcastle upon Tyne, UK*

Critical Care Manual of Clinical Procedures and Competencies, First Edition.
Edited by Jane Mallett, John W. Albarran, and Annette Richardson.
© 2013 John Wiley & Sons, Ltd. Published 2013 by John Wiley & Sons, Ltd.

CLINICAL ASSESSMENT

Chest auscultation

Definition

Auscultation of the lungs is the act of listening with a stethoscope to normal or abnormal breath sounds. This enables assessment of air flow through the tracheobronchial tree.

Indications for chest auscultation

Chest auscultation may be undertaken as a routine baseline assessment, for example preoperative evaluation, or used as part of ongoing assessment with an underlying disease process, for example pneumonia or consolidation. It is part of physical assessment of the respiratory system and is usually undertaken in conjunction with:

- inspection: looking at the chest wall to determine normal and abnormal outlines
- palpation: feeling over the chest wall to identify normal and abnormal structures
- percussion: the chest wall is struck with the fingertips to obtain sounds/vibrations that give indication of the position and consistency of the lungs.

Background

Anatomy and physiology

The lungs are located within the thoracic cavity, with the apex of the lung situated at the 2nd intercostal space and the lung bases at the 6th intercostal space during quiet inspiratory breathing. During deep inspiration the lung bases descend to the 8th intercostal space. The left lung is divided into the left upper and lower lobe by the oblique fissure. The right lung comprises three lobes: the right upper lobe, the middle lobe and the lower lobe, divided by the horizontal and oblique fissures (Figure 5.1).

Key to interpreting chest auscultation findings is the ability to identify and describe where normal and abnormal sounds are located on the chest wall. This is achieved using anatomical landmarks to describe vertical and circumferential chest wall positions. For vertical locations on the anterior surface of the chest, the sternal angle is used to identify the 2nd rib. This allows the remaining intercostal spaces and ribs to be identified enabling practitioners to be specific when describing normal and abnormal physical assessment findings. To locate and describe assessment findings around the circumference of the chest wall, approximated lines are visualized around the chest wall. These include the anterior axillary, mid-axillary, mid-clavicular and scapular landmark lines (Bickley 2010). It is knowledge of these landmark posi-

tions together with understanding of the underlying anatomical lung structures that enables safe technique in chest auscultation.

At its most basic, there are three different types of breath sounds: vesicular, bronchial and bronchiovesicular (Rushforth 2010). Vesicular breath sounds are normal quiet breath sounds, located in the peripheries of the lung fields. The inspiratory and expiratory breath sounds are usually heard as one continuous sound, with expiration heard as a longer phase than inspiration. Bronchial breath sounds are coarse, loud breath sounds which are normally heard over the bronchus but are abnormal if heard elsewhere e.g. if heard over consolidated lung tissue. In bronchial breath sounds there is usually a pause between the inspiratory and expiratory phases. Bronchiovesicular breath sounds are normal sounds heard over lung tissue located between bronchial and peripheral lung tissue, and are a combination of normal bronchial and normal vesicular sounds (Bickley 2010).

Abnormal breath sounds are known as adventitious sounds and include crackles and wheezes (Table 5.1). Wheezes normally occur in obstruction of an airway by bronchospasm or swelling. Crackles may be heard during inspiration or expiration. Fine crackles are often high pitched; they are heard at the end of inspiration and may indicate pulmonary oedema or fibrosis (Jarvis 2008). Coarse crackles are louder bubbling sounds heard on inspiration and expiration and are usually associated with secretions that may clear after coughing (Rushforth 2009). In addition, stridor and rub may also be heard. Stridor is high-pitched inspiration sound caused by laryngeal or tracheal obstruction. A rub is often referred to as a creaking sound caused by pleural friction.

Chest auscultation in critical care

Chest auscultation is a physical assessment skill that is being used by increasing numbers of non-medical health professionals across primary and secondary care settings (Coombs and Morse 2002). Inter-rater reliability in chest auscultation is low at 24%, although this is comparable with inter-rater reliability in interpreting chest radiographs (Mangione 2000). There are websites available to help novice practitioners develop and refine chest auscultation skills (e.g. www.wilkes.med.ucla.edu/intro.html).

Key to undertaking chest auscultation is ensuring that accurate respiratory assessment is made to inform diagnosis, treatment and interventions in care. Therefore knowledge of anatomy and physiology, and correct performance of chest auscultation technique is crucial. Other important aspects to consider in chest auscultation are how to manage dignity and privacy for the patient and how to practise safely within one's own professional practice boundaries, including knowing when and who to refer patient problems on to.

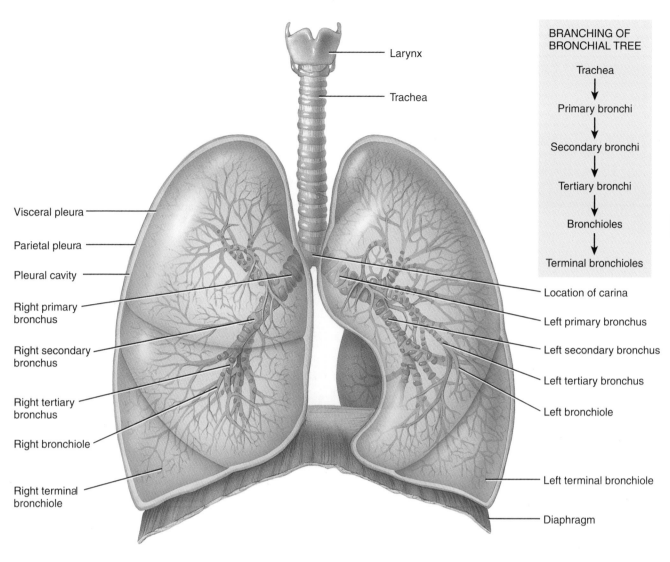

Larynx

Trachea

BRANCHING OF
BRONCHIAL TREE

Trachea
↓
Primary bronchi
↓
Secondary bronchi
↓
Tertiary bronchi
↓
Bronchioles
↓
Terminal bronchioles

Visceral pleura

Parietal pleura

Pleural cavity

Right primary
bronchus

Right secondary
bronchus

Right tertiary
bronchus

Right bronchiole

Right terminal
bronchiole

Location of carina

Left primary bronchus

Left secondary bronchus

Left tertiary bronchus

Left bronchiole

Left terminal bronchiole

Diaphragm

Figure 5.1 Lobes of the lung (from Tortora and Derrickson 2011, reproduced with permission from Wiley).

Table 5.1 Abnormal adventitious (added) breath sounds

Name	Characteristics of sound	Associated patient problems
Wheeze	High pitched, musical sound predominantly in expiration but may occur in inspiration	Asthma, chronic bronchitis, congestive heart failure
Fine crackles	Discontinuous, high-pitched crackling, popping sounds heard during inspiration and not cleared by coughing	Crackles heard early on during inspiration: chronic bronchitis, asthma, emphysema
		Crackles heard late on during inspiration: pneumonia, heart failure, interstitial fibrosis
Coarse crackles	Low-pitched, bubbling sounds in early inspiration. May continue through to expiration. May clear with coughing, suction	Pulmonary oedema, pneumonia, pulmonary fibrosis
Stridor	Breath sounds that are high pitched during inspiration and sound louder in the neck area	Croup, epiglottis in children, inhalation of a foreign object or obstructed airway, laryngeal spasm
Pleural rub	Coarse, low-pitched and grating sound during inspiration and expiration	Pleurisy

Problem-solving table 5.1 Complications: chest auscultation (Procedure guideline 5.1)

Problem	Cause	Suggested actions
Unable to hear breath sounds	Stethoscope bell being used	Use diaphragm of stethoscope
	Stethoscope incorrectly positioned	Reposition stethoscope within normal respiratory landmarks
	Patient not generating sufficient air flow	Get patient to breathe in an out with mouth open – check patient is not becoming dizzy

Arterial blood gas sampling

Definition

An arterial blood gas (ABG) is a test where blood taken from an artery is used to assess the partial pressure of oxygen and carbon dioxide, oxygen saturation and the acidity of the blood.

Indications for arterial blood gas sampling

Information from arterial blood gas and acidity gives information about the patient's respiratory and metabolic function. This information can then be used in conjunction with other respiratory assessment information to inform patient management plans. Sampling of arterial blood is a common investigation undertaken in the critically ill patient (Simpson 2004).

More specifically the indications for arterial blood gas sampling are the monitoring of acid-base balance and respiratory status in:

- acute respiratory failure
- mechanical invasive and non-invasive ventilation therapy (including theatre)
- peri-arrest and cardiorespiratory arrest situations
- severe sepsis and shock
- major trauma
- acute poisoning and other metabolic emergencies, e.g. diabetic ketoacidosis
- acute renal failure.

(Adam and Osbourne 2005)

These conditions all have the potential to either impact on the patient's ability to maintain normal oxygen and carbon dioxide levels (as in respiratory failure) or may potentially impact on the patient's ability to maintain acid-base balance that is key to ensuring healthy cellular functioning (as during prolonged cardiac arrest or other metabolic emergencies).

Background

Anatomy and physiology

Arterial blood sampling can either be accessed by taking blood directly from an artery (arterial stab) or from an indwelling arterial cannula (arterial line). Arterial blood can be taken from major or peripheral arteries for analysis, but the radial and femoral arteries are most commonly used as these are most accessible (Woodrow 2006). If radial artery sampling is undertaken, an Allen test should be undertaken to assess ability of the ulnar artery to supply collateral blood to the hand (Dougherty and Lister 2011). Direct arterial sampling is uncomfortable for the patient and should only be undertaken if infrequent samples (for example less than once every 12 hours) are required. For more frequent serial sampling an arterial cannula should be inserted.

There are several assessments that are important in understanding and interpreting blood gas analysis. These are:

- pH
- measurements of gas exchange (carbon dioxide and oxygen)
- metabolic measures (bicarbonate and base excess)
- assessment of serum electrolytes, including potassium, blood glucose and lactate levels (Woodrow 2006).

pH

Potential hydrogen (pH) is a measure of how acid or alkaline (or base) a substance is. It is a scale that runs from 1 (absolute acid) to 14 (absolute alkali) with 7 being considered 'neutral' (see also Chapter 3). In normal health, blood is slightly alkaline with pH ranging between 7.35 and 7.45 and normal being 7.41. It is kept within this range by central and peripheral chemoreceptors that stimulate the respiratory centres in the pons and medulla in the brain. Acidaemia is when there is an excess of acids in the blood. If blood pH drops below 7.35, it is acidaemic. Alkalaemia occurs when there is too much alkali or too little acid in the blood. If blood pH rises above 7.45, it is alkalaemic.

Gas exchange

In blood gas analysis gas exchange is measured by PaO_2 (partial pressure of arterial oxygen) and $PaCO_2$ (partial pressure of arterial carbon dioxide). The partial pressure of a gas is the pressure exerted by that gas and is measured in units of kilopascals (kPa) or millimetres of mercury (mmHg) (1 kPa is equivalent to 7.5 mmHg). The theory is based on Dalton's Law of Partial Pressures which states that the total pressure of a gaseous mixture is equal to the sum of the partial pressures of each individual component. PaO_2 is a measure of the pressure of oxygen in the blood and has a normal range is 10.0–13.0 kPa (75.0–97.5 mmHg). When oxygen levels fall below this for patients with acute respiratory conditions, the patient is said to be hypoxic. Hypoxia often results from deteriorating lung condition caused by pneumonia, severe lung injury, or pulmonary oedema. Partial pressure of carbon dioxide ($PaCO_2$) has a normal range of 4.7–6.0 kPa (35.3–45.0 mmHg) and is the pressure of carbon dioxide dissolved in the blood. CO_2 is the primary metabolite of cellular respiration and if not cleared from the body will lead to acidosis (Adam and Osbourne 2005; Resuscitation Council 2011).

Metabolic measures

There are two main metabolic measures: bicarbonate and base excess. Bicarbonate (normal range 24–27 mmol/L) is a buffer found in the plasma. Buffers prevent major changes in pH by mopping up excess acid in the blood. Bicarbonate (HCO_3^-) is the major buffer in the plasma and therefore gives indication of a patient's acid-base status. Low levels of bicarbonate (less than 24 mmol/L) in the blood are indicative of a metabolic acidosis and show that the stores of bicarbonate have been used up buffering the acid in the plasma. High levels of bicarbonate (greater than 28 mmol/L) in the blood are indicative of a metabolic alkalosis and may occur due to administration of alkali substances (e.g. sodium bicarbonate) or excessive loss of acids (e.g. high loss of gastric acids in nasogatric aspirates). Base excess (BE) is another measure of the body's acid-base status with a range of +2 to −2. BE is a calculation of the amount of alkali (base) or acid needed to move the pH of the blood to 7.4. Negative base excess indicates that there is an acidosis, while a positive BE indicates an alkalosis (Urden et al. 2005).

Potassium, blood glucose and lactate

There are a number of other measurements available from arterial blood gas analysis that are useful in informing the routine management of critically ill patients. Potassium (normal range 3.5–5.0 mmol/L) is an electrolyte vital for the contraction of myofibres in the heart. Blood glucose control is important for patients with a history of diabetes, and because controlling blood glucose of critically ill patients may improve their chances of survival (van den Berghe et al. 2006). However, more recent research has indicated that intensive glycaemic control may be associated with higher mortality compared to less intensive glycaemic control (NICE SUGAR Study Investigators 2009) (*see* Chapter 8 for details). Lactate (normal value less than 2 mmol/L) is a metabolite produced in cells where there is no oxygen (anaerobic environment). An abnormally high level of lactate (e.g. 6 mmol/L) may indicate that there is insufficient blood flow to perfuse cells (perfusion failure) with a risk of metabolic acidosis (Woodrow 2006).

Arterial blood sampling in critical care

Arterial blood gas analysis provides extremely valuable respiratory assessment data. In applying an understanding of normal and abnormal values, together with knowledge of the patient's symptoms and medical history, and findings from other respiratory assessment (respiratory rate, chest auscultation), an accurate diagnosis can be made and potential interventions identified. However, to obtain accurate arterial blood gas results arterial sampling must occur in a timely manner, i.e. 20 minutes after any intervention in order to accurately reflect respiratory status (Simpson 2004). Adopting a safe and sterile technique is also critical. If the sample is taken from an indwelling, transduced arterial cannula, precautions must be taken to ensure intravenous 0.9% sodium chloride from the flush device does not dilute the sample (*see* Chapter 7 for details and specific complications). Ensuring prompt analysis of the sample is also important so that the blood sample that is analysed gives accurate results on which to base clinical management decisions.

For the majority of patients in critical care areas, arterial blood gas sampling will be undertaken via an indwelling arterial cannula. Whether arterial blood gas sampling is undertaken through direct arterial sampling or via an indwelling arterial cannula, both approaches require skilled personnel to mitigate the associated safety and risk to patient and practitioner. This can be done through regular assessment of the arterial site and patient, and accurate and intelligent interpretation of the arterial blood gas and acidity results. Adherence to infection prevention measures is paramount.

Problem-solving table 5.2: Sampling via arterial puncture

Problem	Cause	Prevention	Action
Arterial spasm and pain	Forceful aspiration when withdrawing blood	The pressure generated in the syringe is higher than that in the artery, causing arterial collapse and irritation. Spasm may leads to arterial thrombosis	Gentle aspiration of sample from artery. Use of local anaesthetic will minimize discomfort
Bruising	Patient anticoagulated or inadequate pressure applied post procedure	Check coagulation status of patient prior to procedure. Securing haemostasis is important as collection of blood in the surrounding tissues may cause compression neuropathy	Ensure pressure applied for a minimum of 5 minutes. Longer may be required if clotting status is abnormal
Local arterial aneurysm	Repeated sampling from the same arterial site	If repeated sampling is required, consider need for an indwelling arterial cannula	Procedure to be undertaken by an experienced practitioner. Proactive use of indwelling arterial cannulae

Problem-solving table 5.3: Sampling via arterial cannula

Problem	Cause	Prevention	Action
Back flow of blood into indwelling cannula	The pressure infusion cuff may not be inflated to the optimal	Ensure that the pressure infusion cuff is inflated to 300 mmHg	Check that the pressure infusion cuff is inflated to 300 mmHg and if not, inflate to correct level
Arterial spasm	Forceful flushing or forceful aspiration when withdrawing blood	This pressure is higher than arterial blood pressure and an automatic flush mode is activated in the system that delivers 3 mL/h. This maintains patency of circuit, cannula and artery (Thompson and Stroud 1984)	Check that the pressure infusion cuff is inflated to 300 mmHg and if not, inflate to correct level
Cerebral embolism	Prolonged, high-pressure flushing can drive a clot or gas bubbles retrograde to produce cerebral embolism	Avoid forceful flushing or aspiration and maintain a slow even pressure when withdrawing blood	Check that the pressure infusion cuff is inflated to 300 mmHg and if not, inflate to correct level

From Dougherty and Lister (2011)

Pulse oximetry

Definition

Arterial oxygen saturation (SaO_2) is a measure of the amount of oxygen attached to haemoglobin molecules as a percentage of the maximum that can be carried in the erythrocytes. Pulse oximetry is a non-invasive method allowing the measurement of the peripheral (capillary) saturation of haemoglobin by oxygen (SpO_2); this is as opposed to direct measurement of blood oxygen saturation (SaO_2) measured via arterial blood gas sampling. Pulse oximetry is non-invasively monitored and measured using a pulse oximeter, which consists of a finger probe and monitor.

Indications for pulse oximetry monitoring

Indications for pulse oximetry monitoring include establishing:

- effectiveness of oxygen therapy
- oxygenation of the unwell patient during inter- and intra-hospital transport
- oxygenation during anaesthesia or administration of sedative, anaesthetic, or analgesic agents with respiratory depressant effects
- oxygenation of patients with respiratory disease, e.g. asthma, chronic obstructive pulmonary diseases, to observe progress and response to treatments
- oxygenation of patients with cardiac dysfunction who may be at risk of developing pulmonary oedema or low cardiac output, e.g. post myocardial infarction.

(Place 2000)

Background

Anatomy and physiology

Oxygen is transported to the body's tissues in blood. Oxygen binds to the haemoglobin molecules in the lungs, forming oxyhaemoglobin. Each haemoglobin molecule has four haem sites to which oxygen can bind. When these four sites are occupied, the haemoglobin is fully saturated with oxygen. The oxygen is transported to the peripheral tissues on the haemoglobin where, due to the presence of lower oxygen partial pressures, the oxygen is released for tissue oxygenation and energy (Tortora and Derrickson 2011).

Blood saturated with oxygen is bright red compared with blood that is low in oxygen, which is more blue in colour. In pulse oximetry, a probe emits and measures light that is absorbed differently by oxygenated and deoxygenated haemoglobin. The probe is typically placed on a translucent part of the patient's body, usually a fingertip or an earlobe. The probe detects the pulse from an arterial (capillary) source using the expansion and contraction of the vessel with each heartbeat. The percentage of oxygen saturation is mathematically calculated by the machine, by combining the value of the reflected light and the detected pulse of the artery.

For healthy patients with a normal haemoglobin level, an optimum oxygen saturation value is 96% and above (Prytherch et al. 2010) (*see also* Chapter 15). The amount of oxygen released from haemoglobin to the tissues is dependent on the affinity of haemoglobin for oxygen. This is often represented diagrammatically as the oxygen dissociation curve (Figure 5.2) and is important in understanding how tissues carry and release oxygen. Oxygen is more readily released to the tissues when:

- pH is decreased
- body temperature is increased
- arterial partial pressure of carbon dioxide ($PaCO_2$) is increased
- 2,3-diphosphoglycerate (2,3-DPG) levels (a by-product of glucose metabolism) are increased.

In critical illness, where patients may have a higher metabolic rate, sepsis with a pyrexia and a lactic acidosis, more oxygen is released to the tissues driven by their underlying physiological state. The converse also applies, in that haemoglobin has an increased affinity for oxygen when:

- pH is increased
- body temperature is decreased
- $PaCO_2$ is decreased
- 2,3-PDG levels are decreased.

Pulse oximetry in critical care

Pulse oximetry is only part of the critical care practitioner's respiratory assessment. Other respiratory parameters, e.g. respiratory rate, tidal volume, partial pressure of oxygen in arterial blood (PaO_2) must also be considered to make comprehensive assessment of patient ventilation. This is particularly important as pulse oximetry readings can be unreliable. For example, haemoglobin binds to carbon monoxide in preference to oxygen forming carboxyhaemoglobin. This makes the blood a bright red colour that transmits increased light from the oximeter probe. As a consequence, levels of SpO_2 can *appear* artificially higher when carboxyhaemoglobin levels are above 3% (Jensen et al. 1998). In cases of carbon monoxide poisoning, blood oxygen saturation analysis is more accurate than SpO_2. Conversely, the SpO_2 can *appear* artificially lower with dark colours on the skin (nail varnish) or bilirubinaemia in the blood where the excessive bilirubin gives an orange/yellow tone.

The main aspects to consider in pulse oximetry are how to manage safety and risk to patient and practitioner through correct probe placement and regular assessment of skin integrity to ensure that the probe gives accurate readings and does not cause tissue damage.

Problem-solving table 5.4: Pulse oximetry

Problem	Possible cause	Suggested actions
Oximeter unable to detect SpO$_2$ due to inadequate light transmission through tissue	Inadequate ambient light detected by the sensor through tissue due to: dark-coloured varnish on nails	Ensure nail beds are clean with any nail varnish removed
	Blue florescent external lighting	Note and minimize environmental conditions
	Blue dye used in imaging investigations	Note possible recent investigations
Unable to register SpO$_2$ reading due to inadequate pulse detection	Probe not well positioned	Reconsider placing on other digits, toes or using other devices
	Patient moving excessively or shivering	Identify cause of excess movement (pain, anxiety, agitation) and treat cause
	Patient has poor peripheral perfusion or inadequate peripheral blood flow, e.g. hypotensive, hypothermic, peripheral vascular disease, atrial fibrillation	Treat underlying cause. Warming the peripheral areas may help

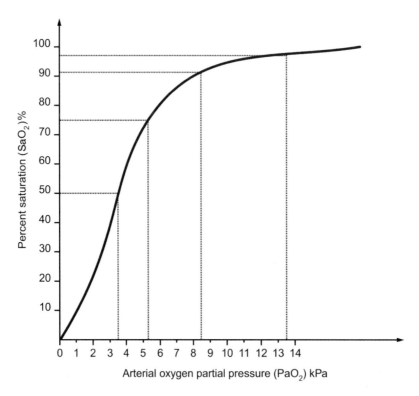

Figure 5.2 Oxygen dissociation curve.

Airway management and care with adjunct airways

Definition

An adjunct airway is a medical device that is positioned in the patient's airway to keep the respiratory tract patent. Airway management is very important in critical care as 20% of all critical incidents are related to situations related to airway management (Needham et al. 2004). Examples of adjunct airways include nasopharyngeal airways, oropharyngeal airways and endotracheal tubes.

Aims and indications

The aims of airway adjuncts include:

- preventing the tongue from falling back and occluding the pharynx
- providing a safe and patent airway channel to aid ventilation and oxygenation
- protecting the respiratory tract from aspiration of stomach contents

- facilitating suction and removal of pulmonary secretions.

Indications for insertion of an airway adjunct include:

- patients with airway obstruction
- patients who cannot protect their own airway, for example due to reduced level of consciousness
- patients who are unable to clear or expectorate pulmonary secretions
- those who require mechanical ventilation, for example peri-operatively or for management of respiratory failure (Joynt 2009).

Background

Anatomy and physiology

In normal breathing, air passes through the nose (or sometimes mouth), nasopharynx, oropharynx, laryngopharynx, trachea, bronchi and then into the lungs (Figure 5.3). An obstruction can occur at any level within the respiratory tract, from the nose or mouth, down to the bronchi. Airway obstruction can be due to a variety of causes, including:

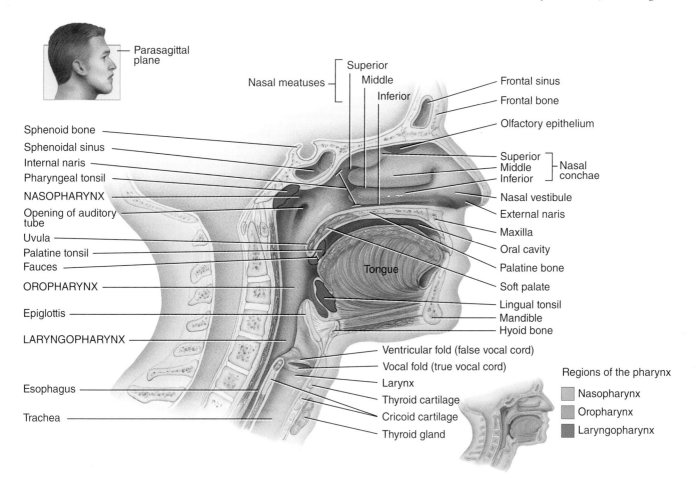

Figure 5.3 Parasagittal section of left side of head and neck (from Tortora and Derrickson 2011, reproduced with permission from Wiley).

- physical blockage of the airway, such as from vomit or a foreign body
- reduced muscle tone within the upper respiratory tract, causing the epiglottis and soft palate to occlude the airway (in unconscious patients)
- laryngeal obstruction in patients with anaphylaxis, laryngeal oedema due to burns, or those who have laryngeal spasm
- bronchial obstruction from respiratory secretions, bronchoconstriction, and less frequently pulmonary oedema or oedema of the lung mucosa.

(Resuscitation Council UK 2011)

Airway obstruction can be classified as either partial or complete. Partial airway obstruction is characterized by reduced air entry and is often associated with noisy breath sounds. In contrast, complete airway obstruction will present with no breath sounds and a grossly abnormal breathing pattern (*see also* Chapter 3).

Airway management in critical care

The most common airway adjunct devices used in critical care are:

- nasopharyngeal airway (NPA)
- oropharyngeal airway (OPA), e.g. Guedel airway
- laryngeal mask airway (LMA)
- endotracheal tube (ETT)
- tracheostomy tube (TT).

Nasopharyngeal airway

A nasopharyngeal airway (NPA) is a curved, hollow, soft plastic tube with a flange that sits against the outside of the nostril and a bevelled end that is positioned in the pharynx. The airway comes in different diameters and lengths (see

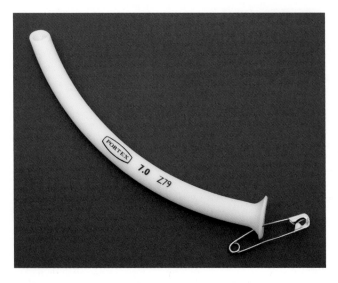

Figure 5.4 Nasopharyngeal airway (from Dougherty and Lister 2011, reproduced with permission from Wiley).

Figure 5.4), the size coding of which varies between manufacturers. The required NPA size for the patient is ascertained by measuring from the nostril to the earlobe or angle of the jaw (Roberts et al. 2005).

Nasopharyngeal airways are suitable for patients who require basic airway management. A correctly placed NPA sits just above the epiglottis and separates the soft palate from the posterior wall of the oropharynx, thereby keeping this part of the airway patent. It also enables nasopharyngeal suctioning to occur. An NPA does not stimulate the gag reflex and is better tolerated than oropharyngeal airways in patients who are awake or conscious. This type of airway is useful in conditions that do not allow for the insertion of an oral airway, such as clenched jaws, trismus (inability to open the mouth), or maxillofacial injuries (Jevon and Pooni 2007). Basal skull fracture remains a relative contraindication for use of an NPA due to the potential risk for perforation through the skull fracture into the cranial cavity (Schade et al. 2000).

The nose and nostrils should be inspected for any obvious blockages or deviation of the septum prior to insertion of the NPA. This will inform whether an NPA is suitable or indicate which nostril may be used. If resistance is detected during placement of an NPA into one nostril, for example due to nasal polyps, the NPA should be withdrawn and inserted via the other nostril. Further complications of NPA insertion include nasal haemorrhage noted in 30% of insertions and stimulation of laryngeal or glossopharyngeal reflexes, causing vomiting or laryngospasm (Resuscitation Council UK 2011).

Oropharyngeal airway

An oropharyngeal airway (OPA), for example a Guedel airway, is a hollow, curved plastic tube with a flanged and reinforced opening at the mouth end. When in place, the OPA sits within the oral cavity over the tongue preventing the tongue falling back and occluding the pharynx (Figure 5.5). OPAs come in a variety of sizes, which are often distinguished by the colour of the flange. Oropharyngeal airways are indicated for those patients who are unconscious and at risk of airway obstruction due to a reduced muscle tone in the airways (Levitan and Ochroch 2000). Use of an OPA in conscious or semi-conscious patients may stimulate glossopharyngeal or laryngeal reflexes causing laryngospasm, coughing or vomiting (Resuscitation Council UK 2011).

Correct sizing of the OPA is vital. If the tube is too short it will not prevent tongue displacement or soft palate obstruction and if it is too long, the distal end may make contact with the epiglottis, causing laryngospasm or coughing (Resuscitation Council UK 2011). The correct size of the OPA is achieved by placing the OPA against the patient's cheek with the flange parallel to the front teeth. If correctly sized the tip of the OPA will reach no further than the angle of the patient's jaw. The OPA is initially inserted upside down with the curvature towards the tongue to prevent pushing the tongue backwards into the pharynx. When the OPA is positioned at the back of the tongue it is rotated 180 degrees so that the curvature follows the contour of the roof of the mouth.

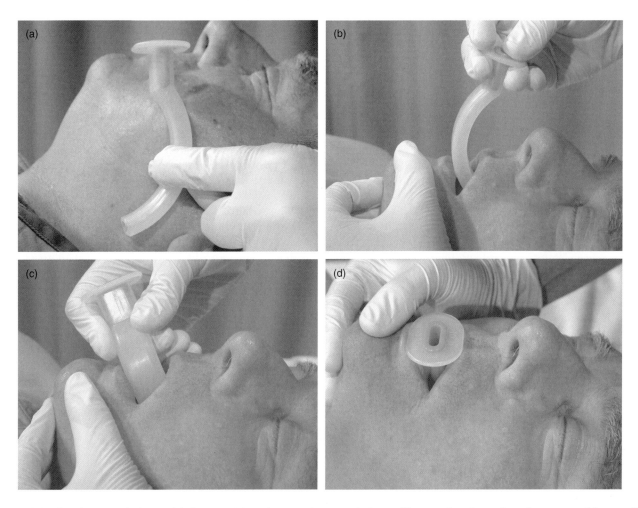

Figure 5.5 Oropharyngeal airway. (a) Correct sizing of an oropharyngeal airway. Measure the airway from the corner of the mouth. (b) Insert the airway in an upside down position to the junction of the hard and soft palate. (c) Rotate the airway 180° once you have reached the junction of the hard and soft palate. (d) Insert the airway until it lies in the oropharynx. (From Moule and Albarran 2009, reproduced with permission from Wiley.)

Problem-solving table 5.5: Oropharyngeal airway (OPA)

Problem	Possible causes	Preventative measures
Patient coughs or gags	The OPA may be stimulating a cough or gag reflex. This may be due to the patient being too awake to tolerate the tube. Alternatively, it could be attributed to insertion of a larger tube than is required or perhaps the presence of a foreign body within the pharynx, for example vomit	Assess consciousness level of patient prior to procedure. If conscious, use a NPA rather than OPA. If patient coughs or gags while the OPA is in situ, remove the OPA and reassess the patient's airway and breathing. If the patient still requires airway support, consider NPA
Patient makes noises in the upper airway, for example gurgling or snoring, that might indicate partial airway obstruction	The OPA may be the incorrect size for the patient, allowing the tongue to partially obstruct the patient's airway. This could be also due to foreign bodies within the pharynx, such as blood or vomit	Remove the OPA and reassess the patient's airway and breathing. Visualize the oropharynx and suction any secretions or vomit using a rigid oropharyngeal suction catheter, such as a Yankauer catheter. Reassess the size required and insert a correctly sized replacement OPA. Reassess the patient and consider airway manoeuvres if upper airway noises continue. That is 'head-tilt-chin-lift' or 'jaw-thrust'. Request expert help or assistance if problem remains

Laryngeal mask airway

A laryngeal mask airway (LMA) consists of a tube, with an elliptical-shaped inflatable cuff at one end (Ramachandran and Kannan 2004). This supraglottic airway adjunct is placed 'blindly' (without the use of a laryngoscope) by insertion into the oropharynx and lower pharynx. When in position it sits overlying the glottis with the inflated cuff forming a seal over the larynx facilitating airway protection and offering some protection from aspiration of stomach contents (Lavery and McCloskey 2008) (Figure 5.6). LMAs come in sizes 1 (neonates to 5 kg) with a 5 mL cuff to a size 5 (70–100 kg adult) with a 45 mL cuff. Following insertion the device can be used to ventilate the patient with gentle positive pressure by connecting the LMA to a bag-valve-mask apparatus or mechanical ventilator.

Compared with invasive airway adjuncts (endotracheal tubes), LMAs cause less pharyngeal stimulation and allow patients to breathe spontaneously with lower requirements for anaesthetic drugs. LMAs can also be placed more rapidly and successfully by healthcare staff with limited advanced airway skills (Choyce et al. 2000). LMAs are useful airway adjuncts where endotracheal intubation has failed and bag-valve-mask ventilation is unsuccessful (Resuscitation Council UK 2011). This has resulted in increasing use of LMAs in the operating theatre, recovery areas and as an airway management option in resuscitation situations. Different types of LMA are now in use including i-gel, Pro-seal and ILMA. As with the placement of any airway adjunct, it is important that continuous assessment of the patient's airway and breathing occurs during and after placement to ensure that correct positioning of the adjunct has occurred and that effective oxygenation is being achieved.

Endotracheal tube

An endotracheal tube (ETT) is a polyvinyl chloride tube with an inflatable cuff at one end that, when correctly positioned, sits above the carina in the trachea. The cuff is inflated via a pilot balloon (Figure 5.7). The ETT provides airway patency and a high degree of protection against aspiration. It also allows positive pressure to be delivered through the device to enable effective ventilation of the lungs and is considered the 'gold standard' airway protection device (Adam and Osbourne 2005; Resuscitation Council UK 2011). An ETT can be placed using the orotracheal or nasotracheal route. In most situations the orotracheal route is used as the approach is simpler and more direct. The nasotracheal approach gives greater patient comfort and is favoured where patients have jaw fractures (Rodricks and Deutschman 2000).

ETTs are available in a variety of sizes, sized according to the inner diameter of the tube. A radio-opaque marker runs the length of the ETT making it visible on X-ray. To reduce the incidence of cuff-related problems (tracheal ischaemia, erosion, laryngeal stenosis, etc.), high-volume low-pressure cuffs are preferred (Sengupta et al. 2004).

The insertion of an ETT is termed intubation and requires advanced ventilation skills, specific airway equipment and close monitoring of the patient during and after the procedure (see Procedure guideline 5.7).

Extubation is the removal of an endotracheal tube from a patient's airway, usually following a period of mechanical ventilation (see Procedure guideline 5.19). Prior to extubation the patient should be assessed for their ability to maintain their own airway (Scales and Pilsworth 2007). Extubation usually occurs after a period of weaning of ventilatory support. This may include the use of a spontaneous weaning trial (see below and Chapter 10).

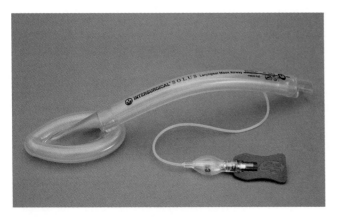

Figure 5.6 Laryngeal mask airway (from Dougherty and Lister 2011, reproduced with permission from Wiley).

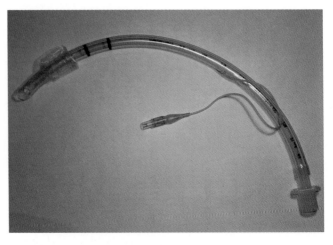

Figure 5.7 Endotracheal tube.

Tracheostomy tube

Definition

A tracheostomy tube is a curved tube that is positioned into the trachea via a stoma in the anterior neck tissues situated below the cricoid cartilage (Tortora and Derrickson 2011). When correctly positioned, the tip of the tracheostomy tube sits above the carina of the trachea. Tracheostomy tubes are made of plastic or metal. They may have a single lumen consisting of the tube, a built-in cuff connected to a pilot balloon for inflation purpose and obdurator that is used during the insertion procedure. Tracheostomy tubes may also have a double lumen consisting of a tube and built-in cuff, and an inner cannula that can be removed for cleaning.

In general, a single tube has a larger inner diameter than the same-sized tube with an inner cannula, allowing greater air flow. However, improvements in modern plastics allow for increased inner–outer diameter ratios. Thus, tubes of the same inner diameter will have different outer diameters depending on the materials used, which has a direct impact on practical management of tracheostomies, particularly if changing tubes (Figure 5.8).

Indications

A tracheostomy may be indicated to:

- facilitate weaning from mechanical ventilation therapy
- bypass an upper airway obstruction, for example, in acute airway obstruction or neoplasm
- aid the removal of respiratory secretions
- reduce the work of breathing, thereby preventing airway obstruction, for example in bulbar palsy.

(Intensive Care Society 2008)

Systematic reviews of the literature have demonstrated the benefits of shorter ventilation periods and reduced length of stays in intensive care for patient with tracheostomies who require long-term ventilation (Griffiths et al. 2005). However, results from more recent large-scale clinical trials are less conclusive (TRACMAN 2009).

A tracheostomy can be inserted via an open procedure that is usually performed in an operating room, or via a percutaneous procedure that can be undertaken by skilled clinicians at the bedside (Pryor et al. 2000). Several complications can occur during tracheostomy insertion, including infection, haemorrhage and laryngeal nerve injury, therefore the clotting status of the patient should be checked prior to procedure, strict aseptic technique should be used during the procedure and close observation of the stoma site for bleeding or infection after the procedure is required. Patients who are unable to tolerate changes or breaks in ventilation, e.g. those requiring high levels of PEEP (greater than 10 cm H_2O) or high levels of inspired oxygen (FiO_2 greater than 0.6) are not suitable for tracheostomy (Intensive Care Society 2008).

When a patient has a tracheostomy in situ, additional patient care is required, including humidification of inspired gases, cuff and tube management, suctioning of secretions and consideration of communication with the patient (see

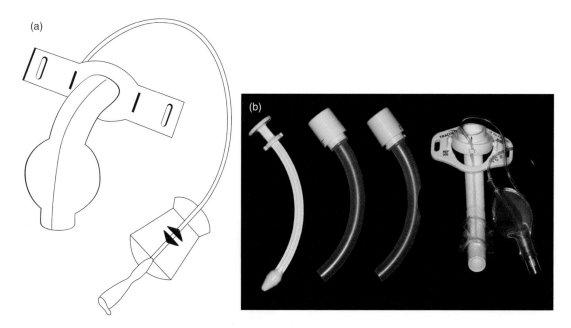

Figure 5.8 (a) Portex cuffed tracheostomy tube. (b) Kapitex Tracheotwist cuffed fenestrated tube (from Dougherty and Lister 2011, reproduced with permission from Wiley).

Procedure guidelines 5.13, 5.20 and 5.21). The timing and technique for removal and decannulation of the tracheostomy tube are also important practice considerations.

MONITORING AIRWAY ADJUNCTS

Partial pressure of end tidal carbon dioxide (ETCO₂) monitoring

Definition

End tidal CO_2 monitoring is the direct continuous measurement of end expired levels of carbon dioxide. Although commonly known in clinical practice as $ETCO_2$, it is more correctly termed partial pressure of end tidal CO_2 ($PETCO_2$).

Indications for end tidal CO_2 monitoring

Measurement of $ETCO_2$ enables breath by breath assessment of adequacy of lung ventilation in critically ill patients and may be measured by a stand-alone system, e.g. colorimetric device or a module within the bedside monitor. Normal $ETCO_2$ values are 4.5–6 kPa (35–45 mmHg). Specific indications for $ETCO_2$ monitoring include:

- respiratory monitoring of the ventilated patient
- monitoring during transport of the critically ill patient
- monitoring during anaesthesia
- assessment following tracheal tube insertion to confirm correct placement.

(Bersten 2004)

As discussed earlier, CO_2 is a metabolite of cellular respiration and if not cleared from the body will lead to acidosis causing respiratory, cardiac and central nervous system problems. $ETCO_2$ monitoring allows assessment of CO_2 levels to inform action required to maintain CO_2 within normal limits.

Background

Anatomy and physiology

Carbon dioxide (CO_2) is the by-product of anaerobic metabolism in cells. In health, CO_2 is transported to the lungs, where it diffuses from the circulation into the alveoli. In patients with normal lung function, $PaCO_2$ and $ETCO_2$ have similar partial pressure values, with $ETCO_2$ usually less than 1 kPa (7.5 mmHg) below $PaCO_2$ (Capovilla et al. 2000). However, in patients with poor lung function, e.g. chronic obstructive airway disease or decreased pulmonary blood flow, $ETCO_2$ may be substantially below $PaCO_2$ (Woodrow 2006).

$ETCO_2$ monitoring in critical care

A capnometer measures the absorption of infrared light by CO_2 in order to calculate the partial pressure of exhaled CO_2. This is achieved by passing an infrared light through expiratory gases and using a photodetector to measure the infrared light. The amount of CO_2 in the gas is calculated using the absorption properties of CO_2 and displayed as a numeric value (mmHg or kPa) and also as a continuous graph called a capnogram. $ETCO_2$ sampling of exhaled gases can occur by side stream method, where a sample of gas is transported by a fine bore tube to the bedside for analysis, or by mainstream sampling, where analysis occurs directly in the patient ventilator system.

The normal capnographic waveform has key characteristics (Figure 5.9), with exhalation represented as the positive upstroke and inspiration as the down stroke. The zero baseline on the capnograph represents the period where gas is exhaled from the anatomical dead space followed by gas from the intermediate airways. The waveform plateaus as the exhaled gas velocity slows as alveolar exhalation is nearly complete. This is then followed by inspiration that is virtually devoid of CO_2, seen on the capnograph as the down stroke returning to baseline. The capnograph should be a square waveform. A sloping upstroke may indicate obstructive lung disease as expiration for these patients takes longer and requires more effort. Presence of any respiratory disease can be confirmed through further patient assessment and history and may be useful to consider when making ventilator-weaning plans for the patient.

The main aspects to consider in monitoring of $ETCO_2$ are how to manage safety and risk to patient and to ensure that the capnometer is correctly placed within the ventilator circuit. Baseline comparison of arterial blood gas analysis is also necessary to assess the accuracy of $ETCO_2$ with $PaCO_2$.

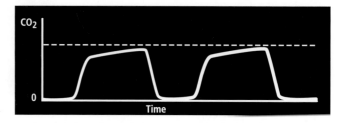

Figure 5.9 Normal capnographic waveform.

Problem-solving table 5.6: Complications of capnography

Problem	Cause	Suggested actions
No ETCO$_2$ reading or inaccurate ETCO2 reading	Mechanical, equipment or replacement failure	Check placements is as per local guidelines Re-check calibration ('zeroing') procedure Change capnometer and cables, etc. If problems continue, seek technical help
ETCO$_2$ high	Consider the presence of the following: ■ hypoventilation or inadequate minute volume ■ obstruction of the airways ■ decreased alveolar ventilation ■ use of respiratory depressant drugs ■ increased metabolism ■ hyperthermia	Treat underlying cause. For example, increase minute volume through increase in rate/tidal volume Inform senior practitioners and continue monitoring arterial blood gases and trend of ETCO$_2$
ETCO$_2$ low	High minute volume or low cardiac output	Treat underlying cause. For example, decrease minute volume through decrease in rate/tidal volume Inform practitioners and continue monitoring arterial blood gas and ETCO$_2$ trend
	A dramatic drop in ETCO$_2$ indicates: ■ cardiac arrest ■ pulmonary embolism A dramatic drop in ETCO$_2$ also occurs in cardiopulmonary bypass	Check other patient observations and follow emergency procedures as required
	A sudden drop in ETCO$_2$ values indicates: ■ mechanical ventilation failure ■ disconnection from the ventilator	Check ventilator Check all equipment connections

Measuring endotracheal/tracheostomy tube cuff pressure

Definition

Endotracheal tube cuff pressure is the pressure exerted within the cuff of a tracheal tube (endotracheal tube, tracheostomy tube) against the mucosal tissue of the trachea to hold the tube in place. The tracheal cuff is an inflatable balloon near the end of the endotracheal and tracheostomy tube that creates a seal against the tracheal wall.

Indications for measuring endotracheal/tracheostomy tube cuff pressure

Any patient who has an endotracheal tube or tracheostomy tube in situ requires regular measurement of the pressure within the cuff. This is to ensure there is an adequate cuff seal to enable effective ventilation without exerting unnecessary pressure on the tracheal mucosa. Too low a cuff pres-

sure may result in air and pressure loss from the lungs during forced ventilation and risk aspiration of saliva and gastric feed or gastric content. Too high a cuff pressure may result in tissue damage and necrosis, tracheal stenosis and trachea-oesophageal fistulas, particularly in vulnerable patients, e.g. those who are hypotensive, undernourished, or on steroid medication (Sengupta et al. 2004).

Background

Anatomy and physiology

For healthy cells, oxygen must be delivered through the arterial tree from major arteries to small capillaries with the capillary network supplying and maintaining a healthy tracheal mucosa. The pressure at which the blood supply to the tracheal mucosa is occluded is 30–32 mmHg (40 cm H$_2$O). However, this is based on research from healthy volunteers (Lowthian 1997). As the blood pressure in critically ill patients is likely to be lower and/or the mucosa more poorly perfused, it is assumed that the capillaries may be occluded at an even lower pressure. Therefore 20 mmHg is considered a safer limit and used as the maximum pressure for tracheal cuff inflation (Lorente et al. 2007).

Endotracheal/tracheostomy tubes in critical care

A range of tracheal cuffs are in use, but the most preferable is the high-volume low-pressure cuff that allows a large surface area of the cuff to come into contact with the tracheal wall while exerting lower pressures compared to standard high-volume cuffs. Cuff manometers are handheld devices that are used to measure tracheal cuff pressures. These measurements should be undertaken during patient assessment, after intubation and if a cuff leak is present.

Recent guidelines by the Department of Health advocate a four-hourly cuff pressure measurement (DH 2011). Most cuff manometers display a safe range (20–25 mmHg). There is still debate whether even high-volume low-pressure cuffs prevent aspiration, and therefore other practices should be considered, including adoption of a ventilator care bundle (NICE/NSPA 2008).

The main aspects to consider in tracheal cuff pressure measurement are how to manage safety and risk to patient and practitioner through safe technique. Cuff leaks and tracheal suctioning can be very frightening to conscious ventilated patients. Practitioners can do much to minimize patient distress by preparing the patient for this procedure and working with patient's breathing to optimize timing of the cuff pressure measurement (Johnson 2004).

Problem-solving table 5.7: Complications of tracheal cuff pressure measurement

Problem	Cause	Suggested actions
Cuff pressure too high – in excess of 25 mmHg	High-pressure low-volume cuffed tube in place	Maintain cuff seal and inform relevant practitioners regarding need to re-intubation with low-pressure high-volume cuffed tube
	High peak airway pressure (in excess of 25 mmHg)	Check cause of high airway pressure. Maintain cuff seal and inform relevant practitioners
	Tracheal tube may be too small for patient	Maintain cuff seal and inform relevant practitioners of the need to insert appropriate-sized tracheal tube
Cuff pressure too low – below 15 mmHg	Low airway peak pressure (under 20 mmHg)	Check cause of low airway pressure and, if required, inform relevant practitioners. Inflate cuff to safe pressure if leak detected
Persistent cuff leak	Cuff pressure too low	Inflate cuff until leak occluded, maintain seal. Inform relevant practitioners
	Tracheal tube displaced, possibly sitting between and or above vocal cords	Inform relevant practitioners. Prepare to check length of ETT on CXR and/or deflate cuff and position tracheal tube further down trachea

INTERVENTIONS FOR THE RESPIRATORY SYSTEM

Ventilatory support

Ventilatory support is where an individual's spontaneous breathing is either mechanically assisted or replaced. There are two types of ventilatory support: non-invasive and invasive ventilatory support (see Table 5.2). Non-invasive ventilation support is used when the individual's airway is patent and only assistance to spontaneous breathing is required. Invasive ventilation support is used when the individual is unable to maintain an airway and either requires assistance in breathing with airway protection or a ventilator to undertake the breathing. A wide range of conditions can result in an individual requiring some form of ventilatory support. There are many therapies available from simple administration of oxygen via nasal cannulae or facemask through to advanced invasive ventilator modes.

Indications for ventilatory support

Ventilatory support is utilized when an individual's ability to undertake pulmonary gas exchange is impaired. The level

Table 5.2 Types of ventilation

Non-invasive ventilatory support (NIV)	Invasive ventilatory support (IV)				
	Pressure mode	**Pressure mode (weaning)**	**Volume mode**	**Hybrid ventilatory support**	**Novel ventilation modes**
Continuous positive airway pressure (CPAP) ventilation	Pressure control ventilation (PCV)	Continuous positive airway pressure (CPAP) ventilation	Volume control ventilation (VCV)	Pressure control ventilation-volume guarantee (PCV-VG)	Extracorporeal membrane oxygenation (ECMO)
Bi-level positive airway pressure (BiPAP) ventilation	Bi-level ventilation (NB also known as BiPAP)	Pressure support (PS)	Synchronized intermittent mandatory ventilation (SIMV-VC)	Synchronized intermittent mandatory ventilation (SIMV-PC)	High-frequency oscillation ventilation (HFOV)
	Bi-level airway pressure release ventilation (BiPAP APRV)			Neurally adjusted ventilatory assist (NAVA)	

of intervention required can be gauged by a robust assessment by the clinical team leading to an informed plan of action for instigating the appropriate level of respiratory support. Using the lowest level of ventilatory support to restore normal gas exchange to the patient condition is important, as use of invasive ventilation is associated with higher risk of ventilator-associated pneumonia (VAP) (NICE/NSPA 2008).

Specific indications for invasive and non-invasive ventilation are listed in the relevant sections below.

Background

Anatomy and physiology

Regulation of normal ventilation is complex. There are two types of sensor that help control ventilation. These are the central (medulla) and peripheral (aortic arch) chemoreceptors that respond to chemical changes in the blood, and mechanoreceptors located in the chest wall that respond to changes in lung volume. If changes are detected in either the chemical or mechanical environment messages, this changes how ventilation is centrally controlled by the brain (Urden et al. 2002). The central nervous system coordinates ventilation. The brainstem regulates involuntary ventilation while the cerebral cortex enables voluntary ventilation to override the brainstem's automatic control. The result of this central control is that the principal muscles of ventilation (intercostals, diaphragm, serratus group and sternocleidomastoid) contract and relax as part of the breathing pattern. This movement of the rib cage and diaphragm increases and decreases the overall size of the thoracic cavity, causing intrapulmonary pressure changes. This causes air to enter and exit the lungs, i.e. inspiration and expiration. Even during normal quiet ventilation, energy must be expended as work of breathing to overcome the normal elastic and resistive properties of the lungs. Respiratory problems significantly increase the work of breathing (Loring et al.

2009). Therefore any preventable or treatable respiratory issues must be resolved before respiratory failure occurs.

The role and transportation of oxygen and carbon dioxide have been detailed previously. However, when considering ventilation support, an understanding is also required of the mechanism whereby oxygen and CO_2 diffuse across the alveoli and capillary membrane. Diffusion is a process where substances are transported from an area of low concentration to an area of high concentration via random movement. Ventilatory support facilitates this process by increasing the level of oxygen and assisting the removal of CO_2. Ventilatory support is therefore used when the breathing function deteriorates or fails.

Alveoli are key structures that enable effective oxygen and CO_2 exchange in the in the lungs. Alveolar cells are a single layer of squamous epithelial cells that are covered with a cobweb of capillaries (Marieb 2008). The thinness of the alveolar cell wall combined with the close proximity of the capillaries allows the diffusion of gases across the membrane. The amount of gas diffused across the alveoli each minute and the amount of blood available to take the oxygen to the cells are important factors in respiration. The amount of gas that reaches the alveoli (V – ventilation) is 4 L/min. The amount of blood that reaches the alveoli (Q – perfusion) is 5 L/min. This can be expressed as a ventilation perfusion (V/Q) ratio. In a healthy adult, the V/Q ratio is 4:5 or 0.8. Perfusion without ventilation is termed a shunt and results in a lower V/Q ratio (for example 0.6). Alveolar changes may result from chronic long-term conditions such as emphysema, or acute illnesses such as pneumonia and adult respiratory distress syndrome (ARDS). Ventilation without perfusion is termed dead space and results in a higher V/Q ratio. Perfusion changes may occur as a result of pulmonary embolism, or reduced pulmonary circulation (Woodrow 2008).

When ventilatory failure is related to lack of oxygen in the blood (hypoxaemia) it is classified as type 1 respiratory failure. Type 1 respiratory failure is most commonly seen in pulmonary oedema and pneumonia (Sharma 2006). However, in many disease processes CO_2 retention (hypercapnia) occurs as well. When hypoxemia with hypercapnia occur, this is classified as type 2 respiratory failure. Type 2 respiratory failure is often seen in patients with chronic respiratory problems including chronic obstructive pulmonary disease (COPD) or acute respiratory problems such as ARDS (Priestley 2006).

Non-invasive ventilation

Definition of non-invasive ventilatory (NIV) support

NIV is the provision of ventilatory support through the patient's upper airway using a tight-fitting mask or similar device attached to a NIV machine. NIV supports breathing in respiratory failure. This is important as work of breathing in respiratory failure can account for 30% of total oxygen consumption (Scottish Intensive Care Society 2010). There are different modes of NIV that can be delivered including:

- continuous positive airway pressure (CPAP) ventilation
- bi-level positive airways pressure (BiPAP) ventilation.

(British Thoracic Society 2008)

NIV in critical care – an overview

The implementation of NIV therapy (CPAP and BiPAP) in acute respiratory failure can be controversial and current debate often centres on setting a clear action plan. The British Thoracic Society (2008) advocates that patients who might be suitable for invasive ventilation if NIV fails should only receive NIV in level 3 critical care facilities. In a study by Roberts et al. (2011), when NIV was used in clinical practice it revealed higher mortality rates than in corresponding randomized clinical trials. This was attributed to NIV being used as the maximum respiratory treatment in patient groups for whom efficacy of NIV is currently uncertain. The need for advanced care planning to identify what treatment options exists for those with end-stage respiratory failure and exacerbation of COPD has been highlighted. It has been suggested that large randomized controlled trials are required to identify variables that accurately predict patient outcomes to inform clinical decisions about escalation of care in this area (Steer et al. 2010).

CPAP

CPAP is a ventilation technique that blows a stream of air into the lungs to keep the airways open. Use of CPAP maintains a positive pressure throughout the whole respiratory

cycle when breathing spontaneously (Keilty and Bott 1992). The positive pressure is achieved by a valve in the CPAP circuit that is set to create a resistance during expiration. This positive pressure keeps the alveoli open for gas exchange at end expiration.

Indications for CPAP

These include:

- acute hypoxemic respiratory failure without hypercapnia
- as a method of gradually reducing ventilation support and enabling development of spontaneous breathing (weaning) from mechanical ventilation
- post-operatively
- sleep apnoea
- pulmonary oedema.

(BTS 2008)

Contraindications for CPAP

- Facial injury or recent facial surgery
- Facial burns
- Inability to protect own airway
- Vomiting or risk of aspiration
- Life-threatening hypoxia
- Recent gastrointestinal surgery
- Copious secretions
- Haemodynamic instability

(British Thoracic Society 2008)

BiPAP

BiPAP is a type of non-invasive ventilation that keeps the airways of the lungs open by delivering air at different pressures. Two gas pressures are used in BiPAP. A higher pressure is used in inspiration (inspiratory positive airway pressure, IPAP) and a lower pressure is used in expiration (expiratory positive airway pressure, EPAP). As the patient breathes in, the BiPAP ventilator detects the drop in pressure during the inspiratory breath and then delivers a flow of air into the patient's airway until the predetermined inspired pressure (IPAP) is reached. This extra pressure augments the breath to create a greater tidal volume. When the patient breathes out, a predetermined pressure is kept in the lungs (EPAP) that maintains the alveoli in an open position facilitating gas exchange (Moore and Woodrow 2009). When using BiPAP, there is also an option to add a back-up supported breathing rate. The machine will then use predetermined regular positive pressure to enable the patient to inspire if the patient has an inadequate respiratory drive or fails to breathe.

Caution should be exercised when using the terms BiPAP, BIPAP and bi-level (*see* Table 5.2) as they are all used to describe different modes of non-invasive and invasive ventilation. Critical care practitioners should ensure they fully understand what each mode of ventilation the patient is receiving and what specific observations and care are required.

Indications for BiPAP

Indications for BiPAP include:

- type 2 respiratory failure
- acute-on-chronic hypercapnic respiratory failure (where there is an acute deterioration in an individual with significant pre-existing hypercapnic respiratory failure (high $PaCO_2$ [above 45 mmHg], low pH [between 7.26 and 7.35] and high bicarbonate [above 28 mmol/L]))
- type 2 respiratory failure where tracheal intubation is not deemed appropriate

- part of a weaning plan from mechanical ventilation
- respiratory failure due to chest wall deformity or neuromuscular disease
- obstructive sleep apnoea if acidosis is present.

(British Thoracic Society 2008)

Contraindications for BiPAP

- Facial injury or recent facial surgery
- Facial burns
- Inability to protect own airway
- Vomiting or risk of aspiration
- Life-threatening hypoxia
- Recent gastrointestinal surgery
- Copious secretions
- Haemodynamic instability

(British Thoracic Society 2008)

81

Problem-solving table 5.8: CPAP and BiPAP

Problem	Cause	Preventative measures
Mask leaks Some leakage is expected but leaks may cause inefficient ventilation, eye irritation, noise, dry mouth and nasal problems	Badly sized mask Nasogatric tube (NGT) in situ	Reassess mask size Readjust head straps Use foam dressing (e.g. Granuflex) to customize the mask for a better fit if possible Adjust flow to allow for leaks
Gastric distension	Positive pressure from the high flow of air may cause stomach insufflation	Reduce flow on CPAP, or IPAP on the on BiPAP machine Place NG tube to decompress stomach
Intolerance/inability to cooperate	Hypoxia or hypercapnia leading to confusion	Undertake arterial blood gas (ABG) analysis to assess adequacy of gas exchange Constant supervision may be necessary until the ABGs are normalized Include patient in plans to facilitate better cooperation with the ventilation strategy (British Thoracic Society 2008)
Persistent hypoxia	Oxygen tubing is not attached or leaking Atelectasis Patient's condition is worsening	Check all connections and oxygen supply Increase flow and or O_2 on CPAP On BiPAP increase EPAP, remembering to increase IPAP to maintain the same level of pressure support Full respiratory review and consideration of escalation of treatment is required
Hypocapnia	Ventilation rate too high Lung condition has improved and the NIV therapy is now over-ventilating the patient	Reduce ventilation rate Reduce flow if on CPAP Reduce IPAP if on BiPAP Assess whether the patient still requires NIV; undertake a reassessment of respiratory function

(Continued)

Problem solving table 5.8: (Continued)

Hypercapnia	Exhalation port blocked	Ensure port is open
	Insufficient tidal volume achieved	Increase IPAP
	Insufficient respiratory drive	Add or increase breath rate
	Poor-fitting mask	Assess mask for leakage
	Circuit set up incorrectly	Check connections and identify leaks
	The patient spending inadequate time periods on the BiPAP system	Encourage more sustained periods of use, particularly during sleep If on CPAP consider commencing BiPAP
Pressure damage to bridge of nose and or chin	Mask fitting too tightly or incorrectly placed leading to pressure damage	Consider nasal mask (if patient breathes through nose). Facemask is recommended by the British Thoracic Society (2008) for first 24 hours to maximize gas flow delivery into the lungs Undertake regular inspection of areas at risk from pressure damage Use transparent or foam dressing to reduce pressure damage
Dry mouth	High flows of air cause dry oral secretions	Considering implementing a wet humidification circuit if the therapy is going to be maintained for longer periods Regular mouth care during breaks from the therapy

Invasive ventilation

Definition of invasive ventilator support

Invasive ventilator support is ventilation delivered via an invasive airway such as an endotracheal tube or tracheostomy tube (Woodrow 2006). It is designed to temporarily replace or support the patient's own ventilation. In most cases positive pressure ventilation will be used to manage invasively ventilated patients within critical care.

Indications for invasive ventilation

Indications for invasive ventilation include:

- impending or existing respiratory failure and inability to sustain adequate gas exchange
- severe cardiovascular instability and inability to sustain adequate gas exchange
- severe neurological dysfunction and inability to sustain adequate gas exchange

- metabolic acidosis with decompensating respiratory function
- postoperatively when inability to maintain airway and respiratory function.

Contraindications for invasive ventilation

Contraindications to invasive ventilation are hard to quantify as intubation (placing of an endotracheal tube in the trachea) is sometimes an emergency and unplanned procedure. However, early consideration must be given as to whether the patient will be able to reduce reliance on ventilation and return to a normal respiratory function before intubation occurs.

Complications of invasive ventilation include:

- aspiration
- tracheal stenosis
- laryngeal oedema
- infection
- barotrauma

- decreased cardiac output, especially with positive end expiratory pressure (monitor BP immediately after commencing ventilation)
- fluid retention
- immobility
- stress ulcer
- paralytic ileus
- inadequate nutrition.

(Woodrow 2006)

Background

Anatomy and physiology

In normal inspiration the diaphragm contracts and moves downwards to generate negative intrapleural pressure. This creates a pressure gradient between the atmosphere and the alveoli, resulting in air being drawn into the lungs. In invasive ventilation, the ventilator pushes air into the lungs under positive pressure (Marieb 2008). Through the ventilator gas flow, gas pressure and ventilator valves can be used to control flow of air in inspiration, lung capacity and speed of expiration. This ability to control ventilation allows the clinician to alter the lung movement thereby improving gas exchange.

Invasive ventilation in critical care

Numerous studies have been undertaken into the use and management of invasive ventilation (Esteban et al. 2002; Burns et al. 2006; Epstein 2006). Such studies have addressed a range of different questions about ventilation modes; situations when invasive ventilation can improve patient outcome; and the ethical and financial issues concerned with using invasive ventilation in complex and long-term cases.

With the increasing numbers of ventilators available for critical care, new modes of ventilation continuing to emerge. Each mode of ventilation requires clinicians to understand:

- the way that the ventilator is working
- how to set up the ventilator to deliver specific modes
- how to set the alarm parameters pertinent to the mode and individual patient requirements
- what ventilator observations should be made.

Local unit guidelines and manufacturers' manuals should be used to inform and support safe practice.

The use of 'care bundles' (a group of evidence-based interventions for specific areas of care) to guide invasive ventilator care and reduce incidence of ventilation associated pneumonias (VAPs) (Berenholtz et al. 2011) has developed widely in recent years. Care bundles covering the following interventions have been shown to reduce VAP in critical care:

- elevating the patient's head to 30 to 45° from horizontal
- therapy aimed at the prophylaxis of stress-related ulcers
- regularly and temporarily withholding sedation to allow any excess to be eliminated
- oral decontamination (NICE/NSPA 2008).

In 2008, NICE and the National Patient Safety Agency (NPSA) reviewed all current evidence on VAP prevention and developed a technical guide that has been adopted in many critical care areas throughout the United Kingdom (NICE/NSPA 2008).

Invasive ventilation modes

Traditionally invasive ventilation modes can be divided into three types. These are pressure, volume and spontaneous modes of ventilation. More recently companies that manufacture mechanical ventilators have developed modes that cross over these traditional boundaries. In this chapter, these will be described as hybrid modes.

Pressure modes of invasive ventilation

In pressure modes of ventilation, the ventilator delivers a flow of air to the lung until the pressure generated in the ventilator circuit reaches the pressure limit set on the ventilator. The benefit of this mode is lung protection, as it prevents the alveoli being over distended (volutrauma) and reduces the risk of excessively high pressures and rupture of the alveoli (barotrauma). Pressure modes of ventilation are mostly commonly used in patients who have stiff lungs, i.e. poor lung compliance such as in acute lung injury or ARDS. There are three main pressure modes:

- pressure control ventilation (PCV)
- bi-level ventilation
- bi-level airway pressure release ventilation (APRV).

Pressure control ventilation (PCV)

PCV is a mode of ventilation where a pressure limit is set for each breath delivered by the ventilator. When this pressure limit is reached, the ventilator then cycles into an expiratory breath. The pressure in the patient's airway therefore determines the volume of each breath. This mode has a fixed breath rate. Patients on this mode are often heavily sedated and may also be receiving muscle relaxants to enable control of their respiratory function. It is important to monitor the size of the breath (tidal volume) as this will be determined by the compliance of the patient's lungs. If the tidal volume is inadequate to maintain adequate patient gas exchange it may be necessary to increase the pressure limit on the ventilator. If compliance is poor so that adequate gas exchange in this mode is not achieved, it may be necessary to use more advanced invasive ventilation strategies such as oscillation ventilation or introducing inhaled nitric oxide (Krishnan and Brower 2000).

Bi-level ventilation – also known as bi-level positive airway pressure (BiPAP)

Bi-level ventilation is a specific mode of pressure control ventilation where a high and a low pressure are set on the ventilator and the machine cycles between the two. The patient can breathe in and out at nearly any point in the respiratory cycle and these breaths will be pressure supported by the ventilator. During inspiration the breath is supported by pressure to the predetermined upper limit. At expiration the predetermined lower pressure is kept in the ventilator circuit and respiratory tract in order to keep the alveoli open. In this way ventilation and gas exchange is improved. The benefits of bi-level ventilation are that patient can receive a pressure-controlled mode of ventilation without requiring heavy sedation. This mode is comfortable for the patient as bi-level offers pressure control ventilation while allowing the patient to take their own breaths. This makes this a versatile mode for patients with a range of conditions from those with extremely compromised lung function through to those who are being assisted to reduce reliance on ventilation support. As a result it is often referred to as the universal mode of ventilation.

Bi-level airway pressure release ventilation (APRV) ventilation – also known as BiPAP APRV

Bi-level APRV is a type of ventilation whereby the ventilator pressure rapidly decreases at the end of an inspiratory phase. The normal inspiratory (I)/expiratory (E) ratio is 1:2. However, in bi-level APRV the ventilator is set to an inverse inspiratory/expiratory ratio mode delivering a breath with a longer inspiratory phase with comparatively short expiratory time. The aim of this mode of ventilation is to allow the lung to remain inflated for a longer period of time to promote the diffusion of oxygen across the alveoli/capillary membrane. The longer period of inspiration may increase the diffusion of oxygen but it reduces the time for CO_2 to be moved out of the lungs during the expiratory phase. For this reason this mode should only be used where PaO_2 levels are excessively low and permissive hypercapnia (low tidal volumes leading to raised CO_2 levels) is acceptable in order to promote patient oxygenation. Close monitoring of arterial blood gases is vital to ensure that the patient's CO_2 levels do not compromise the patient's acid-base balance (Bigatello et al. 2001).

Volume modes of invasive ventilation

Volume modes of ventilation deliver a fixed volume of gas into the lungs. The tidal volume and the respiratory rate are therefore set on the ventilator. It is often adopted for patients with normal compliant lungs undergoing surgery when a simple mode of ventilation is required. However, as this volume of gas is delivered into the patient regardless of the pressure in the patient's airway, monitoring of the patient's airway pressure is important to minimize the risk of barotrauma. There are two main volume modes:

- volume control ventilation (VCV)
- synchronized intermittent mandatory ventilation (SIMV-VC).

Volume control ventilation (VCV)

Volume control ventilation is a mandatory type of ventilation where a fixed volume for inspiration is delivered.

Synchronized intermittent mandatory ventilation (SIMV-VC)

SIMV-VC is a mandatory mode of ventilation where the ventilator synchronizes delivery of the fixed volume of inspiratory breath to any spontaneous breathing effort the patient may make. SIMV-VC is often combined with pressure support to augment the patient's independent breaths.

Hybrid invasive ventilation modes

Over the past decade, ventilators have been developed that combine both pressure and volume modes of ventilation. Such modes have the advantage of delivering the maximum tidal volume in a breath at a lower predetermined airway pressure than if the patient was being ventilated on a volume mode of ventilation. This maximizes gas exchange while minimizing the risk of barotrauma. The main types of hybrid ventilation to date are:

- pressure control ventilation-volume guarantee (PCV-VG)
- synchronized intermittent mandatory ventilation – pressure controlled (SIMV-PC)
- neurally adjusted ventilatory assist (NAVA).

Pressure control ventilation-volume guarantee (PCV-VG)

Pressure control ventilation-volume guarantee ventilation is a mode of ventilation where the inspiratory pressure limit is fixed and the volume of inspiratory breath is controlled. The ventilator attempts to ensure the patient receives the set volume within the set pressure limits. However, this mode does not provide any ventilator support to any spontaneous breathing. It is not therefore comfortable if the patient is waking and attempting to initiate their own breaths.

Synchronized intermittent mandatory ventilation – pressure controlled (SIMV-PC)

Synchronized intermittent mandatory ventilation – pressure controlled is a mandatory mode of ventilation but one where the ventilator synchronizes itself to any spontaneous breathing of the patient. This mode of ventilation is therefore often combined with pressure support.

Neurally adjusted ventilatory assist (NAVA)

During weaning from mechanical ventilation, the overall aim is to reduce the number and degree of mechanically assisted breaths while increasing patient breaths until liberation from ventilator support is achieved. Providing 'too much' support will delay weaning, while providing 'too little' support will simply fatigue the patient (*see* Weaning from mechanical ventilation). Currently, clinician assessment, sometimes aided by clinical practice guidelines, is the main factor determining whether current support is 'too much' or 'too little'.

Although clinical examination and measurement of vital signs during weaning are important, there is current and growing interest in more objectively and continuously measuring the degree of patient effort, and providing the 'right' amount of assistance on a breath-by-breath basis (Moerer 2012). Neurally adjusted ventilatory assist is a method of attempting to quantify and optimize the amount of ventilatory support required as the patient's condition changes.

Assessing respiratory effort may be by detection of neurological activity (e.g. in the respiratory centre, vagus nerve, or diaphragm) or by measurement of lung mechanics and patient effort. Typically, more mechanical support is provided when patients can make only limited respiratory efforts, and the ventilator provides incrementally less support as the patient becomes stronger.

Although this offers significant conceptual advances over traditional ventilation modes (e.g. by reducing ventilator–patient dsysynchrony), this is still a predominantly research-based intervention at present.

Novel invasive ventilation modes
High-frequency oscillation ventilation (HFOV)

HFOV typically uses special ventilators with a respiratory rate of 150–900 breaths/min, each delivering a small tidal volume. This tidal volume (typically less than 100 mL) is much lower than a patient's physiological dead space (typically 150–200 mL), so oxygenation does not occur by direct delivery to the alveoli as with conventional ventilation. Instead, a complex number of factors, including bulk flow

and diffusion of oxygen from the trachea, account for the ability of HFOV to deliver sufficient oxygen to alveoli.

The postulated benefits of HFOV include lower peak, but higher mean, intrathoracic pressures than conventional ventilation. This may permit more rapid healing of bronchopleural fistulae, or facilitate management of patients with severe ARDS by allowing ventilation without derecruitment (Sud et al. 2010b). Several trials (OSCAR, OSCILLATE) are currently under way to better define what benefit, if any, HFOV actually shows over conventional ventilation (Fan and Rubenfeld 2010).

Extracorporeal membrane oxygenation (ECMO)

Conventional or high-frequency ventilation modes require that a patient has at least a minimum of functioning lung tissue to allow gas exchange. In very severe, but reversible, disease, ECMO may be an appropriate means to provide organ support until the lungs recover (Gaffney et al. 2010). A large double-lumen cannula is placed in the venous system (usually superior vena cava, although a variety of ECMO configurations exist). This drains deoxygenated blood, pumps it through a membrane oxygenator and then returns oxygenated blood to the patient via the second lumen. The patient's heart then pumps this oxygenated blood around the body. During this time, the lungs may be almost completely rested, and a variable degree of cardiac output can be provided by the ECMO pump. As the patient recovers, the cardiorespiratory support is gradually removed and conventional ventilation introduced.

This is a high-cost, high-risk intervention (patients require systemic anticoagulation while receiving ECMO) and at present, there is conflicting evidence about the cost-effectiveness of ECMO. In the UK, its use is restricted to specialist centres only (Moran et al. 2010).

Spontaneous invasive ventilation modes

Spontaneous modes of ventilation are when the patient is intubated and instigates the breath, and the ventilator assists the breathing with added pressure or flow. There are two main spontaneous modes of ventilation:

- continuous positive pressure airway pressure (CPAP)
- pressure support (PS) – uses the same principles as BiPAP in non-invasive ventilation.

These modes of ventilation have both been described earlier in the chapter when discussing non-invasive ventilation. However, both CPAP and PS can be delivered via a ventilator or a stand-alone machine to patients with an invasive airway. This enables these spontaneous modes of ventilation to be used as part of a weaning plan for intubated patients.

Problem-solving table 5.9: Problem solving and safety checks for invasive ventilator therapy care

Problem	Cause	Suggested actions
Displacement of ventilation tubing of endotracheal tube (ET) or tracheostomy tube (TT)	Disconnection from the ventilator	Check to make sure that the patient has not become disconnected from the ventilator or that the ventilator tubing has not become detached from the machine. Even small leaks from small connectors will cause the ventilator to alarm
	Migration of ET tube either up or down the airway	Check ET position. Once an ET tube is placed and there is adequate ventilation the ET position should recorded. Note the position of the teeth at the tube using the centimetre markings (Lynn-McHale Wiegand 2011); this indicates how many centimetres of tube have been passed into the trachea If the tube has migrated, the risk is that the tube is either out of the trachea or has moved into the right main bronchus and is only ventilating the right lung. Absence of left-sided movement or breath sounds may indicate right main stem intubation (Lynn-McHale Wiegand 2011) Auscultate lung bases and apices for bilateral chest sounds to assess tube placement in the trachea (Lynn-McHale Wiegand 2011). Observe for symmetrical chest movement and oxygen saturations (Lynn-McHale Wiegand 2011). Prepare to ventilate with 'bag, valve and mask'
	Displacement of the TT	Check TT position; auscultate the chest to assess breath sounds in both lungs. Displacement is rare with tracheostomies; however, due to the variety of tube lengths and patient sizes it does exist. Look for delayed chest motions, bilateral decreased breath sounds, unilateral sounds and excessive coughing (Lynn-McHale Wiegand 2011). Prepare to ventilate with 'bag, valve and mask' If not competent to re-intubate, the assessing practitioner must call for help as a displaced tracheal or tracheostomy tube is an emergency that must be dealt with immediately
Obstruction of airway or ventilator tubing	External sources such as pressure on ventilator tubing or patient biting on endotracheal tube	Check that all tubing is free from any sources of pressure, such as being caught in bed cot sides. Assess patient's endotracheal tube. Inspect all ventilator tubing to ensure there is no visible obstruction. Check any filters for obstruction or water saturation
	Internal sources such as sputum plugs or bronchospasm. This may indicated by secretions in the airway, inspiratory wheeze, expiratory crackles, increased peak airway pressure shallow respirations, SpO_2 changes (Lynn-McHale Wiegand and Carlson 2005)	Auscultate the patient's chest to assess for reduced airflow due to plugs, or wheezes associated with bronchospasm. Prepare the patient for suctioning and possible manual hyperinflation (Lynn-McHale Wiegand and Carlson 2005)
	If a patient is demonstrating signs of obstruction that have not been resolved by the removal of external or internal obstructions as listed, the clinical team may have to investigate whether the patient's lung compliance is deteriorating	A full respiratory review by the clinical team will be required, including a chest X-ray. Ventilation strategies may need to altered to a mode that controls lung pressures in order to provide protection for traumatic damage to the non-compliant lungs

Pneumothorax	A pneumothorax occurs when air is able to enter the potential space between the visceral and parietal pleura (American College of Surgeons 2008). This can cause the lung on the effected side to collapse, pushing the chest contents out of position. The most dangerous type of pneumothorax, a simple pneumothorax, can readily convert to a tension pneumothorax (where air can enter the pleural cavity but cannot escape) where positive pressure ventilation is applied (American College of Surgeons 2008) and can prove fatal. The signs of a tension pneumothorax in a ventilated patient include increased airway pressures, reduced minute volume, tracheal deviation, hyper-resonance with decreased or absent breath sounds over the affected side (Urden et al. 2002) and unequal chest wall movement	Inspect the chest to assess for equal bilateral movement of the chest wall Auscultate the chest to assess for air entry in all zones of the lung. Continuous observations of ventilation measurements and SpO_2 levels, and taking immediate action as required are vital to ensure the patient is being safely managed. A respiratory review may be required If a tension pneumothorax is suspected it is a medical emergency and requires immediate attention
Equipment problems	Although problems with equipment are uncommon, they can and do occur. It is important to know the equipment being used	Have emergency equipment available that can be used to ventilate the patient if the primary machine fails Once the patient is safe, investigate possible equipment problems

Weaning from mechanical ventilation

Definition

Weaning from mechanical ventilation is the process by which a ventilator dependent patient is liberated from mechanical ventilation.

Aim

The weaning process should aim to liberate the patient from mechanical ventilation as rapidly as possible, while maintaining safety and comfort throughout.

Background

Weaning may be a rapid process taking only a few minutes (e.g. following minor elective surgery in a fit patient), or it may be extremely protracted over months (e.g. following multiple organ failure in an elderly patient). These two extreme examples and the spectrum of weaning in between all have similar components:

- the reduction of mechanical support
- testing a patient's readiness for spontaneous ventilation
- extubation or decannulation of the airway.

Although all three elements are required for successful weaning, it is possible to wean from ventilation but still require an artificial airway, or to lead a reasonable quality of life despite requiring long-term ventilator support with or without an artificial airway. Despite weaning from mechanical ventilation comprising a significant part of the work of most critical care level 3 facilities, there is conflicting evidence about what the optimal approach to this is.

Anatomy and physiology

A patient with normal lungs will only require low inflation pressures to generate a good tidal volume. Typically, an inflation pressure of 10–12 cm H_2O will result in a tidal volume of 7–10 mL/kg (around 600–700 mL in an adult). Patients with severe lung pathology have stiffer, less-compliant lungs, so even high inflation pressures, for example 30–35 cm H_2O) may generate only relatively small tidal volumes. Thus, a severely ill patient may initially require high levels of respiratory support but as the underlying condition improves, this support can be removed. Balancing the appropriate degree of support to a patient's needs is sometimes a difficult skill.

Normal breathing requires a patent airway, adequate neurological control of respiratory pattern and respiratory muscles, and good lung function, along with adequate cardiac function. This is to allow transport of oxygen to tissues and CO_2 removal to the lungs for excretion, but also to meet the demands of any additional work imposed as mechanical ventilation is removed. Additionally, nutritional status, electrolyte imbalance (e.g. hypophosphataemia, hypokalaemia), and resolution of underlying diseases such as intra-abdominal sepsis should be addressed to optimize the success of attempted weaning (Macintyre et al. 2001).

Reduction of mechanical support

Traditional weaning methods include:

- spontaneous breathing trial (SBT) using a T piece
- reduction in pressure support ventilation (PSV), also termed assisted spontaneous breathing (ASB)
- reduction in mandatory ventilation breaths (IMV) weaning.

It is likely that IMV-directed weaning is less successful than either SBT- or PSV-directed weaning (Macintyre 2001; Ortiz et al. 2010), but the actual technique used is determined as much by local practices and practitioner preferences as by robust clinical evidence. The difficulties in identifying one particular method as more useful are complex and multiple (Blackwood et al. 2011).

Although weaning guidelines and protocols are in common use, there is conflicting evidence about how helpful they are. For example, some studies indicate that they facilitate more rapid weaning than usual practice (practitioner-directed weaning), while in others they show no benefit (Krishnan et al. 2004; Blackwood 2011). It may simply reflect the reality of critical care that easy-to-wean patients are easy to wean irrespective of protocolized care, and difficult-to-wean patients require individual weaning plans rather than a 'one-size-fits-no-one' plan. A typical weaning guideline or protocol recommends a daily 'sedation hold' (*see also* Chapter 10) and weaning assessment. If successful, the degree of PSV or ASB is incrementally reduced until the next weaning assessment. A failed trial or development of fatigue leads to an increase in PSV and or ASB for 12–24 hours.

Testing patient readiness

Readiness testing has two purposes. First, to identify those who are ready for liberation from ventilator support, and second, to identify those who are not yet ready. Clinical assessment alone is insufficiently robust to define these two groups, and ideally, a set of objective measurements would accurately predict the readiness of a particular patient to manage prolonged removal of ventilator support. Unfortunately, such measurements do not exist. Thus, current assessments of weaning ability rely on a combination of clinical assessment and measurements. A consequence of this is that a proportion of patients will be incorrectly assessed. An unknown proportion of patients receive unnecessarily prolonged ventilation. On the other hand, even planned extubations have a failure rate of 10–15% within the first 72 hours (Frutos-Vivar et al. 2006), but unplanned

extubation leads to re-intubation in only approximately 50% of patients (Chevron et al. 1998). Thus, a significant number of patients expected to succeed extubation actually fail (from fatigue, hypoxaemia, airway compromise, or a combination of these), and a significant number expected to fail (i.e. accidentally extubated) actually succeed.

There are numerous measures of readiness to wean, some of which are listed below:

- maximal inspiratory pressure
- compliance
- minute volume
- occlusion pressure
- work of breathing
- gastric mucosal acidosis
- oxygen cost of breathing
- weaning index
- integrative weaning index (a derived number calculated from other indirect measurements)
- inspiratory effort quotient.

None of these has sufficient sensitivity or specificity to be adequately predictive of weaning success, and they are uncommonly used in routine practice. However, the Rapid Shallow Breathing Index (RSBI) is well known, extensively investigated, simple to calculate and has a higher predictive accuracy than other scores (Tanios 2006). Even so, there remains debate about whether it should be routinely used as a decision-making tool (Macintyre 2001; Tobin and Jubran 2006; Tobin 2011).

The RSBI is the ratio of respiratory rate/tidal volume (f/Vt). A patient taking fewer, larger breaths is more likely to succeed with weaning than a patient taking rapid shallow breaths. A generally accepted indicator of success is an RSBI ratio of less than 105. For example, a patient with a respiratory rate of 30 and tidal volume of 0.4 L has a RSBI ratio of $30/0.4 = 75$, so is likely to succeed with weaning. The same patient breathing tidal volumes of 0.25 L has a ratio of 120, and is likely to fail. Patients with an RSBI less than 105 have a high (approximately 85%) chance of successfully weaning from mechanical ventilation (Bien et al. 2010).

As part of preparation for assessing readiness to wean, a patient should meet various criteria. Traditional optimal criteria for weaning include:

- resolution of underlying disease process
- adequate control of acid-base balance
- haemodynamic stability
- adequate haemoglobin
- appropriate temperature
- appropriate level of consciousness
- adequate nutritional status
- adequate oxygenation (this varies between patients, but is often regarded as an acceptable PaO_2 with an inspired FiO_2 of 0.5 and PEEP below 7 cmH$_2$O).

(ICS 2007)

Knowledge about what constitutes 'appropriate' or 'adequate' changes with increasing scientific knowledge, and will vary from patient to patient, so is generally assessed on a case-by-case basis. For example, some patients will wean well despite haemoglobin levels of 7 g/dL, a level previously considered too low for comfort. Others may require higher (10–12 g/dL) haemoglobin concentrations. Similarly, the use of β-blockers, diuretics and ACE inhibitors to improve fluid balance and cardiac function has varied over the years as evidence from studies and trials has accumulated.

Breathing through an ETT imposes a greater work of breathing than normal respiration. This additional work may be compensated for by applying a low level of ventilator support. Some ventilators incorporate automatic tube compensation (ATC) to adjust for this, although settings of 5 cm H_2O PEEP and 5–7 cm H_2O PSV may be sufficient for other ventilators. Successful respiration for 2 hours with minimal support (e.g. 5 cm H_2O CPAP and 5–7 cm H_2O PSV) is a reasonable indicator of reaching the end of the weaning process, and of ongoing success with spontaneous ventilation (Ely et al. 1996).

Opinions vary regarding the use of periods of complete rest, particularly if a patient has suffered an episode of fatigue related to a weaning attempt. Although superficially attractive, 'resting' the patient may cause more harm than good, with diaphragm dysfunction and atrophy a recognized complication of completely removing any work from the respiratory system (Vassilakopoulos et al. 2006). Overall, it is perhaps more successful to gradually increase a patient's respiratory work until they can manage daily trials of spontaneous breathing (T piece or CPAP). This can be followed by a 2-hour trial of CPAP with extubation considered if successful (Esteban et al. 1995).

Towards the end of the weaning process, a decision must be made about readiness for extubation/decannulation (see below).

Extubation/decannulation

Extubation is the removal of an endotracheal tube, generally considered to be either oral or nasal. Decannulation is the removal of a tracheostomy (or similar) tube from the trachea.

The decision to extubate may be taken once acceptably low levels of respiratory support are achieved (see Readiness to wean).

Prerequisites

Adequate airway control is required to prevent aspiration following extubation. It requires an ability to cough adequately, along with a high enough level of consciousness (often taken to be a Glasgow Coma Score of 8 or more). The acceptable cough quality is partly related to the volume and nature of any respiratory tract secretions: high volumes of tenacious secretions will require a stronger cough to clear, and may delay extubation compared with a similar patient who has little or no secretions.

- The strength of cough may be measured using a peak flow meter attached to the end of the ETT/tracheostomy. A peak expiratory flow rate (PEFR) below 60 L/min markedly increases the chance of re-intubation.
- A reduced level of consciousness causing an inability to follow four simple commands ('open your eyes', 'squeeze my hand', 'stick out your tongue', 'follow object with eyes') also increases the likelihood of re-intubation.
- Combining a PEFR less than 60 L/min with an inability to follow these commands, and in the presence of high sputum volumes (greater than 2.5 mL/h) has a 100% failure of extubation, compared to 3% if none of these factors is present (Rothaar and Epstein 2003).

Another prerequisite for extubation is the absence of significant laryngeal oedema. This may be assessed by the presence of an air leak when the ETT cuff is deflated. If there is no cuff leak, post-extubation stridor (due to laryngeal oedema) is more likely, although not inevitable. This may be prevented by the use of corticosteroids prior to extubation.

Extubation procedure

A variety of extubation techniques have been reported, including the administration of higher levels of positive end expiratory pressure (PEEP) via the mechanical ventilator at the point of extubation, and the delivery of a manual inspiratory breath via a Waters circuit or bag-valve-mask at the point of cuff deflation during extubation. Such manoeuvres act to recruit alveoli and optimize lung functioning at the point of extubation (Hodd et al. 2010). However, Hodd reports that the most commonly employed extubation method utilized in the UK focuses on aspiration of secretions during cuff deflation (Hodd et al. 2010). There is a clear need for comparative research in this area.

Post-extubation management

A proportion of patients will require re-intubation. Close monitoring of vital signs in the post-extubation period is required to detect fatigue, deteriorating respiratory function, or other distress that may force a decision to re-intubate. Most patients requiring re-intubation do so within the first 72 hours, and for unplanned extubations, often much sooner (Penuelas et al. 2011). Although some patients may benefit from non-invasive ventilation (NIV) after extubation, it is unclear how best to select this group. Suggestions include that obese patients and those with known COPD or a high $ETCO_2$ prior to extubation should receive this, although the evidence is incomplete at present (Kallet 2009).

Delayed decision making about re-intubation should be avoided if possible. A patient who is failing a trial of extubation should either receive NIV if appropriate, or be re-intubated promptly rather than waiting for obvious respiratory failure to supervene. This is because delayed re-intubation is associated with higher complication and mortality rates (Epstein 2004).

Problem-solving table 5.10: Extubation

Problem	Possible cause	Prevention	Suggested action
Respiratory distress characterized by tachypnoea, reduction of SpO$_2$ and increased work of breathing	Respiratory muscle fatigue Presence of secretions Presence of bronchoconstriction Increasing airway resistance		Provide reassurance to patient Assess for the presence of secretions or bronchoconstriction and treat as required Pause the weaning process and if required increase ventilator support, i.e. increase positive end expiratory pressure (PEEP) pressure support or inspiratory pressures Discuss with senior practitioners if guidance required Reassess the patient following any chance in weaning plan
Haemodynamic instability, i.e. hypotension or hypertension, rhythm abnormalities	Possible hypoxia Respiratory muscle fatigue. Hypovolaemia Pain or discomfort Underlying pathology, such as sepsis		Discuss with senior practitioners if guidance is required Suspend active weaning and if required increase the ventilator support, i.e. increase positive end expiratory pressure (PEEP) pressure support or inspiratory pressures Assess for and treat any underlying causes for instability, i.e. administration of fluid boluses for hypovolaemia

Other respiratory interventions

Intermittent positive pressure breathing (IPPB, e.g. Bird, Bennett PR2)

Definition

Intermittent positive pressure breathing (IPPB) is a form of assisted breathing whereby positive pressure is maintained throughout inspiration followed by passive expiration. The gas flow is delivered via a pressure-cycled machine.

Indications for intermittent positive pressure breathing

IPPB increases lung expansion thereby improving gas exchange and respiratory function. Specific indications for IPPB include:

- sputum retention
- increased work of breathing
- patients with atelectasis
- decreased lung volumes on auscultation
- patients who are unable to take a deep breath.

(Harden 2004)

Contraindications

- Presence of lung abscess or bullae or proximal lung tumour
- Untreated pneumothorax or surgical emphysema
- Post lung surgery/oesophageal surgery
- Bronchopleural fistula
- Facial fractures/surgery
- Active TB
- Basal skull fractures
- Haemoptysis of unknown cause

(Weber and Pryor 1993)

Complications

- Loss of hypoxic drive in COPD patients
- Reduced BP due to reduction in venous return
- Bronchospasm

Background

Anatomy and physiology

Relevant anatomy and physiology have been detailed in earlier non-invasive and invasive mechanical ventilation sections.

Intermittent positive pressure breathing in critical care

There is variable uptake in the use of IPPB (for example 'Bird') across critical care areas and the evidence base in this area remains inconsistent and inconclusive (Denehy and Berney 2001). There is some evidence demonstrating the use of IPPB in improving lung volumes and cough effectiveness in the acute postoperative recovery phase, although studies on which such claims are made are dated (Weber and Pryor 1993). IPPB (Bird) remains one of several techniques that can promote respiratory function and should be used for short periods of time, e.g. 10 minutes every hour, and not continuously (Harden 2004). The inspiratory pressure, sensitivity, flow rate and air mix needed to deliver IPPB therapy are adjustable by the IPPB controls on the machine (Table 5.3). Patient positioning, incentive spirometry (a technique that encourages patients to breathe deeply by using a spirometer with feedback of tidal volume values) and CPAP can also improve gas exchange, improve secretion clearance and thereby reduce the work of breathing. Problem-solving Table 5.11 covers problem solving with IPPB.

Suctioning via a tracheal tube (endotracheal or tracheostomy)

Definition

Suctioning is the removal of secretions and material using negative pressure. Suctioning of the respiratory tract is usually achieved using a flexible or rigid suction catheter attached via tubing to either a portable suction machine or a wall suction unit that produces negative pressure.

Aim and indications

The primary aim of suctioning is the aspiration and removal of secretions (often pulmonary secretions) to promote airway patency and improve oxygenation.

Signs and indications for suctioning include:

- audible secretions during inspiration
- reduced breath sounds or chest movements
- coarse crackles heard on chest auscultation
- decrease in oxygen saturation (SaO_2)
- deterioration in arterial blood gas values, i.e. an increase in $PaCO_2$ or a reduction in PaO_2
- peripheral or central cyanosis
- a saw tooth pattern on the flow-volume loop on the monitor screen of the ventilator (if available), suggesting impedance to the inspired breath, due to the presence of pulmonary secretions.

91

Table 5.3 IPPB (BIRD) controls

General settings and observations	What it tells us
Inspiratory pressure	The pressure received by the patient when the machine is triggered on inspiration
Sensitivity	The amount of effort required by the patient to trigger the machine. Low sensitivities make it easy for the patient to trigger
Flow rate	Rate at which the gas is delivered to the patient. Higher flow = faster delivery
Air mix	Oxygen drives the machine. For the BIRD machine, if the air mix control is pulled out it gives a 40% oxygen/60% air mix to the patient and if the control is pushed in it gives the patient 100% oxygen

(From Denehy and Berney 2001. Reproduced with permission from European Respiratory Society.)

Problem-solving table 5.11: For IPPB (Bird)

Problem	Cause	Suggested actions
Pressure reading on BIRD not reaching its pre-set level	Patient not creating an adequate seal around the mouthpiece	Reassure the patient to help them understand the purpose of the therapy. Nose clips may enable mouth breathing
Pressure reading on BIRD is exceeding pre-set level	Patient blowing out into the machine	Help patient synchronize with BIRD so that during inspiration the patient is passive
Machine triggering too easily or not at all	Sensitivity level inappropriate for patient	If triggering too easily, then increase level required to trigger. If machine not triggering with patient effort, then decrease trigger level
Patient appears to be air hungry and breathless on the BIRD	Flow rate not set high enough, especially if the patient is tachypnoeic	Increase flow rate until the patient is comfortable

- a sudden increase in peak inspiratory pressure (if on volume controlled ventilation) or a reduced tidal volume (if on pressure controlled ventilation).

(American Association of Respiratory Care 2010)

Background

Anatomy and physiology

The respiratory system anatomy consists of upper respiratory tract structures (mouth, nose, nasal cavities and pharynx) and lower respiratory tract structures (larynx, trachea, main bronchus, bronchioles and alveoli) (Figure 5.10).

The respiratory system can be divided functionally into the 'conducting zone' and the 'respiratory zone'. The conducting zone (from the nose to terminal bronchioles) not only filters and warms inhaled air, it also guides inspired air to the respiratory zone (alveoli and capillaries), the main area of gaseous exchange (Tortora and Derrickson 2011).

In health, particles breathed in from atmospheric air are eliminated during expiration or coughing. Mucus produced by goblet cells lining the respiratory tract trap particulate matter and ciliated cells assist in their removal. In the upper respiratory tract, the mucus-containing material is moved by ciliated cells down towards the pharynx. In the lower tract, the cilia move the mucus up towards the pharynx (Tortora and Derrickson 2011). In the terminal bronchioles, which are mostly lined with non-ciliated simple cuboidal epithelium, inhaled particles are removed by macrophages. A functioning cough reflex ensures that these respiratory secretions are then propelled towards the oropharynx, where they are expectorated or swallowed (Marieb and Hoehn 2007). Disruption of these protective processes or blockage in anatomical structures can cause respiratory compromise or failure.

Patients in critical care may have increased mucus production due to respiratory disease and be less able to clear secretions due to reduced level of consciousness or physiological reserve. Patients with an endotracheal tube may be sedated, thereby reducing the effectiveness of the normal protective mechanism of the cough reflex (Rolls et al. 2007). Mucus viscosity is further increased as a result of breathing inspired air that is not humidified and at temperature lower than normal inspired air (Bersten and Soni 2009). If the resultant sections are not removed, there is risk of infection, atelectasis and alveolar collapse (Day et al. 2002).

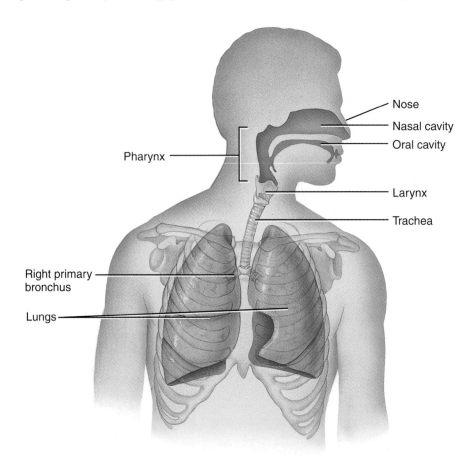

Figure 5.10   Anterior view showing organs of respiration (from Tortora and Derrickson 2011, reproduced with permission from Wiley).

Suctioning through endotracheal and tracheal tubes

Suctioning is a frequent clinical procedure in critical care settings. Open or closed suctioning techniques can be used to remove secretions from intubated patients. Open suctioning involves the disconnection of a patient from ventilatory support to remove the pulmonary secretions. A single-use sterile suction catheter can then be introduced and used in the endotracheal or trachestomy tube (Seckel 2008). Open suctioning can be used to clear secretions in patients breathing unaided, breathing through an artificial airway (OPA, NPA) and in patients who are receiving short-term mechanical ventilation via an ETT. Disconnection from any ventilator support for the purpose of suctioning will result in the loss of positive end expiratory pressure (PEEP) and increase the infection risk to the patient and care giver (Wood 1998; Seckel 2008). A further advancement in suctioning options includes subglottic suctioning, where there is growing evidence for its use to reduce ventilator-associated pneumonia (Gujadhur et al. 2004; Hallais et al. 2011).

Closed endotracheal or tracheal suctioning occurs when suctioning is via a sterile, sheathed suction catheter that is inserted into the respiratory circuit, ensuring that the ventilation support system remains connected during suctioning (Pedersen et al. 2009). This technique, often used in unstable and longer-term ventilated patients, minimizes the risks of cross-infection and maintains ventilatory support (Pedersen et al. 2009).

The removal of secretions through suctioning has associated risks, including:

- hypoxia/hypoxaemia
- bronchoconstriction
- bleeding
- atelectasis (alveoli collapse)
- tracheal ulceration and damage
- haemodynamic instability
- raised intracranial pressure (ICP).

(Pedersen et al. 2009; AARC 2010)

It is important to note the growing evidence base to inform what have been traditional suctioning practices. Studies have demonstrated that instillation of saline into tracheal tubes to loosen secretions prior to suctioning has little benefit other than stimulating a cough reflex (Thompson 2000). Routine manual hyperinflation with 100% oxygen prior to suctioning is also not recommended because it causes significant changes in mean arterial pressure, cardiac output, pulmonary artery pressure and pulmonary airway pressure. The recommended way to pre-oxygenate a patient prior to suction if the patient is hypoxic is to use the ventilator capability to deliver 100% pre-oxygenation (Thomson 2000). Furthermore, the diameter of the suction catheter should be limited to less than 50% of the internal diameter of the tracheal tube. This then allows air to enter the lung during suctioning and avoids the development of atelectasis caused by excessive negative pressure (Day et al. 2002). Frequency of suctioning should be guided by the purulence and viscosity of secretions, airway status and change in respiratory parameters, not by rigid and routine unit practices.

Problem-solving table 5.12: Suctioning difficulties

Problem	Possible causes	Preventative measures
Unable to aspirate secretions effectively	Secretions might be too viscous to be aspirated. Suctioning equipment may be malfunctioning or humidification system incorrectly assembled	Ensure the patient is adequately hydrated. Check that humidification systems are functioning. Check all connections within ventilation circuit and replace suction unit if necessary
Patient instability: oxygen desaturation and haemodynamic deterioration	Patient sensitive to oxygen changes or loss of positive end expiratory pressure (PEEP) May be due to hypoxia-related dysrhythmia or stimulation of the vagus nerve causing bradycardia	Ensure patient is appropriately oxygenated using the ventilator capability to pre-oxygenate with 100% oxygen Ensure patient is cardiovascularly stable prior to procedure. Monitor condition and seek advice from senior practitioner as required
Patient distress	Discomfort and pain associated with insertion of the suction catheter and induction of a cough response	Explain the rationale for the procedure to the patient. Suction when clinically indicated rather than at regular intervals due to the risk of adverse side effects (Rolls et al. 2007). If appropriate, analgesia or sedation may be useful

Humidification

Definition

A gas sample may contain moisture as discrete water droplets (aerosol) or as invisible water vapour. Humidity is the amount of water vapour in a gas sample. There are several measures of humidity, including absolute and relative, but for the purposes of clinical practice, absolute humidity (the mass of water in a volume of gas, measured in mg/L) is most appropriate. The ambient temperature (such as that in a breathing circuit or in the body) is a major determinant of how much water vapour can be carried in a gas. A higher temperature allows for a greater humidity, while a lower temperature results in more condensation forming (Williams 2005).

Aims and indications

Humidification serves two purposes:

- warming inspired air
- adding water to inspired air.

Background

Anatomy and physiology

The conducting structures of the respiratory tract, comprising the nasopharynx and mouth, along with the larynx, trachea and terminal bronchioles, take no part in gas exchange. However, they are important in warming, filtering and humidifying inspired air before it reaches the respiratory part, which consists of the respiratory bronchioles and alveoli.

The mucosa of much of the respiratory tract between the upper airways and bronchioles comprises a ciliated epithelium, the cells of which produce mucus. This mucus has several functions. First, it traps particulate matter, thus protecting the alveoli. Second, it moves trapped matter towards the mouth due to the motions of the cilia 'the mucociliary escalator'. Third, the water contained in the mucus helps to humidify inspired gases.

Drying of the mucosa has been shown to directly injure the ciliated cells with as little as one hour of exposure to cold dry air (Chalon et al. 1972). The mechanism by which this occurs is unclear, although dry, thick mucus is more difficult to move. In addition, some drugs (for example nicotine) can directly impair ciliary function. If very dry and cold air is inspired (such as in the polar regions) (Table 5.4) (Thompson 2010), or if the upper airways are bypassed (such as with tracheostomy or endotracheal tubes), the mucus layer in the airways may dry out, leading to thickened, tenacious secretions.

During normal breathing of dry air at room temperature, the nose, pharynx and tracheal mucosa filter, warm and add moisture to inspired air. Air reaching the alveoli is at body temperature, and contains about 44mg/L (6% by volume) water vapour.

Table 5.4 Variation in water content of air in relation to temperature

Temperature (°C)	0°C	20°C Room temperature	37°C Body temperature
Water content (mg/L)	5	18	44

Medical gases are supplied dry to prevent frosting or corrosion in tubes, valves and other mechanical parts of medical equipment. The clinical requirement to humidify inspired gases has long been recognized (Wilkes 2011a), although the methods used depend on cost, complexity, efficiency and available technology.

Humidifiers

Humidifiers can be classified as either active or passive devices (Wilkes 2005). Active devices are able to humidify the airways irrespective of the patient's ability to do so. Passive devices depend on the patient generating sufficient moisture during expiration to humidify inspired gas. Specifications for humidifier performance are to provide at least 30 mg H_2O/L of delivered gas at 30°C, although there is a significant variability in actual performance (Wilkes 2011a).

Passive humidifiers

The most frequently used device is a heat and moisture exchanger (HME), sometimes combined with a bacterial filter (HMEF). A typical HME is a small plastic casing with a volume of between 3 and 60 mL, containing either a foam or paper membrane through which inspired gases flow. The membrane is impregnated with a salt such as calcium chloride, which enhances the efficiency of the humidification process. When warm, moist expired air flows through the membrane, water condenses out on to the salt. Conversely, cool, dry air flowing in the other direction becomes warmer and humidified during inspiration (Wilkes 2005).

A bacterial filter usually consists of either a mat of densely packed glass fibre strands or a looser membrane of electrostatically charged material. The former acts as a simple physical barrier to particulate matter. The latter forms a physical and functional barrier due to electrical repulsion of any particles in the circuit. Theoretically, the dense glass fibre mat may have a greater resistance to gas flow than the electrostatic membrane, although this is unlikely to have a significant clinical impact.

Active humidifiers

At their most basic, active humidifiers consist of a water container in the inspiratory limb of a breathing circuit through which inspired gas passes. The gas may flow over the water, or bubble through it, becoming humidified en route. These simple systems are inefficient, and most active humidifiers have a mechanism to warm the water as a means of increasing humidity. The water may be directly warmed in the container, usually to 30–37°C (Hess et al. 2003), or the inspiratory limb may contain a heating coil to prevent condensation developing between the container and the patient.

Some systems also have a heated expiratory limb to prevent similar precipitation in the expiratory limb (particularly if the ventilator has an expiratory flow meter which may be damaged by excess water).

An alternative method to moisten inspired gas is by adding small water droplets using nebulization, either by a gas-driven device or an ultrasonic nebulizer (Hess 2000). A gas-driven nebulizer consists of a specifically engineered tube through which the driving gas (usually oxygen) flows. Pressure changes due to the tube shape (the Venturi effect, Figure 5.11) cause entrainment of liquid through a side port. This liquid may be water or drug, e.g. bronchodilators (Hess 2000).

An ultrasonic nebulizer has a rapidly (typically around 2 MHz) vibrating plate or mesh, and any water on this plate is fragmented into droplets. Air passing over this thus becomes humidified, producing an aerosol for inhalation.

Both forms of nebulization result in a range of differently sized water droplets carried in the inspired gas. Most are too large to remain airborne for long periods, and precipitate out into the breathing circuit or proximal airways. Only a small proportion reaches the alveoli (which may be most relevant when considering drug deposition for inhaled therapy in ventilated patients) (Hess et al. 2003).

Problems with humidifiers

Problems with humidifiers include:

- active heating systems may overheat (over 37°C) and cause patient injury
- bacterial colonization of water leading to transmission of infection
- blockage of HME due to excess secretions/water or drugs
- damage to ventilator equipment from excess condensation (particularly flow monitors in the expiratory limb of ventilator circuits)
- increased dead space in the breathing circuit
- increased resistance to gas flow in the breathing circuit from the humidifier (Wilkes 2011b).

Choosing a humidifier

Theoretically, since they can generate higher temperatures, heated humidifiers are more efficient than passive devices. Heated devices also theoretically have less dead space or resistance to airflow in a breathing circuit than HMEs. Additionally, heated circuits reduce condensation, so may decrease the risk of bacterial colonization of condensate. However, a meta-analysis of 13 studies involving almost

95

The Venturi effect in Clinical Practice		
Use	**Carrier Gas**	**Side Port addition**
Controlled Oxygen therapy	Oxygen	Room Air
Drug delivery	Oxygen	Bronchodilators
Humidification	Air/oxygen mix	Water

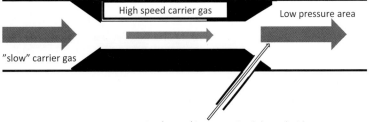

Gas flowing through a constriction will move faster than before the constriction, but immediately after the constriction, will slow down.

This change in velocity is associated with a drop in pressure, which in turn sucks fluid or a second gas through a side port.

High speed carrier gas

Low pressure area

"slow" carrier gas

Gas/water/drug entrained through side port

Figure 5.11 Venturi effect.

3000 patients showed little evidence that the increased cost or complexity of heated humidifiers is justified (Siempos et al. 2007). Rates of ventilator-associated pneumonia, duration of ventilation, mortality and ICU stay were similar with either type of humidifier. It may be appropriate to reserve the use of heated humidifiers for some specific patient groups with contraindications to passive devices, e.g. those with hypothermia, very thick respiratory secretions, haemoptysis, or significant atelectasis. Other patients can be managed adequately with HMEs (Siempos et al. 2007).

Problem-solving table 5.13: **Humidification**

Problem	Cause	Prevention	Action
Damage to ventilator equipment (e.g. flow measurement sensor)	Condensation in expiratory limb	Heated expiratory limb Expiratory limb water trap	Place dependent part of expiratory circuit below any equipment at risk
Thick, tenacious secretions	Inadequate humidification	Ensure adequate heating and water delivery to circuit	
Patient burns	Overheated circuit	Functioning heated humidifier	Avoid active heater
Ventilator acquired pneumonia	Possible bacterial colonization of circuit	Avoid prolonged pooling of water in circuits	
Inadequate patient ventilation	Blockage of circuit or humidifier/filter	Regular checking of circuit and ancillaries	

Manual hyperinflation and hyperoxygenation

Definition

Manual hyperinflation is the technique of disconnecting the patient from the ventilator and inflating the lungs with larger volumes than ventilator breaths in order to improve oxygenation, prevent atelectasis and improve lung compliance (Paratz et al. 2002). It has been historically defined as delivering tidal volumes to airway pressures of 40 cm H_2O (Rothen et al. 1993) or a tidal volume (Vt) that is 50% greater than that delivered by the ventilator (Singer et al. 1994).

Manual hyperinflation is delivered using a circuit that delivers 100% oxygen and a self-inflating bag such as a Mapleson C circuit and reservoir bag (see Figure 5.12). A manual hyperinflation breath usually consists of a slower, deeper inspiration, an inspiratory hold and a quick release of the reservoir bag to increase the expiratory flow rate. Most modern-day ventilators can also deliver ventilator hyperinflation breaths with similar effect (Berney and Denehy 2002).

Aims and indications

The aim of manual hyperinflation is to restore alveoli volume by inflating collapsed alveoli through collateral channels of ventilation and to facilitate the removal of pul-

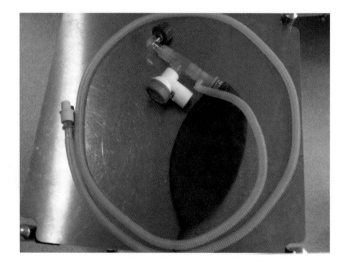

Figure 5.12   Mapleson C circuit and reservoir bag.

monary secretions (Stiller 2000). It is indicated for intubated, ventilated patients who require:

- improved levels oxygenation, e.g. post procedures
- increased clearance of pulmonary secretions
- improved lung compliance and reversal of atelectasis.

(Hodgson et al. 2000; Choi and Jones 2005)

Background

Anatomy and physiology

The respiratory lobes, bronchioles and alveoli are important respiratory structures in maintaining pulmonary ventilation, external respiration and the transportation of respiratory gases (Tortora and Derrickson 2011). In patients with respiratory disorders, or those receiving sedation/general anaesthetic, lung function and lung mechanics can become altered. Lung tissue can become compressed, alveolar air can be reabsorbed and surfactant function can become impaired (Hedenstierna and Lennart 2010). These are all causes of atelectasis.

The development of atelectasis leads to decreased lung compliance, impaired oxygenation and increased pulmonary resistance that further contributes to lung injury. Therefore manoeuvres that recruit alveoli, such as hyperinflation, may be of use in atelectasis. The use of some form of hyperinflation seems to be beneficial over simple suctioning alone (Blattner et al. 2008; Dennis et al. 2012). Although manual hyperinflation has been the traditional method to achieve this, and is common practice in some institutions, on balance, adjustments to a mechanical ventilator provide a more effective, stable method of recruiting atelectatic lung.

Manual hyperinflation and hyperoxygenation in critical care

The short-term effects of manual hyperinflation on pulmonary compliance and resolution of atelectasis have been well documented (Hodgson et al. 2000). Patients requiring this intervention are likely to be ventilated. When performing hyperinflation, the patient is either disconnected from the ventilator and manual hyperinflation and hyperoxygenation breaths are delivered via a Mapleson C circuit and reservoir bag, or the ventilator is adjusted to deliver larger volumes. The temporary removal from positive pressure ventilation can result in a loss of PEEP (positive end expiratory pressure) within the lungs, and subsequent alveolar derecruitment. Therefore for patients being ventilated and receiving more than 10 cm H_2O PEEP, use of a PEEP valve within the circuit should be considered to maintain PEEP during manual hyperinflation.

Furthermore, to prevent barotrauma in critically ill patients who are at high risk of further lung injury, it is recommended that a pressure gauge (manometer) is placed in the circuit to minimize the risk of barotrauma by ensuring that inspiratory pressures do not rise above 40 cm H_2O.

A ventilator should be used in most circumstances to prevent the loss of PEEP and barotrauma associated with manual hyperinflation (Choi and Jones 2005; Savian et al. 2006; Maxwell and Ellis 2007).

Due to the physiological changes that manual hyperinflation can cause, this manoeuvre should not be used in patients with:

- large emphysematous bullae
- subcutaneous emphysema
- undrained pneumothorax
- recent lung surgery with bronchial resection
- open bronchopulmonary fistula
- bronchospasm or peak airway pressures greater than 40–50 cm H_2O
- complex ventilation needs, e.g. inverse ratio ventilation
- cardiovascular instability
- agitation/aggression or acute head injury.

(Northern Health and Social Care Trust 2007)

Problem-solving table 5.14: Manual hyperinflation

Problem	Possible cause	Preventative measures
Hypotension or haemodynamic instability during the manual hyperinflation procedure	Possible hypoxia associated with a break in mechanical ventilation Increased intrathoracic pressure inhibiting venous return to the heart	Discontinue procedure, reattach patient to the mechanical ventilator and provide additional oxygen therapy if required
Patient agitation or restlessness	Discomfort from the procedure, or inadequate analgesia or sedation	Discontinue procedure, reattach patient to the mechanical ventilator. Explain the reason for the procedure to the patient. Provide additional analgesia or sedation if indicated

Prone ventilation

Definition

Prone ventilation is ventilating a patient in a face-down position, rather than in the usual supine position.

Aims and indications

The aims of prone ventilation are to:

- facilitate particular surgical interventions (e.g. spinal operations)
- improve oxygenation in severely hypoxaemic patients (e.g. acute respiratory distress syndrome [ARDS]).

Indications for prone ventilation in critically ill patients include:

- to improve oxygenation in patients with severe hypoxaemic respiratory failure who have failed to respond positively to conventional ventilator management techniques.

Background

Anatomy and physiology

An understanding of the mechanisms of action and the benefits and risks of placing critically ill patients in the prone position are necessary for appropriate decision making and management. A common cause of severe hypoxaemia in critical care is acute lung injury (ALI) or acute respiratory distress syndrome (ARDS). These exhibit a similar pathological appearance, but ARDS represents a more severe manifestation of the disease. ALI is partly defined by a PaO_2 below 42 kPa, and ARDS by a PaO_2 below 27 kPa while breathing 100% oxygen. Other defining criteria include an acute duration of onset, a non-cardiogenic but recognized cause and typical bilateral infiltrative appearances on chest X-ray. ALI and ARDS may be due to a primary lung insult (e.g. pneumonia, aspiration pneumonitis) or secondary to extrapulmonary disease (e.g. sepsis, trauma, acute pancreatitis).

In each case, the lung shows alveolar infiltration, congestion and reduced compliance. Fibrotic scarring may develop with ALI/ARDS, especially if persistent for several weeks. All these changes cause V/Q mismatch with impaired oxygen transfer from alveoli to pulmonary capillaries, with resultant hypoxaemia. In severe disease, up to 70% of lung tissue may be abnormal, leaving only 30% to meet the often increased demands of critical illness. Thus, an adult patient has only a small amount of normal lung available for respiration. This 'baby lung' concept of ARDS leads to the requirement for careful management of mechanical ventilation to protect the remaining normal lung tissue, while not further injuring abnormal lung tissue (Gattinoni and Pesenti 2005).

Prone ventilation is one element of such management (along with low tidal volume ventilation, permissive hypercapnia, pressure-limited ventilation and careful fluid balance). The mechanisms by which prone ventilation improves oxygen

are still incompletely understood (Sud et al. 2010b), but are multifactorial, and include:

- more uniform ventilation from ventral to dorsal areas of lung compared to supine positioning
- reduced alveolar collapse
- reduced alveolar over-distension
- reduced lung compression by the heart and mediastinum
- reduced lung compression by the diaphragm
- possibly greater postural drainage of secretions allowing alveolar expansion
- altered chest wall compliance.

Perhaps surprisingly, placing patients prone does not improve functional residual capacity significantly, and distribution of pulmonary blood flow is only minimally altered by prone ventilation. Prone positioning improves oxygenation in about 75% of patients, and this effect may persist following a return to the supine position. The best predictor of a sustained response (longer than 2 hours) is an improvement in oxygenation of greater than 1 kPa during the first 30 minutes (Sud et al. 2010b). It is unclear with current evidence how long patients should be placed prone for, although many authors (McAuley et al. 2002) recommend relatively long periods prone (greater than 18 hours). A practical compromise may be to schedule positioning with other required clinical interventions as long as gas exchange is deemed adequate.

Although oxygenation is improved in many patients placed prone, the effects on requirements for organ support, length of stay in a critical care level 3 facility and mortality are less clear. Studies in this area are not directly comparable, but it seems likely that prone ventilation reduces mortality by around 15% in patients with the most severe hypoxaemia (PaO_2 less than 13 kPa with FiO_2 of 1.0), but not for those with less severe disease (Sud et al. 2010b). Likewise, patients may demonstrate improvements in oxygenation with repeated episodes of prone positioning if hypoxaemia recurs over days or weeks.

Risks of prone ventilation

As with most procedures and interventions in critically ill patients, there are disadvantages and risks associated with the use of prone ventilation. Problems related to prone positioning include:

- facial and orbital oedema (due to dependent positioning)
- pressure area breakdown (as for any critically ill patient)
- endotracheal tube obstruction or accidental extubation (although this is not necessarily more likely than for supine patients)
- dislodgement of vascular catheters or wound drains, particularly during repositioning
- difficulty with enteral tube feeding because of increased gastro-oesophageal reflux (patients' heads are often lower than their stomachs during prone positioning)

- occasionally, haemodynamic instability, including cardiac arrest (a multifactorial problem, including cytokine-induced myocardial dysfunction, peripheral vasoplegia and problems associated with wide variation in venous return during patient movement).

Obesity makes prone positioning technically more difficult, but is not associated with an increase in complications.

Relative contraindications to prone positioning include:

- raised intracranial pressure
- spinal or pelvic instability
- pregnancy
- extreme haemodynamic instability and shock, due to the risk of cardiac arrest

- patients regarded as 'not for attempted resuscitation'.

(Ball et al. 2001)

Caution should be shown with patients who have undergone recent abdominal or thoracic surgery because of the risk of dislodging drains, dressings and potential disruption to organ function or blood flow due to pressure. However, the overall risks of prone ventilation are less common than generally perceived. Published reviews (Gattinoni et al. 2001; Ward 2002) provide contradictory information, with both increased or decreased rates of the above complications when supine and prone ventilation were compared.

In summary, it is reasonable to consider prone ventilation for patients with refractory severe hypoxaemia following best conventional ventilation strategies.

Problem-solving table 5.15: Prone ventilation

Problem	Cause	Action
Inadequate ventilation while prone	Inappropriate ventilator settings Obstruction of endotracheal tube due to position Patient–ventilator dysynchrony	Alter to appropriate ventilation settings Check endotracheal tube position and reposition if obstructed Increase sedation or consider use of neuromuscular blocking agents
Pressure area breakdown	Reduced mobility due to sedation/paralysis Abnormal distribution of pressure/weight while in prone position	Change patient's position regularly Use a pressure redistribution mattress (see also Chapter 12)
Gastro-oesophageal reflux	Reduced gastric motility due to critical illness	Consider prokinetics, alter position Consult dietician urgently. Stop or reduce the rate of nasogastric feed Consider introduction of a gastric motility agent, for example metoclopramide
Haemodynamic instability	Changes in venous return Reduced vasomotor tone	Ensure adequate fluid loading before positioning changes Ensure availability of vasoconstrictors Consider return to supine position
Corneal abrasions and peri-orbital oedema	Use of pharmacological paralysis agents (for example atracurium) will result in total muscle paralysis, including the ocular muscles responsible for blinking. Reduced eye movement, can lead to dry ocular membranes and corneal abrasions. Direct trauma to the cornea due to prone position	Regular eye care, as directed (see Chapter 12). Possible use of hydrocolloid dressings, polyethylene or swabs soaked in sterile water (for details see Chapter 12) (Koroloff et al. 2004; Sivasankar et al. 2006)
Cardiorespiratory arrest	Due to hypoxia or the underlying cause of the respiratory failure, i.e. sepsis and hypovolaemia	Immediately return patient to the supine position, using the appropriate number of assistants. Commence cardiopulmonary resuscitation following current resuscitation guidelines (see Chapter 18)
Accidental disconnection of intravenous access device and/or tubing	Loose connections	Reconnect intravenous access device or tubing Ensure all tubing is correctly secured and connections tight. Monitor the patient for any complications or abnormalities

Chest drains

Definition

A chest drain is a tube inserted through the skin and sub-cutaneous tissues into either the pleural space or the mediastinum.

The majority of chest drains encountered in critical care are intercostal drains placed between the ribs into the pleural space. Mediastinal drains are in many respects similar to wound drains in other sites, so will not be considered further here.

Insertion of chest drains is usually performed as an aseptic technique.

Aims and indications

Chest drains may be inserted for a variety of indications, principally:

- pneumothorax drainage
- removal of pleural fluid or pus
- postoperative wound management.

These abnormalities may occur in combination, e.g. traumatic haemopneumothorax.

Background

Anatomy and physiology

Each lung is normally enclosed in a layer of pleura tightly adherent to the lung itself – the visceral pleura. Another layer of pleura, the parietal pleura, lines the inside of the chest cavity. The space between these two layers is the pleural space. In health, this space has no air and only a small amount of fluid within it to aid lubrication of the lungs during breathing. The presence of air in this space is termed a pneumothorax. The presence of blood is a haemothorax, of pus is an empyema and of excess other fluid is a pleural effusion.

Pneumothorax

A pneumothorax is a collection of air inside the chest, but outside the lung itself. Commonly, this is caused by damage to the pleura overlying the lung, from trauma, surgical intervention, or rupture of alveoli during mechanical ventilation. Pneumothoraces may also arise spontaneously. A pneumothorax may be described as simple, open, or tension.

An open pneumothorax has a connection between the outside air and the pleural space, e.g. stab wound, intraoperative thoracotomy. Treatment of this involves closing the defect in the chest wall, thus converting the pneumothorax to a simple pneumothorax (see below), which can then be managed with a chest drain.

In a simple pneumothorax, the air that has leaked into the pleural space is not under pressure, usually because there is no ongoing leak between the lung tissue and pleural space, and the pneumothorax therefore does not expand with each breath. A small simple pneumothorax may resolve spontaneously or with needle aspiration (Aguinagaldea et al. 2010). Larger pneumothoraces (perhaps greater than 20% of lung volume) usually require an intercostal drain to aid resolution.

However, particularly in a patient receiving mechanical ventilation, there is a significant risk of conversion from a simple to a tension pneumothorax, where a proportion of each inspired breath escapes through a leak between the lung and the pleural space, and increases the size of the pneumothorax. This incremental expansion of the pneumothorax increases the gas pressure within that side of the chest. This increasing pressure collapses the lung and twists the mediastinum and great veins, with detrimental effects on both gas exchange and haemodynamics. This may be fatal if untreated or unrecognized, and this may be a particularly rapid process (a few minutes) for patients receiving mechanical ventilation.

The identification of which type of pneumothorax is present is therefore important, since it will affect the urgency and nature of required treatment.

Signs and symptoms of pneumothorax

Classically, a pneumothorax will present with:

- tachypnoea
- dyspnoea
- hypoxaemia
- reduced air entry on the affected side
- tracheal shift away from the affected side (in a tension pneumothorax)
- tachycardia and hypotension, followed by shock and cardiac arrest, particularly with a tension pneuomothorax.

Pleural fluid

As noted above, the pleural space normally contains only a small amount of fluid. This fluid volume is determined by the interaction of a number of complex factors, and pathological increases in the volume of this fluid may be due to a variety of causes, including:

- cardiac failure
- fluid overload
- chyle (fluid leakage from damage to the thoracic duct, usually in the right hemithorax)
- parapneumonic fluid collection (due to infection)
- pus (empyema)
- capillary leak syndrome
- blood.

Chest drain insertion

There are several types of chest drain, used for different purposes, each with specific characteristics (Shalli et al. 2009; Havelock et al. 2010). They are shown in Table 5.5.

The insertion technique has relevance for the equipment required, patient comfort, and for the management of drain removal. Small-bore drains tend to be better tolerated by patients. Large-bore chest drain insertion is often a painful procedure. Fifty per cent of patients in one study reported pain scores of 9 or 10 on a scale of 1 to 10 (Luketich et al. 1998). Adequate analgesia and, if required, sedation, should be provided in a timely manner. Large-bore chest drains are often supplied with a metal trocar. This should be removed prior to drain insertion. Simply using the trocar to blindly find the pleural space is associated with an unacceptably high complication rate (up to 30%), including lung, liver or even cardiac perforation (Haron et al. 2010; Havelock et al. 2010).

Small-bore drains inserted using the Seldinger technique also carry a risk of accidental organ puncture or lung laceration, but this may be reduced using real time ultrasound imaging to direct the needle during insertion (Havelock et al. 2010). Most drains are inserted in the 4th or 5th intercostal space in the mid-axillary line, but occasionally drains may be placed in the anterior chest wall or other sites (e.g. for loculated collections or pneumothoraces).

Once the drain is inserted, it should be secured. Purse string sutures should not be used because they convert a linear wound into a painful, unsightly scar. Simple interrupted sutures are recommended to close the wound and to secure the drainage tube (Havelock et al. 2010).

Large amounts of tape and padding to dress the site are also unnecessary, particularly for small-bore drains. A simple occlusive dressing, with a mesentery or omental dressing to stabilize the tube several inches from the insertion site is usually sufficient (Figure 5.13). The position of the drain is usually confirmed using a chest X-ray.

Management of chest drains

The chest drain is connected to a one-way valve system. In some situations, a simple Heimlich-type flutter valve is used, such as when an underwater seal drain is not available or transport of the patient with an underwater seal drain is difficult. A Heimlich-type flutter valve is a one-way valve consisting of a plastic tube with a flexible, flattened inner latex tube attached internally at one end. Air, blood, or fluid flows into the latex tube and out at the other end. The latex tube collapses on itself at rest, thus preventing any backflow of air or fluid into the chest (Heimlich 1983) (Figure 5.14).

Table 5.5 Types of chest drain

	Small bore	Large bore
Size	8–14 French gauge	greater than 14 French gauge
Typical indications	Pneumothoraces Watery fluid collections	Blood Empyema Thicker, viscous fluid collections
Insertion technique	Guidewire through needle (Seldinger)	Blunt dissection or direct vision
Securing technique	Suture or simple dressing	Sutures and dressing
Removal technique	Single operator	Two-person technique
Patient discomfort	Low	Higher

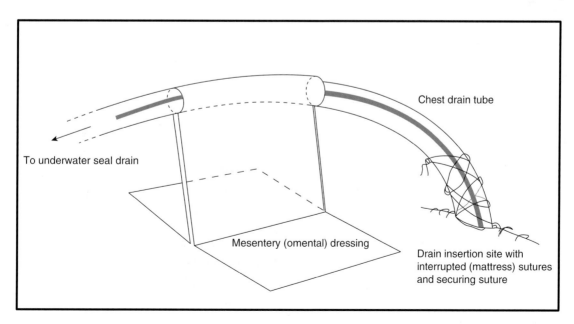

Figure 5.13 Mesentery or omental dressing.

101

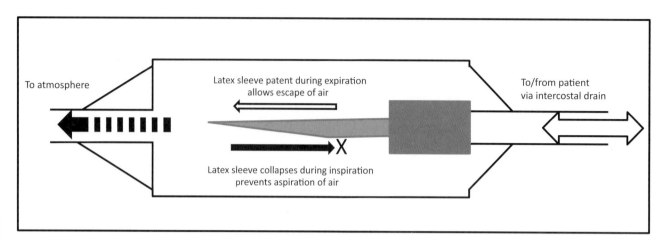

To atmosphere

Latex sleeve patent during expiration
allows escape of air

To/from patient
via intercostal drain

Latex sleeve collapses during inspiration
prevents aspiration of air

X

Figure 5.14 Heimlich flutter valve.

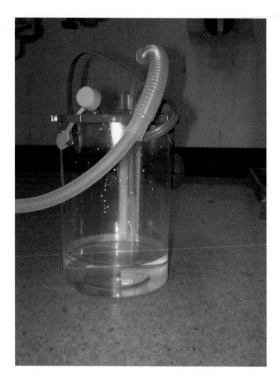

Figure 5.15 Underwater seal system.

However, most chest drains in critical care are managed using an underwater seal system. This allows drainage of air and fluid from the pleural space into a container, while preventing any backflow of fluid or air into the pleural space (Figure 5.15). Obviously, if the drainage container is held above the level of the insertion point, such backflow becomes more likely.

Variations on the standard single bottle underwater seal system include a second bottle and the addition of suction.

- A second bottle (Figure 5.16) is typically added when significant fluid drainage is anticipated. The first bottle collects the fluid, while the second provides the underwater seal. This prevents a large amount of fluid collecting in a single bottle, which may impede further drainage.
- Suction is generally added to a drainage system to help resolve persistent pneumothoraces (often due to a bronchopleural fistula). Suction is obtained by connecting the drain to a high-volume, low-pressure wall suction, typically at between 10 and 20 cm H_2O (Laws 2003).

Fluid in a drain that is patent, correctly placed in the pleural space and connected to an underwater seal should 'swing'. This means the fluid in the chest drain tubing rises and falls with respiration. For a spontaneously breathing patient, inspiration should make the fluid rise towards the patient and expiration should make it fall. The converse is true for a patient receiving positive pressure ventilation. This is because, during positive pressure ventilation, inspiration is due the generation of a positive pressure within the chest, while spontaneous inspiration is a result of a negative pressure developing within the chest.

If a drain is placed for a pneumothorax, it should 'bubble'. This is the air of the pneumothorax being displaced from the pleural space into the drain. The degree of bubbling will depend on the size of air leak. A large leak may persist throughout the respiratory cycle, while a smaller leak may only occur during expiration. Resolution of the pneumothorax will lead to cessation of bubbling.

A non-bubbling drain may be one that has corrected the underlying pneumothorax, or it may be malfunctioning, perhaps because it is blocked or kinked. Likewise, a drain that does not swing may be blocked or kinked. Identification of the problem should lead to appropriate management – drain removal, unblocking, or possibly replacement.

As a general principle, chest drains should not be clamped, especially for patients receiving mechanical ventilation. The

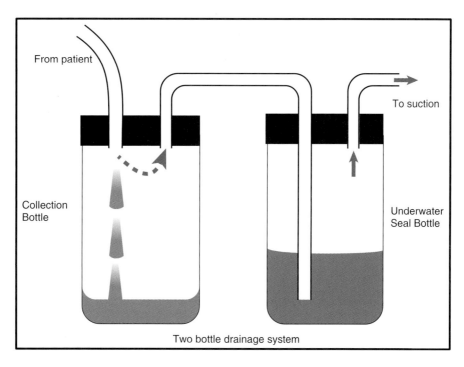

Figure 5.16 Two-bottle drainage system.

risk in this group is of developing a tension pneumothorax (see above). Drains should only be clamped under the direction of senior experienced staff (Havelock et al. 2010).

Vital signs should be observed and recorded for patients with intercostal drains in place, and any deterioration should alert practitioners to the possibility of a problem with the drain. The volume of fluid draining should also be recorded, since this will have a bearing on clinical decisions about the need for surgery or timing of drain removal.

Chest drain removal

A chest drain is removed when it has resolved the underlying problem, and the decision to do so typically involves reviewing the patient's clinical status and chest X-ray appearances. A drain volume less than 200 mL in 24 hours, with no ongoing air loss or bubbling, is often regarded as an acceptable limit (Havelock et al. 2010). A large-bore drain site should be examined to ensure that the wound can be closed by the existing suture following drain removal. If not, an additional suture may be required before drain removal.

Clamping of the drain before removal is generally unnecessary, and may be dangerous due to the risk of causing or worsening a tension pneumothorax. Removing the drain with a simple pneumothorax, as long as it is small enough to resolve, rarely causes a clinical problem. It is common to remove the drains from mechanically ventilated patients following treatment of simple pneumothoraces or drained tension pneumothoraces. However, if the patient has a tension pneumothorax draining air through the drain, and that drain is then clamped, the escaping air will stay in the chest cavity and cause the physiologically disturbances of an untreated tension pneumothorax.

Chest drain removal should be carried out by two practitioners, one to remove the drain, the other to secure the site and apply a dressing (Havelock et al. 2010). Chest drain removal may be briefly painful, so adequate explanation, analgesia and sedation if required should be provided.

When removing a chest drain, the lung should be expanded to prevent generation of a pneumothorax. Thus, the timing of removal is different for a spontaneously breathing patient and a mechanically ventilated patient.

- If a patient is breathing spontaneously, the chest tube should be removed either while the patient performs a Valsalva manoeuvre (expiration against a closed glottis) or with a brisk, firm movement during expiration. For large-bore drains, the assistant ties the previously placed closure suture as the drain is removed. For small-bore drains, an occlusive dressing can be placed as the drain is removed.
- If a patient is mechanically ventilated, the drain can be removed during inspiration using the same technique.

Chest X-ray post removal is unlikely to change management, but is an established tradition. Any residual pneumothorax, subcutaneous emphysema and absence of fluid or blood collections would be noted.

Problem-solving table 5.16: Chest drain insertion

Problem	Possible cause	Prevention	Suggested action
Surgical emphysema	Worsening pneumothorax, a blocked chest drain or possibly a side hole in the chest drain lying outside the pleural cavity	Ensure sufficient drain is within the pleural cavity. Ensure drain is adequately secured to patient, particularly during repositioning	Inform senior practitioner immediately if required. Monitor patient for any signs of respiratory distress. Undertake urgent chest X-ray to confirm chest drain position. Insert a further chest drain if required
Haemorrhage	Pre-existing untreated coagulopathy at time of drain insertion. Possible trauma to intercostal blood vessels	Consider checking clotting profile if coagulopathy suspected prior to insertion	Inform senior practitioner immediately if required. Monitor patient's vital signs. Administer fluid replacement if indicated
Acute respiratory distress following insertion	Worsening pneumothorax or development of a tension pneumothorax. Possible direct trauma to underlying lung or other organs. Possible re-expansion pulmonary oedema, particularly if large chronic effusion drained too rapidly	Correct insertion technique. Consider ultrasound guidance for insertion. Consider limiting volume drained initially to 1500 mL/h (Havelock et al. 2010)	Inform senior practitioner immediately if required. Monitor patient's vital signs. Prepare for urgent chest drain insertion or thoracocentesis
Pain	Insufficient or short-acting analgesia during procedure		Administer additional analgesia as prescribed
Non-bubbling drain	No pneumothorax. Drain blocked (for example, with thrombus). Kinked drain	Regularly monitor drain tubing for patency. Ensure that drain tubing is not kinked when the patient is positioned	Remove drain – if initially inserted for a pneumothorax. Replace tubing. Unkink tubing. Tube may require flushing or reinsertion. Seek advice from senior practitioner

Problem-solving table 5.17: Chest drain removal

Problem	Possible cause	Prevention	Suggested action
No closure suture noted at time of drain removal	Clinician error or displacement of suture		Inform senior practitioner immediately if required. Prepare equipment for insertion of a replacement closure suture. Remove drain as planned, once suture in place
Respiratory distress following chest drain removal	Development of a pneumothorax or tension pneumothorax		Monitor patient's vital signs. Administer oxygen. Prepare for insertion of chest drain or for needle thoracocentesis
Continued leakage from chest drain site	Inadequate wound closure. Haemorrhage or wound infection. Pleural effusion		Remove dressing and inspect wound site. Clean and dress wound site. Inform senior practitioner immediately if required. Monitor wound site and leakage

Flexible fibreoptic bronchoscopy

Definition

Bronchoscopy is a technique of visualizing the inside of airways by inserting a probe with a miniature camera (bronchoscope) into the airways usually through the nose or mouth, or occasionally through a tracheostomy (Urden et al. 2005).

Indications for flexible bronchoscopy

A bronchoscopy is used to make a diagnosis (examine airways, take specimens) or as a therapy (to inflate a collapsed lung, remove secretions). More specifically the indications for undertaking a bronchoscopy are:

- haemoptysis (NB In large haemorrhage a rigid bronchoscope is more suitable; see below)
- infectious pneumonia
- complex intubations
- pulmonary injury following chest trauma
- undiagnosed pulmonary infiltrates
- lung masses
- mediastinal lymphadenopathy
- airway disorder
- endobronchial lesions
- therapeutic suctioning
- collection of diagnostic material.

(British Thoracic Society 2001)

Contraindications and complications

- Sedation management
- Hypoxaemia
- Bronchospasm
- Haemorrhage
- Infections
- Pneumothorax
- Haemodynamic instability
- Not recommended within 6 weeks post myocardial infarction as it can lead to ischaemic changes

(British Thoracic Society 2001)

Background

Anatomy and physiology

There are two types of bronchoscope. One type is hard and rigid, the other a flexible fibreoptic bronchoscope. The lumen of a flexible bronchoscope is narrower than that of a rigid bronchoscope. This allows the flexible bronchoscope to pass within an established invasive manufactured airway (such as an ET or TT) making it more suitable for assessment of critically ill patients. The flexible bronchoscopy uses a fibreoptic system to visualize the nasal passages, pharynx, larynx, vocal cords and tracheal bronchial tree. In this way, all airway structures and passages used to move air from the atmosphere into the small airways can be visualized and inspected.

Bronchoscopy in critical care

The British Thoracic Society (BTS) has developed comprehensive evidenced-based bronchoscopy guidelines that can be used to guide practice. These are recommended to the reader where the key issues considered include:

- complications, contraindications and precautions
- sedation and anaesthesia/analgesia
- cleaning and decontamination
- infection prevention measures, including PPE
- staff training to undertake this procedure.

(BTS 2001)

Competency and troubleshooting

Due to ongoing infection prevention and decontamination developments, readers are directed to the BTS website (www.brit-thoracic.org.uk) for the most current practice guidelines and competencies.

Summary

Assistance for breathing is important for critically ill patients whose respiration is compromised. Accurate assessment and ongoing monitoring of lung function and underlying pathology using a range of methods is crucial to choosing the most appropriate ventilation technique to meet the patient's requirements. The team of practitioners caring for the patient, therefore, are required to be competent in assessing, monitoring and providing ventilator support cognisant of other patient co-morbidities and risks. This must be delivered within a holistic package of care in order to improve the physiological status and comfort of the patient.

105

Procedure guideline 5.1: Chest auscultation

Equipment

- Stethoscope
- Alcohol swab and gel

Procedure

Action	Rationale
1 Where possible, explain and discuss the procedure with the patient. If the patient lacks the capacity to make decisions the practitioner must act in the patient's best interests.	To ensure that the patient understands the procedure and gives their valid consent. To ensure the patient's best interests are maintained (Mental Capacity Act 2005).
2 Wash and gel hands and use personal protective equipment.	To minimize risk of cross-infection (DH 2008).
3 Clean stethoscope head with alcohol swab.	To minimize risk of cross-infection (DH 2008).
4 Draw curtains around patient and only expose patient's chest.	To maintain patient dignity, privacy, comfort and confidentiality.
5 Ensure the best position for the patient, and for the clinician, to be able to fully assess both anterior and posterior lung sounds.	To ensure patient and personal comfort during auscultation.
6 Using diaphragm of the stethoscope, assess anterior and posterior chest wall.	To ensure a comprehensive assessment by using knowledge of underlying lung structure and a range of auscultation positions.
7 Listen for one inspiratory and expiratory breath cycle across a range of chest wall positions (2nd intercostal space to 8th intercostal space).	To obtain an overall understanding of the airflow across the lungs.
8 Start by listening to the lung apexes, moving down the intercostal spaces to the lung bases.	To facilitate a complete assessment by use of a systematic approach.
9 First assess for vesicular or bronchial breathing, then assess for adventitious sounds.	To identify normal sounds prior to ascertaining abnormal sounds to facilitate accurate assessment.
10 Always compare sounds on the right side to those on the left side.	To identify any differences and similarities between the two lungs.
11 After auscultation ensure that the patient is comfortable.	Moving the patient to listen to the lungs might have placed them in an uncomfortable position. In addition, it might be a good opportunity to move the patient to reduce pressure on vulnerable areas.
12 Remove personal protective equipment. Wash hands and apply alcohol gel to hands and clean stethoscope.	To minimize risk of cross-infection (DH 2008).
13 Document normal and abnormal assessment findings in the patient's notes.	To: - provide an accurate record - monitor effectiveness of procedure - reduce the risk of duplication of treatment - provide a point of reference or comparison in the event of later questions - acknowledge accountability for actions - facilitate communication and continuity of care. (NMC 2008; GMC 2013; HCPC 2012)
14 Make referral to a senior practitioner with any new findings.	To work within professional role boundaries to safeguard the patient and practitioner. Unless diagnosis and intervention is part of the role, referral is important.

Procedure guideline 5.2: Arterial puncture: radial artery (adapted with permission from the Royal Marsden Hospital Manual of Clinical Nursing Procedures)

Essential equipment

- Intravenous sterile dressing pack
- Sterile gloves
- Hypoallergenic tape

- 2% chlorhexidine in 70% alcohol
- Heparinized arterial blood gas syringe
- 18 G needle

Procedure

Action	Rationale
1 Where possible, explain and discuss the procedure with the patient. If the patient lacks the capacity to make decisions the practitioner must act in the patient's best interests.	To ensure that the patient understands the procedure and gives their valid consent. To ensure the patient's best interests are maintained (Mental Capacity Act 2005). To minimize anxiety, which may distort analysis or exacerbate symptoms.
2 Check the concentration of oxygen the patient is breathing and body temperature at time of sampling.	Inspired oxygen concentration and temperature parameters are required to interpret arterial blood gases accurately.
3 Check the patient's current coagulation screen, platelet count, medical history and prescription chart for anticoagulation therapy.	To identify possible risk of bleeding and haematoma formation post procedure and, where appropriate, to prevent puncture until coagulation is corrected.
4 Prepare trolley.	To reduce the risk of cross-infection.
5 Wash hands with bactericidal soap and water or bactericidal alcohol hand rub.	To reduce the risk of cross-infection.
6 Perform the Allen test.	To confirm patency of ulnar artery circulation and assess collateral circulation to the hand in the event of radial artery damage, for example thrombosis.
7 Locate and palpate the radial artery with the middle and index fingers of the non-dominant hand.	To assess maximum pulsation to ensure radial artery is optimum site for successful puncture. The dominant hand will be used to perform puncture.
8 Inspect and assess the surrounding tissues and anatomical structures.	Check and assess surrounding tissues for excoriation/infection, poor perfusion or other puncture sites. If any of these are present the site should not be used.
9 Prepare the patient position: gently extend the wrist over a rolled towel (ask for assistance if required).	To reduce the risk of the patient moving unexpectedly, which could result in through puncture. To flex the hand/foot slightly to facilitate insertion.
10 Open the pack and equipment onto it. Withdraw the plunger of the syringe 1–2 mL before the puncture.	To reduce blood haemolysis. Arterial pressure causes a brisk pulsatile reflux of blood into the syringe (unless the patient is severely hypotensive).
11 Place a sterile field under the patient's wrist and maintain aseptic technique throughout the procedure.	To minimize the risk of infection.
12 Clean site with chlorhexidine in 70% alcohol.	To minimize the risk of infection.
13 Administer subcutaneous local anaesthetic.	To minimize pain during the procedure. Local vasodilation effects of the local anaesthetic may reduce vasospasm, making for a successful puncture.

(Continued)

Procedure guideline 5.2: *(Continued)*

14 Clean hands with bactericidal skin cleaning solution.	To minimize the risk of infection.
15 Apply sterile gloves.	To minimize the risk of infection and prevent contamination of hands with blood.
16 Re-identify the point of maximum pulsation, hold position with index/middle finger.	To guide position of radial artery and aid successful puncture.
17 Angle the needle at a 30–45° angle, with the bevel of the needle up just distal to the finger position. Advance needle slowly into the artery until a flashing pulsation is seen in the hub of the needle.	To minimize trauma to the artery. Rapid insertion may result in a through puncture Pulsatile flow indicates access to radial artery Arterial pressure causes blood to pulsate spontaneously back into the syringe.
18 Slowly aspirate by gently pulling the plunger of the arterial gas syringe to a minimum of 0.6 mL of blood for the sample (check recommended amount of blood as directed by manufacturer's guidelines).	To minimize vasospasm. To ensure optimal volume is obtained in order to ensure an appropriate mix of blood with heparin (*see* manufacturer's guidelines).
19 Withdraw the needle, immediately followed by application of pressure using a low-linting dressing. Promptly return the wrist to the neutral position following sampling.	To prevent haematoma formation and excessive bleeding. Prolonged hyperextension may be associated with changes in median nerve conduction.
20 Apply pressure for a minimum of 5 minutes or until no signs of bleeding are observed. Ask for assistance from another practitioner if necessary.	To minimize blood loss and to ensure pressure exerted to prevent haematoma formation and blood loss. Assistance with pressure application enables the sample to be analysed swiftly.
21 Dispose of equipment safely.	To prevent contamination of others.
22 Expel any air bubbles from the syringe, and cap the arterial syringe and label according to hospital policy.	To keep sample airtight and avoid inaccuracies.
23 Check puncture site and apply a clean, sterile, low-linting gauze dressing using a non-touch technique. Secure with tape.	To maintain pressure and prevent haematoma formation.
24 Clearly document procedure and rationale for procedure in the patient's notes and verbally communicate arterial analysis findings to relevant clinical teams.	To: ■ provide an accurate record ■ monitor effectiveness of procedure ■ reduce the risk of duplication of treatment ■ provide a point of reference or comparison in the event of later questions ■ acknowledge accountability for actions, and ■ facilitate communication and continuity of care. (NMC 2008; GMC 2013; HCPC 2012)

Procedure guideline 5.3: Arterial blood gas sampling: arterial cannula (adapted with permission from the Royal Marsden Hospital Manual of Clinical Nursing Procedures)

Essential equipment

- Intravenous sterile pack
- 5 mL luer-lock syringe (if required)
- Gloves
- Heparinized arterial blood gas syringe
- 2% chlorhexidine in 70% alcohol
- Bactericidal alcohol handrub

Procedure

Action	Rationale
1 Where possible, explain and discuss the procedure with the patient. If the patient lacks the capacity to make decisions the practitioner must act in the patient's best interests.	To ensure that the patient understands the procedure and gives their valid consent. To ensure the patient's best interests are maintained (Mental Capacity Act 2005).
2 Wash hands with bactericidal soap and water or bactericidal alcohol hand rub.	To minimize the risk of cross-infection.
3 Clean hands with bactericidal alcohol handrub.	To prevent cross-infection.
4 Prepare equipment and micro-field.	Minimize the risk of cross-infection.
5 Press silence button on arterial monitor for the duration of sampling.	The continual alarm disturbs both the patient and others in the unit. Alarms of no clinical significance should be minimized.
6 Apply personal protective equipment.	To prevent contamination of practitioner with blood.
7 Clean sampling port with chlorhexidine 70% and allow to dry.	To minimize the risk of infection.
8 Prepare system according to manufacturer's guidelines. Draw back on any fluid in the cannula in preparation to take arterial sample. This may include use of a blood reservoir system or a 5 mL screw connecting syringe (such as a Luer-Lock syringe).	To remove any fluid (such as 0.9% sodium chloride flush), old blood and small emboli) from the cannula in order obtain an uncontaminated specimen of arterial blood.
9 Check the cannula contains only undiluted, uncontaminated arterial blood by sampling from the port.	To prevent contamination of blood with flush solution.
10 Attach heparinized blood gas syringe and slowly withdraw recommended volume of blood (as specified in manufacturer's instructions).	To prevent the artery going into spasm. To ensure the correct volume of blood mixes with the recommended heparin in the gas syringe.
11 Remove the gas syringe safely as per manufacturer's guidelines.	To prevent haemorrhage or blood spillage.
12 Clean port with chlorhexidine 70%.	To minimize the risk of infection.
13 Gently rotate arterial blood gas syringe.	To ensure the blood and heparin contained within the syringe are mixed in order to appropriately preserve the blood for analysis.
14 If a blood reservoir system is used, return reserve blood to the patient. Using a flush device, flush arterial cannula tubing until clear.	To clear blood from the cannula and arterial tubing to maximize patency.

(Continued)

Procedure guideline 5.3: (Continued)

15 As cannula is flushed observe digits for signs of blanching, discoloration, or complaints of pain from the patient. Ensure the patient is comfortable.	To enable early recognition of proximal or distal embolism.
16 Check pressure infuser cuff is inflated to 300 mm Hg.	To prevent backflow of blood into cannula and circuit.
17 Analyse arterial blood gas results, document result and report abnormalities.	To obtain results to optimize patient management. To: ■ provide an accurate record ■ monitor effectiveness of procedure ■ reduce the risk of duplication of treatment ■ provide a point of reference or comparison in the event of later questions ■ acknowledge accountability for actions ■ facilitate communication and continuity of care. (NMC 2008; GMC 2013; HCPC 2012)

Procedure guideline 5.4: Pulse oximetry (adapted with permission from the Royal Marsden Hospital Manual of Clinical Nursing Procedures)

Essential equipment
■ Pulse oximeter
■ Power source
■ Cleaning materials (according to manufacturer's recommendations and local policy)
■ Sensor applicable to the chosen site
■ Appropriate method of documentation

Optional equipment

■ Variety of sensors available for different sites

Procedure

Action	Rationale
1 Wash hands thoroughly with soap and water and dry and apply personal protective equipment.	To reduce the risk of cross-contamination.
2 Where possible, explain and discuss the procedure with the patient. If the patient lacks the capacity to make decisions the practitioner must act in the patient's best interests.	To ensure that the patient understands the procedure and gives their valid consent. To ensure the patient's best interests are maintained (Mental Capacity Act 2005).
3 While talking to the patient, assess their respiratory condition, including their ability to talk in full sentences, the colour of their skin, whether they appear to be in distress, and whether they are alert and orientated.	This initial assessment can give important information about the patient's respiratory function and any potential problems.
4 Determine the site to be used to perform pulse oximetry. The site should have a good blood supply, determined by checking it is warm, with a proximal pulse and brisk capillary refill.	The sensor requires a well-perfused area or it will not get strong enough signals to produce a result.
5 Select the correct pulse oximeter sensor for each site.	To ensure good contact and not apply too much pressure.

6 Clean the sensor as per manufacturer's instructions. Clean the area to be used and ensure that it is free from dirt. If using the patient's fingers ensure that all nail polish has been removed.	Dirt or nail polish may interfere with the transmission of the light signals, causing inaccurate results.
7 Position the sensor securely but do not secure it with tape, unless specifically recommended by the manufacturer. If the pulse oximetry is to be continuous then the site needs to be changed at least every 4 hours.	If it is too tight it may impede the blood flow, leading to inaccurate results. Changing the site reduces the risk of pressure ulcer formation.
8 Turn the pulse oximeter on and set the alarms on the device dependent on the patient's condition and within locally agreed limits.	To ensure that it is ready to use.
9 Check that the pulse reading on the device corresponds with patient's palpated pulse.	Any large deviations in pulse measurements may indicate that the device is not measuring accurately or is being affected by movement.
10 Document results clearly, including the time and date of the reading together with the level of any supplemental oxygen.	To: ■ provide an accurate record ■ monitor effectiveness of procedure ■ reduce the risk of duplication of treatment ■ provide a point of reference or comparison in the event of later questions ■ acknowledge accountability for actions ■ facilitate communication and continuity of care. (NMC 2008; GMC 2013; HCPC 2012) Detail about the level of additional oxygen provides more comprehensive clinical information to guide treatment decision making.
11 Remove personal protective equipment and dispose of per national guidelines. Clean the pulse oximeter according to manufacturers recommendations and local policy.	To reduce the risk of cross-infection. Equipment may become colonized and be a source of infection to another patient.

111

Procedure guideline 5.5: Insertion and removal of a nasopharyngeal (NP) tube

Equipment

- Selection of nasopharyngeal tubes (to include sizes 6 and 7)
- Sachet of sterile lubrication gel
- Gloves
- Disposable apron
- Eye protection (visor or goggles)

Procedure

Action	Rationale
1 Where possible, explain and discuss the procedure with the patient. If the patient lacks the capacity to make decisions the practitioner must act in the patient's best interests.	To ensure that the patient understands the procedure and gives their valid consent. To ensure the patient's best interests are maintained (Mental Capacity Act 2005).

(Continued)

Procedure guideline 5.5: (*Continued*)

2 Wash hands or decontaminate with alcohol gel and adopt personal protective equipment including eye protection.	To prevent cross-contamination of infection and to protect the practitioner.
3 Select a nasopharyngeal tube for insertion. For most adults a size 6 or size 7 is suitable (Jevon and Pooni 2007). Sizing techniques, such as matching a tube's internal lumen diameter to the patient's little finger are now discouraged.	Correct sizing of tube will ensure a satisfactory lumen size and diameter to facilitate respiration, administration of oxygen and aspiration of respiratory secretions, while preventing the tube from being displaced into the pharynx.
4 Prepare the NP airway according to manufacturer instructions, some NP airway have a safety pin to insert across the flange while other NP's have a large flange.	Following the manufacturer's guidance in preparing the NP airway flange is a precautionary measure to prevent inhalation of the airway (Jevon and Pooni 2007).
5 Lubricate the shaft of the nasopharyngeal tube with a small amount of lubricant gel.	To facilitate a smooth insertion of the tube into the nasal passage.
6 Pass the airway vertically along the floor of the nose, using a slight twisting action, into the posterior pharynx. If there is resistance remove the airway and try the left nostril (Resuscitation Council UK 2011).	Following the natural contour of the nasal passage will reduce trauma.
7 Evaluate correct tube placement and comfort. Assess for signs suggesting an improvement in the patient's condition or their tolerance of the adjunct: ■ absence of upper airway obstruction noises, such as gurgling or snoring ■ absence of coughing or gagging, indicating tube tolerance.	To assess patency and ensure that the airway is maintained.
8 Removal of the tube. While the patient is breathing out, hold the flange and pull out the nasopharyngeal airway in one smooth downward motion. Gently clean the nostril and examine nostril for signs of local trauma, injury or erosion.	Withdrawal during expiration prevents aspiration. Assessing for signs of damage as a result of tube placement will allow treatment and documentation.
9 Document care and any abnormalities.	To: ■ provide an accurate record ■ monitor effectiveness of procedure ■ reduce the risk of duplication of treatment ■ provide a point of reference or comparison in the event of later questions ■ acknowledge accountability for actions ■ facilitate communication and continuity of care. (NMC 2008; GMC 2013; HCPC 2012)

112

Procedure guideline 5.6: Insertion and removal of an oropharyngeal airway

Equipment

- Selection of oropharyngeal tubes (to include sizes 2, 3 and 4)
- Non-sterile gloves
- Disposable apron
- Eye protection, i.e. visor or goggles

Procedure

Action	Rationale
1 Where possible, explain and discuss the procedure with the patient. If the patient lacks the capacity to make decisions the practitioner must act in the patient's best interests.	To ensure that the patient understands the procedure and gives their valid consent. To ensure the patient's best interests are maintained (Mental Capacity Act 2005).
2 Wash hands or decontaminate with alcohol gel and adopt personal protective equipment, including eye protection.	To prevent cross-contamination of infection and to protect the practitioner.
3 The most common sizes are 2 for small adults, 3 for medium adults and 4 for large adults (Resuscitation Council UK 2011). Estimate the correct size of the airway by placing it against the patient's face and measuring it from the angle of the jaw to the incisors (Jevon and Pooni 2007).	An inappropriately sized oropharngeal tube could easily become displaced, cause an obstruction, or could stimulate a cough or gag reflex.
4 Open and inspect the patient's mouth. If debris or excessive secretions present remove these.	Insertion of an oropharngeal tube in the presence of a foreign body or excessive secretions would cause these to be displaced into the larynx, causing an obstruction (Resuscitation Council UK, 2011).
5 Turn the tube upside down and insert gently into the patient's mouth until it reaches the junction between the hard and soft palate. Rotate the tube 180° and advance it into position within the pharynx.	Insertion of the tube in an upside down position and rotation once in the mouth reduces the chance of tongue displacement backwards and possible airway obstruction (Resuscitation Council UK 2011).
6 Evaluate tube placement for correctness and comfort. Assess for signs suggesting an improvement in the patient's condition or their tolerance of the adjunct: ■ absence of upper airway obstruction noises, such as gurgling or snoring ■ absence of coughing or gagging, indicating tube tolerance.	To ensure that the tube has improved the patient's airway patency and respiratory function. To ascertain whether the tube is causing the patient any distress or discomfort.
7 Removal of the OP airway. Grasp flange and guide the OPA out by directing airway down towards chin. Suction oropharynx – if indicated.	Removal may be required if the patient: ■ is not tolerating the OPA ■ is vomiting ■ regains consciousness ■ regains a gag reflex ■ moves to more advanced airway management.
8 Document care and any abnormalities.	To: ■ provide an accurate record ■ monitor effectiveness of procedure ■ reduce the risk of duplication of treatment ■ provide a point of reference or comparison in the event of later questions ■ acknowledge accountability for actions ■ facilitate communication and continuity of care. (NMC 2008; GMC 2013; HCPC 2012)

Procedure guideline 5.7: Endotracheal tube insertion

Equipment

- Selection of cuffed endotracheal tubes (sizes 6, 6.5, 7, 7.5, 8, 8.5 and 9)
- Rigid oropharyngeal suction catheter, such as a Yankauer sucker, attached to high-flow suction
- 10 mL syringe
- Laryngoscope, with a size 3 Macintosh blade
- Bag-valve-mask device attached to oxygen supply
- Bougie
- Length of endotracheal tube tape or bandage
- Intubation medications as prescribed
- Capnography device
- Stethoscope
- Emergency resuscitation equipment
- Personal protective equipment

Procedure

Action	Rationale
1 Where possible, explain and discuss the procedure with the patient. If the patient lacks the capacity to make decisions the practitioner must act in the patient's best interests.	To ensure that the patient understands the procedure and gives their valid consent. To ensure the patient's best interests are maintained (Mental Capacity Act 2005).
2 Wash hands or decontaminate hands with alcohol gel. Adopt personal protective equipment including eye protection.	To prevent cross-contamination of infection and to protect the practitioner.
3 Ensure safety checks are carried out prior to commencement, these include: ■ check that the oxygen supply is functioning and attached to a bag-valve-mask device ■ check that the suction is functioning and attached to a rigid oropharyngeal suction catheter (such as a Yankauer catheter) ■ ensure that the laryngoscope has a functioning light source and a chosen lubricated endotracheal tube is prepared ■ check that emergency resuscitation equipment is nearby and accessible.	To enable swift treatment in an emergency situation associated with intubation, for example cardiac arrest.
4 Ensure that the patient has patent intravenous access, prepare the intravenous medications required for the intubation. These may include a sedative and a muscle relaxant.	Venous access is necessary for the prompt and safe administration of medications utilized during endotracheal intubation. These will anaesthetize and paralyse the patient, allowing the practitioner to insert the endotracheal tube through the patient's larynx into the trachea.
5 Ensure the patient is adequately monitored, to include: ECG, SpO$_2$ and blood pressure monitoring. Position the monitoring, so that is it visible while performing the procedure.	So that any procedure related complications can be detected promptly, for example hypotension, dysrhythmia, or hypoxemia.
6 Ensure that there is adequate space at the head of the bed. If required, move bed out from the wall and remove bed headboard if present. Ensure that the patient is lying in the supine position.	To provide adequate space to perform the procedure and manoeuvre the airway effectively. The practitioner conducting the procedure usually stands behind the patient's head.
7 Give the patient 85% via bag-valve-mask for a minimum of 15 seconds (Jevon and Pooni 2007).	To maximize oxygenation of the patient prior to the intubation procedure; this aims to prevent complications associated with hypoxia that may occur during the procedure.
8 Administer prescribed intravenous medications prior to intubation.	To facilitate an appropriate level of sedation and muscle paralysis that will allow manipulation of the airway and passage of the endotracheal tube through the vocal cords into the trachea.

9 Position the patient's airway by extending the neck and flexing the head. A pillow kept in situ under the patient's head and shoulders can facilitate this positioning (Jevon and Pooni 2007).

This position, along with the use of a laryngoscope, will allow for a clear view of the patient's larynx.

10 Hold the laryngoscope in your left hand and advance the blade into the patient's mouth, then use the laryngoscope to lift the epiglottis to enable visualization of the vocal cords. Use right hand to advance the lubricated endotracheal tube through the vocal cords and into position within the trachea.

This approach facilitates intubation of the trachea with the endotracheal tube.

11 Attach the endotracheal tube to a bag-valve-mask or the ventilator utilizing a catheter mount. Initially ventilate the patient with the highest oxygen concentration available (Resuscitation Council UK 2011), and then reduce the oxygen concentration as guided by the patient's condition.

To resume the administration of oxygen to the patient and ensure adequate oxygenation of the patient.

12 Inflate the endotracheal tube cuff with sufficient air so that an audible leak is no longer heard around the cuff during ventilation; 7–10 mL is the usual volume of air required (Jevon and Pooni 2007). Keep the patient informed throughout the procedure.

Inflation of the endotracheal tube cuff will establish a seal. Cuff pressure should be measured 4 hourly, maintained between 20 and 30 cm H_2O or 2 cm H_2O above peak inspiratory pressure (NICE 2009).

13 Confirm tube position by examining the patient:
  ■ attach a capnography device
  ■ observe for bilateral chest movement
  ■ auscultation over the chest and epigastrium.

To confirm correct endotracheal tube position, as incorrect position could result in significant risk to the patient, i.e. hypoxia.
A CO_2 detector can confirm the position of the ET tube in the airway (American College of Surgeons Committee on Trauma 2008).

14 Assess for clinical stability by reviewing the patient's ECG, SpO_2 and blood pressure. Secure endotracheal tube with tape or tube-fastening device. A bite block or an oropharyngeal airway may also be required to prevent tube damage if the patient is noted to be biting the endotracheal tube.

To detect any complications associated with intubation, i.e. hypoxia, hypotension and dysrhythmia. Securing the endotracheal tube in place will prevent accidental displacement and installation of a bite block will ensure that the patient does not bite through the endotracheal tube.

15 Request a portable chest X-ray.

To gain radiographic confirmation of endotracheal tube position and to evaluate the effectiveness of mechanical ventilation.

16 When convenient, an arterial blood sample should be obtained to assess gas exchange.

To evaluate the effect of mechanical ventilation on the patient's gaseous exchange.

17 Dispose of gloves and apron. Wash hands.

To prevent cross-contamination of pathogens.

18 Document care.

To:
  ■ provide an accurate record
  ■ monitor effectiveness of procedure
  ■ reduce the risk of duplication of treatment
  ■ provide a point of reference or comparison in the event of later questions
  ■ acknowledge accountability for actions
  ■ facilitate communication and continuity of care.

(NMC 2008; GMC 2013; HCPC 2012)

Procedure guideline 5.8: Tracheostomy formation and tube insertion

Equipment

- Two competent practitioners, one being an anaesthetist
- Pillow and/or sandbag to aid appropriate positioning
- Laryngoscope
- Rigid oropharyngeal suction catheter, such as a Yankauer catheter, attached to high-flow suction
- Sterile gown and sterile and non-sterile gloves
- Surgical mask
- Eye protection, i.e. goggles or visor

- Surgical drapes
- Skin disinfectant, i.e. 2% chlorhexidine or iodine preparation
- Percutaneous tracheostomy set, including tube and dilators
- Bronchoscope
- Resuscitation trolley and equipment

Procedure

Action	Rationale
1 Where possible, explain and discuss the procedure with the patient. If the patient lacks the capacity to make decisions the practitioner must act in the patient's best interests.	To ensure that the patient understands the procedure and gives their valid consent. To ensure the patient's best interests are maintained (Mental Capacity Act 2005).
2 Wash hands or decontaminate hands with alcohol gel. Adopt personal protective equipment including eye protection.	To prevent cross-contamination of infection and to protect the healthcare professional.
3 Ensure safety checks are carried out prior to commencement. These include checking that the oxygen and suction supplies are functioning. Also that emergency resuscitation equipment is nearby and accessible.	To enable swift treatment in an emergency situation associated with intubation, i.e. cardiac arrest.
4 Ensure that NG feed has been discontinued for several hours prior to the procedure.	To prevent aspiration of stomach contents during the procedure.
5 Check that the patient's blood results are within acceptable ranges. Correct coagulation or postpone procedure if values are abnormal.	Abnormal coagulation values may put the patient at risk of haemorrhage or haematoma formation during the procedure.
6 Oxygenate the patient to 1.0 FiO_2 via their mechanical ventilator. If not mechanically ventilated administer high-flow oxygen at 15 L/min via a bag-valve-mask device.	To prevent periods of hypoxia that may be associated with this procedure.
7 Ensure that the patient is in a supine position, with their head slightly extended. The use of a pillow or sandbag under their shoulders may facilitate this (ICS 2008).	This position will allow for clear visualization of the patient's airway with a laryngoscope.
8 Administer the prescribed anaesthetic and paralysing agents.	To facilitate an appropriate level of sedation and muscle paralysis that will allow manipulation of the airway and passage of the tracheostomy into the trachea.
9 Suction the patient's pharynx under direct laryngoscopy and also suction via the endotracheal tube (if in situ).	To remove secretions that could easily be aspirated into the lungs.
10 If the patient already has an endotracheal tube in situ, deflate the endotracheal tube cuff and pull back the tube under direct visualization with the laryngoscope, so that the tip of the tube now lies within the larynx and at the level of the cricoid cartilage (ICS 2008). Alternatively, fully remove the endotracheal tube and replace it with a laryngeal mask airway (ICS 2008).	Pulling back the endotracheal tube to the level of the cricoid cartilage allows the tracheostomy stoma to be formed and the tracheostomy tube to be introduced while still allowing mechanical ventilation and oxygenation to continue. To maintain oxygenation and ventilation during the procedure.

11 Observe the endotracheal tube and tracheal anatomy using a bronchoscope (ICS 2008).	To confirm appropriate endotracheal tube positioning (if present) within the larynx and to explore the internal anatomy of the trachea prior to cannulation, stoma dilation and tracheostomy tube insertion.
12 Wash hands and put on a sterile gown, sterile gloves and eye protection.	To promote asepsis during the procedure and to prevent the transmission of pathogens.
13 Utilize an assistant to assemble a sterile procedure trolley, with all required equipment laid out, including the percutaneous tracheostomy tube, dilators, cannulation needle and sutures. The practitioner should check that the tracheostomy tube is functional and intact (ICS 2008).	Equipment is to hand and remains sterile.
14 Clean the incision site using a chlorhexadine- or iodine-based preparation. Drapes should then be applied over the patient.	To decontaminate the patient's skin and to ensure a sterile field is prepared prior to the procedure.
15 Identify the incision site (which correlates to the T2-T3 thoracic vertebrae) and inject local anaesthetic around the area (ICS 2008).	To prevent pain during and following the procedure.
16 The trachea is cannulated at the identified incision site using a cannulation needle, which is part of the percutaneous tracheostomy kit.	Cannulation of the trachea allows access to the tracheal cavity and will facilitate insertion of dilators.
17 Once this cannulation has been achieved, correct position should be confirmed by aspiration of air or pulmonary secretions via the needle. Alternative strategies to confirm cannulation position include the use of capnography attached to the needle or the observation of bubbles at the hub of the needle after water or saline has been injected into the needle itself (ICS 2008).	To prevent inadvertent cannulation of neck tissues (ICS 2008), which could lead to the development of surgical emphysema on commencement of mechanical ventilation.
18 Percutaneous tracheostomy kit dilators are used to form the stoma and facilitate insertion of a tracheostomy tube. The dilators are introduced to the stoma in increasing sizes to dilate the stoma gently to an appropriate size to hold the airway.	Dilation of incision site will establish a tracheostomy stoma.
19 Appropriate tube position can be confirmed using a bronchoscope allowing direct visualization of the position in the bronchus or capnogragh (ICS 2008).	Confirmation of tracheostomy tube will ensure that the tube is appropriately inserted into the trachea prior to connection to mechanical ventilation (ICS 2008).
20 If tracheostomy tube positioning is correct, the cuff should be inflated and the patient attached to a mechanical ventilator. The endotracheal tube can then be removed.	To avoid periods of hypoxia and to allow for normal mechanical ventilatory support to continue.
21 Secure the tracheostomy tube with tracheostomy tapes (ICS 2008).	To prevent inadvertent tube displacement.
22 Recheck the patient's monitoring: ECG, SpO_2 and blood pressure. Perform an arterial blood gas.	To detect any complications associated with tracheostomy insertion, i.e. hypoxia, hypotension and dysrhythmia. Utilize an arterial blood gas to evaluate the effectiveness of mechanical ventilation and oxygenation.

(Continued)

Procedure guideline 5.8: *(Continued)*

23 Evaluate the patient's ongoing sedative requirements utilizing local sedation scoring tool.	Effective sedation management and review is a clearly identified aspect in the prevention of the ventilator-acquired pneumonia (NICE/NSPA 2008). Scoring and management will be following local practice but aiming to minimize sedation where the clinical condition allows is advocated.
24 Document care.	To: ■ provide an accurate record ■ monitor effectiveness of procedure ■ reduce the risk of duplication of treatment ■ provide a point of reference or comparison in the event of later questions ■ acknowledge accountability for actions ■ facilitate communication and continuity of care. (NMC 2008; GMC 2013; HCPC 2012)

Procedure guideline 5.9: Tracheostomy care: stoma care and dressing changes (adapted with permission from the Royal Marsden Hospital Manual of Clinical Nursing Procedures)

Equipment

- Non-sterile gloves, disposable apron and protective eye wear
- Sterile dressing pack, which includes sterile gloves
- 0.9% sodium chloride

- Replacement tracheostomy dressing
- Replacement tracheostomy tapes
- Additional assistance from a member of the clinical team

Procedure

Action	Rational
1 Where possible, explain and discuss the procedure with the patient. If the patient lacks the capacity to make decisions the practitioner must act in the patient's best interests.	To ensure that the patient understands the procedure and gives their valid consent. To ensure the patient's best interests are maintained (Mental Capacity Act 2005).
2 Wash hands with soap and water or decontaminate with alcohol gel. Put on non-sterile gloves, apron and eye protection.	To prevent cross-contamination of pathogens and to protect the clinician from potential harm.
3 Utilize an assistant to support the tracheostomy tube during the procedure.	To avoid accident tube displacement when the tracheostomy ties have been removed.
4 Assemble material required for the dressing change on a cleaned dressing trolley.	To maintain asepsis during the procedure.
5 Remove the tracheostomy ties and dressing. Dispose of these in a suitable waste container.	

6 Remove non-sterile gloves, decontaminate hands and put on sterile gloves contained within dressing pack.	To promote asepsis during the procedure (Dougherty and Lister 2011).
7 Inspect the tracheostomy stoma site, noting any abnormalities, i.e. signs of infection or wound breakdown.	To detect complications early and facilitate prompt treatment.
8 Cleanse around the stoma with 0.9% sodium chloride-soaked sterile gauze. Dispose of soiled gauze in a suitable clinical waste container.	To facilitate removal of secretions and debris from around the stoma site.
9 Insert a new sterile tracheostomy dressing around stoma site and tube.	To absorb secretions from stoma and to prevent pressure damage from tube.
10 Attach new tracheostomy tapes, ensuring that 1–2 fingers can be placed between the tapes and the patient's neck.	To ensure that the tube stays in place and to prevent complications associated with the tapes being too tight, i.e. skin damage and possible reduced cerebral blood flow.
11 Reassess patient's condition and offer reassurance if required.	To detect any signs of deterioration or discomfort associated with manipulation of the tube during the procedure.
12 Document care.	To: ■ provide an accurate record ■ monitor effectiveness of procedure ■ reduce the risk of duplication of treatment ■ provide a point of reference or comparison in the event of later questions ■ acknowledge accountability for actions ■ facilitate communication and continuity of care. (NMC 2008; GMC 2013; HCPC 2012)

Procedure guideline 5.10: Inner cannula care (adapted with permission from the Royal Marsden Hospital Manual of Clinical Nursing Procedures)

Equipment

■ Non-sterile gloves, disposable apron and protective eye wear

■ Replacement inner cannula (of the same size as the cannula currently in situ)
■ Access to warm running tap water

Procedure

Action	Rationale
1 Where possible, explain and discuss the procedure with the patient. If the patient lacks the capacity to make decisions the practitioner must act in the patient's best interests.	To ensure that the patient understands the procedure and gives their valid consent. To ensure the patient's best interests are maintained (Mental Capacity Act 2005).
2 Wash hands with soap and water or decontaminate with alcohol gel. Apply personal protective equipment including eye protection.	To prevent cross-contamination of pathogens and to protect the clinician from potential harm.
3 Ensure the replacement inner cannula is easily accessible.	To facilitate a swift inner cannula change.

(Continued)

Procedure guideline 5.10: (Continued)

4 Obtain access to the patient's tracheostomy tube, by either disconnecting their ventilator tubing (if mechanically ventilated) or removing their tracheostomy mark or Swedish nose (Figure 5.17a) and HME if self-ventilating.	To facilitate access to the tracheostomy inner tube.

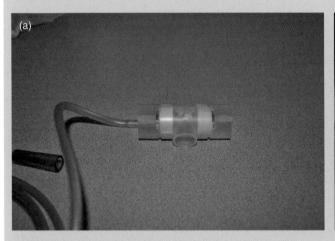 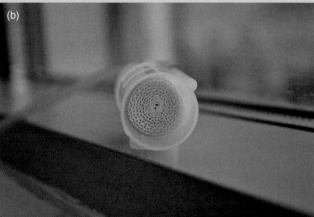

Figure 5.17   (a) and (b) Swedish nose.

5 Using a sterile technique remove the current inner cannula and insert the replacement cannula. Reconnect the patient to their oxygen or ventilator tubing.	To ensure that the patient's prior oxygen or ventilation therapy resumes.
6 Using a sterile technique, remove or change inner cannula. If non-disposable, clean cannula with sterile 0.9% sodium chloride or water and dry thoroughly. Do not leave inner cannula to soak (ICS 2008).	To facilitate secretion and debris removal of the inner cannula. Brushes have been associated with creation of transmission of pathogens and possible excoriation of the tube plastic (Russell 2005). Soaking also increses the risk of exposure to pathogens.
7 The inner tube should be left to air dry and left accessible in anticipation of the next inner tube change (ICS 2008).	
8 Reassess the patient's condition.	To detect any possible complications associated with the inner tube change and to maintain a legal record of care delivered.
9 Document care.	To: ▪ provide an accurate record ▪ monitor effectiveness of procedure ▪ reduce the risk of duplication of treatment ▪ provide a point of reference or comparison in the event of later questions ▪ acknowledge accountability for actions ▪ facilitate communication and continuity of care. (NMC 2008; GMC 2013; HCPC 2012)

120

Procedure guideline 5.11: Tracheostomy removal (decannulation)

Equipment

- 10 mL syringe for cuff deflation if still inflated
- Non-sterile gloves
- Disposable apron
- Eye protection
- Suction equipment

- Face mask with oxygen supply
- Semi-permeable dressing
- Emergency intubation kit in case of a failed decannulation, including a range of tracheostomy tubes

Action	Rationale
1 Review the need for tracheostomy. Decisions to remove a tracheostomy should be made as soon as the tracheostomy is no longer required. However, the Intensive Care Society (2008) suggests that the following factors should be considered: - the pathological process necessitating the insertion of a tracheostomy has resolved - the patient is able to cough and swallow effectively and protect their airway - ventilatory reserve is adequate (decannulation increases anatomical dead space and may increase the work of breathing) - reversible bronchopulmonary infection or pathology has been treated and is resolving - pulmonary secretions are not excessive - nutritional status is adequate - patient is comfortable with the cuff deflated - the airway is patent above the level of the stoma.	Successful decannulation is more likely if all aspects of assessment have been considered and managed.
2 If a decision to remove the tracheostomy is made, where possible explain and discuss the procedure with the patient. If the patient lacks the capacity to make decisions the practitioner must act in the patient's best interests.	To ensure that the patient understands the procedure and gives their valid consent. To ensure the patient's best interests are maintained (Mental Capacity Act 2005).
3 Stop NG feeding at least 2 hours before removal – review when to recommence with medical team.	To prevent aspiration of stomach contents.
4 Wash hands with soap and water or decontaminate with alcohol gel. Apply personal protective equipment including eye protection.	To prevent cross-contamination of pathogens and to protect the clinician from potential harm.
5 Sit the patient into an upright position.	To maximize respiratory function.
6 Deflate the cuff and carry out tracheal suction. Assess that patient remains comfortable and maintains good respiratory function.	To assess the patient's ability to breath around the tube to ensure they will cope with the decannulation procedure. If secretions are present this may lead to patient distress and cause the procedure to fail. Allow for patient recovery.
7 Apply decannulation cap, apply facial oxygen supply and encourage the patient to take deep breaths and cough.	To provide supplementary oxygen and to help them begin to feel the change in breathing and ensure they are strong enough to clear secretions to avoid complications associated with suctioning and decannulation, and related hypoxia.

(Continued)

121

Procedure guideline 5.11: (*Continued*)

8 If the patient has appropriate respiratory function remove ties or Velcro fastener. Pull the tracheostomy out and down towards the chest in a curved manner.	To allow the tracheostomy to be removed. To follow the natural passage of the trachea and to minimize local trauma.
9 Cover the stoma site with a sterile semi-permeable dressing (ICS 2008).	Coverage of the stoma site will redirect the breaching through the upper airways.
10 Dispose of the tracheostomy tube and the suction catheter in an appropriate clinical waste receptacle.	To prevent cross-contamination or transmission of pathogens.
11 Remove eye protection and dispose of apron and gloves.	To prevent cross-contamination or transmission of pathogens.
12 Wash hands with soap and water or decontaminate with alcohol gel.	To prevent cross-contamination or transmission of pathogens.
13 Assess patient for any changes in vital signs and respiratory function. Undertake an arterial blood gas if able. Instruct the patient to alert the nurse if they experience any difficulty in breathing following the procedure.	To ensure that any complications associated with extubation are noted promptly and the appropriate interventions implemented.
14 Document care.	To: ■ provide an accurate record ■ monitor effectiveness of procedure ■ reduce the risk of duplication of treatment ■ provide a point of reference or comparison in the event of later questions ■ acknowledge accountability for actions ■ facilitate communication and continuity of care. (NMC 2008; GMC 2013; HCPC 2012)

Procedure guideline 5.12: End tidal CO_2 monitoring

Equipment	
■ Capnographic device ■ Any airway adaptor or monitoring cables	■ Protective equipment, etc.

Procedure

Action	Rationale
1 Where possible, explain and discuss the procedure with the patient. If the patient lacks the capacity to make decisions the practitioner must act in the patient's best interests.	To ensure patient understands the procedure and gives their valid consent. To ensure the patient's best interests are maintained (Mental Capacity Act 2005).
2 Wash and gel hands and use personal protective equipment. Clean equipment.	To minimize risk of cross infection (DH 2008).

3 Place capnometer into the patient's ventilator circuit in line with local clinical guidelines and manufacturer's recommendations.	To ensure accurate sampling and analysis of gas is achieved. It is important to place the capnometer probe as per manufacturer's instructions.
4 Ensure the ventilator tubing is well supported.	To ensure that the ventilator tubing does not cause dragging on the tracheal tube. This may cause the tracheal tube to dislodge or cause pressure damage to the patient's mouth or trachea.
5 Take any precautions necessary to minimize disruption in the patient's ventilation by having all equipment required and making as short a break in the circuit as possible.	To reduce the risk of patient not receiving enough oxygen via the ventilator.
6 Undertake calibration ('zeroing') procedures as per manufacturer's recommendations. If calibration fails, seek technical support.	To ensure accurate measurements appropriate calibration ('zeroing') procedures are required.
7 Once $ETCO_2$ is continuously reading, compare $ETCO_2$ reading with $PaCO_2$ on blood gas analysis and note any major discrepancies.	To assess whether the capnometer is calibrated appropriately. The cause of any major discrepancies in $ETCO_2$ and $PaCO_2$ needs to be investigated.
8 Note shape of capnograph waveform. Use knowledge of underlying lung physiology and pathology to understand anomalies in the capnogaph and the impact this may have on the patient's ventilation and respiratory management (see Figure 5.9).	To review and amend treatment with clinical team.
9 Set alarms parameters as per local guidelines.	Alarms must be set to alert the practitioner to any potential patient ventilation problem.
10 On completion, ensure the patient is comfortable.	
11 Remove personal protective equipment. Wash hands and use apply alcohol gel to hands and clean cuff manometer.	To minimize risk of cross infection (DH 2008).
12 Document findings as per local policy.	To: ■ provide an accurate record ■ monitor effectiveness of procedure ■ reduce the risk of duplication of treatment ■ provide a point of reference or comparison in the event of later questions ■ acknowledge accountability for actions ■ facilitate communication and continuity of care. (NMC 2008; GMC 2013; HCPC 2012)
13 Make referral to senior practitioner with any new findings.	To work within professional role boundaries to safeguard patient and practitioner. Unless diagnosis and intervention is part of role, referral is important.

123

Procedure guideline 5.13: Tracheal cuff pressure measurement

Equipment

- Cuff pressure manometer (NB check stethoscope and emergency oxygen)
- 10 mL syringe (dependent on manometer)
- Suction available

Procedure

Action	Rationale
1 Where possible, explain and discuss the procedure with the patient. If the patient lacks the capacity to make decisions the practitioner must act in the patient's best interests.	To ensure that the patient understands the procedure and gives their valid consent. To ensure the patient's best interests are maintained (Mental Capacity Act 2005).
2 Wash and gel hands and use personal protective equipment. Clean equipment.	To minimize risk of cross-infection (DH 2008).
3 Draw curtains around patient.	To maintain patient dignity, privacy, comfort and confidentiality.
4 Auscultate chest.	To undertake basic initial checks, e.g. tube placement.
5 Check availability of oxygen and suction. Suction if required.	To ensure emergency equipment is nearby.
6 Attach manometer to pilot cuff of the endotracheal/tracheostomy tube.	To enable the pressure in the pilot cuff to be measured on the manometer.
7 Note pressure reading and adjust within safe range by inflating/withdrawing air from cuff.	To ensure the cuff is at the correct pressure (20–25 mmHg).
8 Assess for noise of air escaping from around the tube cuff.	To ensure that the cuff is sealed against the tracheal mucosa. If air can be heard escaping the seal is not complete. To ensure a comprehensive assessment is made using knowledge of underlying lung structure and a range of auscultation positions.
9 Ensure the patient is comfortable.	
10 Remove personal protective equipment and dispose of as per local policy. Wash hands and apply alcohol gel to hands.	To minimize risk of cross-infection (DH 2008).
11 Clean cuff manometer as per local guidelines.	To minimize risk of cross-infection (DH 2008).
12 Document findings as per local policy.	To: <ul><li>provide an accurate record</li><li>monitor effectiveness of procedure</li><li>reduce the risk of duplication of treatment</li><li>provide a point of reference or comparison in the event of later questions</li><li>acknowledge accountability for actions</li><li>facilitate communication and continuity of care.</li></ul>(NMC 2008; GMC 2013; HCPC 2012)
13 Make referral to senior practitioner team with any new findings.	To work within professional role boundaries to safeguard patient and clinician. Unless diagnosis and intervention is part of role, referral is important.

Procedure guideline 5.14: Continuous positive airway pressure (adapted with permission from the Royal Marsden Hospital Manual of Clinical Nursing Procedures)

Essential equipment

- High-flow CPAP delivery system, e.g. Drager bellows
- Suitable gas supply +/– flow meter
- CPAP helmet or mask
- CPAP circuit

- Humidification system (mask only) with temperature control
- Oxygen analyser
- Pulse oximetry
- Nasogastric tube

Procedure

Action	Rationale
1 Assess patient's conscious level.	To obtain a baseline and to be able to assess for change in condition.
2 Where possible, explain and discuss the procedure with the patient. If the patient lacks the capacity to make decisions the practitioner must act in the patient's best interests.	To ensure that the patient understands the procedure and gives their valid consent. To ensure the patient's best interests are maintained (Mental Capacity Act 2005).
3 Observe and record the following: ■ patient's respiratory function, including respiratory rate, work of breathing and tissue oxygen saturation (SaO_2) ■ colour, skin and mental status.	To obtain a baseline of respiratory function. A reduction in level of consciousness or altered mental status may indicate hypoxaemia.
4 Decide whether it is appropriate to insert an arterial cannula in order to monitor the acid-base balance.	To avoid any unnecessary procedures.
5 Observe and record the patient's cardiovascular, function and fluid balance status.	To obtain a baseline in order to assess any change in conditions.
6 Assess patient's level of anxiety and compliance with treatment (the patient's ability to cope with the treatment).	To enable an assessment to be made and an evaluation of the suitability of CPAP therapy.
7 Wash and gel hands and use personal protective equipment.	To minimize risk of cross-infection (DH 2008).
8 Set up CPAP circuit, CPAP valve, oxygen and flow as discussed with clinical team.	To ensure CPAP parameters optimize patient's ventilation and comfort.
9 Ensure patient is in a comfortable position, sitting up in bed at a 45° angle or more or in a chair well supported by a pillow.	To promote comfort and aid lung expansion and breathing.
10 Explain to patient how the helmet or mask is to be applied.	To relieve anxiety and to reassure patient. To aid patient's compliance with CPAP.
11 Apply helmet/mask gently, applying pressure as the patient adapts to the tight-fitting mask. Hold mask until patient is comfortable and settled.	To relieve anxiety and to reassure patient. To aid patient's compliance with CPAP.
12 Once the patient is settled with mask/helmet, apply the head strap or shoulder straps. Ensure mask/helmet and head strap are comfortable for the patient; alter position as required.	To retain mask in place and aid patient comfort.

125

(Continued)

Procedure guideline 5.14: (*Continued*)

13 Ensure a good seal and that no leaks are present.	To ensure a tight seal in order that the system functions optimally.
14 Apply tissue protective dressing around vulnerable pressure points: nose, ears, back of head and neck, if required.	To alleviate pressure and prevent tissue breakdown.
15 Remove personal protective equipment and wash hands.	To minimize risk of cross-infection (DH2008).
16 Document care in clinical notes.	To: ■ provide an accurate record ■ monitor effectiveness of procedure ■ reduce the risk of duplication of treatment ■ provide a point of reference or comparison in the event of later questions ■ acknowledge accountability for actions ■ facilitate communication and continuity of care. (NMC 2008; GMC 2013; HCPC 2012)
17 Give further explanation to family/next of kin of how CPAP works and the importance of their presence and participation in communication.	To relieve anxiety and support and reassure family and patient.
18 Reassure the patient constantly. Discuss with clinical team the management of any undue anxiety.	To relieve patient anxiety and promote cooperation.
19 Continue observation of vital signs and work of breathing. If patient is tiring, notify senior practitioner.	To prevent acute respiratory deterioration or to inform competent practitioner in a timely manner in order to intubate the patient to avoid a respiratory arrest.

Procedure guideline 5.15: BiPAP

Equipment

- BiPAP machine
- Suitable gas supply
- BiPAP circuit
- Correctly sized facemask as per manufacturer's instructions
- Foam adherent dressing dressing (e.g. Granuflex) to protect areas where facemask may cause pressure damage
- Humidification system if suitable
- Oxygen analyser
- Saturation probe

A full respiratory plan should have been made by the clinical team, including plans for prescribed oxygen and decisions around an escalation plan if NIV fails.

Procedure

Action	Rationale
1 Where possible, explain and discuss the procedure with the patient. If the patient lacks the capacity to make decisions the practitioner must act in the patient's best interests.	To ensure that the patient understands the procedure and gives their valid consent. To ensure the patient's best interests are maintained (Mental Capacity Act 2005).
2 Explain the sensation of BiPAP and the tight-fitting mask.	Explanation of the therapy will reduce the patient's anxiety.
3 Wash and gel hands and use personal protective equipment.	To minimize risk of cross-infection (DH 2008).

4 Observe and record the following: ■ assess patient's conscious level	To obtain a baseline and to be able to assess for change in condition. To obtain a baseline of respiratory function.
■ patient's respiratory function including respiratory rate, work of breathing and tissue oxygen saturation (SaO_2) ■ colour, skin, and mental status.	A reduction in level of consciousness or altered mental status may indicate hypoxaemia.
5 Decide whether it is appropriate to insert an arterial cannula to monitor the acid-base balance.	To avoid unnecessary procedures.
6 Observe and record the patient's cardiovascular, function and fluid balance status.	To obtain a baseline in order to assess any change in conditions.
7 Set up the circuit switch on the machine, set pressure and oxygen levels. Initially set the IPAP at a lower level than required while getting the patient comfortable on this mode.	To ensure the machine is set at an appropriate level for the patient. Initial IPAP of 10 cm H_2O and EPAP of 4–5 cm H_2O are recommended by the BTS (2008). This lower level enables to patient to get used to the experience of BiPAP before it is increased to a therapeutic level.
8 Ensure patient in a comfortable position sitting up in bed at a 45° angle or more or in a chair, well supported by a pillow.	To promote comfort and aid lung expansion and breathing.
9 Hold face mask up to the patient's face, allowing them to adjust to the mask and the flow of air. Once the patient has adjusted to the flow fasten head straps and assess the patient's mask for comfort and any air leakage.	To ensure the patient is comfortable, as use of high-flow gases can be uncomfortable.
10 Increase the IPAP and EPAP to desired level until a therapeutic response is achieved or patient tolerability has been reached.	To facilitate tolerability of BiPAP. The BTS (2008) advocates a gradual increase of 2–5 cm increments at a rate of approximately 5 cm H_2O each 10 minutes. The patient should be maintained on the therapy as much as possible for the first 24 hours from initiation to provide the maximum affect and reduce the risk of treatment escalation (BTS 2008). A 'pressure escalation plan' will increase tolerability and allow the greatest chance of success.
11 If the patient is finding the therapy uncomfortable, discuss the therapy management plan with the patient. For example, planning with the patient when they can have breaks from the therapy. Timing NIV breaks around medication administration and meal times will minimize the time off therapy.	To enable the patient to have more control over therapy, reduce anxiety and facilitate acceptability of BiPAP. Often patients will be very anxious because of their breathing difficulties. Spending time with them and creating a treatment plan that is fully inclusive may make the difference between the failure or success in this therapy.
12 Apply tissue protective dressing around vulnerable pressure point, e.g. nose, ears and back of head, if required.	To alleviate pressure and prevent tissue breakdown.
13 Once established on BiPAP assess the patient's respiratory and cardiovascular status by reassessing: ■ continuous SpO_2 ■ respiratory rate ■ auscultation ■ chest wall movement ■ heart rate ■ blood pressure ■ ABG (post-therapy instigation).	To assess the effectiveness of the therapy and also to recognize if the therapy is causing any other physiological compromise. Haemodynamic instability is a contraindication to BiPAP, as increased intrathoracic pressure created by the positive pressure pushed into the lungs may reduce cardiac output and venous return.

127

(Continued)

Procedure guideline 5.15: (*Continued*)

14 Remove personal protective equipment, dispose of as national policy and wash hands.	To minimize risk of cross-infection (DH 2008).
15 On completion of assessment, document findings as per local policy.	To: ■ provide an accurate record ■ monitor effectiveness of procedure ■ reduce the risk of duplication of treatment ■ provide a point of reference or comparison in the event of later questions ■ acknowledge accountability for actions ■ facilitate communication and continuity of care. (NMC 2008; GMC 2013; HCPC 2012)
16 Maintain regular observations of the patient as detailed in patient care plan.	BiPAP is a complex therapy with several risk factors; close observation is vital to ensure positive therapeutic effect and patient safety. Regular observation is also important to prevent acute respiratory deterioration or to inform senior practitioners in a timely manner in order to intubate the patient to avoid a respiratory arrest.

Procedure guideline 5.16: Invasive ventilator therapy care

Equipment

■ Invasive airway, either endotrachael tube or tracheostomy
■ Positive pressure ventilator (many models are available)
■ Ventilation circuit appropriate to the airway in situ

■ Bacterial filters and humidification systems either heat and moisture exchange humidifiers (HME) or wet circuit dependant on local policy for humidification management

The clinical team should have undertaken a full review setting out plans for modes, settings and oxygen. The team should be available for constant review in the early stages of positive pressure mechanical ventilation as this may be a dynamic and changing situation requiring instant decision making and fine tuning of settings.

Procedure

Action	Rationale
1 Where possible, explain and discuss the procedure with the patient. If the patient lacks the capacity to make decisions the practitioner must act in the patient's best interests. Introduce self to patient explaining the need for ventilation. Explain the sensations that may be experienced and that the patient will not be able to speak.	To ensure that the patient understands the procedure and gives their valid consent. To ensure the patient's best interests are maintained (Mental Capacity Act 2005). To reduce anxiety. There is no clear evidence to support the effect of talking to a sedated or comatose patient when undertaking therapeutic interventions but it is felt to be good practice to try and communicate with your patient whatever their sedation score or conscious level. Knowledge of anticipated sensory experiences reduces stress (Lynn-McHale Wiegand 2011).
2 Wash and gel hands and use personal protective equipment.	To minimize the risk of cross-infection (DH 2008).
3 Set up ventilator circuit as per manufacturer's instructions and undertake ventilator checks. All ventilators have a system of safety checks that should be undertaken prior to use.	To assess gas flows and valves within the ventilation system. Testing the machine and equipment before use is a vital aspect of safe ventilation. NB Training on this should be provided by the manufacturers of the ventilation or competent practitioners in the department.

4 Ensure humidification equipment is in place and functioning correctly.	To ensure the patient receives humidified air or gas. To prevent drying of the airways. The decision on which type of humidification to use is a departmental one and may be affected by the expected ventilation time frame. However, NICE/NSPA (2008) and the DH high impact interventions (2007) set out that appropriate humidification of inspired gas is a vital aspect in ventilator-acquired pneumonia prevention.
5 Set mode, settings and ventilator alarms as agreed in respiratory plan, and assess the ventilator is working using a test lung.	To immediately alert practitioners of any patient-related respiratory and/or ventilator problem. Ventilator alarms are a vital safety component in the care of ventilated patients as they sense changes in the patient's respiratory function or ventilation flows. Identification of the alarm will allow the practitioner to assess the problem and react appropriately. The use of the test lung allows a physical assessment of the gas flow prior to patient connection.
6 Following all safety checks connect the patient to the ventilator.	To initiate ventilation support and in accordance with prescribed guidance and to the patient's needs.
7 Provide support to the ventilator tubing connected to the patient's airway while connecting to the ventilator.	To prevent airway migration. Ventilator tubing can be heavy and dislodge airways if incorrectly managed. Careful positioning and use of tubing stabilization arms will prevent risk to the patency of the patient's airway.
8 Remove personal protective equipment and dispose of according to local policy. Wash hand and apply alcohol gel.	To minimize the risk of cross-infection (DH 2008).
9 Once patient is established on the ventilator undertake a full respiratory assessment, starting with chest wall movement and auscultation, to establish adequate movement of air in the patient's lungs. Also consider: ■ continuous SpO_2 ■ respiratory rate ■ heart rate ■ blood pressure ■ ABG ■ adequacy of tidal volume achieved ■ adequacy of minute volume achieved ■ mean and peak pressures.	To assess the effectiveness of the therapy and recognize any physiological compromise. Caution should be taken in patients with haemodynamic instability as the increased intrathoracic pressure created by the positive pressure being pushed into the patient's lungs may reduce cardiac output and venous return.
10 Once safely established on ventilation aim to position your patient with a head elevation of 30-45°.	To prevent micro-aspiration (small amounts of fluid tracking from the stomach to the lung) which is associated with VAPS. Head elevation for ventilated patients is advocated by NICE/NSPA (2008).
11 Document findings in patient notes and patient observations charts as per local unit policy.	To: ■ provide an accurate record ■ monitor effectiveness of procedure ■ reduce the risk of duplication of treatment ■ provide a point of reference or comparison in the event of later questions ■ acknowledge accountability for actions ■ facilitate communication and continuity of care. (NMC 2008; GMC 2013; HCPC 2012)

129

(Continued)

Procedure guideline 5.16: (Continued)

12 Maintain regular observations of the patient as detailed in their care plan.	To monitor condition of patient and revise care plan with clinical team as necessary. NB Ventilated patients should have a minimum of one nurse to one patient (BACCN 2010).
13 Follow ventilation care bundles or guidelines with consideration of: ■ positioning ■ mouth care ■ sedation levels as per local policy sedation holding ■ stress ulcer prophylaxis.	Care bundles are advocated by the NICE and NPSA 2008 technical guideline and aim to minimize the risks of VAPS.

Procedure guideline 5.17: Weaning from mechanical ventilation

Action	Rationale
1 Where possible, explain and discuss the procedure with the patient. If the patient lacks the capacity to make decisions the practitioner must act in the patient's best interests.	To ensure that the patient understands the procedure and gives their valid consent. To ensure the patient's best interests are maintained (Mental Capacity Act 2005).
2 Consult best practice and/or local guidelines relating to weaning strategies. The content below is intended to highlight issues that should be considered during the weaning process.	To ensure that local guidelines are being followed and adhered to.
3 Assess the patient for suitability to commence weaning from mechanical ventilation. The patient should meet the following: ■ have a normal I:E (inspiratory:expiratory) ratio (ICS 2007) ■ have reducing inhaled oxygen requirement (FiO_2 less than 0.5 or less than 50%) (ICS 2007) ■ acceptable respiration rate, tidal volumes and airway pressures (ICS 2007) ■ evidence of resolution or reversal of the original cause of respiratory failure (MacIntyre 2001) ■ haemodynamic stability (MacIntyre 2001).	To ensure that it is appropriate to commence the withdrawal from mechanical ventilator support and to avoid complications associated with inappropriate weaning.
4 Utilize a local weaning protocol or guideline to facilitate the gradual reduction in ventilator support.	To ensure that the weaning process is standardized and evidence based for the local patient population.
5 Monitor the patient closely for complications associated with weaning. These could include respiratory distress, an increased work of breathing or haemodynamic changes (i.e. change in blood pressure, pulse). If adverse signs are noted, consider pausing the weaning process.	To facilitate prompt detection and treatment complications associated with the weaning process.
6 Document care.	To: ■ provide an accurate record ■ monitor effectiveness of procedure ■ reduce the risk of duplication of treatment ■ provide a point of reference or comparison in the event of later questions ■ acknowledge accountability for actions ■ facilitate communication and continuity of care. (NMC 2008; GMC 2013; HCPC 2012)

Procedure guideline 5.18: Intermittent positive pressure breathing (Bird)

Equipment

- Disposable HME
- IPPB machine, e.g. Bird

- Disposable circuit

Procedure

Action	Rationale
1 Where possible, explain and discuss the procedure with the patient. If the patient lacks the capacity to make decisions the practitioner must act in the patient's best interests.	To ensure that the patient understands the procedure and gives their valid consent. To ensure the patient's best interests are maintained (Mental Capacity Act 2005).
Introduce self to patient and explain the need for IPPB (Bird) therapy. Explain to the patient what the machine does, how it may feel, and gain their consent to use the machine.	Explanation of the therapy will reduce the patient's anxiety.
2 Wash and gel hands and use personal protective equipment.	To minimize risk of cross-infection (DH 2008).
3 Position the patient with the area of lung volume loss or retained secretions uppermost if possible.	To optimize the impact of the therapy.
4 Assess whether 100% oxygen or an air/oxygen mix (40% oxygen and 60% air) is most appropriate to drive the machine.	To match patient's current oxygen need and compensate for increased respiratory effort during therapy.
5 Fit the disposable circuit (with filter in situ) to the IPPB machine.	To minimize risk of cross-infection (DH 2008).
6 Set sensitivity, flow rate and inspiratory pressure controls as appropriate. There are no standardized values but common settings are: ■ sensitivity 5–7 ■ flow rate set at level that is most comfortable for the patient ■ inspiratory pressure – start on 10 and increase to between 15 and 20 as patient tolerates.	To ensure the patient receives therapy that is comfortable and that can be tolerated. Settings are chosen for patient comfort while maximizing impact of the therapy.
7 Instruct patient to close lips around the mouthpiece and breath in through their mouth. The machine will be triggered and gives the patient a deep breath as the Bird blows air into the chest. Once the inspiratory pressure is reached the machine will turn off and expiration is passive.	A good seal around the mouthpiece ensures maximum pressure is reached.
8 Wipe down the IPPB machine after treatment, e.g. with a disinfecting sanitizing wipe. Clean the disposable (single patient use) circuit and then put in a clear bag labelled and stored in the patient's locker. When the patient no longer requires the disposable circuit dispose of as per hospital procedure. Remove personal protective equipment. Wash hands and use apply alcohol gel to hands.	To minimize risk of cross-infection (DH 2008).
9 Ensure the patient is comfortable.	

131

(Continued)

10 Document findings as per local policy.	To: ■ provide an accurate record ■ monitor effectiveness of procedure ■ reduce the risk of duplication of treatment ■ provide a point of reference or comparison in the event of later questions ■ acknowledge accountability for actions ■ facilitate communication and continuity of care. (NMC 2008; GMC 2013; HCPC 2012)
11 Make referral to senior clinical team with any new findings.	To work within professional role boundaries to safeguard patient and practitioner. Unless diagnosis and intervention is part of role, referral is important.

Procedure guideline 5.19: Endotracheal extubation

Equipment

■ Sterile and non-sterile gloves.
■ Disposable apron
■ Eye protection

■ Functioning suction and oxygen supply
■ Two appropriately trained practitioners

Procedure

Action	Rationale
1 Where possible, explain and discuss the procedure with the patient. If the patient lacks the capacity to make decisions the practitioner must act in the patient's best interests.	To ensure that the patient understands the procedure and gives their valid consent. To ensure the patient's best interests are maintained (Mental Capacity Act 2005).
2 Wash hands with soap and water or decontaminate with alcohol gel. Adopt personal protective equipment including eye protection.	To prevent cross-contamination of pathogens and to protect practitioners.
3 Prior to the procedure, the patient's identity should be confirmed.	To ensure that the procedure is being carried out on the correct patient.
4 Undo or cut the tapes that are securing the endotracheal tube. Ensure that the practitioner assisting with the extubation procedure holds the tube.	Utilizing a colleague to hold the endotracheal tube following removal of the securing tapes may help to avoid accidental displacement of the endotracheal tube prior to the extubation procedure.
5 Select the appropriate-sized suction catheter for the procedure. Utilize the following equation to guide catheter selection: (Size of endotracheal/tracheostomy tube − 2) × 2 = size of suction catheter (French gauge).	The suction catheter should occlude less than half of the internal lumen of the endotracheal tube (Pedersen et al. 2009). Suctioning using a larger-sized catheter is thought to cause an increased negative pressure within the alveoli, causing potential alveolar collapse and atelectasis (Wood 1998; Pedersen et al. 2009).
6 Attach the proximal end of the catheter to the suction tubing, ensuring that the catheter stays within the sterile packaging.	
7 Turn on the high-flow suction at the suction meter. Set the suction level to 80–120 mmHg or 10.6–16 kPa.	Atelectasis, hypoxia and mucosal damage have attributed to the use of excessive suction pressures (Wood 1998; Pedersen et al. 2009). To avoid these suction-related complications lower suction pressures that still facilitate secretion removal are recommended.

8 Place one hand into a sterile glove and maintain the sterility of this hand.	To reduce the risk of infection and introduction of pathogens into the airway.
9 Disconnect the ventilator tubing from the end of the endotracheal tube. Silence the mechanical ventilator alarms or place into stand-by mode.	To avoid unnecessary audible alarms that might be distressing to the patient.
10 Remove suction catheter from packaging, ensuring that only the sterile gloved hand comes into contact with the catheter.	So that the sterility of the catheter is maintained and contamination of the airway is avoided.
11 Gently insert and advance the catheter into the patient's endotracheal tube until resistance is felt, signifying the catheter reaching the carina. Withdraw the suction catheter by 1–2 cm.	Applying suction after withdrawing the catheter by 1–2 cm avoids mucosal damage to the carina (Pedersen et al. 2009).
12 Apply suction by occluding the suction port located at the proximal end of the suction catheter. Suction should be applied continuously rather than intermittently.	Occluding the suction port will direct the negative pressure down the suction catheter, aiding aspiration of secretions during the procedure. Continuous suction during the extubation procedure is considered to be more effective, and in addition will cause less pulmonary tissue damage.
13 The practitioner assisting with the procedure should now fully deflate the endotracheal tube cuff with a 10 mL syringe.	Deflation of the endotracheal tube cuff will allow the tube to be removed from the trachea without causing any trauma to the vocal cords or airway structures.
14 Maintain suction and gently withdraw the endotracheal tube with the suction catheter in situ from the patient's airway. Suction should only be applied during catheter withdrawal and for no more than 15 seconds in duration.	Lengthy suction attempts are associated with increased adverse complications, such as hypoxia and mucusal damage (Pedersen et al. 2009).
15 Encourage the patient to cough and suction any expectorated secretions from their oral cavity with a rigid oropharyngeal suction catheter, such as a Yankauer catheter.	To ensure that any retained pulmonary secretions are removed from the patient's upper airway.
16 Commence the patient on oxygen therapy via a mask device. Ensure oxygen dosage is prescribed and signed for on the patient's medication chart.	To avoid complications associated with suctioning and extubation-related hypoxia. To continue oxygen therapy that the patient may have been receiving while mechanically ventilated.
17 Dispose of the endotracheal tube and the suction catheter in an appropriate clinical waste receptacle. Remove eye protection and dispose of apron and gloves. Wash hands with soap and water or decontaminate with alcohol gel.	To prevent cross-contamination or transmission of pathogens.
18 Assess patient for any changes in observations. Undertake an arterial blood gas if able. Instruct the patient to alert the nurse if they experience any difficulty in breathing following the procedure.	To ensure that any complications associated with extubation are noted promptly and the appropriate interventions implemented.
19 Document care.	To: ■ provide an accurate record ■ monitor effectiveness of procedure ■ reduce the risk of duplication of treatment ■ provide a point of reference or comparison in the event of later questions ■ acknowledge accountability for actions ■ facilitate communication and continuity of care. (NMC 2008; GMC 2013; HCPC 2012)

Procedure guideline 5.20: Suctioning (adapted with permission from the Royal Marsden Hospital Manual of Clinical Nursing Procedures)

(a) Open endotracheal suctioning

Equipment

- Disposable apron
- Sterile gloves
- Eye protection, such as a facial visor or goggles

- Selection of suction catheters (10, 12 and 14 French gauge)
- Suction unit, canister and tubing
- Disposable receptacle or clinical waste bag

Procedure

Action	Rationale
1 Where possible, explain and discuss the procedure with the patient. If the patient lacks the capacity to make decisions the practitioner must act in the patient's best interests.	To ensure that the patient understands the procedure and gives their valid consent. To ensure the patient's best interests are maintained (Mental Capacity Act 2005).
2 Observe and assess the patient for signs and symptoms that might indicate the need for endotracheal suctioning. A full respiratory assessment should be undertaken, including chest auscultation. The need for suction may be confirmed by audible or visible secretions, a change in respiration rate, SpO_2/PaO_2, cough, or work of breathing. Peripheral or central cyanosis, tachycardia or falling SaO_2 may override the need for auscultation.	To facilitate the prompt removal of pulmonary secretions from the patient's respiratory tract.
3 Wash hands with soap and water or decontaminate hands with alcohol gel. Put on gloves, disposable apron and eye protection.	To reduce cross-contamination and to protect the practitioner performing the procedure.
4 Oxygenate the patient with 100% oxygen for 30 to 60 seconds prior to suctioning.	Endotracheal suctioning is known to cause hypoxia/hypoxaemia, which in turn can predispose to dysrhythmia. Oxygenation is recommended to prevent these possible complications (AARC 2010).
5 Select the appropriate-sized suction catheter for the procedure. Utilize the following equation to guide catheter selection: (Size of ETT/tracheostomy tube (mm) −2) × 2 = size of suction catheter (French gauge).	The suction catheter should occlude less than half of the internal lumen of the endotracheal tube (Pedersen et al. 2009). Suctioning using a larger-sized catheter is thought to cause an increased negative pressure within the alveoli, causing potential alveolar collapse and atelectasis (Wood 1998; Pedersen et al. 2009).
6 Attach plastic connector end of the catheter to the suction tubing, ensuring that the catheter stays within the sterile packaging.	To ensure the catheter remains sterile; this will reduce the risk of iatrogenic introduction of pathogens into the patient's respiratory tract during the suction procedure.
7 Turn on the suction at the suction meter. Set the suction level to 10.6–16 kPa (80–120 mmHg).	Atelectasis, hypoxia and mucosal damage have been attributed to the use of excessive suction pressures (Wood 1998; Pedersen et al. 2009). To avoid these suction-related complications, lower suction pressures that still facilitate secretion removal are recommended.

8	Remove suction catheter from packaging, ensuring that the sterile catheter is not touched.	So that the sterility of the catheter is maintained and contamination of the airway is avoided.
9	Disconnect the endotracheal or tracheostomy tube from the attachment (ventilator tubing or tracheostomy mask) if required.	To facilitate the introduction of a suction catheter into the endotracheal or tracheostomy tube.
10	Gently insert and advance the catheter into the patient's endotracheal or tracheostomy tube until resistance is felt, signifying the catheter reaching the carina (the junction between the left and right main bronchi). Withdraw the suction catheter by 1–2 cm.	Applying suction after withdrawing the catheter by 1–2 cm avoids mucosal damage to the carina (Pedersen et al. 2009).
11	Apply suction by occluding the suction port located at the connector end of the suction catheter. Suction should be applied continuously, rather than intermittently.	To facilitate the removal of pulmonary secretions. There is no evidence that suction applied intermittently rather than continuously causes less mucosal trauma within the respiratory tract.
12	Withdraw the suction catheter slowly, while maintaining suction.	Application of suction only on catheter withdrawal will minimize mucosal damage within the respiratory tract (Wood 1998).
13	Suction should only be applied during catheter withdrawal and for no more than 15 seconds in duration. The whole procedure should be smooth and quick.	Lengthy suction attempts are associated with increased adverse complications, such as hypoxia and mucosal damage (Pedersen et al. 2009).
14	Reattach the ventilator tubing or tracheostomy mask to the patient's endotracheal or tracheostomy tube.	To resume ventilator support or oxygen therapy.
15	Dispose of the used suction catheter. This could be achieved by wrapping the used suction catheter around the gloved hand. Remove the glove, with the used suction catheter contained within it. Dispose of glove and catheter into an appropriate waste receptacle.	To facilitate removal of soiled and contaminated clinical equipment and also to prevent cross-contamination or transmission of pathogens.
16	If further suction attempts are required, repeat the above stages utilizing a fresh glove and suction catheter.	Utilizing a fresh suction catheter and glove will ensure that pulmonary secretions and pathogens are not reintroduced into the respiratory tract.
17	Reassess the patient and evaluate the effectiveness of the procedure.	To evaluate the effectiveness of the procedure and to direct future interventions.
18	Suction patient as required, rather than at regular timed intervals.	To avoid the potential adverse complications and risks associated with endotracheal suctioning, i.e. dysrhythmia, tracheal trauma and hypoxaemia, routine suctioning should be avoided (Van de Leur et al. 2003).
19	Document care.	To: <ul><li>provide an accurate record</li><li>monitor effectiveness of procedure</li><li>reduce the risk of duplication of treatment</li><li>provide a point of reference or comparison in the event of later questions</li><li>acknowledge accountability for actions</li><li>facilitate communication and continuity of care.</li></ul> (NMC 2008; GMC 2013; HCPC 2012)

(Continued)

Procedure guideline 5.20: (Continued)

(b) Closed endotracheal suctioning

Equipment

- Disposable apron
- Non-sterile gloves
- Closed endotracheal suctioning system
- Vial of 0.9% sodium chloride (if required for catheter irrigation)
- Suction unit, canister and tubing

Procedure

Action	Rationale
1 Where possible, explain and discuss the procedure with the patient. If the patient lacks the capacity to make decisions the practitioner must act in the patient's best interests.	To ensure that the patient understands the procedure and gives their valid consent. To ensure the patient's best interests are maintained (Mental Capacity Act 2005).
2 Observe and assess the patient for signs and symptoms that might indicate the need for endotracheal suctioning. A full respiratory assessment should be undertaken, including chest auscultation. The need for suction may be confirmed by audible or visible secretions, a change in respiration rate, SpO_2 PaO_2, cough, or work of breathing. Peripheral or central cyanosis, tachycardia or falling SaO_2 may override need for auscultation.	To detect any possible need for suctioning and to facilitate prompt removal of respiratory secretions.
3 Wash hands with soap and water or decontaminate hands with alcohol gel. Put on non-sterile gloves and disposable apron.	To reduce cross-contamination and infection, plus to protect the practitioner performing the procedure.
4 Oxygenate the patient with 100% oxygen for at least 30 seconds prior to suctioning.	Endotracheal or tracheal suctioning is known to cause hypoxia/hypoxaemia, which in turn can predispose to dysrhythmia. Oxygenation is recommended to prevent these possible complications (AARC 2010).
5 Closed suction catheters have two sizing mechanisms: the length is defined according to the nature of airway (i.e. tracheostomy versus endotracheal) and also the width of the airway. Ensure that the appropriate length and has been selected as demonstrated by the guidance on the manufacturer's packaging. To select the correct width utilize the following equation to guide catheter selection: (Size of ETT/tracheostomy tube −2) × 2 = size of suction catheter (French gauge).	During a routine suction procedure, trauma to and stimulation of the carina should be minimized, therefore the suction catheter should only be inserted down a tracheal tube until it just emerges out of the lumen of the tube (Rolls et al. 2007). The suction catheter should occlude less than half of the internal lumen of the endotracheal tube (Pedersen et al. 2009). Suctioning using a larger-sized catheter is thought to cause an increased negative pressure within the alveoli, causing potential alveolar collapse and atelectasis (Wood 1998; Pedersen et al. 2009).
6 Unlock the thumb control valve (located where the closed suction system meets the tubing from the suction meter). Turn on the suction meter. Set the suction level to 80–120 mmHg or 10.6–16 kPa.	Atelectasis, hypoxia and mucosal damage have attributed to the use of excessive suction pressures (Wood 1998; Pedersen et al. 2009). To avoid these complications, lower suction pressures that still facilitate secretion removal are recommended.
7 Ensure the thumb control valve aspect of the closed suction system and endotracheal or tracheostomy tube are held secure.	To prevent accidental tube displacement during the suctioning procedure. Applying suction after withdrawing the catheter by 1–2 cm avoids trauma and mucosal damage to the carina (Pedersen et al. 2009).

8 (a) Grasp the suction catheter through the protective sheath and gently advance the catheter into the endotracheal or tracheostomy tube until resistance is felt, signifying the catheter reaching the carina.
(b) Withdraw the suction catheter by 1–2 cm.

(a) To facilitate advancement of the suction catheter and to ensure that suction is applied at the appropriate depth within the respiratory tract.

(b) Applying suction after withdrawing the catheter by 1–2 cm avoids mucosal damage to the carina (Pedersen et al. 2009).

9 Apply suction by depressing the thumb control valve. Suction should be applied continuously, rather than intermittently. Withdraw the suction catheter slowly, while maintaining suction. Suction should only be applied during catheter withdrawal and for no more than 15 seconds in duration.

Application of suction only on catheter withdrawal will minimize mucosal damage within the respiratory tract (Wood 1998). Lengthy suction attempts are associated with increased adverse complications, such as hypoxia and mucusal damage (Pedersen et al. 2009).

10 Ensure that the suction catheter is fully retracted into the protective sheath. Correct withdrawal may be confirmed by a black stripe on the catheter, which should be seen within the protective sheath (Kimberly-Clark 2003).

A catheter left within the endotracheal or tracheostomy tube may cause increased airway resistance (Kimberly-Clark 2003).

11 Irrigate the suction catheter by attaching a sterile vial of 0.9% sodium chloride to the irrigation port (located next to the thumb control valve). Ensure the catheter has been fully retracted into the protective sheath. Depress the thumb control valve while injecting 0.9% sodium chloride into the catheter via the irrigation port, until the catheter is clear of secretions and debris (Kimberly-Clark 2003).

Irrigation will promote catheter patency and prevent reintroduction of secretions and debris retained within the catheter.

12 Ensure the thumb control valve is locked at the end of the suction procedure.

Locking of the thumb control valve prevents accidental application of suction.

13 Reassess the patient and evaluate the effectiveness of the procedure.

To evaluate the effectiveness of the procedure and to direct future interventions.

14 Remove eye protection and dispose of apron and gloves in an appropriate waste receptacle. Wash hands or use alcohol gel.

To prevent cross-contamination or transmission of pathogens.

15 Suction patient as required, rather than at regular timed intervals.

To avoid the potential adverse complications and risks associated with endotracheal suctioning, i.e. dysrhythmia, tracheal trauma and hypoxaemia, routine suctioning should be avoided (Van de Leur et al. 2003).

16 Document care.

To:
- provide an accurate record
- monitor effectiveness of procedure
- reduce the risk of duplication of treatment
- provide a point of reference or comparison in the event of later questions
- acknowledge accountability for actions
- facilitate communication and continuity of care.

(NMC 2008; GMC 2013; HCPC 2012)

Procedure guideline 5.21: Humidification (adapted with permission from the Royal Marsden Hospital Manual of Clinical Nursing Procedures)

Equipment

As a variety of humidification systems exist, equipment will vary and specific items are not, therefore, included here. In addition, as different humidification systems require specialized procedures, please consult the manufacturer's instructions in addition to the guideline outlined below.

Procedure

Action	Rationale
1 Discuss the choice of humidification device with the multidisciplinary team.	To ensure that the patient receives optimum and appropriate humidification therapy.
2 Where possible, explain and discuss the procedure with the patient. If the patient lacks the capacity to make decisions the practitioner must act in the patient's best interests.	To ensure that the patient understands the procedure and gives their valid consent. To ensure the patient's best interests are maintained (Mental Capacity Act 2005).
3 Follow manufacturer's instructions to assemble the chosen humidification device.	To facilitate safe and appropriate assembly of the humidification device.
4 Inspect the apparatus or device at regular intervals. That is: ■ inspect the HME for internal obstruction from secretions ■ confirm the set temperature on water bath humidifiers is set appropriately ■ check for any build-up of condensate within the ventilator or oxygen tubing.	To avoid possible complications associated with humidification devices, such as: ■ soiling from secretions with HMEs ■ inappropriate temperature settings ■ condensate within the tubing.
5 Inspect the water reservoir at regular intervals and ensure adequate levels of water within this. Do not allow the device to run empty of water.	To ensure that the patient receives continued appropriate levels of humidification.
6 Ensure that the ventilator or oxygen tubing is positioned at a level lower than the patient (Dougherty and Lister 2011).	To facilitate drainage of condensate away from the patient and into a water trap (if present).
7 Provide reassurance to the patient and family as required (Dougherty and Lister 2011).	The device may be uncomfortable, distressing and noisy to the patient and their family.
8 Change humidification tubing as per hospital and manufacturer's instructions.	To reduce possible complications associated with bacterial contamination within the circuit.
9 Monitor effectiveness of therapy and document. In particular note amount and viscosity of secretions.	To: ■ provide an accurate record ■ monitor effectiveness of procedure ■ reduce the risk of duplication of treatment ■ provide a point of reference or comparison in the event of later questions ■ acknowledge accountability for actions ■ facilitate communication and continuity of care. (NMC 2008; GMC 2013; HCPC 2012)

138

Procedure guideline 5.22: Manual hyperinflation

Equipment

- 2-litre Mapleson C bagging system (also referred to as a Waters' circuit) with integrated adjustable pressure-limiting (APL) valve and pressure manometer or a bag-valve-mask device, with the mask removed
- Functioning oxygen supply
- Suction apparatus (closed suction system is preferable) and a functioning suction supply.
- Disposable apron
- Non-sterile gloves

Procedure

Action	Rationale
1 Where possible, explain and discuss the procedure with the patient. If the patient lacks the capacity to make decisions the practitioner must act in the patient's best interests.	To ensure that the patient understands the procedure and gives their valid consent. To ensure the patient's best interests are maintained (Mental Capacity Act 2005).
2 Wash hands with soap and water or decontaminate with alcohol gel. Put on apron and non-sterile gloves.	To reduce cross-contamination and infection, and to protect the practitioner performing the procedure.
3 If appropriate, administer sedation or analgesia to the patient.	Analgesia and sedative medications may be used to minimize discomfort or distress.
4 Ensure that the patient is being monitored: ECG, SpO$_2$ and blood pressure.	To detect any complications during the procedure and to monitor effectiveness.
5 Attach the oxygen tubing element of the bagging system to the oxygen supply. Select 15 L/min on the oxygen flow meter.	So that the patient will continue to receive oxygen during the procedure.
6 Silence the ventilator alarms and promptly transfer the patient from the ventilator circuit to the bagging system. Place the ventilator into standby mode if available.	So to not alarm or distress the patient and to avoid excessive background noise within the critical care unit.
7 Give 3–4 gentle normal tidal volume breaths, by squeezing the bag element of the circuit. Attempt to synchronize these with the patient's own respiratory effort.	To allow the patient to become accustomed to breathing through the bagging circuit.
8 To deliver the hyperventilation breaths, squeeze the bag element of the system, giving the patient a slow inspiratory breath. Ensure that the breath is held for 1–2 seconds and then allow a rapid exhalation. Aim to give the patient tidal volumes 50% greater than their normal ventilator tidal volume (Maa et al. 2005). If a manometer is present in the circuit, during inspiration ensure that the peak inspiratory pressure does not rise above 40 kPa.	The use of larger-than-normal tidal volume is based on the hypothesis that by delivering a larger volume breath over time the expiratory flow rate may increase and assist in moving secretions towards more proximal airways (Maa et al. 2005). It is reasonable and prudent to minimize the peak airway pressure as much as possible during manual hyperinflation to prevent barotrauma (Maa et al. 2005).
9 Administer 3–4 hyperventilation breaths, followed by normal tidal volume breaths. Suction the patient after 6–8 hyperventilation breaths or when pulmonary secretions are audible in the upper airway. Use of a closed suction system is preferable.	To facilitate movement of retained secretions and then allow these to be aspirated from the patient's respiratory tract.
10 Repeat the above sequence until secretions have been cleared or until breath sounds have improved on auscultation.	To ensure that remaining secretions have been aspirated.

139

(Continued)

Procedure guideline 5.22: (Continued)

11 Reattach the patient to the ventilator circuit and resume mechanical ventilation.	To enable prior mechanical ventilation to resume.
12 Reassess the patient.	To evaluate the effectiveness of the manual hyperinflation procedure.
13 Wash hands with soap and water or decontaminate with alcohol gel. Dispose of gloves and apron in an appropriate waste container.	To prevent cross-contamination of pathogens.
14 Document care.	To: <ul><li>provide an accurate record</li><li>monitor effectiveness of procedure</li><li>reduce the risk of duplication of treatment</li><li>provide a point of reference or comparison in the event of later questions</li><li>acknowledge accountability for actions</li><li>facilitate communication and continuity of care.</li></ul> (NMC 2008; GMC 2013; HCPC 2012)

Procedure guideline 5.23: Prone positioning

Equipment

- Non-sterile gloves
- Disposable apron
- Appropriate number of practitioners to move patient (depending on assessment and treatment), including the availability of an anaesthetist in case of need for reintubation
- Pressure-relieving mattress
- Sheets
- Pillows

Procedure

Action	Rationale
1 Where possible, explain and discuss the procedure with the patient. If the patient lacks the capacity to make decisions the practitioner must act in the patient's best interests.	To ensure that the patient understands the procedure and gives their valid consent. To ensure the patient's best interests are maintained (Mental Capacity Act 2005).
2 Ensure that the risk of developing pressure ulcers is calculated, that the patient is on a suitable pressure-relieving mattress, with a sliding sheet in situ under the patient's sheet prior to commencing the procedure. Assess pressure areas, including groin areas, knees and abdomen. Provide support for feet to prevent foot drop. Document findings in notes prior to prone positioning.	To prevent the development of pressure ulcers and soft tissue damage. A sliding sheet will minimize manual handling risks to the patient and practitioners during the manoeuvre.
3 Ensure that the eyelids are covered by appropriate dressing (see Chapter 12) and gently lubricated with simple eye ointment prior to changing position. Suction oral secretions. Document in notes.	The patient's eyes are vulnerable to corneal abrasions and dryness during and after the manoeuvre (Ball et al. 2001 Rowe 2004). Secretions may pool inside the oral cavity, turning the patient may cause these secretions to move.

4 Assess all vascular access device sites:
  (a) check for signs of infection or inflammation, which might prompt need for vascular access device change prior to the manoeuvre. Change vascular access device if required and in accordance with local guidelines.
  (b) ensure that all vascular access devices and infusion tubing are suitably secured.

  (a) To enable relatively easy access to the vascular access device. Changing a vascular access device may be extremely difficult once the patient has been turned into the prone position.
  (b) To reduce the risk of accidental displacement during the manoeuvre.

5 Assess the endotracheal or tracheostomy tube:
  (a) check that the dressings and tapes holding the ETT or tracheostomy tube are secure. Change the dressings and tapes as required. For an endotracheal tube note the length of the tube in cm at the patient's teeth and document this.
  (b) insert a closed suction system if one is not already in place (see Suction section of this chapter).

  (a) To reduce the risk of accidental tube displacement.

  (b) Placement of the patient into prone position may increase drainage of oral and pulmonary secretions due to movement; a closed suction system will allow prompt aspiration of secretions if required.

6 If appropriate, change any dressing, especially those located on the patient's chest or abdomen.

Dressings on the patient's front may be difficult to assess and access once the patient has been placed prone.

7 Remove all chest electrodes prior to positioning and replace on the dorsal surface of the chest (Ball et al. 2001).

ECG electrodes, especially those on the patient's anterior chest, could cause tissue damage if left in place following the manoeuvre.

8 Assess level of sedation and need for analgesia prior to turning the patient prone.

Bolus of prescribed analgesia and sedation may be administered during the procedure – follow local guidance.

9 Stop any nasogastric feed and aspirate stomach contents. Spigot the nasogastric tube while conducting the manoeuvre, recommence feed once patient is prone.

To reduce the risk of aspiration during the manoeuvre.

10 Undertake any required investigations prior to the manoeuvre, including chest X-rays, 12-lead ECGs. Obtain an arterial blood gas to compare with post-prone results.

Performing an arterial blood gas will provide a baseline measurement and will allow the affect of the manoeuvre to be evaluated. Chest X-rays and 12-lead ECGs will be difficult to do once the patient has been placed into the prone position.

11 Disconnect all non-essential intravenous infusions (ensuring that these are 'Leur locked') and haemodynamic monitoring. Ensure that remaining intravenous infusion tubing and haemodynamic monitoring lines have sufficient length.

To reduce the risk of accidental tubing displacement during the manoeuvre.
Recommence infusions once patient is prone.

Performing the manoeuvre (based on Ball et al. 2001; Rowe 2004)
12 Lead practitioner:
  (a) assemble the clinical team who are assisting with the manoeuvre

  (b) allocate roles and brief the team on their responsibilities during the turn
  (c) maintain responsibility for protecting the patient's airway and safety.

  (a) To ensure that there is an adequate number of competent practitioners to undertake the manoeuvre in a safe manner. The procedure should only be undertaken when there are adequate staffing levels.
  (b) So that all practitioners have knowledge of their role and duties during the manoeuvre.
  (c) To ensure that the patient's airway and safety is being managed throughout the procedure.

(Continued)

Procedure guideline 5.23: (Continued)

13 Lead practitioner: (a) direct the team in their responsibilities and positions (b) ensure airway safety and maintenance.	(a) To enable the manoeuvre to be conducted in a safe and controlled manner. (b) To help to avoid accidental displacement of the endotracheal or tracheostomy tube. This may involve taking position at the top of the patient's head.
14 Ensure the patient is positioned in the supine position, with the arms positioned by their sides and their palms facing in.	Keeping the patient's arms close to their body will help prevent harm and or injury in the process of turning prone.
15 Position pillows (in pillow cases) onto the patient's chest, pelvis and across their knees.	To help cushion these bony prominences during the manoeuvre and once the patient is in the prone position.
16 Ensure that all monitoring cables, invasive monitoring, or infusion tubing are secured and trailed up towards the patient's head.	To help prevent accidental dislodgement and to keep the equipment accessible once the patient is in the prone position.
17 Ensure that the sheet under the patient is pulled tight and place a second sheet over the patient. Match up the corners of the top and bottom sheet, leaving the patient's face and head uncovered. The edges of the sheets should now be rolled together tightly, leaving the patient cocooned in the sheets (Rowe 2004).	Utilizing these two sheets to cocoon the patient will ensure that all limbs, tubing and monitoring are safely secured during the manoeuvre.
18 With the support of practitioners, gently move the patient away from the ventilator and position them near to the edge of the bed as is safely possible (Rowe 2004).	To reduce the sheer forces associated with patient repositioning, so reducing the risk of injury to team members undertaking the manoeuvre. To ensure their central position once they have been turned on to their front.
19 Roll the patient into the lateral position, facing the centre of the bed. Gently lay the patient on to their front, with pillows placed to support the chest, pelvis and knees.	To position the patient in the prone position, at the same time cushioning the bony prominences.
20 If appropriate, position the patient in the middle of the bed.	So that the patient is in a central position within the bed.
21 (a) Once settled, turn the patient's head to either the right or left. If the head if turned to the right, raise the patient's right arm and flex their elbow flexed to 90° (Rowe 2004) with their right hand pointing toward the head. Position the left arm by the patient's side. Complete the opposite actions if the patient's head is facing the left. Alternate the direction of the head and limbs every 2 hours. (b) Place bed into reverse-Trendelenberg position (horizontal angle of the bed tilted downwards at an angle of 30–45°; Rowe 2004).	(a) Alternating the direction of the head and limbs will reduce the risk of pressure damage to the facial structures and also limit the development of facial oedema (McCormick and Blackwood 2001). (b) Positioning the bed into a reverse-Trendelenberg position will prevent aspiration of gastric contents into the lungs.
22 Reattach all patient monitoring, which may have been disconnected during the prone positioning manoeuvre, i.e. arterial pressure, central venous pressure and ECG.	To resume normal patient monitoring and to facilitate early detection of physiological changes or deterioration that may be due to the pronation manoeuvre or the patient's underlying pathology.

23	Prone positioning should last between 3 and 6 hours (Crowe 2004) and episodes should be planned carefully in accordance with other patient care interventions, i.e. chest X-rays.	Some research indicates that patients should spend at least 6 hours in the prone position, as they can show a delayed beneficial response (McCormick and Blackwood 2001; McAuley et al. 2002; Crowe 2004). Patient care and interventions should be planned carefully, as certain procedures would require the patient to be supine, rather than in the prone position, i.e. vascular access changes or chest X-rays.
24	Document care.	To: ■ provide an accurate record ■ monitor effectiveness of procedure ■ reduce the risk of duplication of treatment ■ provide a point of reference or comparison in the event of later questions ■ acknowledge accountability for actions ■ facilitate communication and continuity of care. (NMC 2008; GMC 2013; HCPC 2012)

Procedure guideline 5.24: Insertion of a chest drain

Equipment

■ Sterile and non-sterile gloves and sterile gown
■ Sterile drapes
■ Skin antiseptic solution, i.e. iodine or chlorhexidine in alcohol
■ Local anaesthetic, i.e. 1% or 2% lidocaine
■ Selection of sterile syringes and needles
■ Sterile gauze swabs
■ Scalpel with blade

■ Forceps (round tipped) or 'Kelly clamp' for blunt dissection
■ Chest drain
■ Suture
■ Dressing
■ Closed drainage system with connecting tubing
■ Sterile water if required for an underwater seal drain
■ Guideline and dilators for Seldinger type drains
■ Cut-down theatre instrument set

The above equipment may be available in a kit form, which simplifies the preparation prior to the procedure

Procedure

Action	Rationale
1 Where possible, explain and discuss the procedure with the patient. If the patient lacks the capacity to make decisions the practitioner must act in the patient's best interests.	To ensure that the patient understands the procedure and gives their valid consent. To ensure the patient's best interests are maintained (Mental Capacity Act 2005).
2 Prior to the procedure, the patient's identity should be confirmed.	To ensure that the procedure is being carried out on the correct patient.
3 Confirm the site intended for drain insertion by reviewing the patient's clinical signs and chest X-ray. Ultrasound may be a useful adjunct for bedside drain insertion.	To ensure that the procedure is being carried out on the correct site.
4 Wash hands, put on non-sterile gloves and disposable apron.	To prevent cross-contamination of pathogens. Non-sterile gloves can be used to prepare and position the patient. The practitioner inserting the drain later in the procedure will require sterile gloves and gown.
5 Assess patient's requirement for sedation and analgesia during the procedure. Liaise with practitioner undertaking the procedure regarding the need and choice of sedatives or analgesics.	To avoid causing pain to the patient. Chest drain insertion has been reported as being extremely painful and the cause of great discomfort.

(Continued)

6 Place the patient into a position that will facilitate drain insertion. That is, in bed, rotated slightly away from the intended insertion site. Pillows can be positioned under the patient's shoulder to help achieve this slight rotation. The arm from the same side as the lesion should then be lifted up above the patient's head and kept in that position. This may require the assistance of another practitioner.	To allow clear access to the intended insertion site. If the patient is sedated they may be unable to maintain their arm in this position, so will require assistance.
7 Select the appropriate size chest drain. Smaller-size drains are recommended; however, for acute haemothorax, large-bore drains are preferable.	Patients have reported less discomfort from smaller-size chest drains. When rapid evacuation of a haemothorax and close monitoring of blood loss is required, the increased lumen size of a larger-bore drain may be more effective.
8 Wash hands and put on sterile gown and sterile gloves.	To ensure that the procedure is conducted in an aseptic manner and to reduce the risk of a secondary wound infection or an empyema.
9 Position a dressing trolley by the bedside and prepare a sterile field prepared on it. All required equipment should be emptied on to the sterile draped trolley, ensuring that asepsis is maintained.	To ensure that all the required sterile equipment is available.
10 Cleanse the insertion site with iodine or chlorhexadine.	To reduce the risk of infection of the drain insertion site.
11 Place sterile drapes over the patient, with the intended insertion site remaining exposed.	To reduce the risk of infection of the drain insertion site.
12 Infiltrate local anaesthetic around the intended drain site. First into the dermal layer of the skin and then into the deeper tissues, such as the intercostal muscles and pleura. Up to 3mg/kg of lidocaine 1% or 2% is usually administered.	To reduce the significant pain and discomfort associated with this procedure. This method allows the superficial layers of tissue to be anaesthetized while the deeper layers are being anaesthetized, thus reducing the pain and discomfort to the upper layers of tissues. This also ensures that all the layers through which the drain is to be inserted are anaesthetized.
13 (a) Insert smaller bore drains (8–14 French gauge) using a guide-wire (Seldinger) technique. (b) Insert medium bore drains (16–24 French gauge) using blunt dissection or a Seldinger technique. (c) Insert large-bore drains (above 24 French gauge) using blunt dissection. That is, make a small incision through the skin and dissect a channel through the subcutaneous tissue and intercostal muscles with forceps. Insert the chest drain tube into the tract, aided by a trocar or clamps.	(a) Blunt dissection is not required for smaller-bore drains. This method utilizes guide-wires and dilators to facilitate insertion of a drain into the pleural cavity. (b) To facilitate insertion of the medium-bore tube. The choice of technique depends on a number of factors, including the size of the patient, anticipated drain position and purpose of the drain. (c) To facilitate the insertion of the large-bore drain. Large drains cannot be pushed through the tissue with a guide wire without causing kinking of the wire and damage to the drain.
14 (a) Insert two sets of sutures for large-bore drains. One suture is intended to secure the drain in place and the other is utilized following drain removal to facilitate wound closure. (b) A small-bore drain may only require a single suture.	(a) The anchoring suture ensures that the drain remains secure and in position, while the closure suture is utilized following drain removal to achieve closure of the insertion site wound. The use of purse-string closure sutures has been noted to turn a linear wound into a circular shaped one, which can be painful and cause an unsightly scar. (b) A drain inserted with a guide-wire (Seldinger) technique is usually a snug fit in the skin and subcutaneous tissues, so does not require a suture to close the wound.

15 Attach the drain to the preassembled drainage system. If required, the drain should be attached to a high-volume/low-pressure suction unit, with suction usually set between 5 to 20 cmH$_2$O.	Suction may be required to treat a persistent pneumothorax or following pleurodesis.
16 Cover the insertion site in a transparent dressing. Avoid a large amount of padding and tape over the site. Use a mesentery or omental dressing (a looped portion of tape) to provide extra support to the drain tubing (see Figure 5.13).	A transparent dressing will allow observation of the drain insertion site for signs of infection or leakage (Laws et al. 2003). Thick padding and dressings over drain insertion sites may restrict chest expansion (Laws et al. 2003). A mesentery or omental dressing (looped portion of tape) may prevent accidental tube displacement and prevent tube kinking.
17 Dispose of all procedure waste in an appropriate clinical waste reciprocal.	To promote a safe working environment.
18 Wash hands and remove gloves and apron.	To reduce the risk of cross-contamination and infection.
19 Reassess the patient, noting vital signs, respiratory function, pain and sedation levels.	To enable early detection of complications associated with chest drain insertion, such as pain, haemorrhage, or a further pneumothorax.
20 Request a portable chest X-ray and ensure a member of a medical team reviews this promptly.	To confirm tube position, evaluate intervention and to detect possible complications.
21 Document care and any abnormalities.	To: ■ provide an accurate record ■ monitor effectiveness of procedure ■ reduce the risk of duplication of treatment ■ provide a point of reference or comparison in the event of later questions ■ acknowledge accountability for actions ■ facilitate communication and continuity of care. (NMC 2008; GMC 2013; HCPC 2012)

145

Procedure guideline 5.25: Chest drain removal on a ventilated patient (adapted with permission from the Royal Marsden Hospital Manual of Clinical Nursing Procedures)

Equipment

- Non-sterile gloves
- Disposable apron
- Eye protection
- Sterile stitch-cutter blade

- Spencer Wells clamps
- Sterile gauze swabs
- Two appropriately trained practitioners

Procedure

Action	Rationale
1 Where possible, explain and discuss the procedure with the patient. If the patient lacks the capacity to make decisions the practitioner must act in the patient's best interests.	To ensure that the patient understands the procedure and gives their valid consent. To ensure the patient's best interests are maintained (Mental Capacity Act 2005).

(Continued)

Procedure guideline 5.25: (Continued)

2 Wash hands with soap and water or decontaminate with alcohol gel. Put on non-sterile gloves, apron and eye protection.	To prevent cross-contamination of pathogens and to protect clinicians.
3 Ensure that the patient has adequate analgesia prior to chest drain removal.	Chest drain removal is associated with significant discomfort and pain for the patient (Laws et al. 2003).
4 Position the patient so that the drain insertion site is visible and accessible. Remove any dressings that are covering the drain insertion site.	To allow sufficient access to the chest site.
5 Place a large absorbent pad underneath the drain insertion site.	To absorb any blood or pleural fluid that may be displaced during drain removal.
6 Disconnect the chest drain from suction, if suction has been utilized.	Removal of chest drains while still on suction may cause the development of a tension pneumothorax (Hunter 2008).
7 (a) Locate and identify the anchoring sutures and any closure sutures around the drain insertion site. Using the sterile stitch-cutter blade cut and remove the anchoring sutures. (b) Also cut any closure sutures present to a length of 5 cm.	(a) Cutting the anchoring sutures will allow the chest drain to be removed from the patient's thorax. (b) To prepare closing sutures for tying following the drain removal.
8 Allocate roles. Practitioner 1: remove the chest drain. Practitioner 2: tie the closure suture.	To enable all team members to be aware of their role and responsibility during the chest drain removal procedure.
9 At the appropriate point in the respiratory cycle, swiftly remove the chest drain and the suture tied to close the skin incision. A small-bore drain may simply need removal and covering with an appropriate dressing.	To facilitate smooth removal of drain and closure of wound site to prevent occurrence of pneumothorax. Small-bore drains are likely to have been used with simple pneumothoraces or pleural effusions. Any remaining air is likely to resolve following removal of drain.
10 Tie the closure suture, cut off and discard any excess thread.	Tying the suture closes the insertion site and prevents air entering the pleural cavity from outside.
11 Clean the drain site with 0.9% sodium chloride.	To remove any clots or debris, which could cause a wound infection.
12 Apply a suitable adhesive dry dressing, such as gauze covered with a transparent waterproof dressing.	A transparent waterproof dressing will prevent air leaking into the pleura if the drain site has not been closed adequately.
13 Discard the tubing and chest drain in a suitable clinical waste receptacle.	To ensure workplace safety and to reduce the risk of infection or cross-contamination.
14 Wash hands or decontaminate with alcohol gel. Dispose of gloves and apron in a clinical waste bin. Remove eye protection.	To ensure workplace safety and to reduce the risk of infection or cross-contamination.
15 Assess patient for any abnormal changes in observations, i.e. desaturation or tachypnea. If able, instruct the patient to alert the nurse if they experience any difficulty in breathing following the procedure.	To ensure that any complications associated with chest drain removal are noted promptly and the appropriate interventions implemented.

16	Request a portable chest X-ray and ensure the medical team has reviewed this.	To evaluate therapy and to detect any possible complications associated with chest drain removal, such as pneumothorax.
17	Document the procedure in the patient's notes, including the amount of drainage contained within the drain prior to disposal.	To: ■ provide an accurate record ■ monitor effectiveness of procedure ■ reduce the risk of duplication of treatment ■ provide a point of reference or comparison in the event of later questions ■ acknowledge accountability for actions ■ facilitate communication and continuity of care. (NMC 2008; GMC 2013; HCPC 2012)

Competency statement 5.1: Specific procedure competency statements for chest auscultation

Complete assessment against relevant fundamental competency statements (*see* Chapter 2, pp. 20, 21)	Evidence
Specific procedure competency statements for chest auscultation	**Evidence of competency for chest auscultation**
Demonstrate ability to: ■ teach and assess or ■ learn from assessment.	Examples of evidence of teaching, assessing and learning.
Identify reason(s) for chest auscultation.	Able to discuss aim and rationale with mentor.
Identify risks, potential problems and complications of chest auscultation.	Can give two examples of potential risks, problems and complications associated with chest auscultation.
Demonstrate knowledge and understanding of local and national policies, guidance and procedures in relation to chest auscultation including: ■ hospital policy and procedure.	Able to debate own practice with regard to chest auscultation at advanced level, e.g. DH (2010a).
Demonstrate knowledge and understanding of underpinning evidence base in relation to chest auscultation, including: ■ reason for chest auscultation ■ differences and origins of vesicular, bronchial and adventitious noises ■ clinical significance of stridor, wheeze, fine and coarse crackles, pleural rub.	Can present and cite evidence base to underpin normal and abnormal chest assessment findings.
Demonstrate correct technique in relation to chest auscultation, including: ■ appropriate infection control precautions ■ preparation and positioning of patient ■ assessing for vesicular, bronchial and adventitious sounds ■ comparison of left and right side of chest ■ accurate documentation.	Under direct observation, able to perform correct examination technique, identify correct landmark positions and the underlying lung anatomy.
Demonstrate correct care of patient before, during and after chest auscultation, including: ■ ensuring the patient is comfortable ■ ensuring the patient's privacy and dignity.	Able to undertake a reflective discussion with mentor with regards to patient care in relation to *Essence of Care* 2010 (DH 2010b).

Competency statement 5.2: Specific procedure competency statements for arterial blood sampling

Complete assessment against relevant fundamental competency statements (*see* Chapter 2, pp. 20, 21)	Evidence
Specific procedure competency statements for arterial blood sampling	**Evidence of competency for arterial blood sampling**
Demonstrate ability to: ■ teach and assess or ■ learn from assessment.	Examples of evidence of teaching, assessing and learning.
Identify reason(s) for arterial blood sampling, including: ■ acute respiratory failure ■ peri-arrest and cardiorespiratory arrest situations ■ severe sepsis and shock.	Can undertake a teaching session with junior practitioners identifying three main aims for arterial blood sampling.
Identify risks, potential problems and complications with arterial blood sampling, including: ■ median nerve injury ■ haemorrhage from puncture site.	Can identify key risk factors, problems and complications associated with arterial blood sampling through discussion with mentor.
Demonstrate knowledge and understanding of local and national policies, guidance and procedures for arterial blood sampling.	Able to debate own practice with regard to arterial blood sampling via arterial puncture in light of local practice documents.
Demonstrate knowledge and understanding of underpinning evidence base of arterial blood sampling including: ■ principles of asepsis.	Can present and cite evidence base to demonstrate understanding of acid-base balance.
Prepare equipment required for procedure of arterial blood sampling.	Can supervise junior practitioners undertaking this procedure, ensuring that universal precautions and personal protective equipment is used.
Demonstrate correct technique in relation to procedure of arterial blood sampling, including: ■ use of correct sampling port ■ taking the correct volume for the sample ■ analysing the sample in a timely manner.	Under direct observation, is able to perform correct sampling and processing technique.
Demonstrate correct care of patient before, during and after the procedure of arterial blood sampling, including: ■ gaining consent from patient ■ maintaining patient comfort.	Can undertake a reflective discussion with mentor with regard to patient care in relation to *Essence of Care 2010* (DH 2010b).

148

Competency statement 5.3: Specific procedure competency statements for pulse oximetry

Complete assessment against relevant fundamental competency statements (*see* Chapter 2, pp. 20, 21)	Evidence
Specific procedure competency statements for pulse oximetry	**Evidence of competency for pulse oximetry**
Demonstrate ability to: ■ teach and assess or ■ learn from assessment.	Examples of evidence of teaching, assessing and learning.
Identify reason(s) for pulse oximetry, including: ■ effectiveness of oxygen therapy ■ oxygenation of the unwell patient during inter- and intra-hospital transport ■ oxygenation of patients with respiratory disease, e.g. asthma, chronic obstructive pulmonary diseases.	Can identify three reasons for use of pulse oximetry with mentor.
Identify risks, potential problems and complications with pulse oximetry, including: ■ tissue damage with prolonged placement of probe in one place.	Can make contribution to an education package, including key risk factors, problems and complications associated with pulse oximetry.
Demonstrate knowledge and understanding of local and national policies, guidance and procedures for pulse oximetry.	Able to debate own practice with regard to pulse oximetry in light of local practice documents.
Demonstrate knowledge and understanding of underpinning evidence base of pulse oximetry, including: ■ scientific knowledge of oxygen saturation.	Can present and cite evidence base to demonstrate underpinning knowledge of the role of pulse oximetry in patient assessment.
Prepare equipment required for procedure of pulse oximetry.	Can demonstrate to mentor how to use pulse oximetry.
Demonstrate correct technique in relation to procedure of pulse oximetry, including: ■ correct placement of probe.	Under direct observation, is able to perform correct technique.
Demonstrate correct care of patient before, during and after pulse oximetry, including: ■ ensuring patient comfort.	Can undertake a reflective discussion with mentor with regard to patient care in relation to *Essence of Care 2010* (DH 2010b).

Competency statement 5.4: Specific procedure competency statements for nasopharyngeal airway and oropharyngeal airway

Complete assessment against relevant fundamental competency statements (*see* Chapter 2, pp. 20, 21)	Evidence
Specific procedure competency statements for insertion of a nasopharyngeal tube	**Evidence of competency for insertion of a nasopharyngeal tube**
Demonstrate ability to: ■ teach and assess or ■ learn from assessment.	Examples of evidence of teaching, assessing and learning.
Identify reason(s) for insertion of a nasopharyngeal/oropharyngeal tube: ■ facilitate the removal of pulmonary secretions, by passing a suction catheter through the adjunct into the patient's respiratory tract ■ provision of airway support.	*May be demonstrated by*: ■ discussion with supervisor/mentor ■ teaching session for peers ■ completion of a reflective text, workbook or educational package to test knowledge.

(Continued)

Identify risks, potential problems and complications associated with insertion of a nasopharyngeal/oropharyngeal tube and how to prevent or manage them: ■ incorrect size inserted ■ incorrect insertion technique ■ inappropriate usage and use when contraindicated ■ risk of trauma, gagging, vomiting, or haemorrhage.	*May be demonstrated by*: ■ discussion with supervisor/mentor ■ teaching session for peers ■ completion of a reflective text, workbook, or educational package to test knowledge.
Demonstrate knowledge and understanding of local and national policies, guidance and procedures in relation to insertion of a nasopharyngeal oropharyngeal tube: ■ national guidance surrounding the insertion of nasopharyngeal/ oropharyngeal airways by the Resuscitation Council UK (2011) ■ local or hospital guidelines on the insertion of nasopharyngeal airways.	*May be demonstrated by*: ■ discussion with supervisor/mentor ■ teaching session for peers ■ completion of a reflective text, workbook, or educational package to test knowledge.
Demonstrate knowledge and understanding of evidence base in relation to insertion of a nasopharyngeal/oropharyngeal tube.	*May be demonstrated by*: ■ discussion with supervisor/mentor ■ teaching session for peers ■ completion of a reflective text, workbook, or educational package to test knowledge.
Demonstrate skills that are required in relation to insertion of a nasopharyngeal/oropharyngeal tube: ■ basic respiratory assessment and awareness of signs or symptoms of respiratory distress or deterioration ■ universal precautions.	*May be demonstrated by*: ■ direct observation of procedure ■ teaching session for peers, utilizing an airway manikin ■ practical assessment.
Prepare equipment according to local policies for the insertion of a nasopharyngeal/oropharyngeal tube:	*May be demonstrated by*: ■ direct observation of procedure ■ teaching session for peers, utilizing an airway manikin ■ practical assessment.
Demonstrate the correct technique for the insertion of a nasopharyngeal/oropharyngeal tube: ■ correct selection of tube size ■ correct insertion technique ■ evaluation of intervention.	*May be demonstrated by*: ■ direct observation of procedure. ■ teaching session for peers, utilizing an airway manikin ■ practical assessment.

Competency statement 5.5: Specific procedure competency statements for insertion of an endotracheal tube

Complete assessment against relevant fundamental competency statements (*see* Chapter 2, pp. 20, 21)	Evidence
Specific procedure competency statements for assisting with the insertion of an endotracheal tube	**Evidence of competency for insertion of an endotracheal tube**
Demonstrate ability to: ■ teach and assess or ■ learn from assessment.	Examples of evidence of teaching, assessing and learning.
Identify reason(s) for insertion of an endotracheal tube: ■ to secure and maintain a patient's airway ■ to prevent and guard against aspiration of stomach contents ■ to facilitate removal of pulmonary secretions ■ to facilitate the delivery of positive pressure ventilation.	*May be demonstrated by*: ■ discussion with supervisor/mentor ■ teaching session for peers ■ completion of a reflective text, workbook, or educational package to test knowledge.

Identify risks, potential problems and complications associated with insertion of an endotracheal tube and how to prevent or manage them:
- trauma within the oropharynx or trachea
- hypoxia
- dysrhythmia
- cardiac arrest
- haemodynamic instability
- intubation of right or left main bronchi
- intubation of oesophagus.

May be demonstrated by:
- discussion with supervisor/mentor
- teaching session for peers
- completion of a reflective text, workbook, or educational package to test knowledge.

Demonstrate knowledge and understanding of local and national policies, guidance and procedures in relation to insertion of an endotracheal tube:
- national guidelines from the Resuscitation Council UK or the Royal College of Anaesthetists
- local or hospital guidelines concerning the use of endotracheal tubes.

May be demonstrated by:
- discussion with supervisor/mentor
- teaching session for peers
- completion of a reflective text, workbook, or educational package to test knowledge.

Demonstrate knowledge and understanding of evidence base in relation to insertion of an endotracheal tube.

May be demonstrated by:
- discussion with supervisor/mentor
- teaching session for peers
- completion of a reflective text, workbook, or educational package to test knowledge.

Demonstrate skills that are required in relation to assisting with the insertion of an endotracheal tube:
- basic respiratory assessment and awareness of signs or symptoms of respiratory distress or deterioration
- universal precautions
- suctioning of oropharyngeal secretions, vomit, or blood using a rigid oropharyngeal suction catheter, such as a Yankauer catheter
- use of a bedside patient monitor (with SpO_2, ECG and blood pressure) and interpretation of values.

May be demonstrated by:
- direct observation of procedure
- teaching session for peers, utilizing an airway manikin
- practical assessment.

Prepare equipment required in relation to insertion of an endotracheal tube.
- selection of cuffed endotracheal tubes (to include sizes 6, 6.5, 7, 7.5, 8, 8.5 and 9)
- rigid oropharyngeal suction catheter, such as a Yankauer catheter.
- 10 mL syringe
- laryngoscope, with a size 3 Macintosh blade
- bag-valve-mask device attached to oxygen supply
- bougie
- length of tape, bandage, or tube stabilizing device
- intravenous medications required for intubation
- capnography device
- emergency resuscitation equipment.

May be demonstrated by:
- direct observation of procedure
- teaching session for peers, utilizing an airway manikin
- practical assessment.

Demonstrate the correct technique for the insertion of an endotracheal tube:
- correct selection of endotracheal tube size
- correct assembly of tube insertion apparatus
- appropriate device insertion technique
- evaluation of intervention.

May be demonstrated by:
- direct observation of procedure
- teaching session for peers, utilizing an airway manikin
- practical assessment.

Competency statement 5.6: Specific procedure competency statements for tracheostomy formation and tube insertion auscultation

Complete assessment against relevant fundamental competency statements (*see* Chapter 2, pp. 20, 21)	Evidence
Specific procedure competency statements for assisting with the insertion of a tracheostomy tube	**Evidence of competency for insertion of a tracheostomy tube**
Demonstrate ability to: ■ teach and assess or ■ learn from assessment.	Examples of evidence of teaching, assessing and learning.
Identify reason(s) for insertion of a tracheostomy tube: ■ to facilitate respiratory weaning from mechanical ventilation ■ to bypass an upper airway obstruction, i.e. neoplasm or an acute airway obstruction ■ to prevent an airway obstruction, i.e. in Bulbar palsy.	*May be demonstrated by*: ■ discussion with supervisor/mentor ■ teaching session for peers ■ completion of a reflective text, workbook. or educational package to test knowledge.
Identify risks, potential problems and complications associated with insertion of a tracheostomy tube and how to prevent or manage them: ■ hypoxia ■ dysrhythmia ■ cardiac arrest ■ haemodynamic instability ■ inadvertent insertion into neck tissues ■ aspiration of gastric contents.	*May be demonstrated by*: ■ discussion with supervisor/mentor ■ teaching session for peers ■ completion of a reflective text, workbook, or educational package to test knowledge.
Demonstrate knowledge and understanding of local and national policies, guidance and procedures in relation to insertion of a tracheostomy tube: ■ national guidelines from the Resuscitation Council UK or the Royal College of Anaesthetists ■ local or hospital guidelines concerning the use of tracheostomy tubes.	*May be demonstrated by*: ■ discussion with supervisor/mentor ■ teaching session for peers ■ completion of a reflective text, workbook, or educational package to test knowledge.
Demonstrate knowledge and understanding of evidence base in relation to insertion of a tracheostomy tube.	*May be demonstrated by*: ■ discussion with supervisor/mentor ■ teaching session for peers ■ completion of a reflective text, workbook, or educational package to test knowledge.
Demonstrate skills that are required in relation to assisting with the insertion of a tracheostomy tube: ■ basic respiratory assessment and awareness of signs or symptoms associated with respiratory distress or deterioration ■ universal precautions ■ suctioning of oropharyngeal secretions, vomit, or blood using a rigid oropharyngeal suction catheter, such as a Yankauer catheter ■ use of a bedside patient monitor (with SpO_2, ECG and blood pressure) and interpretation of values.	*May be demonstrated by*: ■ direct observation of procedure ■ teaching session for peers, utilizing an airway manikin ■ practical examination.

Prepare equipment required in relation to insertion of a tracheostomy tube:
- pillow and/or sandbag
- laryngoscope
- rigid oropharyngeal suction catheter, such as a Yankauer catheter, attached to high-flow oxygen
- sterile gown and sterile and non-sterile gloves
- surgical mask
- eye protection
- surgical drapes
- skin disinfectant, i.e. 2% chlorhexadine or iodine preparation
- percutaneous tracheostomy set, including tracheostomy tube and dilators
- bronchoscope
- resuscitation trolley and equipment.

May be demonstrated by:
- direct observation of procedure
- teaching session for peers, utilizing an airway manikin
- practical examination.

153

Demonstrate the correct technique for the procedure in relation to assisting with the insertion of a tracheostomy tube:
- correct assembly of tube insertion apparatus
- appropriate device insertion technique
- evaluation of intervention.

May be demonstrated by:
- direct observation of procedure
- teaching session for peers, utilizing an airway manikin
- practical examination.

Competency statement 5.7: Specific procedure competency statements for tracheostomy removal/decannulation

Complete assessment against relevant fundamental competency statements (*see* Chapter 2, pp. 20, 21)	Evidence
Specific procedure competency statements for endotracheal tube extubation	**Evidence of competency for endotracheal tube extubation**
Demonstrate ability to: ■ teach and assess or ■ learn from assessment.	Examples of evidence of teaching, assessing and learning.
Identify reason(s) for tracheostomy removal: ■ patient now able to maintain own airway, i.e. following a period of reduced conscious level or an episode of upper airway obstruction/swelling.	*May be demonstrated by*: ■ discussion with supervisor/mentor ■ teaching session for peers ■ completion of a reflective text, workbook, or educational package.

(Continued)

Competency statement 5.7: (*Continued*)

Identify risks, potential problems and complications associated with tracheal tube removal and how to prevent or manage them:
■ laryngospasm
■ aspiration of gastric contents
■ inadequate airway patency due to:
   ■ insufficient reversal of sedative or paralysing agents
   ■ oropharyngeal oedema or haemotoma
■ insufficient ventilatory stimuli, i.e. respiratory depression due to opioids
■ increased coughing immediately following procedure
■ cardiovascular effects, i.e. hypertension and tachycardia
■ raised intracranial pressure (ICP).
	May be demonstrated by:
	■ discussion with supervisor/mentor
	■ teaching session for peers
	■ completion of a reflective text, workbook. or educational package.

Demonstrate knowledge and understanding of local and national policies, guidance and procedures in relation to tracheal tube removal: ■ local or hospital guidelines concerning the removal of endotracheal tubes.	*May be demonstrated by*: ■ discussion with supervisor/mentor ■ teaching session for peers ■ completion of a reflective text, workbook, or educational package.
Demonstrate knowledge and understanding of evidence base in relation to tracheostomy removal.	*May be demonstrated by*: ■ discussion with supervisor/mentor. teaching session for peers ■ completion of a reflective text, workbook, or educational package.
Demonstrate skills that are required in relation to tracheostomy removal: Basic respiratory assessment and awareness of signs or symptoms of respiratory distress or deterioration ■ universal precautions ■ use of suction apparatus ■ use of a bedside patient monitor (with SpO_2, ECG and blood pressure) and interpretation of values.	*May be demonstrated by*: ■ direct observation of procedure ■ teaching session for peers, utilizing an airway manikin ■ practical examination.
Prepare equipment required in relation to tracheostomy removal: ■ non-sterile gloves ■ disposable apron ■ eye protection ■ a functioning suction and oxygen supply ■ two appropriately trained practitioners.	*May be demonstrated by*: ■ direct observation of procedure ■ teaching session for peers, utilizing an airway manikin ■ practical examination.
Demonstrate the correct technique for the procedure in relation to tracheostomy removal: ■ correct assembly of tracheostomy removal apparatus ■ appropriate tracheostomy removal technique ■ evaluation of intervention.	*May be demonstrated by*: ■ direct observation of procedure ■ teaching session for peers, utilizing an airway manikin. ■ practical examination.

Competency statement 5.8: Specific procedure competency statements for end tidal CO$_2$ (ETCO$_2$) monitoring

Complete assessment against relevant fundamental competency statements (*see* Chapter 2, pp. 20, 21)	Evidence
Specific procedure competency statements for end tidal CO$_2$ monitoring	**Evidence of competency for end tidal CO$_2$ monitoring**
Demonstrate ability to: ■ teach and assess or ■ learn from assessment.	Examples of evidence of teaching, assessing and learning.
Identify reason(s) for ETCO$_2$ monitoring, including: ■ respiratory monitoring of the ventilated patient ■ monitoring during transport of the critically ill patient ■ assessment following tracheal tube insertion to confirm correct placement.	Can identify three reasons for use of ETCO$_2$ monitoring with mentor.
Identify risks, potential problems and complications of ETCO$_2$ monitoring, including: ■ incorrect placement of ETCO$_2$ in ventilator circuit.	Able to explore with a junior practitioner the key risk factors, problems and complications associated with ETCO$_2$.
Demonstrate knowledge and understanding of local and national policies, guidance and procedures of ETCO$_2$ monitoring.	With mentor can explore the relevance of the document Standards in Capnography in Critical Care (ICS 2009).
Demonstrate knowledge and understanding of underpinning evidence base of ETCO$_2$ monitoring, including: ■ CO$_2$ production and removal from the body.	Can present and cite evidence base to demonstrate underpinning knowledge of the role of ETCO$_2$ in patient assessment.
Prepare equipment required for procedure of ETCO$_2$ monitoring.	Can teach a student practitioner how to prepare equipment.
Demonstrate correct technique in relation to procedure of ETCO$_2$ monitoring including: ■ correct and safe placement of the ETCO$_2$ monitor.	Under direct observation, is able to perform correct technique.
Demonstrate correct care of patient before, during and after ETCO$_2$ monitoring, including: ■ checking ventilator observations after placement of ETCO$_2$ monitor.	Can undertake a reflective discussion with mentor with regard to patient care in relation to *Essence of Care 2010* (DH 2010b).

155

Competency statement 5.9: Specific procedure competency statements for tracheal cuff pressure measurement

Complete assessment against relevant fundamental competency statements (see Chapter 2, pp. 20, 21)	Evidence
Specific procedure competency statements for tracheal cuff pressure measurements	**Evidence of competency for tracheal cuff pressure measurements**
Demonstrate ability to: ■ teach and assess or ■ learn from assessment.	Examples of evidence of teaching, assessing and learning.
Identify reason(s) for tracheal cuff pressure measurement, including: ■ maintaining cuff seal around tracheostomy tube.	Able to prepare a teaching plan for orientation programme to intensive care that includes indications for tracheal cuff pressure measurement.
Identify risks, potential problems and complications of tracheal cuff pressure measurement, including: ■ maintaining pressure within range to prevent damage to tracheal mucosa.	Is able to explore with mentor the key risk factors, problems and complications associated with tracheal cuff pressure measurement.
Demonstrate knowledge and understanding of local and national policies, guidance and procedures of tracheal cuff pressure measurement.	For new members of staff is able to identify and locate key clinical policies and resources.
Demonstrate knowledge and understanding of underpinning evidence base of tracheal cuff pressure measurement, including: ■ physiology of capillary blood flow.	Can present and cite evidence base to specific to tracheal damage in long-term patients.
Prepare equipment required for procedure of tracheal cuff pressure measurement.	Is able to assemble correct equipment.
Demonstrate correct technique in relation to procedure of tracheal cuff pressure measurement, including: ■ knowledge of safety equipment required.	Can demonstrate safe practice when supervising junior/non-registered staff in tracheal cuff pressure measurement.
Demonstrate correct care of patient before, during and after tracheal cuff pressure measurement, including: ■ keeping the patient informed throughout the procedure.	Can undertake a reflective discussion with mentor with regard to patient care in relation to *Essence of Care 2010* (DH 2010b).

Competency statement 5.10: Specific procedure competency statements for non-invasive ventilator (NIV) therapy

Complete assessment against relevant fundamental competency statements (see Chapter 2, pp. 20, 21)	Evidence
Specific procedure competency statements for non-invasive ventilator therapy	**Evidence of competency for non-invasive ventilator therapy**
Demonstrate ability to: ■ teach and assess or ■ learn from assessment.	Examples of evidence of teaching, assessing and learning.
Identify reason(s) for implementing NIV therapy, including: ■ type 1 and 2 respiratory failure ■ part of a weaning plan from mechanical ventilation ■ obstructive sleep apnoea if acidosis is present.	Provides a teaching session to junior practitioners considering indications for and contraindications to NIV therapy. Explains the differences between type 1 and 2 respiratory failure.
Identify risks, potential problems and complications of NIV therapy when utilized for: ■ type 1 and 2 respiratory failure ■ type 2 respiratory failure where tracheal intubation is not deemed appropriate ■ part of a weaning plan from mechanical ventilation.	Is able to explore with mentor the key risk factors, problems and complications associated with NIV therapy.
Demonstrate knowledge and understanding of local and national policies, guidance and procedures of NIV therapy.	Is able to locate and discuss local policy and BTS (2008) guidance to support evidenced-based knowledge.
Demonstrate knowledge and understanding of underpinning evidence base of NIV therapy, including: ■ principles of gas exchange at alveolar level.	As above.
Prepare equipment required for NIV therapy.	Is able to prepare equipment according to local policy and procedural guideline.
Demonstrate correct technique in relation to implementing and maintaining NIV therapy, including: ■ most appropriate choice of mode.	Is able to implement therapy according to local policy and procedural guideline.
Demonstrate correct care of patient before, during and after NIV therapy, including: ■ assess for skin integrity at all pressure points.	Can undertake a reflective discussion with mentor with regard to patient care in relation to *Essence of Care 2010* (DH 2010b).

157

Competency statement 5.11: Specific procedure competency statements for invasive ventilator therapy care

Complete assessment against relevant fundamental competency statements (*see* Chapter 2, pp. 20, 21)	Evidence
Specific procedure competency statements for invasive ventilator therapy care	**Evidence of competency for invasive ventilator therapy care**
Demonstrate ability to: ■ teach and assess or ■ learn from assessment.	Examples of evidence of teaching, assessing and learning.
Identify reason(s) for implementing invasive ventilation, including: ■ inability to sustain adequate gas exchange.	Can teach junior practitioner or learner about indications for and complications of invasive ventilation.
Identify risks, potential problems and complications of invasive ventilation, including: ■ potential for reduced cardiac output.	Is able to explore with mentor the key risk factors, problems and complications associated with invasive ventilations.
Demonstrate knowledge and understanding of local and national policies, guidance and procedures of invasive ventilation.	Is able to locate and discuss local policy in relation to invasive ventilation. Is able to locate guidance from NICE and NPSA in relation to VAPs preventions and explain the reasoning behind the recommendations.
Demonstrate knowledge and understanding of underpinning evidence base of invasive ventilation, including: ■ principles of ventilation and respiration.	Can explain the risk factors of ventilation and related evidence related to VAP prevention.
Prepare equipment required for procedure of implementation and ongoing care of patients receiving invasive ventilation.	Can prepare equipment according to local policy and procedural guideline. Demonstrate pre-ventilation checks undertaken with manufacturer checklists. Able to relate six examples of safety checks and troubleshooting.
Demonstrate correct technique in relation to implementation and ongoing care of patients receiving invasive ventilation, including: ■ knowledge and understanding of ventilator/ventilator mode ■ knowledge and understanding of ventilator settings and patient observations.	Is able to implement therapy according to local policy and procedural guideline. Is able to discuss ventilator settings and observations in line with local policy.
Demonstrate correct care of patient before, during and after invasive ventilation therapy, including: ■ safe care of the endotracheal tube ■ psychological support of the intubated patient.	Can undertake a reflective discussion/diary with mentor input with regard to patient care in relation to *Essence of Care 2010* (DH 2010b).

Competency statement 5.12: Specific procedure competency statements for intermittent positive pressure breathing (IPPB) (Bird)

Complete assessment against relevant fundamental competency statements (see Chapter 2, pp. 20, 21)	Evidence
Specific procedure competency statements for intermittent positive pressure breathing (IPPB) (Bird)	**Evidence of competency for intermittent positive pressure breathing (IPPB) (Bird)**
Demonstrate ability to: ■ teach and assess or ■ learn from assessment.	Examples of evidence of teaching, assessing and learning.
Identify reason(s) for implementing IPPB (Bird), including: ■ sputum retention ■ patients with atelectasis.	Able to provide a teaching session to junior practitioners considering indications and contra indications to IPPB therapy.
Identify risks, potential problems and complications of IPPB (Bird) including: ■ Reduced BP due to reduction in venous return ■ Bronchospasm.	Able to explore with mentor the key risk factors, problems and complications.
Demonstrate knowledge and understanding of local and national policies, guidance and procedures of IPPB (Bird).	Able to locate and discuss local policy.
Demonstrate knowledge and understanding of underpinning evidence base of IPPB (Bird), including: ■ impact of increasing positive intrathoracic pressure.	Able to teach a junior practitioner the reason for using IPPB (Bird) therapy.
Prepare equipment required for procedure of implementation and ongoing care of patients receiving IPPB (Bird).	Able to prepare equipment according to local policy and procedural guideline.
Demonstrate correct technique in relation to implementation and ongoing care of patients receiving IPPB (Bird), including: ■ ensuring seal around mouthpiece.	Able to implement therapy according to local policy and procedural guideline.
Demonstrate correct care of patient before, during and after IPPB (Bird) including: ■ patient education to improve compliance with IPPB therapy.	Can undertake a reflective discussion with mentor with regard to patient care in relation to *Essence of Care 2010* (DH 2010b).

159

Competency statement 5.13: Specific procedure competency statements for endotracheal tube extubation

Complete assessment against relevant fundamental competency statements (*see* Chapter 2, pp. 20, 21)	Evidence
Specific procedure competency statements for endotracheal tube extubation	**Evidence of competency for endotracheal tube extubation**
Demonstrate ability to: ■ teach and assess or ■ learn from assessment.	Examples of evidence of teaching, assessing and learning.

(*Continued*)

Competency statement 5.13: (*Continued*)

Identify reason(s) for endotracheal tube extubation:
- patient no longer requiring mechanical ventilation, i.e. improving respiratory function
- patient now able to maintain own airway, i.e. following a period of reduced conscious level or an episode of upper airway obstruction/swelling.

May be demonstrated by:
- discussion with supervisor/mentor
- teaching session for peers
- completion of a reflective text, workbook, or educational package.

Identify risks, potential problems and complications associated with endotracheal tube extubation and how to prevent or manage them:
- laryngospasm
- aspiration of gastric contents
- inadequate airway patency due to:
  - insufficient reversal of sedative or paralysing agents
  - oropharyngeal oedema or haemotoma
- insufficient ventilatory stimuli, i.e. respiratory depression due to opioids
- increased coughing immediately following procedure
- cardiovascular effects, i.e. hypertension and tachycardia
- raised intracranial pressure (ICP).

May be demonstrated by:
- discussion with supervisor/mentor
- teaching session for peers
- completion of a reflective text, workbook, or educational package.

Demonstrate knowledge and understanding of local and national policies, guidance and procedures in relation to endotracheal tube extubation:
- local or hospital guidelines concerning the removal of endotracheal tubes.

May be demonstrated by:
- discussion with supervisor/mentor
- teaching session for peers
- completion of a reflective text, workbook, or educational package.

Demonstrate knowledge and understanding of evidence base in relation to ETT extubation.

May be demonstrated by:
- discussion with supervisor/mentor
- teaching session for peers
- completion of a reflective text, workbook, or educational package.

Demonstrate skills that are required in relation to ETT extubation:
- basic respiratory assessment and awareness of signs or symptoms of respiratory distress or deterioration
- universal precautions
- use of suction apparatus
- use of a bedside patient monitor (with SpO_2, ECG and blood pressure) and interpretation of values.

May be demonstrated by:
- direct observation of procedure
- teaching session for peers, utilizing an airway manikin
- practical examination.

Prepare equipment required in relation to ETT extubation:
- sterile and non-sterile gloves
- disposable apron
- eye protection
- a functioning suction and oxygen supply
- two appropriately trained practitioners.

May be demonstrated by:
- direct observation of procedure
- teaching session for peers, utilizing an airway manikin
- practical examination.

Demonstrate the correct technique for the procedure in relation to endotracheal extubation:
- correct assembly of extubation apparatus
- appropriate extubation technique
- evaluation of intervention.

May be demonstrated by:
- direct observation of procedure
- teaching session for peers, utilizing an airway manikin
- practical examination.

Competency statement 5.14: Specific procedure competency statements for suctioning

Complete assessment against relevant fundamental competency statements (*see* Chapter 2, pp. 20, 21)	Evidence
Specific procedure competency statements for open and closed endotracheal suctioning	**Evidence of competency for open and closed endotracheal suctioning**
List the reason(s) for using either open or closed endotracheal suctioning: ■ to facilitate the removal of pulmonary secretions ■ to promote tube patency ■ to improve oxygenation.	*May be demonstrated by*: ■ discussion with supervisor/mentor ■ teaching session for peers ■ completion of a reflective text, workbook, or educational package.
Discuss the risks, potential problems and complications associated with open and closed endotracheal suctioning and how to prevent or manage them: ■ hypoxia and/or hypoxaemia ■ haemodynamic instability ■ raised intracranial pressure (ICP) ■ bronchoconstriction ■ bleeding ■ atelectasis ■ cardiac dysrhythmias ■ cardiac arrest ■ potential death ■ tracheal ulceration or damage ■ patient pain or discomfort.	*May be demonstrated by*: ■ discussion with supervisor/mentor ■ teaching session for peers ■ completion of a reflective text, workbook, or educational package.
Demonstrate knowledge and understanding of local and national policies, guidance and procedures in relation to open and closed endotracheal suctioning: ■ local or hospital guidelines concerning the use of use of open or/and closed suctioning.	*May be demonstrated by*: ■ discussion with supervisor/mentor ■ teaching session for peers ■ completion of a reflective text, workbook, or educational package.
Demonstrate knowledge and understanding of evidence base in relation to open and closed endotracheal suctioning.	*May be demonstrated by*: ■ discussion with supervisor/mentor ■ teaching session for peers ■ completion of a reflective text, workbook, or educational package.
Demonstrate skills that are required in relation to open and closed endotracheal suctioning: ■ basic respiratory assessment and awareness of signs or symptoms associated with respiratory distress or deterioration ■ universal precautions ■ use of a bedside patient monitor (with SpO_2, ECG and blood pressure) and interpretation of values.	*May be demonstrated by*: ■ direct observation of procedure ■ teaching session for peers, utilizing an airway manikin ■ practical examination.
Prepare equipment required in relation to open and closed endotracheal suctioning: ■ disposable apron ■ sterile or non-sterile appropriately sized gloves ■ eye protection, such as a facial visor or goggles ■ a selection of suction catheters (10, 12 and 14 French gauge) for open suctioning ■ closed endotracheal suctioning system for closed suctioning ■ vial of 0.9% sodium chloride (if required for catheter irrigation) for closed suctioning ■ functioning suction unit, canister and tubing ■ disposable receptacle or clinical waste bag.	*May be demonstrated by*: ■ direct observation of procedure ■ teaching session for peers, utilizing an airway manikin ■ practical examination.
Demonstrate the correct and safe technique in relation to open and closed endotracheal suctioning: ■ correct selection of suction catheter size ■ correct assembly of suction apparatus ■ appropriate device insertion technique ■ evaluation of intervention.	*May be demonstrated by*: ■ direct observation of procedure. ■ teaching session for peers, utilizing an airway manikin ■ practical examination.

Competency statement 5.15: Specific procedure competency statements for humidification

Complete assessment against relevant fundamental competency statements (*see* Chapter 2, pp. 20, 21)	Evidence
Specific procedure competency statements for humidification	**Evidence of competency for humidification**
Demonstrate ability to: ■ teach and assess or ■ learn from assessment.	Examples of evidence of teaching, assessing and learning.
Identify reason(s) for humidification: ■ patients with an endotracheal tube ■ patients with a tracheostomy tube ■ laryngectomy patients ■ those receiving highflow or high-concentration oxygen therapy.	*May be demonstrated by*: ■ discussion with supervisor/mentor ■ teaching session for peers ■ completion of a reflective text, workbook, or educational package to test knowledge.
Identify risks, potential problems and complications associated with humidification and how to prevent or manage them: ■ insufficient water to achieve optimum humidification ■ insufficient temperature setting to achieve optimum humidification ■ temperature set too high ■ potential for bacterial contamination of humidification apparatus ■ risk of electrical malfunction.	*May be demonstrated by*: ■ discussion with supervisor/mentor ■ teaching session for peers ■ completion of a reflective text, workbook, or educational package to test knowledge.
Demonstrate knowledge and understanding of local and national policies, guidance and procedures in relation to humidification: ■ local or hospital guidelines concerning the use of humidification therapy.	*May be demonstrated by*: ■ discussion with supervisor/mentor ■ teaching session for peers ■ completion of a reflective text, workbook, or educational package to test knowledge.
Demonstrate knowledge and understanding of evidence base in relation to humidification, including: ■ mucociliary escalator ■ absolute humidity.	*May be demonstrated by*: ■ discussion with supervisor/mentor ■ teaching session for peers ■ completion of a reflective text, workbook, or educational package to test knowledge.
Demonstrate skills that are required in relation to humidification: ■ basic respiratory assessment and awareness of signs or symptoms of respiratory distress or deterioration ■ universal precautions ■ use of a bedside patient monitor (with SpO_2, ECG and blood pressure measurement capabilities) and interpretation of values.	*May be demonstrated by*: ■ direct observation of procedure ■ teaching session for peers ■ practical examination.
Prepare equipment required in relation to humidification: ■ humidification device ■ water supply if required.	*May be demonstrated by*: ■ direct observation of procedure ■ teaching session for peers ■ practical examination.
Demonstrate the correct technique for the procedure in relation to humidification: ■ correct assembly of humidification apparatus ■ appropriate monitoring and maintenance of humidification device ■ evaluation of intervention.	*May be demonstrated by*: ■ direct observation of procedure ■ teaching session for peers ■ practical examination.

Competency statement 5.16: Specific procedure competency statements for manual hyperinflation

Complete assessment against relevant fundamental competency statements (*see* Chapter 2, pp. 20, 21)	Evidence
Specific procedure competency statements for manual hyperinflation	**Evidence of competency for manual hyperinflation**
Demonstrate ability to: ■ teach and assess or ■ learn from assessment.	Examples of evidence of teaching, assessing and learning.
Identify reason(s) for manual hyperinflation: ■ to hyperoxygenate patient's pre- and post-endotracheal or tracheal suctioning ■ to assist in the mobilization of respiratory secretions ■ to correct atelectasis.	*May be demonstrated by*: ■ discussion with supervisor/mentor ■ teaching session for peers ■ completion of a reflective text, workbook, or educational package to test knowledge.
Identify risks, potential problems and complications associated with manual hyperinflation and how to prevent or manage them: ■ haemodynamic instability ■ influence on intracranial pressure ■ risks associated with volutrauma or barotrauma.	*May be demonstrated by*: ■ discussion with supervisor/mentor ■ teaching session for peers ■ completion of a reflective text, workbook, or educational package to test knowledge.
Demonstrate knowledge and understanding of local and national policies, guidance and procedures in relation to manual hyperinflation. ■ local policies or hospital guidelines concerning the use of manual hyperinflation.	*May be demonstrated by*: ■ discussion with supervisor/mentor ■ teaching session for peers ■ completion of a reflective text, workbook, or educational package to test knowledge.
Demonstrate knowledge and understanding of evidence base in relation to manual hyperinflation.	*May be demonstrated by*: ■ discussion with supervisor/mentor ■ teaching session for peers ■ completion of a reflective text, workbook, or educational package to test knowledge.
Demonstrate skills that are required in relation to manual hyperinflation: ■ basic respiratory assessment and awareness of signs or symptoms of respiratory distress or deterioration ■ universal precautions ■ use of suction apparatus ■ use of a bedside patient monitor (with SpO_2, ECG and blood pressure) and interpretation of values.	*May be demonstrated by*: ■ direct observation of procedure ■ teaching session for peers, utilizing an airway manikin and bagging circuit ■ practical examination.
Prepare equipment required in relation to manual hyperinflation as detailed in the procedural guideline.	*May be demonstrated by*: ■ direct observation of procedure ■ teaching session for peers, utilizing an airway manikin and bagging circuit ■ practical examination.
Demonstrate the correct technique for the procedure in relation to manual hyperinflation: ■ correct assembly of manual hyperinflation apparatus ■ correct assembly of suction apparatus ■ appropriate manual hyperinflation technique ■ evaluation of intervention.	*May be demonstrated by*: ■ direct observation of procedure ■ teaching session for peers, utilizing an airway manikin and bagging circuit ■ Practical examination.

163

Competency statement 5.17: Specific procedure competency statements for prone positioning

Complete assessment against relevant fundamental competency statements (*see* Chapter 2, pp. 20, 21)	Evidence
Specific procedure competency statements for prone positioning	**Evidence of competency for prone positioning**
Demonstrate ability to: ■ teach and assess or ■ learn from assessment.	Examples of evidence of teaching, assessing and learning.
Identify reason(s) for prone positioning: ■ ARDS or ALI ■ mechanically ventilated patients with high PEEP requirements ■ patients with basal collapse and consolidation that would benefit from postural drainage to aid secretion removal ■ patients with a respiratory acidosis.	*May be demonstrated by*: ■ discussion with supervisor/mentor ■ teaching session for peers ■ completion of a reflective text, workbook, or educational package.
Identify risks, potential problems and complications associated with prone positioning and how to prevent or manage them: ■ wound considerations, i.e. anterior chest or abdominal wounds ■ haemodynamic instability, prior to and due to the procedure ■ logistical considerations, i.e. number of staff available, equipment and expertise to perform procedure safely ■ anatomical considerations, i.e. pregnant or abdominally obese patients, presence of external fixators.	*May be demonstrated by*: ■ discussion with supervisor/mentor ■ teaching session for peers ■ completion of a reflective text, workbook, or educational package.
Demonstrate knowledge and understanding of local and national policies, guidance and procedures in relation to prone positioning: ■ local or hospital guidelines concerning prone positioning.	*May be demonstrated by*: ■ discussion with supervisor/mentor ■ teaching session for peers ■ completion of a reflective text, workbook, or educational package.
Demonstrate knowledge and understanding of evidence base in relation to prone positioning.	*May be demonstrated by*: ■ discussion with supervisor/mentor ■ teaching session for peers ■ completion of a reflective text, workbook, or educational package.
Demonstrate skills that are required in relation to prone positioning: ■ basic respiratory assessment and awareness of signs or symptoms of respiratory distress or deterioration ■ universal precautions ■ awareness and knowledge of safe manual handling practices ■ use of a bedside patient monitor (with SpO_2, ECG and blood pressure) and interpretation of values.	*May be demonstrated by*: ■ direct observation of procedure ■ teaching session for peers ■ practical examination.
Prepare equipment required in relation to prone positioning: ■ non-sterile gloves ■ disposable apron ■ a minimum of five practitioners, including one anaesthetist ■ pressure-relieving mattress ■ sheets ■ pillows.	*May be demonstrated by*: ■ direct observation of procedure ■ teaching session for peers ■ practical examination.
Demonstrate the correct technique for the procedure in relation to prone positioning: ■ correct assembly of required equipment/personnel ■ performs the prone positioning manoeuvre ■ evaluation of intervention.	*May be demonstrated by*: ■ direct observation of procedure ■ teaching session for peers ■ practical examination.

Competency statement 5.18: Specific procedure competency statements for insertion of a chest drain

Complete assessment against relevant fundamental competency statements (*see* Chapter 2, pp. 20, 21)	Evidence
Specific procedure competency statements for chest drain insertion	**Evidence of competency for chest drain insertion**
Demonstrate ability to: ■ teach and assess or ■ learn from assessment.	Examples of evidence of teaching, assessing and learning.
Identify reason(s) for chest drain insertion: ■ pneumothorax in a mechanically ventilated patient ■ following needle thoracocentesis for a tension pneumothorax ■ persistent or recurrent pneumothorax following simple needle decompression/aspiration ■ large secondary spontaneous pneumothorax in patients over 50 years of age ■ malignant pleural effusion ■ empyema and complicated parapneumonic pleural effusion ■ traumatic haemopneumothorax ■ postoperative, i.e. following cardiothoracic surgery.	*May be demonstrated by*: ■ discussion with supervisor/mentor ■ teaching session for peers ■ completion of a reflective text, workbook, or educational package to test knowledge.
Identify risks, potential problems and complications associated with chest drain insertion and how to prevent or manage them: ■ surgical emphysema ■ haemorrhage ■ acute respiratory distress following procedure ■ pain or discomfort.	*May be demonstrated by*: ■ discussion with supervisor/mentor ■ teaching session for peers ■ completion of a reflective text, workbook, or educational package to test knowledge.
Demonstrate knowledge and understanding of local and national policies, guidance and procedures in relation to chest drain insertion: ■ national guidelines from the British Thoracic Society (BTS) ■ local or hospital guidelines concerning the insertion of chest tubes.	*May be demonstrated by*: ■ discussion with supervisor/mentor ■ teaching session for peers ■ completion of a reflective text, workbook, or educational package to test knowledge.
Demonstrate knowledge and understanding of evidence base in relation to chest drain insertion.	*May be demonstrated by*: ■ discussion with supervisor/mentor ■ teaching session for peers ■ completion of a reflective text, workbook, or educational package to test knowledge.
Demonstrate skills that are required in relation to chest drain insertion: ■ basic respiratory assessment and awareness of signs or symptoms of respiratory distress or deterioration ■ universal precautions ■ pain assessment and management ■ use of a bedside patient monitor (with SpO_2, ECG and blood pressure measurement capabilities) and interpretation of values.	*May be demonstrated by*: ■ direct observation of procedure ■ teaching session for peers ■ practical examination.

165

(Continued)

Competency statement 5.18: *(Continued)*

Prepare equipment required in relation to chest drain insertion: ■ sterile and non-sterile gloves and sterile gown ■ sterile drapes ■ skin antiseptic solution, i.e. iodine or chlorhexidine in alcohol ■ local anaesthetic, i.e. 1% or 2% lidocaine ■ selection of sterile syringes and needles ■ sterile gauze swabs ■ scalpel with blade ■ forceps (round tipped) or 'Kelly clamp' for blunt dissection ■ chest drain.	*May be demonstrated by*: ■ direct observation of procedure ■ teaching session for peers ■ practical examination.
Demonstrate the correct technique for the procedure in relation to chest drain insertion: ■ correct selection of chest drain tube ■ correct assembly of chest drain insertion apparatus ■ correct assembly of chest drain canister and tubing ■ appropriate device insertion technique ■ evaluation of intervention.	*May be demonstrated by*: ■ direct observation of procedure ■ teaching session for peers ■ practical examination.

166

Competency statement 5.19: Specific procedure competency statements for removal of a chest drain

Complete assessment against relevant fundamental competency statements (*see* Chapter 2, pp. 20, 21)	Evidence
Specific procedure competency statements for chest drain removal	**Evidence of competency for chest drain removal**
Demonstrate ability to: ■ teach and assess or ■ learn from assessment.	Examples of evidence of teaching, assessing and learning.
Identify reason(s) for chest drain removal: ■ following successful drainage of a pleural effusion ■ following successful drainage of pneumothorax and lung re-expansion.	*May be demonstrated by*: ■ discussion with supervisor/mentor ■ teaching session for peers ■ completion of a reflective text, workbook, or educational package.
Identify risks, potential problems and complications associated with chest drain removal and how to prevent or manage them: ■ development of a pneumothorax ■ development of a tension pneumothorax ■ continued leakage or haemorrhage from drain incision ■ wound infections surrounding the chest drain incision.	*May be demonstrated by*: ■ discussion with supervisor/mentor ■ teaching session for peers ■ completion of a reflective text, workbook, or educational package.
Demonstrate knowledge and understanding of local and national policies, guidance and procedures in relation to chest drain removal: ■ national guidelines from the British Thoracic Society (BTS) ■ local or hospital guidelines concerning the insertion of chest tubes.	*May be demonstrated by*: ■ discussion with supervisor/mentor ■ teaching session for peers ■ completion of a reflective text, workbook, or educational package.

Demonstrate knowledge and understanding of evidence base in relation to chest drain removal.	*May be demonstrated by*: ■ discussion with supervisor/mentor ■ teaching session for peers ■ completion of a reflective text, workbook, or educational package.
Demonstrate skills that are required in relation to chest drain removal: ■ basic respiratory assessment and awareness of signs or symptoms of respiratory distress or deterioration ■ universal precautions ■ pain assessment and management ■ use of a bedside patient monitor (with SpO_2, ECG and blood pressure measurement capabilities) and interpretation of values.	*May be demonstrated by*: ■ direct observation of procedure ■ teaching session for peers ■ practical examination.
Prepare equipment required in relation to chest drain removal: ■ non-sterile gloves ■ disposable apron ■ eye protection ■ sterile stitch-cutter blade ■ forceps/clamps, i.e. Spencer Wells clamps ■ sterile gauze swabs ■ manual inspiratory hold function on the patient's mechanical ventilator ■ two appropriately trained healthcare practitioners.	*May be demonstrated by*: ■ direct observation of procedure ■ teaching session for peers ■ practical examination.
Demonstrate the correct technique for the procedure in relation to chest drain removal.	*May be demonstrated by*: ■ direct observation of procedure ■ teaching session for peers ■ practical examination.

167

References and further reading

Adam S and Osbourne S (2005) *Critical Care Nursing: science and practice*. Oxford: Oxford University Press.

Aguinagaldea B, Zabaletaa J, Fuentesa M et al. (2010) Percutaneous aspiration versus tube drainage for spontaneous pneumothorax: systematic review and meta-analysis. *European Journal of Cardiothoracic Surgery* 37(5): 1129–1135.

American Association of Respiratory Care (2010) AARC clinical practice guidelines: endotracheal suctioning of mechanically ventilated patients with artificial airways 2010. *Respiratory Care* 55(6): 758–764.

American College of Surgeons Committee on Trauma (2008) *Advanced Trauma Life Support Student Course Manual* (8e). Chicago: ACS.

Ball C, Adams J, Boyce S and Robinson P (2001) Clinical guidelines for the use of the prone position in acute respiratory distress syndrome. *Intensive and Critical Care Nursing* 17(2): 94–104.

Berenholtz SM, Pham JC, Thompson DA et al. (2011) Collaborative cohort study of an intervention to reduce ventilator associated pneumonia in an intensive care unit. *Infection Control Hospital Epidemiology* 32: 305–314.

Berney S and Denehy L (2002) A comparison of the effects of manual and ventilator hyperinflation on static lung compliance and sputum production in intubated and ventilated intensive care patients. *Physiotherapy Research International* 7(2): 100–108.

Bersten A (2004) Respiratory monitoring. In: Bersten A and Soni N (eds) *Oh's Intensive Care Manual* (5e). Oxford: Butterworth-Heinnemann.

Bickley L (2010) *Bates Guide to Physical Examination and History Taking* (10e). Philadelphia: Lippincott, Williams and Wilkins.

Bien M-Y, Lin YS, Shie H-G et al. (2010) Rapid shallow breathing index and its predictive accuracy measured under five different ventilatory strategies in the same patient group. *Chinese Journal of Physiology* 53(1): 1–10.

Bigatello LM, Patroniti N and Sangalli F (2001) Permissive hypercapnia. *Current Opinion in Critical Care* 7(1): 34–40.

Blackwood B, Alderdice F, Burns K et al. (2011) Use of weaning protocols for reducing duration of mechanical ventilation in critically ill adult patients: Cochrane systematic review and meta-analysis. *British Medical Journal* 342: c7237.

Blattner C, Guaragna JC and Saadi E (2008) Oxygenation and static compliance is improved immediately after early manual hyperinflation following myocardial revascularisation: a randomised controlled trial. *Australian Journal of Physiotherapy* 54: 173–178.

British Association of Critical Care Nurses (2010) *Standards for Nurse Staffing in Critical Care*. London: BACCN.

British Thoracic Society (2001) *BTS Guidelines on Diagnostic Flexible Bronchoscopy*. London: BTS.

British Thoracic Society (2008) *The use of non-invasive ventilation in the management of patients with chronic obstructive pulmonary disease admitted to hospital with acute type II respiratory failure (with particular reference to Bilevel positive pressure ventilation)*. London: BTS.

Burns KEA, Adhikari NKJ and Meade MO (2006) Metanalysis of non-invasive weaning to facilitate liberation form mechanical ventilation. *The Canadian Journal of Anaesthesia* 53: 305–315.

Capovilla J, Van Couwenberghe C and Miller WA (2000) Non-invasive blood gas monitoring. *Critical Care Nursing Quarterly* 23(2): 79–86.

Chalon J, Loew DA and Malebranch J (1972) Effect of dry anaesthetic gas on tracheobronchial ciliated epithelium. *Anesthesiology* 37: 338–343.

Chevron V, Ménard JF, Richard JC et al. (1998) Unplanned extubation: risk factors of development and predictive criteria for reintubation. *Critical Care Medicine* 26(6): 1049–1053.

Choi JS and Jones AY (2005) Effects of manual hyperinflation and suctioning in respiratory mechanics in mechanically ventilated patients with ventilator-associated pneumonia. *Australian Journal of Physiotherapy* 51(1): 25–30.

Choyce MS, Avidan C, Patel A et al. (2000) Comparison of laryngeal mask and intubating laryngeal mask insertion by the naive intubator. British Journal of *Anaesthesia* 84: 103–105.

Coombs MA and Morse SE (2002) Physical assessment skills: a developing dimension of clinical nursing practice. *Intensive and Critical Care Nursing* 18: 200–210.

Day T, Farnell S and Wilson-Barnett J (2002) Suctioning: a review of current research recommendations. *Intensive and Critical Care Nursing* 18: 79–89.

Denehy L and Berney S (2001) The use of positive pressure devices by physiotherapists. *European Respiratory Journal* 17: 821–829.

Dennis D, Jacob W and Budgeon C (2012) Ventilator versus manual hyperinflation in clearing sputum in ventilated intensive care unit patients. *Anaesthesia and Intensive Care* 40(1): 142–149.

Department of Health (2007) *Saving Lives: reducing infection, delivering clean and safe care*. London: DH.

Department of Health (2008) *The Health and Social Care Act 2008: Code of Practice for health and adult social care on the prevention and control of infections and related guidance*. London: DH.

Department of Health (2008) *Clean, Safe Care, Reducing Infection and Saving Lives*. London: DH.

Department of Health (2010a) *Advanced Level Nursing: a position statement*. London: DH.

Department of Health (2010b) *Essence of Care: 2010*. London: DH.

Department of Health (2011) High impact intervention care bundle to reduce ventilation associated pneumonia.hcai.dh.gov.uk/. . ./2011-03-14-HII-Ventilator-Associated-Pneumonia-FINAL.1. PDF. [accessed 13 June 2011].

Dougherty L and Lister S (2011) *The Royal Marsden Hospital Manual of Clinical Nursing Procedures* (8e). Oxford: Wiley-Blackwell. The Royal Marsden Hospital.

Ely EW, Baker AM, Dunagan DP et al. (1996) Effect on the duration of mechanical ventilation of identifying patients capable of breathing spontaneously. *New England Journal of Medicine* 335: 1864–1869.

Epstein SK (2004) Putting it all together to predict extubation outcomes. *Intensive Care Medicine* 30(7): 1255–1257.

Epstein SK (2004) Extubation failure: an outcome to be avoided. *Critical Care* 8(5): 310–312.

Epstein S (2006) Complications in ventilator supported patients. In; Tobin M (ed.) *Principles and Practice of Mechanical Ventilation* (2e). New York: MacGraw Hill.

Esteban A, Frutos, Tobin MJ et al. (1995) A comparison of four methods of weaning patients from mechanical ventilation. *New England Journal of Medicine* 332: 345–350.

Esteban A, Anzueto A, Frutos F et al. (2002) Characteristics and outcomes in adult patients receiving mechanical ventilation; a 28 day international study. *Journal of American Medical Association* 287: 345–355.

Fan E and Rubenfeld GD (2010) High frequency oscillation in acute lung injury and ARDS. *British Medical Journal* 340: c2315.

Frutos-Vivar F, Ferguson ND, Esteban A et al. (2006) Risk factors for extubation failure in patients following a successful spontaneous breathing trial. *Chest* 130(6): 1664–1671.

Gaffney AM, Wildhirt SM, Griffin MJ et al. (2010) Extracorporeal life support. Clinical Review. *British Medical Journal* 341: c5317.

Gattinoni L and Pesenti A (2005) The concept of 'baby lung'. *Intensive Care Medicine* 31(6): 776–784.

Gattinoni L, Tognoni G, Pesenti A et al. (2001) Effect of prone positioning on the survival of patients with acute respiratory failure. *New England Journal of Medicine* 345(8): 568–573.

General Medical Council (2013) *Good Medical Practice*. London: GMC. http://www.gmc-uk.org/gmp2013 [accessed 25 March 2013].

Griffiths J, Barber VS, Morgan L and Young JD (2005) Systematic review and meta-analysis of studies of the timing of tracheostomy in adult patients undergoing artificial ventilation. *British Medical Journal* 330(7502): 1243. doi:10.1136/bmj.38467.485671.E0.

Gujadhur R, Helme BW, Sanni A and Dunning J (2005) Continuous subglottic suction is effective for prevention of ventilator associated pneumonia. *Interactive Cardiovascular and Thoracic Surgery* 4(2): 110–115. doi: 10.1510/icvts.2004.100149.

Hallais C, Merle V, Guitard PG et al. (2011) Is continuous subglottic suctioning cost-effective for the prevention of ventilator-associated pneumonia? *Infection Control and Hospital Epidemiology* 32(2): 13115.

Harden B (2004) *Emergency Physiotherapy*. London: Churchill Livingstone.

Haron H, Rashid NA, Dimon MZ et al. (2010) Chest tube injury to left ventricle: complication or negligence? *Annals of Thoracic Surgery* 90: 308–309.

Havelock T, Teoh R, Laws D et al. on behalf of the BTS Pleural Disease Guideline Group (2010) Pleural procedures and thoracic ultrasound: British Thoracic Society pleural disease guideline. *Thorax* 65(Suppl 2): ii61–eii76.

Health and Care Professions Council (2012) *Standard of Conduct, Performance and Ethics*. London: HCPC. http://www.hcpc-uk.org/assets/documents/10003B6EStandardsofconduct,performanceandethics.pdf [accessed January 2013].

Hedenstierna G and Lennart E (2010) Mechanisms of atelectasis in the perioperative period. *Clinical Anaesthesiology* 24(2): 157–169.

Heimlich HJ (1983) Heimlich valve for chest drainage. *Medical Instrumentation* 17(1): 29–31.

Hess DR (2000) Nebulizers: principles and performance. *Respiratory Care* 45(6): 609–622.

Hess DR, Kallstrom TJ, Mottram CD et al. (2003) AARC Clinical practice guideline. Care of the ventilator circuit and its relation to ventilator-associated pneumonia. *Respiratory Care* 48(9): 869–879.

Hodd J, Doyle A, Carter J, Albarran J and Young P (2010) Extubation in intensive care units in the UK: an online survey. *Nursing in Critical Care* 15(6): 281–284.

Hodgson C, Denehy L, Ntoumenopoulos G, Santamaria J and Carroll S (2000) An investigation of the early effects of manual lung hyperinflation in critically ill patients. *Anaesthesia and Intensive Care* **28**: 255–261.

Hunter J (2008) Chest drain removal. *Nursing Standard* **22**: 45, 35–38.

Intensive Care Society (2007) When and how to wean [online]. http://www.ics.ac.uk/intensive_care_professional/standards_and_guidelines/weaning_guidelines_2007_ [accessed 30 January 2013].

Intensive Care Society (2008) Standards for the care of adult patients with a temporary tracheostomy [online]. Available from: http://www.ics.ac.uk/intensive_care_professional/standards_and_guidelines/care_of_the_adult_patient_with_a_temporary_tracheostomy_2008 [accessed 1 April 2011].

Intensive Care Society (2011) Capnography Guidelines. [online]. Available from: http://www.ics.ac.uk/professional/standards_safety_quality/standards_and_guidelines/capnography_guidelines [Accessed 25 January 2013].

Jarvis C (2008) *Physical Examination and Health Assessment (6e)*. Missouri, USA: Elsevier Saunders.

Jensen LA, Onyskiw JE and Prasad NGN (1998) Meta-analysis of arterial oxygen saturation monitoring by pulse oximetry in adults. *Heart and Lung* **27**(6): 387–408.

Jevon P and Pooni JS (2007) *Treating the Critically Ill Patient*. Oxford: Blackwell Publishing.

Johnson P (2004) Reclaiming the everyday world: how long term patients in critical care seek to gain aspects of power and control over their environment. *Intensive and Critical Care Nursing* **20**(4): 190–199.

Joynt GM (2009) Airway management and acute upper-airway obstruction. In: Oh TE (ed.) *Intensive Care Manual (6e)*. Oxford: Butterworth-Heinemann.

Kallet RH (2009) Noninvasive ventilation in acute care: controversies and emerging concepts. *Respiratory Care* **54**(2): 259 –263.

Keilty S and Bott J (1992) Continuous positive airways pressure. *Physiotherapy* **78**(2): 90–92.

Khan FM, Bokhamsin A and Carol J (2011) Application of VAP bundles resulting in low incidence of VAP in ICU. *BMC Proceedings* **5**(Suppl 6): P68.

Kimberly-Clark (2003) *Ballard TRACH CARE closed suction system for adults* [Online]. Available from: http://www.vap.kchealthcare.com/media/62888/trach%20care%2072%20hour%20css%20dfu.pdf [Accessed 25 January 2013].

Koroloff N, Boots R, Lipman J et al. (2004) A randomised controlled study of the efficacy of hypromellose and Lacri-Lube combination versus polyethylene/cling wrap to prevent corneal epithelial breakdown in the semiconscious intensive care patient. *Intensive Care Medicine* **30**(6): 1122–1126.

Krishnan JA, Moore D, Robeson C et al. (2004) A prospective, controlled trial of a protocol-based strategy to discontinue mechanical ventilation. *American Journal of Respiratory and Critical Care Medicine* **169**(6): 673–678.

Krishnan JA and Brower RG (2000) High-frequency ventilation for acute lung injury and ARDS. *Chest* **118**(3): 795–807.

Lavery GG and McCloskey BV (2008) The difficult airway in adult critical care. *Critical Care Medicine* **36**(7): 2163–2173.

Laws D, Neville E and Duffy J (2003) British Thoracic Society guidelines for the insertion of a chest drain. *Thorax* **58**(Suppl II): ii53–59.

Levitan R and Ochroch EA (2000) Airway management and direct laryngoscopy: a review and update. *Critical Care Clinics* **16**: 373.

Lorente L, Lecuona M, Jiménez A et al. (2007) Influence of an endotracheal tube with polyurethane cuff and subglottic secretion drainage on pneumonia. *American Journal of Respiratory and Critical Care Medicine* **176**: 1079–1083.

Loring SH, Garcia-Jacques M and Malhotra A (2009) Pulmonary characteristics in COPD and mechanisms of increased work of breathing. *Journal of Applied Physiology* **107**: 309–314.

Lowthian P (1997) Notes on the pathogenesis of serious pressure sores. *British Journal of Nursing* **6**(16): 344–353.

Luketich JD, Kiss MD, Hershey J et al. (1984) Chest tube insertion: a prospective evaluation of pain management. *Clinical Journal of Pain* **14**: 152–154.

Lynn-McHale Wiegand DJ (2011) *American Association of Critical Care Nurses (AACCN) Procedure Manual for Critical Care*. 6th edition. St Louis: Saunders Elsevier.

Maa S-H, Hung T-J and Hsu K-H (2005) Manual hyperinflation improves alveolar recruitment in difficult-to-wean patients. *Chest* **128**: 2714–2721.

MacIntyre NR (2001) Evidence-based guidelines for weaning and discontinuing ventilatory support: A collective task force facilitated by the American College of Chest Physicians; the American Association for Respiratory Care; and the American College of Critical Care Medicine. *Chest Journal* **120**(suppl 6): 375S–496S http://journal.publications.chestnet.org/issue.aspx?journalid=99&issueid=21971&direction=P [accessed 30 January 2013].

Mangione S (2000) *Physical Diagnosis Secrets*. Philadelphia: Hanley and Belfus Inc.

Marieb E (2008) *Human Anatomy and Physiology (9e)*. California: Addison Wesley.

Marieb EN and Hoehn K (2007) Human Anatomy and Physiology (7e). San Francisco: Pearson Benjamin Cummings. Maxwell LJ and Ellis ER (2007) Pattern of ventilation during manual hyperinflation performed by physiotherapists. *Anaesthesia* **62**: 27–33.

McAuley DF, Giles S, Fichter H et al. (2002) What is the optimal duration of ventilation in the prone position in acute lung injury and acute respiratory distress syndrome? *Intensive Care Medicine* **28**(4): 414–418.

McCormick J and Blackwood B (2001) Nursing the ARDS patient in the prone position: the experiences of qualified ICU nurses. *Intensive & Critical Care Nursing* **17**: 331–340.

Mental Capacity Act (2005) http://www.legislation.gov.uk/ukpga/2005/9/pdfs/ukpga_20050009_en.pdf [accessed 9 February 2012].

Moerer O (2012) Effort-adapted modes of assisted breathing. *Current Opinion in Critical Care* **18**(1): 61–66.

Moore T and Woodrow P (2009) *High Dependency Nursing Care. Observation intervention and support for level 2 patients* (2e). London: Routledge Taylor and Francis.

Moran JL, Chalwin RP and Graham PL (2010) Extracorporeal membrane oxygenation (ECMO) reconsidered. *Critical Care and Resuscitation* **12**: 131–135.

Moule P and Albarran J (2009) *Practical Resuscitation for Healthcare Professionals*. 2nd edition. Oxford: Wiley-Blackwell.

National Institute for Health and Clinical Excellence/National Patient Safety Agency (2008) *Technical patients safety solutions for ventilator associated pneumonia in adults. Alert reference NICE/NPSA/2008/PSG002*. London: DH.

Needham DM, Thompson DA, Holzmueller CG et al. (2004) A system factors analysis of airway events from the Intensive Care Unit Safety Reporting System (ICUSRS). *Critical Care Medicine* **32**: 2227–2233.

NICE-SUGAR Study Investigators (2009) Intensive versus conventional glucose control in critically ill patients. *New England Journal of Medicine* **360**: 1283–1297.

Northern Health and Social Care Trust (2007) *Manual Hyperinflation of Adult Patients in Critical Care. A guideline*. Northern Health and Social Care Trust, Northern Ireland.

Nursing and Midwifery Council (2008) *The Code: standards of conduct, performance and ethics for nurses and midwives*.

London: NMC. http://www.nmc-uk.org/Documents/Standards/The-code-A4-20100406.pdf [accessed 15 February 2012].

Ortiz G, Frutos-Vivar F, Ferguson ND et al. Outcomes of patients ventilated with synchronized intermittent mandatory ventilation with pressure support. A comparative propensity score study. *Chest* 137(6): 1265–1277.

Paratz J, Lipman J and McAuliffe M (2002) Effect of manual hyperinflation on hemodynamics, gas exchange, and respiratory mechanics in ventilated patients. *Intensive Care Medicine* 17(6): 317–324.

Pedersen CM, Rosendahl-Nielsen M, Hjermind J and Egerod I (2009) Endotracheal suctioning of the adult intubated patient – what is the evidence? *Intensive and Critical Care Nursing* 25: 21–30.

Penuelas O, Frutos-Vivar F, Fernandez C et al. (2011) Characteristics and outcomes of ventilated patients according to time to liberation from mechanical ventilation. *American Journal of Respiratory and Critical Care Medicine* 184(4): 430–437.

Place B (2000) Pulse oximetry: benefits and limitations. *Nursing Times* 96(26): 42.

Priestley MA (2006) Respiratory failure. www.emedicine.com/med/topic1994.htm [accessed 16 July 2011].

Pryor JP, Reilly PM and Shapiro MB (2000) Surgical airway management in the intensive care unit. *Critical Care Clinics* 16: 473.

Prytherch DR, Smith GB, Schmidt P and Featherstone PI (2010) ViEWS – Towards a national early warning score for detecting adult inpatient deterioration. *Resuscitation* 81: 932–937.

Ramachandran K and Kannan S (2004) Laryngeal mask airway and the difficult airway. *Current Opinion in Anaesthesiology* 17: 491–493.

Resuscitation Council UK (2011) *Advanced Life Support* (6e). London: Resuscitation Council UK.

Roberts CM, Stone RA, Buckingham RJ et al. (2011) Acidosis, non-invasive ventilation and mortality in hospitalised COPD exacerbations. *Thorax* 66: 43e8.

Roberts K Whally H and Bleetman A (2005) The nasopharyngeal airway: dispelling myths and establishing the facts. *Emergency Medicine Journal* 22: 394–396.

Rodricks MB and Deutschman CS (2000) Emerging airway management: Indications and methods in the face of confounding conditions. *Critical Care Clinics* 16: 389.

Rolls K, Smith K, Jones P et al. (2007) *Suctioning an adult with a tracheal tube*. NSW Guidelines for Intensive Care. New South Wales Intensive Care Co-ordination and Monitoring Unit (ICCUM).

Rothaar RC and Epstein SK (2003) Extubation failure: magnitude of the problem, impact on outcomes, and prevention. *Current Opinion in Critical Care* 9(1): 59–66.

Rothen H, Sporre B, Engberg G, Wegenius G and Hedenstierna G (1993) Re-expansion of atelectasis during general anaesthesia: a computed tomography study. *British Journal of Anaesthesia* 71: 788–795.

Rowe C (2004) Development of clinical guidelines for prone positioning in critically ill adults, *Nursing in Critical Care* 9 (2): 50–57.

Rushforth H (2009) *Assessment Made Incredibly Easy!* London: Lippincott, Williams and Wilkins.

Russell C (2005) Providing the nurse with a guide to tracheostomy care and management. *British Journal of Nursing* 4(8): 428–433.

Savian C, Paratz J and Davies A (2006). Comparison of the effectiveness of manual and ventilator hyperinflation at different levels of positive end-expiratory pressure in artificially ventilated and intubated intensive care patients. *Heart & Lung: The Journal of Acute and Critical Care* 35(5): 334–341.

Scales K and Pilsworth J (2007) A practical guide to extubation. *Nursing Standard* 22(2): 44–48.

Schade K, Borzotta A and Michaels A (2000) Intracranial malposition of nasopharyngeal airway. *Journal of Trauma* 49(5): 967–968.

Scottish Intensive Care Society (2010) ICM induction programme. www.scottishintensivecare.org.uk

Seckel MA (2008) Ask the experts. *Critical Care Nurse* 28 (1): 65–66.

Sengupta P, Sessler DI Magliner P et al. (2004) Endotracheal tube cuff pressure in three hospitals, and the volume required to produce an appropriate cuff pressure. *BMC Anaesthesiology* 4: 8doi:10.1186/1471-2253-4-8.

Shalli S, Saeed D, Kiyotaka Fukamachi K et al. (2009) Chest tube selection in cardiac and thoracic surgery: a survey of chest tube-related complications and their management. *Journal of Cardiac Surgery* 24(5): 503.

Sharma S (2006) Respiratory failure. www.emedicine.com/med/topic2011.htm [accessed 16 July 2011].

Siempos II, Vardakas KZ, Kopterides P et al. (2007) Impact of passive humidification on clinical outcomes of mechanically ventilated patients: a meta-analysis of randomized controlled trials. *Critical Care Medicine* 35(12): 2843–2851.

Simpson H (2004) Interpretation of arterial blood gases: a clinical guide for nurses. *British Journal of Nursing* 13(9): 522–528.

Singer M, Vermaat J, Hall G et al. (1994) Haemodynamic effects of manual hyperinflation in critically ill mechanically ventilated patients. *Chest* 106: 1182–1187.

Sivasankar S, Jasper S, Simon S et al. (2006) Eye care in ICU. *Indian Journal of Critical Care Medicine* 1 (1): 11–14.

Steer J, Gibson G and Bourke S (2010) Predicting outcomes following hospitalization for acute exacerbations of COPD. *Quarterly Journal of Medicine* 103(11): 817–829.

Stiller K (2000) Physiotherapy in intensive care. *Chest* 118: 1801–1813.

Sud S, Friedrich JO, Taccone P et al. (2010a) Prone ventilation reduces mortality in patients with acute respiratory failure and severe hypoxemia: systematic review and meta-analysis. *Intensive Care Medicine* 36: 585–599.

Sud S, Sud M, Friedrich JO et al. (2010b) High frequency oscillation in acute lung injury and acute respiratory distress syndrome (ARDS): systematic review and meta-analysis. *British Medical Journal* 340: c2327.

Tanios MA, Nevins ML, Hendra KP et al. (2006) A randomized, controlled trial of the role of weaning: predictors in clinical decision making. *Critical Care Medicine* 4: 2530–2535.

Thompson C (2010) *Virtual Anaesthesia Textbook*. http://www.anaesthesia.med.usyd.edu.au/resources/lectures/humidity_clt/humidity.html [accessed June 2012].

Thompson L (2000) Suctioning adults with an artificial airway. In: *A Systematic Review* – Number 9. Australia: The Joanna Briggs Institute for Evidence Based Nursing and Midwifery.

Thompson CE and Stroud SD (1984) Allen's test: a tool for diagnosing ulnar artery trauma. *Nurse Practitioner* 9: 16–17.

Tobin MJ (2011) The new irrationalism in weaning. *Jornal Brasileiro de Pneumologia* 37(5): 571–573.

Tobin MJ and Jubran A (2006) Variable performance of weaning-predictotests: role of Bayes' theorem and spectrum and test-referral bias. *Intensive Care Medicine* 32: 2002–2012.

Tortora B and Derrickson GJ (2011) *Principles of Anatomy and Physiology* (13e). New Jersey: John Wiley and Sons.

TRACMAN (2009) Tracheostomy management in critical care. http://tracman.org.uk

Urden LD, Stacy KM and Lough ME (2002) *Thelan's Critical Care Nursing. Diagnosis and management.* St Louis, MO: Mosby.

Urden L, Stacey K and Lough M (2005) *Thelans Critical Care Nursing (5e)*. St Louis, MO: Mosby.

Van den Berghe G, Wilmer A, Hermans G et al. (2006) Intensive insulin therapy in the ICU. *New England Journal of Medicine* **354**(5): 449–461.

Van de Leur JP, Zwavering JH, Loef BG, Van de Schans CP (2003) Patient recollection of airway suctioning in the ICU: routine versus a minimally invasive procedure. *Intensive Care Medicine* **29**(3): 433–436.

Vassilakopoulos T, Zakynthinos S and Roussos C (2006) Bench-to-bedside review: weaning failure – should we rest the respiratory muscles with controlled mechanical ventilation? *Critical Care* **10**: 204.

Ward NS (2002) Effects of prone position ventilation in ARDS. An evidence-based review of the literature. *Critical Care Clinics* **18**(1): 35–44.

Weber BA and Pryor JA (1993) Physiotherapy skills: techniques and adjuncts. In: Weber BA and Pryor JA (eds) *Physiotherapy for Cardiac and Respiratory Problems*, pp. 113–172. London: Churchill Livingstone.

Wilkes AR (2005) Breathing filters, humidifiers and nebulizers. In: Davey AJ and Diba A (eds) Ward's Anaesthetic Equipment (5e). Philadelphia: Elsevier Saunders.

Wilkes AR (2011a) Heat and moisture exchangers and breathing system filters: their use in anaesthesia and intensive care. Part 1 – history, principles and efficiency. *Anaesthesia* **66**: 31–39.

Wilkes AR (2011b) Heat and moisture exchangers and breathing system filters: their use in anaesthesia and intensive care. Part 2 – practical use, including problems, and their use with paediatric patients. *Anaesthesia* **66**: 40–51.

Williams T (2005) Humidification in intensive care. *South African Journal of Critical Care* **21**(1): 26–31.

Wood C (1998) Endotracheal suctioning: a literature review. *Intensive and Critical Care Nursing* **14**: 124–136.

Woodrow P (2008) *Intensive Care Nursing. A framework for practice* (2e). Abingdon: Routledge Taylor Francis.

Chapter 6

Monitoring of the cardiovascular system: insertion and assessment

Alan T. Platt,[1] Sarah Conolly[2] and Jonathan Round[3]

[1]Northumbria University, Newcastle upon Tyne, UK
[2]James Cook University Hospital, Middlesbrough, UK
[3]Northern Deanery, UK

Critical Care Manual of Clinical Procedures and Competencies, First Edition.
Edited by Jane Mallett, John W. Albarran, and Annette Richardson.
© 2013 John Wiley & Sons, Ltd. Published 2013 by John Wiley & Sons, Ltd.

Introduction

Monitoring the dynamic nature of the cardiovascular system is central to the care of all critically ill patients (Jevon et al. 2007), and practitioners need to possess the knowledge and skills to provide this care in a competent and effective manner. Essential skills include the monitoring of the electrocardiogram, invasive and non-invasive blood pressure, central venous pressure and advanced haemodynamic monitoring techniques (*see also* Chapter 3 for immediate care).

Electrocardiogram monitoring

Definition

An electrocardiogram (ECG) is a recording of the voltage variations within the heart (arising from the atria and ventricles) plotted against time. Duration is measured on the ECG paper on the horizontal axis and amplitude (voltage) measured on the vertical axis.

Aims and indications

The ECG is used to monitor:

- heart rate
- myocardial ischaemia or infarction
- arrhythmias
- conduction defects.

Background

Anatomy and physiology

The contraction and relaxation of cardiac muscle (*see* Figure 6.1) is due to depolarization and repolarizsation of cardiac cells. It is the passage of these electrical signals through the heart that is recorded on the ECG. The conduction pathway is summarized in Figure 6.2. The depolarization begins at the sinoatrial (SA) node, which is located in the right atrium near to where the superior vena cava (SVC) enters. The SA node is a collection of modified myocardial pacemaker cells, which maintain the resting heart rate at between 60 and 100 beats per minute. The rate is mainly controlled through the

174

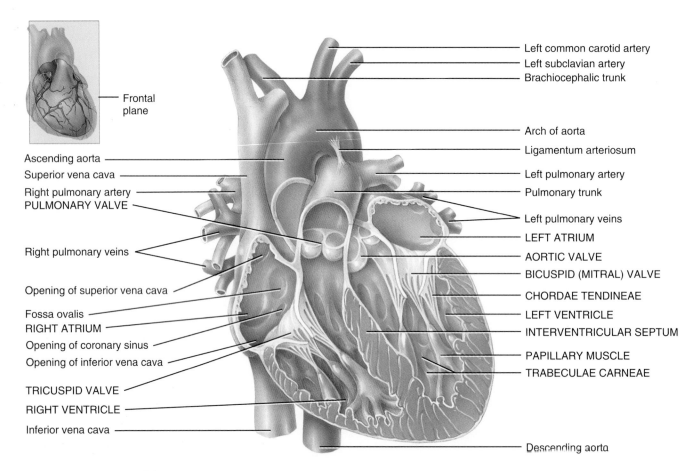

Frontal plane

Ascending aorta
Superior vena cava
Right pulmonary artery
PULMONARY VALVE

Right pulmonary veins

Opening of superior vena cava

Fossa ovalis
RIGHT ATRIUM
Opening of coronary sinus
Opening of inferior vena cava

TRICUSPID VALVE

RIGHT VENTRICLE

Inferior vena cava

Left common carotid artery
Left subclavian artery
Brachiocephalic trunk

Arch of aorta
Ligamentum arteriosum
Left pulmonary artery
Pulmonary trunk

Left pulmonary veins
LEFT ATRIUM
AORTIC VALVE
BICUSPID (MITRAL) VALVE
CHORDAE TENDINEAE
LEFT VENTRICLE
INTERVENTRICULAR SEPTUM
PAPILLARY MUSCLE
TRABECULAE CARNEAE

Descending aorta

Figure 6.1 Structure of the heart: anterior view of frontal section showing internal anatomy (from Tortora and Derrickson 2011, reproduced with permission from Wiley).

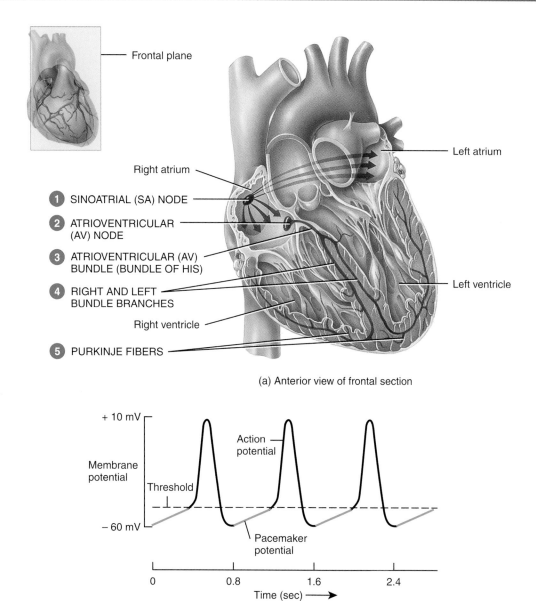

(a) Anterior view of frontal section

+ 10 mV

Membrane potential

Threshold

Action potential

− 60 mV

Pacemaker potential

0   0.8   1.6   2.4

Time (sec)

(b) Pacemaker potentials and action potential in autorhythmic fibres of SA node

Figure 6.2   The conduction system of the heart (from Tortora and Derrickson 2011, reproduced with permission from Wiley).

autonomic nervous system but can be affected by drugs and electrolyte changes (Pinnock et al. 2006).

The electrical impulse then passes through the atria to the atrioventricular (AV) node, which is located posteriorly in the right atrium near to the tricuspid valve and coronary sinus. Here there is a pause to allow the atria to finish contracting before the ventricles begin to contract. From the AV node the impulse travels down conducting fibres called the 'bundle of His' found in the interventricular septum. The bundle of His divides into right and left bundles. The left bundle divides further into anterior and posterior fascicles. These bundles allow transmission of the electrical impulse down the interventricular septum and into the Purkinje system. The Purkinje system is a collection of nerve fibres

that allow the impulse to be carried to the rest of the ventricles (Hampton 1998; Pinnock et al. 2006).

An ECG consists of a series of graphic deflections described as P, Q, R, S, T and U waves that represent events in the cardiac cycle. The normal ECG pattern is illustrated in Figure 6.3.

The P wave represents atrial depolarization and contraction. Delay in conduction between the SA node and AV node is detected by a lengthening of the PR interval. The QRS waves are generally considered together and called a complex. The QRS complex represents ventricular depolarization, so occurs just before ventricular contraction. The duration of the complex indicates if there is any delay in conduction in the bundle of His. The ST segment represents

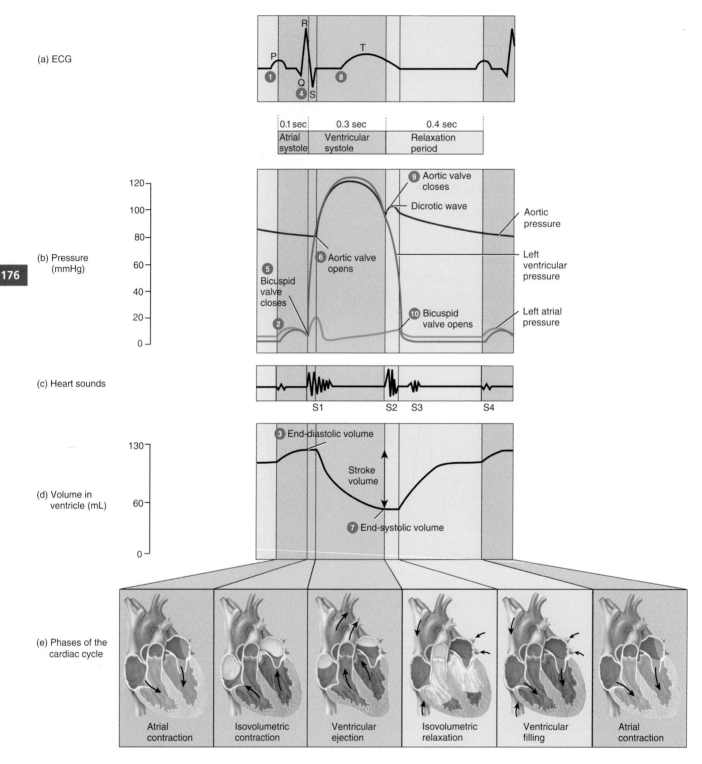

(a) ECG

0.1 sec | 0.3 sec | 0.4 sec
Atrial systole | Ventricular systole | Relaxation period

(b) Pressure (mmHg)

9 Aortic valve closes
Dicrotic wave
Aortic pressure
6 Aortic valve opens
Left ventricular pressure
5 Bicuspid valve closes
10 Bicuspid valve opens
Left atrial pressure

(c) Heart sounds

S1   S2   S3   S4

(d) Volume in ventricle (mL)

3 End-diastolic volume
Stroke volume
7 End-systolic volume

(e) Phases of the cardiac cycle

Atrial contraction | Isovolumetric contraction | Ventricular ejection | Isovolumetric relaxation | Ventricular filling | Atrial contraction

Figure 6.3 Cardiac cycle (from Tortora and Derrickson 2011, reproduced with permission from Wiley).

repolarization of the ventricle (Hampton 1998; Pinnock et al. 2006). The ECG displays the above deflections as leads showing the heart from different directions.

The electrocardiogram is obtained by placing electrodes on the patient's skin in specific positions on the chest. These positions are described later. The electrode is made from silver and silver chloride held on an adhesive disc. The electrode itself is separated from the skin by a foam pad containing a conducting gel. This is illustrated in Figure 6.4. The electrical activity picked up by the electrode is transmitted via a wire to an amplifier, where the signal is boosted and then transformed into a visual display either continuously on a monitor or printed intermittently onto paper (Al-Shaikh and Stacey 2002). The term 'lead' is used in ECG monitoring and often causes confusion, as in some circumstances it is used to describe the wire connecting the electrode on the patient to the machine. However, its correct use is as an electrical image of the heart (Hampton 1998). For example, a 12-lead ECG shows 12 different electrical images of the heart but uses only 10 wires to obtain the images.

The 12-lead ECG

A routine 12-lead ECG is used in a variety of settings and it provides baseline data on cardiac functioning. Importantly, the 12-lead ECG can provide detailed information on the electrical activity of the heart from more directions than a 3- or 5-lead ECG, including from an anterior, inferior, lateral and posterior angles, offering a more comprehensive assessment.

To obtain a 12-lead ECG 10 electrodes are attached to the patient; four sited on the limbs provide the limb leads and six on the chest wall provide the chest or precordial leads. The positioning of the electrodes is shown in Box 6.1.

The electrical activity detected by the electrodes is converted into graphic images known as leads. The electrodes placed on the limbs provide leads I, II, III, aVR, aVF and aVL, and those on the chest wall provide V1, V2, V3, V4, V5 and V6. Each lead represents electrical activity at a specific area of the heart:

- I and aVL focus on the left lateral wall of the heart
- II, III and aVF focus on the inferior wall
- aVR focuses on the right atrium
- V1 and V2 focus on the anterior wall
- V3 and V4 focus on the septum
- V5 and V6 focus on the lateral wall of the left ventricle.

When assessing myocardial ischaemia and infarction, the development of ST changes in certain leads enables the affected area of the heart to be identified (Hampton 1998; Pinnock et al. 2006). The orientation of the leads is shown in Figure 6.5.

Continuous cardiac monitoring

An ECG trace can be continuously displayed on a bedside monitor or transmitted to a distant monitor, where it is termed telemetry. Continuous monitoring can be obtained using a combination of three or five leads; however, setting the monitor to lead II provides optimal visualization of the P wave and QRS complex. In addition, this allows prompt discovery and management of changes in rhythm and (in the case of five leads) development of ischaemia.

Box 6.1 Position of electrodes for a 12-lead ECG

V1	4th intercostal space on the right side of sternum
V2	4th intercostal space on the left side of sternum
V4	5th intercostal space in the left mid-clavicular line
V3	Midway between V2 and V4
V5	5th intercostal space in the left anterior axillary line
V6	5th intercostal space in the left mid-axillary line
VR	Right wrist
VL	Left wrist
VF	Left foot
N	Right foot

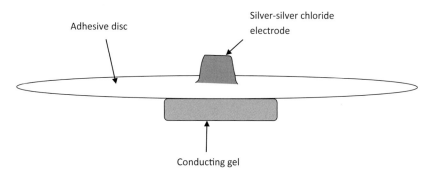

Figure 6.4 Components of an ECG electrode (reproduced with permission from Elsevier).

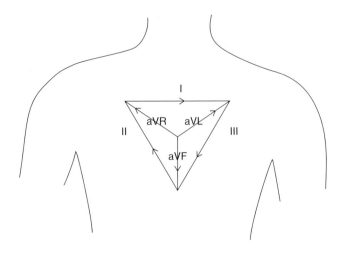

Figure 6.5 Orientation of limb leads.

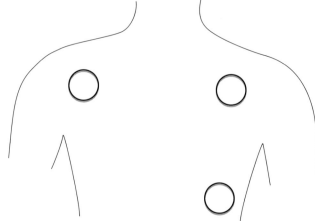

Figure 6.6 Position of 3-lead ECG electrodes.

A printout of the trace can also be obtained at any time from a 3-, 5- or 12-lead ECG. However, it is more common to use a 12-lead ECG if further analysis of the trace is required.

It should be noted that there is very little evidence on the use of the ECG for cardiac monitoring (Drew et al. 2004). The 3-lead ECG is the most basic form and is useful for measuring heart rate and changes in rhythm.

Applying ECG monitoring

To monitor the ECG, electrodes need to be applied in specific positions on the patient's chest wall. The position varies depending on whether a 3-, 5- or 12-lead ECG is being obtained. In addition, it is important not to attach electrodes where defibrillation pads might be placed in the event of a cardiac arrest.

It is important that the electrodes make good contact with the skin to obtain a clear ECG trace. This may require cleaning of the skin and/or shaving the area where the electrodes are to be placed.

When performing a 12-lead ECG, each of the wires to be connected to the electrodes are labelled so they can be connected to the correct electrode (*see* Box 6.1). The wires are then connected to a machine (which is usually portable) where the electrical signals obtained are transformed into the electrocardiogram. This can then be printed off.

The positioning of electrodes for the 3-lead ECG is less important than for the 12-lead ECG, as the former is mainly used for assessment of rate and rhythm. The position of the electrodes for the 3-lead ECG is shown in Figure 6.6. The wires are attached to the monitor displaying the haemodynamic data for that patient, so the ECG is displayed continuously.

If a 5-lead ECG is required for monitoring of cardiac ischaemia, then the leads are positioned as shown in Figure

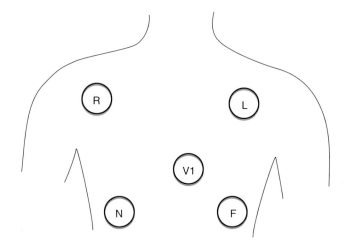

Figure 6.7 Position of 5-lead ECG electrodes.

6.7. When these electrodes are attached to the monitor, two leads are displayed continuously instead of just one (as with the 3-lead ECG), showing one limb lead and one chest lead. The lead displayed can be changed using the monitor's set-up function.

Assessing an ECG

Calculation of heart rate

A 12-lead ECG is printed out on squared paper with the width of each large square (5 mm) representing 0.2 seconds (when the recording is at a standard rate of 2.5 cm/s). This allows calculation of heart rate by measuring the time interval between two consecutive beats, such as the R-R interval, and dividing into 60 seconds (Pinnock et al. 2006).

For example, if the R-R interval is 1 second:

heart rate = 60/1 = 60 beats per minute

Continuous ECG monitoring displays the heart rate and ECG trace simultaneously. However, caution should be used, as the heart rate reading can be inaccurate due to artefact on the trace. This is addressed in Problem-solving table 6.1.

Sinus bradycardia and tachycardia

Continuous ECG monitoring allows the determination of whether a patient is in sinus rhythm or if there has been a change in rhythm. Sinus rhythm is defined as each P wave being followed by a QRS complex at a regular rate. If this is less than 60 beats per minute it is described as sinus bradycardia and more than 100 beats per minute as sinus tachycardia (Pinnock et al. 2006).

Atrial fibrillation

A common arrhythmia (i.e. not in sinus rhythm) in critical care is atrial fibrillation. This is diagnosed by a lack of P waves on the ECG and an irregularly irregular rate. The rate can be fast or slow. This is shown in Figure 6.8.

Cardiac ischaemia

Cardiac ischaemia can be detected using continuous 5-lead ECG monitoring. The 3-lead ECG is insufficient for detecting ischaemia as the chest leads (V1-V6 are the most sensitive for demonstrating ischaemia) are not used. The 5-lead ECG is more accurate as it monitors all the limb leads in addition to one of the chest leads (Drew et al. 2004).

Cardiac ischaemia is demonstrated by elevation or depression of the ST segment from the baseline. If ischaemia appears to develop a 12-lead ECG should be performed to confirm this and determine the areas of the heart involved as described above (see also Chapter 18).

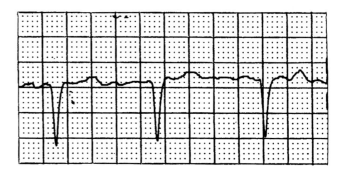

Figure 6.8 ECG demonstrating atrial fibrillation.

Conduction defects

A delay in conduction from the atria to the ventricles (but where all impulses are conducted) is known as first degree heart block. This is detected on the ECG as a prolonged PR interval (more than 0.2 s).

There are two types of second degree heart block: Mobitz type 1 (or Wenckebach phenomenon) and Mobitz type 2. In Mobitz type 1 there is progressive lengthening of the PR interval until a beat is dropped and the cycle then recommences. In Mobitz type 2 there is a normal PR interval but intermittently there is no ventricular contraction (QRS complex) following the atrial contraction (P wave).

Third degree or complete heart block occurs when there is no conduction between the atria and ventricles. Therefore the P waves will be at a normal heart rate but the ventricles will contract at their own inherent rate. This is usually only about 30 beats per minute. This produces an ECG where there is no relationship between the P waves and QRS complexes.

Delays in conduction down the right and left bundle divisions of the bundle of His are known as right and left bundle branch block respectively. Both have a widened QRS complex (greater than 0.12 s). In right bundle branch block, as contraction occurs in the left ventricle first there is a characteristic RSR[1] pattern in V1. In left bundle branch block this RSR[1] pattern is seen in V6.

179

Problem-solving table 6.1: Continuous ECG monitoring

Problem	Cause	Prevention	Suggested action
Electrodes failing to attach properly	Skin too sweaty, oily or excess hair preventing good contact between electrode and skin	Preparation of skin prior to application of electrodes	Skin should be clean and dry prior to applying the electrodes. This may require the use of an alcohol-based skin wipe. Excess hair should be shaved from the area where the electrodes are to be sited to allow good contact of the electrodes with skin. Replace electrode

(Continued)

Problem solving table 6.1: *(Continued)*

Poor-quality ECG trace	Poor electrode contact (see above), artefact from patient movement or electrical equipment. This may prevent accurate interpretation of the ECG	Position the electrodes on skin overlying bone. Switch on the monitor's electrical filter	The electrodes can be repositioned on skin overlying bone rather than muscle to minimize the effect of patient movement or tremor. Many monitors have an electrical filter that can be switched on to minimize the interference from surrounding electrical equipment on the monitor display. Consider replacing electrode
Heart rate reading is wrong	The monitor may be double counting the ECG by misinterpreting the QRS complex and P wave as the same if their amplitude is similar	Monitor heart rate from the arterial pressure monitor if one has been inserted	By increasing or decreasing the gain of the ECG in the set up in the monitor, the difference in height between the P wave and QRS complex may be increased to allow differentiation between the two and correct counting of the heart rate. Displaying another lead may give a better ECG trace allowing correct counting. If an arterial cannula is in situ for invasive blood pressure monitoring this also displays heart rate and so an accurate heart rate can be achieved from this
There is a flat line on the ECG trace	This may be asystole but if the line is perfectly flat it is likely to be due to an electrode disconnection or faulty cable connecting the electrodes to the monitor	Check all electrodes and wires are attached and connected securely	Check the patient for signs of life (are they awake and responsive? Do they have a pulse? Is there an arterial pressure trace if an arterial cannula has been inserted?). If no signs of life then start management for cardiac arrest. If patient is alert, check that the electrodes are fully attached to the skin and the wires are all firmly clipped onto them. If this doesn't solve the problem change the electrodes as the gel may have dried out. If this doesn't work then change the cable and wires attaching the electrodes to the monitor as they may be faulty
The patient has a skin reaction to the electrodes	Patients can develop a skin reaction after prolonged exposure to the electrodes due to either the adhesive or gel on the electrodes	Use hypoallergenic electrodes	Changing the position of the electrodes may help, but the patient is likely to develop irritation at the new area. Hypoallergenic electrodes may reduce the chance of the reaction occurring at the new site

Arterial blood pressure monitoring

Blood pressure monitoring in critical care can be achieved by non-invasive or invasive methods. However, in patients requiring critical care it is normally measured invasively.

Non-invasive arterial blood pressure monitoring

Definition

Non-invasive arterial blood pressure monitoring is measuring the arterial blood pressure without penetrating the surface of the skin.

Aims and indications

Non-invasive blood pressure measurement is used to provide intermittent measurement of arterial blood pressure in patients where there is not expected to be rapid changes in their blood pressure. All patients in acute and community hospitals should have observations, including blood pressure monitoring, undertaken on admission and at least 12 hourly. The frequency with which it is performed should be increased or decreased based on the patient's condition and recommendations of physiological track and trigger systems in place locally (NICE 2006) (*see also* Chapter 3). In critical care this can be every 5 minutes on admission while invasive blood pressure monitoring is being established, but in patients who are in the recovery phase and no longer require invasive monitoring this may be reduced to 1 to 2 hourly.

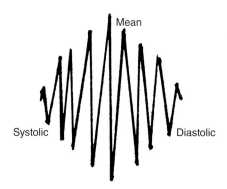

Figure 6.9 Diagram of oscillations from non-invasive blood pressure measurement.

Background

Non-invasive blood pressure monitoring involves the inflation of a cuff around a limb to achieve compression of the artery passing through the limb. The cuff is then deflated and the pressure at which the return of flow through the artery is detected is measured to obtain the blood pressure reading. The return of flow can be detected by manual palpation of the artery, listening for the return of sounds (known as Korotkoff sounds) through a stethoscope or by the use of a pressure transducer to detect changes in amplitude of pressure oscillations known as oscillometry (Hutton et al. 2002). Oscillometry is the most commonly used method of non-invasive blood pressure measurement and is the method used by the DINAMAP (device for indirect non-invasive automatic mean arterial pressure). The cuff is inflated to a pressure estimated to be above the systolic pressure and then slowly deflated at a rate of 3 mmHg/s. When blood begins to flow again, oscillations are detected in the pressure transducer. Systolic pressure is the start of rapidly increasing oscillations; the point of maximum amplitude of the oscillations is the mean arterial pressure and the start of rapidly decreasing oscillations is the diastolic pressure (Figure 6.9) (Al-Shaikh and Stacey 2002). Blood pressure is usually measured in millimetres of mercury (mmHg).

Invasive arterial blood pressure monitoring

Definition

Invasive arterial blood pressure monitoring is measuring the arterial blood pressure by a device inserted into the circulation of a patient.

Aims and indications

An invasive arterial blood pressure system enables beat-to-beat, continuous measurement of blood pressure. It also provides some indication of cardiac contractility through the slope of the upstroke on the arterial pressure waveform, where the more vertical the upstroke the better the contractility (Al-Shaikh and Stacey 2002). Invasive arterial blood pressure monitoring is indicated in those patients who:

- require inotropic or vasopressor drug support so rapid titration of blood pressure can be achieved
- are likely to have significant changes in circulating blood volume either through blood loss or movement of fluid between body fluid compartments
- require frequent arterial blood gas measurement to guide ventilatory management or to monitor acid-base balance (Pinnock et al. 2006).

Background

Invasive blood pressure monitoring is achieved by the insertion of a cannula, usually 20G in size, into an artery of a patient. The artery most commonly used is the radial but the brachial, femoral and dorsal pedis are also used (Bersten et al. 2004). The cannula is attached to a pressure monitoring system consisting of a bag of fluid (usually 0.9% sodium chloride) in a pressure bag set to 300 mmHg (which is commonly called the flush bag), an infusion set and pressure transducer (Figure 6.10).

Anatomy and physiology

The radial artery is located on the lateral aspect of the forearm and is a continuation of the brachial artery. The brachial artery is found in the forearm and is a continuation of the axillary artery (Figure 6.11) (Moore 1985; Erdmann 2004). The radial artery is usually cannulated at the wrist and brachial artery at the elbow, as they are the most superficial and easily palpated sites.

The femoral artery is a continuation of the external iliac artery commencing at the inguinal ligament (Figure 6.12). It is most easily palpated in the femoral triangle. The dorsalis pedis is a continuation of the anterior tibial artery and commences between the two malleoli. It is palpated on the dorsum of the foot.

With each cardiac contraction a volume of blood (stroke volume) is ejected from the left ventricle into the aorta at a pressure of approximately 120 mmHg. During diastole there is no ejection of blood from the left ventricle and the pressure in the aorta drops to approximately 80 mmHg. Blood flow round the body however is kept continuous despite intermittent ejection from the heart. This is due to the elastic nature of the aorta, which allows some of the kinetic energy of the ejected blood to be stored as potential energy during systole. Then, during diastole, the walls of the aorta contract and the potential energy is converted back to kinetic energy maintaining blood flow. As people age, the aorta becomes less elastic and this transfer of energy becomes less efficient. The efficiency of the system is also reduced if the peripheral vessels are dilated, as the reduced resistance to flow makes flow less constant through the cardiac cycle. If the aortic

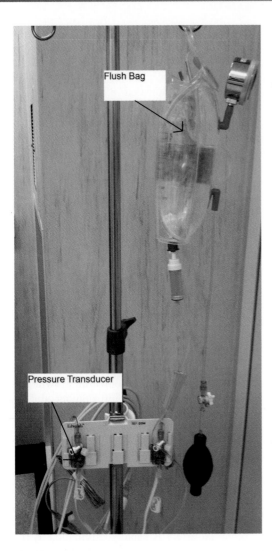

182

Figure 6.10 Arterial and central venous pressure transducer sets (from Al-Shaikh and Stacey 2002, reproduced with permission from Elsevier).

valve is incompetent and allows flow back into the left ventricle during diastole, then flow is also less constant (Power and Kam 2008).

In addition to measurement of systolic and diastolic blood pressure, the pulse pressure and mean arterial pressure (MAP) both give information about the haemodynamic status of the patient.

Pulse pressure (mmHg)

= systolic pressure (mmHg) – diastolic pressure (mmHg).

The pulse pressure is affected by stroke volume and compliance of the arteries. If the stroke volume is increased but the compliance is reduced then the pulse pressure will increase due to the increase in systolic pressure from the larger volume of blood in the aorta and the reduction in diastolic pressure due to the reduced elasticity of the arterial system (Power and Kam 2008).

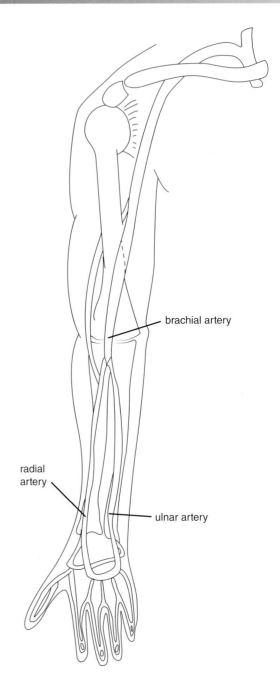

Figure 6.11 Anatomy of the radial and brachial arteries.

MAP (mmHg) = diastolic pressure (mmHg)

$$+ \frac{1}{3}(\text{systolic pressure} - \text{diastolic pressure})\,(\text{mmHg})$$

MAP is the mean arterial pressure throughout the cardiac cycle and is determined by the volume of blood in the arteries at any point in time (*see also* Chapter 3). This is affected by the amount of blood entering the arterial system (cardiac output) and how much leaves and enters the peripheries (peripheral runoff).

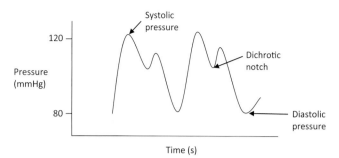

Figure 6.13   Arterial pressure waveform.

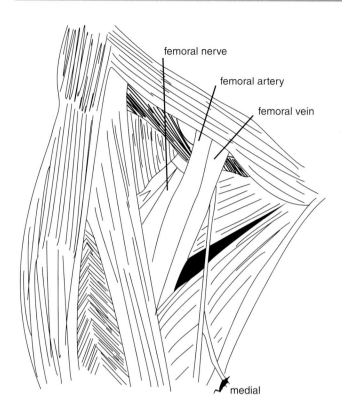

Figure 6.12   Anatomy of the femoral artery and vein.

$$\text{MAP (mmHg)} = \text{total peripheral resistance (mmHg/mL/min)}$$
$$\times \text{peripheral run off (mL/min)}$$

The usual peripheral resistance is 0.02 mmHg/mL/min and peripheral runoff is usually equal to the cardiac output (approximately 5 L/min). Arterial compliance does not affect MAP but it will influence how quickly a change in one of the contributing factors leads to a change in MAP. A lack of compliance in the arterial system explains why some older patients and those with significant arterial disease show rapid changes in MAP (Power and Kam 2008).

The arterial pressure trace is typically as shown in Figure 6.13.

Evidence and current debates

Choice of method of monitoring

Invasive blood pressure monitoring is thought to be more accurate than non-invasive measurement performed using oscillometry, particularly in the critically ill (Mireles et al. 2009). This is because oscillometry tends to overestimate low pressures (less than 60 mmHg) and underestimate high pressures, and it is these extremes of pressure that are more common in the critical care setting. In normotensive patients, oscillometry provides 95% confidences interval of ±15 mmHg (Bersten et al. 2004). Oscillometry is also less accurate in those patients with arrhythmias due to the potentially wide variety of pressures between beats (Al-Shaikh and Stacey

2002; Bersten et al. 2004). The accuracy of oscillometry is also dependent on the use of an appropriate-sized cuff. The cuff should cover two-thirds of the upper arm with the width of the bladder in the cuff being 40% the mid-circumference of the limb. A cuff that is too small will overestimate the blood pressure and too large a cuff will underestimate the pressure (Al-Shaikh and Stacey 2002; Bersten et al. 2004).

Treatment can be guided by aiming to achieve either a certain systolic arterial pressure or a MAP. The further away from the aorta the pressure reading is taken, the higher the systolic pressure reading. This is due to arterial pressure waves reflecting back to the heart combining with further waves transmitted from the heart being added together (Hutton et al. 2002). As MAP remains constant throughout the arterial tree it can be argued that it is a more accurate value for targeting treatment. MAP also remains constant when the invasive arterial pressure trace is 'damped' (see below). Another reason that MAP should be used to monitor and guide treatment is that it is MAP not systolic pressure that determines blood flow to the tissues through autoregulation (Bersten et al. 2004).

Use of heparin in a pressured 'flush bag'

The pressure monitoring system used in measuring arterial blood pressure invasively contains a pressurized bag of 0.9% sodium chloride (flush bag). Previously, 2–3 units of heparin per mL of 0.9% sodium chloride were added to the flush bag to reduce the risk of thrombosis of the arterial cannula (Al-Shaikh and Stacey 2002; Hutton et al. 2002). Following concerns that the addition of heparin to the 0.9% sodium chloride may increase the risk of patients developing coagulpathy, research was undertaken to establish whether 0.9% sodium chloride alone in the flush bag was just as effective at maintaining patency of the arterial cannula as when heparin was added. It has been shown that there is no increase in the incidence of arterial cannula thrombosis with the use of 0.9% sodium chloride compared with heparinized 0.9% sodium chloride (Tuncali et al. 2005; Kannan 2008). In addition, patients were shown to be at risk of developing heparin-induced thrombocytopenia following exposure to heparin in the 0.9% sodium chloride (Selleng et al. 2007). It is now common practice for 0.9% sodium chloride to be used without the addition of heparin to the flush bag.

Insertion of and monitoring using an invasive blood pressure monitoring system

Prior to insertion of the arterial cannula, the pressure monitoring system should be prepared. This consists of a 500 mL bag of 0.9% sodium chloride attached to a specific infusion set containing a pressure transducer. The bag of 0.9% sodium chloride is placed inside a pressure bag that is inflated to 300 mmHg (the 'flush bag') (Figure 6.10). When attached to the arterial cannula this maintains a flow of 3 mL/h of 0.9% sodium chloride to prevent thrombosis of the system. The infusion set usually contains a three-way tap near the arterial cannula to allow blood samples to be taken.

The appropriate site for arterial cannulation is then chosen (usually the radial artery). Performing the modified Allen's test to establish whether the ulnar artery is able to provide adequate blood flow when the radial artery is cannulated is a matter of debate. Its value in assessing how likely a patient is to suffer ischaemic complications from insertion of a radial arterial cannula are not proven (Brzezinski et al. 2009). To perform a modified Allen's test the patient is asked to clench and unclench their fist several times while both the radial and ulnar arteries are occluded by pressure at the wrist. The hand is then unclenched (which should have blanched) and pressure released from the ulnar artery. The time taken for the hand to regain its normal colour is recorded. The value of this figure is also a matter for debate with figures from 3 to 15 seconds described as demonstrating adequate blood flow in the ulnar artery (Brzezinski et al. 2009).

The insertion of the cannula is performed using an aseptic technique. The artery to be cannulated is located by palpation of the pulse and is cannulated using a device similar to an intravenous cannula or by passing a guide wire through a needle that has located the artery and threading the cannula over the guide wire into the artery. The cannula is then connected to the pressure monitoring system.

There is a connector that comes from the pressure transducer, allowing it to be connected via a cable to the monitor. Once the system is connected to the monitor an arterial waveform should appear on the monitor. To allow an accurate recording of the blood pressure to be obtained, the pressure transducer should be at the same level as the patient's right atrium (Al-Shaikh and Stacey 2002) and then calibrated (or 'zeroed'). This involves turning the tap at the transducer so it is 'off to the patient and open to air'. This means the fluid from the flush bag no longer goes down to the cannula but is directed to the opening in the tap to air. A button on the monitor is pressed to calibrate the system to zero and when this is achieved the tap is returned to its usual position.

The monitor will now display the arterial waveform and the numerical readings for systolic, diastolic and mean blood pressure. Appropriate alarm limits for the patient should be set for these parameters. For example, if the systolic pressure is less than 90 mmHg or the mean pressure less than 60 mmHg. If there is thrombus or air in the pressure monitoring system or the flush bag has deflated, then the arterial waveform will appear damped. A damped appearance is when the waveform has a more rounded appearance, with the peak of the pressure trace not as sharp.

The appearance of the arterial waveform also provides data about myocardial contractility. A rapid rise in the upstroke of the arterial waveform indicates good contractility whereas a slower rise may indicate the need for inotropic support. If the dicrotic notch (point where the aortic valve closes) is low on the downstroke this indicates the patient may be vasodilated (Al-Shaikh and Stacey 2002).

Problem-solving table 6.2: Arterial cannulae

Problem	Cause	Prevention	Suggested action
Risk of air emboli	Air bubbles left in the infusion set of the pressure monitoring system	Ensure the infusion set is completely flushed through when initially setting up the pressure monitoring system	When flushing the infusion set ensure the flush bag is kept upright. Visually inspect the system for air bubbles and keep flushing the tubing until there are none visible
	Three-way taps on the infusion set are opened to air allowing entrainment of air into the system	Ensure the three-way taps on the infusion set aren't open to air	Whenever the three-way tap is moved ensure it is never opened to air. If a blood sample is to be taken, attach the syringe before opening the tap
Thrombus forming in the arterial cannula	The pressure bag has deflated below 300 mmHg	Ensure the pressure on the flush bag is maintained at 300 mmHg	As in prevention

	There is no fluid left in the flush bag	Ensure there is adequate fluid left in the flush bag	As in prevention
	The tubing was not flushed adequately following blood sampling	Whenever a blood sample is taken from the arterial cannula ensure the system is fully flushed afterwards so no blood is left in the system	
Ischaemia distal to the arterial cannula	There is insufficient blood flow past the arterial cannula to perfuse the limb distal to it as the cannula occupies the majority of the arterial lumen	Consider performing an Allen test prior to deciding on the site for the cannula Observe the limb distal to the cannula for signs of ischaemia which include: ■ the limb looking paler than the opposite side ■ reduced capillary refill ■ the limb is colder than the opposite side ■ black areas on the skin distal to the cannula ■ the patient complains of altered sensation	If there are any signs of ischaemia and it appears the cannula is responsible for this, the cannula should be removed and the limb observed for recovery. If the limb remains ischaemic further advice should be sought
Inadvertent injection of drugs into the arterial cannula	Inadequate labelling of the arterial cannula Insufficient care when checking where the drugs are being injected	The infusion set in the arterial pressure monitoring system can usually be identified by the red stripe running down the tubing Labels stating 'arterial' can be attached to the infusion set, particularly near the taps that can be used to inject into The practitioner should always check where drugs are being injected	If still injecting the drug when the error is realized, stop injecting immediately and get help from a senior practitioner. This is a potentially catastrophic occurrence and can lead to limb ischaemia and loss of the limb. Management includes intra-arterial injection of lidocaine and papaverine, and intravenous injection of heparin to attempt to maintain blood flow in the artery. The limb should be kept warm and analgesia given as required. Consideration may be given to a sympathetic block
Infection	Inadequate asepsis during insertion of the cannula	Follow the Department of Health (2007) guidelines on preventing infection from intravascular devices	Always clean hands and put on gloves before touching the cannula or area around it
	Inadequate care of the cannula site and maintenance of a clean transparent dressing while in situ		Cover the cannula with a transparent semipermeable dressing. Change dressing every 7 days or whenever it is soiled or damaged
	Prolonged time arterial cannula in situ	Regularly review the need for the arterial cannula and check the site for signs of infection such as redness or pus	Use VIP scoring to monitor regular surveillance of the cannula site
Haemorrhage from the invasive arterial pressure monitoring system	Disconnection or loose connection of the infusion set to the cannula One of the taps allowing sampling is left open The cannula is removed accidently without being noticed	Always check the connections carefully in the arterial monitoring system and ensure taps are closed after sampling	As soon as the haemorrhage is noticed, establish the cause (i.e. disconnection, tap open or cannula removed) and deal with appropriately – reconnect, close tap or apply pressure (until bleeding stops and no evidence of haematoma formation) to where the cannula has been removed

(Continued)

Problem solving table 6.2: (*Continued*)

Arterial injury such as development of a pseudoaneurysm or arteriovenous fistula	Injury can be caused due to trauma to the artery during insertion or due to the effect of prolonged presence of the cannula	Continually reassess the need for an arterial cannula Care taken during insertion of the cannula	If an arterial injury occurs, referral to a vascular surgeon for consideration of surgical intervention

Problem-solving table 6.3: Arterial and central venous pressure monitoring systems

Problem	Cause	Prevention	Suggested action
No waveform appears on the monitor	The cable connecting the pressure transducer to the monitor may not be inserted properly	Check all the connections when setting up the arterial or CVP pressure monitoring system	Check the cable from the pressure transducer to the monitor is inserted properly at both ends
	The arterial cannula or CVC may be blocked either by blood or due to positioning of the cannula. That is the lumen of the arterial cannula or CVC may be against the wall of the blood vessel		Try flushing the arterial cannula or CVC, or altering the position of the limb containing the arterial cannula, or attaching the infusion set to a different lumen of the CVC
	The tap on the pressure transducer may not be in the correct position		Check the tap on the transducer is in the correct position
	The cable may be faulty		Try a new transducer cable
Damped arterial pressure waveform	There may be air bubbles in the infusion set	Ensure the infusion set is adequately flushed prior to attaching to the arterial cannula	Flush the infusion set
	There may be a thrombus in the arterial cannula	Ensure the infusion set is adequately flushed after aspirating from the cannula	Flush the infusion set
	The pressure bag may have deflated or the flush bag may be empty	Regularly check the pressure in the pressure bag and how much fluid remains in the flush bag	Check the pressure bag is set to 300 mmHg and the fluid bag inside is not empty
The arterial cannula or CVC cannot be aspirated or flushed	There may be a thrombus in the cannula or CVC. This can be due to inadequate flushing of the system after aspirating blood	Ensure the infusion set is adequately flushed after aspirating blood	If the cannula or CVC can be flushed but not aspirated try flushing the infusion set
	The opening of that CVC lumen may be against the vein wall		Try aspirating from a different lumen
	The arterial cannula may be kinked or be affected by positioning of the limb	Ensure the arterial cannula and tubing are appropriately tethered and the limb positioned to allow infusion to flow through tubing and cannula	Check for evidence of kinking of the cannula at the skin. Try altering the limb position

	The pressure bag may have deflated or the flush bag may be empty	Regularly check the pressure in the pressure bag and how much fluid remains in the flush bag	Check the pressure bag is set to 300 mmHg and the fluid bag inside is not empty
			The arterial cannula may need to be resited
Abnormal arterial blood pressure or CVP readings	The transducer may be set at the wrong height	The position of the transducer should be checked regularly	Ensure the transducer is set at the correct height (at the level of the right atrium)
	The system may need to be recalibrated (re-zeroed)	Recalibrate transducer (re-zero)	Calibrate (zero) the transducer
	The opening of that CVC lumen may be against the vessel wall		Try attaching the infusion set to a different CVC lumen
	The arterial pressure waveform may be damped		See the advice for a damped waveform in this table

Central venous pressure monitoring

Definition

The purpose of central venous pressure monitoring is to measure the patient's circulating volume. It is a direct index of changes in the pressure of blood returning to the right atrium (pre-load). To measure this requires the insertion of a central venous catheter (CVC).

A CVC is a wide-bore tube that is inserted into a major vein such as the internal jugular, subclavian, or femoral vein. The device can have one to five lumens.

Aims and indications

CVC insertion is indicated in patients who:

- are critically ill and require additional monitoring to guide fluid administration
- have poor peripheral venous access
- require administration of drugs such as inotropes and vasopressors which should be given into a central rather than peripheral vein
- require the administration of long-term antibiotics and parenteral nutrition.

CVP directly measures the pressure in the superior vena cava. This pressure is then used as an indication of filling in the right ventricle, which in turn can be used to guide fluid management in those patients who cannot be managed by clinical examination findings alone. This includes patients with cardiac disease requiring significant fluid replacement who may struggle to cope with large fluid volumes. (The assumptions leading to this are described in more detail in the physiology section.)

Some patients have very poor peripheral venous access making it nearly impossible to insert a peripheral venous catheter. These patients may require insertion of a CVC purely for administration of intravenous drugs. This is also the case in patients who require prolonged courses of intravenous antibiotics. In addition, certain drugs such as inotropes and vasopressors should be administered into a central rather than peripheral vein due to their irritant nature. The comparatively larger volume of blood in central veins results in the drug having less contact with the endothelium of the vein wall, reducing the irritant effect of the drug.

To be used to monitor central venous pressure, the CVC is connected to a system identical to that used for the arterial pressure monitoring system. This consists of a 500 mL bag of 0.9% sodium chloride in a pressure bag (commonly referred to as a 'flush bag') attached to an infusion set.

Background

Anatomy

The internal jugular vein is a continuation of the sigmoid sinus starting at the jugular foramen. It is found in the anterior triangle of the neck within the carotid sheath, usually lateral to the carotid artery. It joins with the subclavian vein at the clavicle to form the brachiocephalic vein. The brachiocephalic vein then becomes the superior vena cava and enters the right atrium. The subclavian vein is a continuation of the axillary vein and commences at the lateral border of the first rib (Moore 1985; Erdmann 2004) (see Figure 6.14).

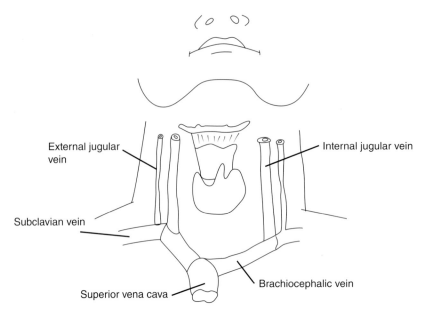

Figure 6.14   Anatomy of the internal jugular and subclavian veins.

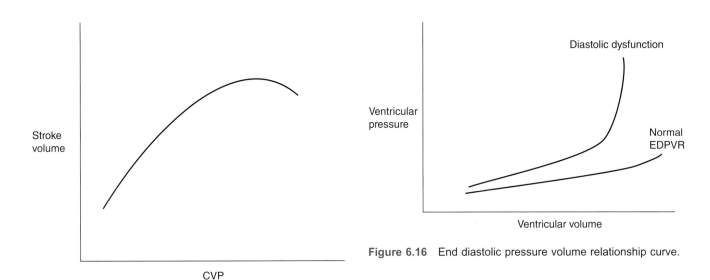

Figure 6.15   Frank–Starling curve.

Figure 6.16   End diastolic pressure volume relationship curve.

The femoral vein is located in the femoral triangle medial to the femoral artery. It is a continuation of the popliteal vein and drains into the external iliac vein (Moore 1985; Erdmann 2004) (*see* Figure 6.12).

Physiology

As ventricular filling is increased, the force of contraction generated by the ventricle is also increased. This is demonstrated by the Frank-Starling curve illustrated in Figure 6.15 (Pinnock et al. 2006). The stretching of the ventricular muscle fibres and subsequent increase in end diastolic volume is described as preload. The CVP is used as a surrogate measure of preload on the right side of the heart as it is not practical to measure the end diastolic volume. The rationale behind this is that end diastolic pressure and end diastolic volume have a linear relationship in a normal heart, as shown in Figure 6.16. Caution then has to be used in interpreting the CVP measurement if the ventricle has decreased compliance due to ischaemia or hypertrophy, as it is likely that higher pressures will be needed to achieve an adequate preload (Pinnock et al. 2006). It has to be remembered that CVP is measuring pressure in the right side of the heart and does not necessarily reflect those in the left side

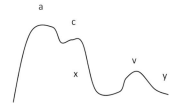

Figure 6.17 Central venous pressure waveform.

of the heart. This occurs, for example, if the left ventricle is impaired and not the right or there are changes in pulmonary pressures.

CVP trace

The CVP trace produces a characteristic waveform as illustrated in Figure 6.17. The 'a' wave corresponds with atrial contraction; the 'c' wave relates to isovolumetric contraction (the heart is contracting but the blood volume in the ventricles remains unchanged as the valves have yet to open) causing the tricuspid valve to bulge into the right atrium; and the 'v' wave is due to the increase in atrial pressure before the tricuspid valve opens. The 'x' descent is due to atrial relaxation and the 'y' descent is due to atrial emptying (Pinnock et al. 2006).

Efficacy of CVP monitoring

The central venous catheter is routinely used in critical care but there is doubt as to its efficacy in monitoring and managing fluid therapy. Some studies have shown that CVP is a poor predictor of a patient's fluid responsiveness (Kumar et al. 2004; Marik et al 2008). It appears to be more useful to consider the trends in the CVP reading than absolute values (Bersten et al. 2004). Nevertheless, the value of the CVP was demonstrated in a study examining early goal-directed therapy which showed a reduction in mortality from sepsis when a series of interventions including volume replacement guided by CVP was undertaken (Rivers et al. 2001). As with any piece of monitoring equipment, the CVP measurement used in isolation is unlikely to be of significant benefit. However, it can provide additional guidance on fluid management when combined with other measurements and clinical examination.

Insertion of and monitoring using a CVP monitoring system

The pressure monitoring system should be prepared prior to insertion of the CVC in an identical way to that of the invasive blood pressure monitoring system.

The site of the CVC is chosen based on the considerations of safety and infection control. Central venous access can be obtained using the landmark technique, where the vein is located using anatomical landmarks, or by using an ultrasound machine to visualize the vein during insertion of the needle. Currently the internal jugular vein is the most commonly used site due to a lower incidence of complications despite the increased infection risk compared to subclavian vein insertion. The National Institute of Clinical Excellence (NICE) has produced guidelines that recommend the use of ultrasound as the preferred method for insertion of a central venous catheter into the internal jugular vein in an elective situation. They state that its use should be considered for the insertion of all central venous catheters electively or in the emergency situation as it reduces the risk of complications such as arterial puncture and pneumothorax (NICE 2002).

Insertion of the CVC should be performed under full aseptic conditions (Pratt et al. 2007). The vein is located using ultrasound guidance (NICE 2002) and punctured using a needle. A guide wire is threaded through the needle into the vein. This technique is known as the Seldinger technique. The needle is removed leaving the guide wire in the vein. A dilator is then passed over the wire into the vein. This is to enlarge the hole in the skin sufficiently to allow the CVC to pass easily over the wire into the vein. The dilator is removed and the CVC placed over the wire. When the CVC is in the vein the guide wire is removed. All the lumens of the CVC are aspirated to ensure blood is drawn back, and then flushed with 0.9% sodium chloride. This is to check that the CVC is in the correct position and to prevent blockage of the CVC by blood left in the catheter to clot.

The CVC is then connected to the pressure monitoring system in the same way the invasive blood pressure monitoring system is set up. The waveform that appears is shown in Figure 6.17. The usual value for CVP is between 0 and 5 mmHg in spontaneously breathing patients and 5–10 mmHg in ventilated patients due to the use of PEEP (Bersten et al. 2004). However, it is not the absolute value of the CVP but the trend that occurs and the response to a fluid bolus that is of most value.

If a fluid bolus is given and there is no change in CVP it is likely the patient is still hypovolaemic (underfilled). If the CVP rises by 1 or 2 mmHg and then rapidly decreases back to baseline when filling stops, this also indicates that the patient is still hypovolaemic but less so than in the first case. If the CVP increases when fluid is given and then stays at the new value when filling is stopped, this indicates that the patient is normovolaemic. A rapidly rising CVP indicates that the patient may be reaching the point where they are becoming hypervolaemic (overfilled) (the top of the curve on Starling's curve). Beyond this point the muscle fibres can become overstretched and contractility decreases (Figure 6.15) (Pinnock et al. 2006). The information from the CVP should also be used in conjunction with blood pressure changes and findings from clinical examination. This will enable a decision to be made as to whether fluid, inotropes, or vasopressors are required to obtain adequate perfusion for a particular patient.

Safety and risk issues

Infection risk

Catheter-related bloodstream infections are an important cause of mortality and morbidity, particularly in critical care. This has led to recent interest in finding ways to reduce these infections. The most important work has come from Pronovost in Michigan, USA (Pronovost et al. 2006) and the 'epic2' guidelines from the UK (Pratt et al. 2007). Pronovost developed five evidence-based recommendations aimed at reducing catheter-related bloodstream infections and implemented a training programme to aid their uptake. The five recommendations were:

- hand washing prior to insertion
- use of full barrier precautions during insertion
- cleaning the skin with chlorhexidine prior to insertion
- avoidance of the femoral vein if possible (this is the site most likely to become infected, with the subclavian vein least likely to become infected)
- the removal of unnecessary catheters.

The implementation of these recommendations led to a significant reduction in catheter-related bloodstream infections in the critical care units that took part (Pronovost et al. 2006). The success of this strategy led to the development of the Matching Michigan work by the National Patient Safety Agency (NPSA), aimed at producing similar reductions in catheter-related bloodstream infections in the UK.

The epic2 project developed evidence-based guidelines to reduce hospital-acquired infections, including those from CVC insertion (Pratt et al. 2007). Their advice was very similar to that of Pronovost (2006) and included:

- use of a single-lumen CVC if possible
- tunnelling the CVC if likely to be required for 3–4 weeks or more

- use of the subclavian vein (the increased risk of pneumothorax during insertion of a subclavian CVC should be balanced against infection risk when choosing between that and the internal jugular vein)
- during insertion maximal sterile barrier precautions should be used (sterile gown, gloves, drape, hat and mask)
- the skin should be cleaned with 2% chlorhexidine gluconate in 70% isopropyl gluconate prior to insertion
- the CVC should be covered with a sterile, transparent semipermeable polyurethane dressing and changed every 7 days or sooner if it is no longer intact
- the injection ports should be decontaminated with alcoholic chlorhexidine gluconate solution before use
- the CVC only needs to be changed if there is evidence of infection or suspicion of a catheter-related bloodstream infection
- antimicrobial-impregnated catheters should be considered for those needing the CVC for 1–3 weeks due to the increased risk of catheter-related infection.

Other evidence states that the use of antimicrobial-impregnated catheters does reduce infection rates but is only of significance in units with high baseline infection rates (Casey et al. 2008). There is some evidence that the use of chlorhexidine-impregnated sponges over the CVC insertion site reduces the risk of catheter-related infection (Timsit et al. 2009) but it is not conclusive enough to have been included in the epic2 or Matching Michigan guidelines.

On the background of this work (Pronovost et al. 2006; Pratt et al. 2007) the Department of Health has published a central venous catheter care bundle that incorporates the above recommendations (DH 2007).

As with invasive blood pressure monitoring, care should be taken when flushing the infusion set, ensuring all taps are closed, the catheter is flushed adequately to prevent thrombosis and the catheter insertion site is monitored for signs of infection. *See* Problem-solving table 6.4 for other problems that may arise.

Problem-solving table 6.4: Central venous catheter insertion

Problem	Cause	Prevention	Suggested action
Arrhythmias	During CVC insertion the guide wire can enter the right atrium and cause arrhythmias	Be aware of how much guide wire has been threaded into the vein to try and ensure it doesn't reach the right atrium Use ECG monitoring during insertion so if arrhythmias occur the wire can be pulled back immediately	If arrhythmias are noted on the ECG on insertion of the guide wire immediately pull back the guide wire until the arrhythmia stops. Usually withdrawal of the guide wire will terminate the arrhythmia, but in rare cases it may need to be treated by cardioversion or anti-arrhythmic medication

Pneumothorax or haemothorax	The needle used for locating the vein during CVC insertion can breach the pleura and cause a pneumothorax. If there is additional vascular injury this will cause a haemothorax	Use ultrasound to guide insertion of the CVC as this should minimize the risk of pneumothorax and haemothorax due to more accurate location of the vein to be cannulated	A chest X-ray should be performed if pneumothorax or haemothorax is suspected. That is, if the patient's oxygen saturation levels decrease, or they become hypotensive, develop respiratory distress or – in ventilated patients – develop high airway pressures. Sometimes a pneumothorax or haemothorax is asymptomatic and only identified following routine chest X-ray post insertion. When a pneumothorax or haemothorax is identified it will often require treatment by insertion of a chest drain into the affected side
Arterial puncture	The artery is located adjacent to the vein in all sites used for insertion of a CVC and so can be punctured accidentally instead of the vein	Use of ultrasound to locate the vein to be used for CVC insertion	Assess if it is likely that the artery has been punctured. If the artery is punctured instead of the vein then the blood will come back out of the needle much quicker than if it was in the vein and will be pulsatile. The blood is usually bright red rather than the dark red of venous blood (arterial blood is better oxygenated than venous blood). On identifying an arterial puncture the needle should be removed and pressure applied until the bleeding has stopped. This is to try and prevent development of a haematoma, which, if in the neck, can lead to airway compromise due to compression of the trachea by the haematoma. If the carotid artery is punctured accidentally then there is the risk of stroke if the artery contains atheromatous plaques
Nerve injury	Nerves are found in close proximity to all the veins used for CVC insertion and so can be damaged during insertion of the needle to locate the vein	Use of ultrasound to locate the vein to minimize the risk of damaging a nerve	If the patient is awake during insertion they may complain of numbness or pins and needles if the nerve is touched. The needle should be removed immediately if this is the case. In sedated patients this may only become apparent at a later date. The area of altered sensation or weakness should be evaluated and documented and may require referral to a neurologist to evaluate further
Air embolism	This is a risk during CVC insertion using the internal jugular vein and to a lesser extent the subclavian vein. If a patient is hypovolaemic the venous pressure at the insertion site may be less than atmospheric pressure and so air can be sucked in via the needle or catheter	The patient's bed is placed head down so that the pressure in the vein to be cannulated is increased, hopefully to a level above atmospheric pressure In addition, when the syringe is taken off the needle cannulating the vein, the end of the needle should be occluded by a finger prior to threading the guide wire to prevent air being entrained. When the catheter is inserted it should be ensured that none of the lumens are left open to air	The signs of a significant air embolism are cardiovascular collapse and cardiac arrest. If air embolism occurs, the patient's bed should be placed head down if not done so already and the patient tilted onto their right side. Attempts should be made to aspirate the air via the CVC if inserted or through the needle if only at that stage of insertion. Cardiopulmonary resuscitation should be commenced if cardiac output is lost. Large air embolism has a poor prognosis

(Continued)

Problem solving table 6.4: *(Continued)*

| Thrombosis of vein | The presence of a catheter in a vein for a prolonged period of time can lead to thrombosis of the vein. This can lead to problems in the long term for vascular access if a patient has required a CVC for an extended period of time and when different sites have been used | Only have a CVC in situ for as long as is clinically indicated | Remove the CVC as soon as it is no longer required |

Advanced haemodynamic monitoring

Introduction

The purpose of the cardiovascular system is to support homeostasis by providing a transport system that continuously perfuses the vital organs with blood (Marieb and Hoehn 2007). Numerous control mechanisms help to regulate the various components of this system to ensure adequate perfusion is maintained (Thibodeau and Patton 2007). The function of monitoring this system is to establish a diagnosis, determine appropriate therapy and monitor the patient's response to treatment (Adam and Osborne 2005). The term haemodynamic monitoring is used to describe this activity.

Definition

Advanced haemodynamic monitoring is the study of the circulation using complex monitoring. Thibodeau and Patton (2007: 734) describe the term haemodynamics as 'a collection of mechanisms that influence the active and changing, or dynamic, circulation of blood'.

Aims and indications

The aim of advanced haemodynamic monitoring is to provide more detailed data and analysis of parameters to:

- aid in the diagnosis of various cardiovascular disorders
- guide therapies to optimize cardiac function
- minimize cardiovascular dysfunction or treat disorders
- evaluate the patient's response to therapy (Morton et al. 2009).

Indications for haemodynamic monitoring include conditions in which cardiac output is insufficient to deliver oxygen to cells as a result of alterations in intravascular volume, vascular resistance and myocardial contractility (Morton et al. 2009).

Background

Advanced haemodynamic monitoring may be either continuous or intermittent (Adam and Osborne 2005). As a patient's condition deteriorates and the body's normal homeostatic mechanisms cannot maintain vital organ perfusion, it is usually necessary to increase the complexity and invasiveness of the monitoring device and the frequency of data sampling (Morgan 2003). Conversely, these can be reduced as a patient's condition improves. Individual haemodynamic readings can be significant in guiding the treatment of a patient, but it is also important to analyse trends from serial data. In addition, it is necessary to assimilate and interpret information from all forms of patient monitoring including clinical observation, e.g. skin colour and temperature (Morgan 2003; Adam and Osborne 2005).

Optimization of haemodynamic status is a key goal in the management of a critically ill patient (Whiteley et al. 2010). This includes achieving optimal cardiac output, oxygen delivery and maintaining adequate organ perfusion (Morton et al. 2009; Whiteley et al. 2010). To achieve this in critically ill patients a number of methods have been developed to monitor their cardiovascular status. These include the pulmonary thermodilution approach, the transpulmonary dilution approach and the use of Doppler ultrasound.

Anatomy and physiology

A detailed understanding of the anatomy and physiology is fundamental to understanding the principles of haemodynamic monitoring, diagnosis and subsequent management.

Cardiac cycle

A cardiac cycle is one complete mechanical cycle of the heart (Figure 6.3) and consists of both the systolic and diastolic phases of the atria and ventricles (Urden et al. 2010; Tortora and Derrickson 2011). During atrial diastole the right atrium fills passively with deoxygenated blood returning from the upper and lower body via the superior and inferior vena cava. At this point the tricuspid valve is closed. Oxygenated blood returns via the pulmonary veins and fills the left atrium, and the bicuspid valve is forced closed. During atrial systole, and ventricular diastole, the tricuspid and the bicuspid valves open, the atria contract and the right and left ventricles begin to fill. This is completed through the contraction of both atria. In ventricular systole the tricuspid and the bicuspid valves close as both ventricles contract and the force of blood opens the pulmonary and aortic valves and blood is ejected into the pulmonary and systemic circulations (Marieb and Hoehn 2007; Urden et al. 2010; Tortora and Derrickson 2011).

This continuous circulation of blood enables it to perform its critical homeostatic function of maintaining the mean arterial pressure (MAP) to preserve tissue perfusion (Morgan 2003; Marieb and Hoehn 2007). Maintaining this pressure is therefore essential and it is influenced by a number of factors, including cardiac output and peripheral resistance (Thibodeau and Patton 2007).

Cardiac output

Cardiac output (CO) is the amount of blood ejected out of the left or right ventricle each minute (Tortora and Derrickson 2011). It is calculated by multiplying the patient's heart rate in beats per minute by their stroke volume, which is defined as the volume of blood pumped out by one ventricle (*see also* Chapter 7). The stroke volume (SV) for each beat is approximately 60–70 mL (Marieb and Hoehn 2007).

Heart rate (beats/min) × stroke volume (mL)

= cardiac output (L/min)

Measured in L/min, this volume is close to the total blood volume, of approximately 5 L. As a result, nearly the entire circulatory volume flows through the pulmonary and systemic circulations each minute (Tortora and Derrickson 2011). Cardiac output is highly variable and changes markedly in response to alterations in the heart rate (HR) and stroke volume (Marieb and Hoehn 2007; Tortora and Derrickson 2011). Cardiac output is the term traditionally used when discussing the effectiveness of the heart (Morton and Fontaine 2009), but all three factors (the HR, SV and CO) must be individually assessed in order to attain a comprehensive assessment of cardiac function (Urden et al. 2010). For example, a patient may have a CO of 5.4 L/min calculated from the following parameters:

- HR of 77 beats per minute and SV of 70 mL

or

- HR rate of 150 beats per minute and SV of 36 mL.

The latter is abnormal due to both values being outside normal parameters. The stroke volume is further influenced by three other factors: preload, afterload and contractility. Preload is discussed earlier in this chapter in the section on CVP monitoring.

Afterload

Afterload refers to the resistance or pressure that the ventricle has to overcome to effectively eject blood into the circulatory system (Marieb and Hoehn 2007). In relation to the left ventricle the afterload is the systemic vascular resistance (SVR) and for the right ventricle it is the pulmonary vascular resistance (PVR). An increase in afterload usually means an increase in the work of the heart (Morton and Fontaine 2009).

Contractility

Contractility is defined as the contractile strength achieved at a given muscle length and, as discussed, can be affected by Frank–Starling mechanisms. However, it can be affected independently of these mechanisms (Marieb and Hoehn 2007; Urden et al. 2010) through stimulation of the sympathetic branch of the autonomic nervous system and the resulting affects of direct neural stimuli and the release of catecholamines on the heart (Morton and Fontaine 2009).

Haemodynamic monitoring

Haemodynamic monitoring is at a critical juncture as the technology that launched invasive haemodynamic monitoring is more than 30 years old. The search to find improved and viable replacement monitoring technologies that are minimally or non-invasive is intense (Urden et al. 2010). Key to these haemodynamic monitoring technologies is the measurement of cardiac output.

The measurement of cardiac output

There are three main techniques to measure cardiac output.

1 The pulmonary thermodilution method: a known amount of cold fluid is injected into the right atrium via a pulmonary artery catheter and the subsequent change in temperature is measured over time and used to calculate the cardiac output.
2 The transpulmonary dilution method: this includes two techniques:
   (i) the thermodilution method – a known amount of cold fluid (indicator) is injected into the blood, usually via a central venous catheter, and the subsequent

dilution of the indicator is measured over time (via change in temperature) and used to calculate the cardiac output

(ii) the dilution method – a dye or chemical (indicator) is injected into the blood and the subsequent dilution of the indicator is measured over time and used to calculate the cardiac output.

3 Oesophageal Doppler monitoring: a probe is inserted into the oesophagus that continuously emits ultrasound waves that measure the flow of blood down the descending thoracic aorta (Adam and Osborne 2005).

Measurement devices

Classically, the pulmonary artery (PA) catheter has been used to measure CO using the pulmonary thermodilution method. The PA catheter is the most invasive of the critical care monitoring catheters (Urden et al. 2010). Since it was first described by Swan and Ganz in the 1970s, it has been widely used for the diagnosis and treatment of critically ill patients (Jevon et al. 2007), and has been seen as the gold standard in cardiovascular monitoring in critical care (Whiteley et al. 2010). Due to a range of complications associated with PA catheters (such as catheter-related sepsis) and the risk of pulmonary artery rupture, their use has been questioned. This has been followed by the advent of less invasive cardiac output monitoring devices (e.g. the oesophageal Doppler), and the widespread use of PA catheters has subsequently diminished (Whiteley et al. 2010).

A number of studies (Harvey et al. 2005, 2006a) have investigated the effect of the use of PA catheters on patient mortality and found no clear evidence of benefit or harm to patients. The lack of clear benefit has nevertheless resulted in less reliance on this device to measure CO in the critically ill (Urden et al. 2010). Harvey et al. (2006b) also found that PA catheters were not cost-effective when used in adult general intensive care patients. Another reason for the reduced usage is the view that PA catheters are a diagnostic rather than a therapeutic tool (Chatterjee 2009). However, a number of clinical circumstances exist where the use of a PA catheter should be considered, for example haemodynamic instability or when shock is unresponsive to treatment that was guided by more conventional means (Roizen et al. 2003; Whiteley et al. 2010).

Subsequently the development and introduction of newer, less invasive techniques that utilize the transpulmonary dilution method of measuring CO has occurred. These are commercially available as a range of different devices, e.g. LiDCO™plus (Lithium Dilution Cardiac Output; LiDCO Limited, Cambridge, UK) and PiCCO® (Pulse induced Continuous Cardiac Output System; Pulsion Medical Systems, Munich, Germany). A further method of measuring CO is through the use of an oesophageal Doppler, and this is commercially available as the CardioQ™ system (Deltex Medical Limited, Chichester, UK). A systematic review (Abbas and Hill 2008) and a meta analysis (Walsh et al. 2008) on the use of an oesophageal Doppler found a link to improved

patient outcomes following major intra-abdominal surgery. In 2011 NICE published guidelines on the use of an oesophageal Doppler in healthcare settings (NICE 2011). These recommend their use in patients who are either undergoing major or high-risk surgery or those patients where invasive cardiovascular monitoring would be considered. However, within the critical care environment there was insufficient evidence to recommend use in preference to other techniques for monitoring CO.

Although many studies (Hamilton et al. 2002; Combes et al. 2004; Costa et al. 2008; Kemps et al 2008; Ritter et al. 2009) have been undertaken to explore the effectiveness of the available CO measurement techniques, insufficient evidence has been uncovered to validate their use so further research is recommended (Morgan 2003; Harvey et al. 2006a; Hadian et al; 2010 NICE 2011). Despite these concerns monitoring should remain as low risk as possible yet be sufficient to provide early warning of circulatory dysfunction, determine appropriate interventions and track responses to therapy (Morgan 2003). The potential value of each technique must be carefully considered prior to insertion (Adam and Osborne 2005). The ideal requirements for a CO monitoring device include:

- accuracy
- precision
- rapid response time
- continuous 'real-time' updating of data
- minimal risk to the patient
- maximal provision of information
- cost-effectiveness.

(Burtenshaw and Isaac 2006)

The benefits, limitations and complications of CO measurement devices can be found in Table 6.1. Users of CO measurement devices must be familiar with their operation and how to troubleshoot problems (Jevon et al. 2007).

Pulmonary thermodilution method

The thermodilution technique is used with pulmonary artery catheters and this can be either intermittent through bolus injection or continuous (Urden et al. 2010). The bolus thermodilution method involves a rapid injection of a measured amount of cold fluid (usually 5–10mL of 0.9% sodium chloride) into the right atrium. This is achieved via a primed intravenous administration set tubing attached to the proximal port of the PA catheter (proximal refers to the closest opening in the PA catheter to the external hub). The 0.9% sodium chloride is injected into the proximal port and mixes with blood, cooling it temporarily. The temperature of the blood is measured using a thermistor near the tip of the PA catheter and the changes in temperature plotted as a time–temperature curve or CO curve (Morgan 2003; Adam and Osborne 2005; Jevon et al. 2007; Urden et al. 2010) CO is inversely proportional to the area under the time–temperature curve, so when the CO is high the injectate will have less

Table 6.1 Benefits, limitations and complications

	PiCCO	LiDCO	ODM
Complications	**Venous/arterial access**	**Venous/arterial access**	■ Dislodgement of probe
(See arterial and CVC complications; Adam and Osborne 2005; Pulsion Medical Systems 2009)	■ Bleeding at site ■ Pneumo +/- haemothorax ■ Air embolism ■ Arterial puncture ■ Nerve injury ■ Venous thrombosis **In use** ■ Incorrect calibration ■ Erroneous data ■ Misinterpretation of data	■ Bleeding at site ■ Pneumo +/- haemothorax ■ Air embolism ■ Arterial puncture ■ Nerve injury ■ Venous thrombosis **In use** ■ Incorrect calibration ■ Erroneous data ■ Misinterpretation of data	■ Damage to oesophageal mucosa and oesophageal bleeding ■ Oesophagotracheal perforation ■ Dysphagia ■ Endobronchial placement **In use** ■ Incorrect positioning ■ Erroneous data ■ Misinterpretation of data
Benefits	■ Minimally invasive ■ No additional invasive catheters ■ Real time: ■ beat-to-beat cardiac output ■ preload and afterload values ■ Simple and quick to set up	■ Minimally invasive ■ No additional invasive catheters ■ Real time: ■ beat-to-beat cardiac output ■ preload and afterload values ■ oxygen delivery ■ Simple and quick to set up	■ Continuous ■ Non-invasive ■ Ease of insertion ■ Decreased risk of arrhythmias ■ Decreased risk of infection
(Ott et al. 2001; Cottis et al. 2003; Singer and Webb 2009; Urden et al. 2010)			
Limitations and contraindications	■ Peripheral arterial vasoconstriction ■ Damped arterial trace ■ CVP in femoral vein (overestimate) ■ Aortic balloon pumps ■ Inaccurate readings ■ Intra-aortic aneurysm ■ Pneumonectomy ■ Aortic stenosis	■ Cannot be used on patients receiving lithium ■ Muscle relaxants (vecuronium, atracurium and pancuronium) may cause inaccurate measurements. ■ Severe peripheral arterial vasoconstriction ■ Severely damped arterial trace ■ Intra-aortic balloon pumps ■ Aortic valve regurgitation ■ Patients under 40kg (paediatric patients) ■ Patients during first trimester of pregnancy	Do not use in patients: ■ Under 16 years ■ With apparent nasal injuries, facial trauma, nasal polyps, a risk of brain injury ■ Undergoing intra-aortic balloon pumping ■ With carcinoma of the pharynx, larynx or oesophagus, aneurysms of the thoracic aorta, severe coarctation of the aorta ■ With tissue necrosis of the oesophagus or nasal passages ■ Severe bleeding diatheses ■ Cross-sectional area must be accurate ■ Ultrasound beam must be parallel – blood flow ■ Beam direction cannot move between measurements
(Ott et al. 2001; Cottis et al. 2003; Morgan 2003; Adam and Osborne 2005; Singer and Webb 2009; Urden et al. 2010)			

time to be warmed by the blood and so the measured temperature at the thermistor will be lower. When the CO is low the blood flow is much slower giving more time for the injectate to warm and be nearer to the blood temperature. This can be calculated by using the modified Stewart–Hamilton equation (Morgan 2003):

$$CO = \frac{V \times (Tb - Ti)}{A} \times \frac{(SI \times CI)}{(SB \times CB)} \times \frac{60 \times CT \times K}{1}$$

where CO = cardiac output; V = volume of injectate (mL); Tb = temperature of blood (B); Ti = injectate temperature; A = area of thermodilution curve in square mm divided by paper speed (mm/s); K = calibration constant in mm/°C and injectate (I); SB, SI = specific gravity of blood and injectate; CB, CI = specific heat of blood and injectate; (SI × CI)/(SB × CB) = 1.08 when 5% dextrose is used; 60 = 60 s/min; CT = correction factor for injectate warning.

This is based on the use of a known indicator (dye, chemical or thermal) as a signal and the determination of its dilution over a given period of time. The analysis of the dilution curve allows cardiac output to be calculated (Morton and Fontaine 2009: 313). If the CO is within normal limits (4–8 L/min) the use of injectate that is iced or at room temperature is equally accurate. However, if the CO is extremely high or low, iced 0.9% sodium chloride may be more accurate (Urden et al. 2010). Three calibrations should be undertaken to obtain a higher level of accuracy.

The continuous technique can be achieved through 'warm' thermodilution cardiac output techniques using a modified PA catheter. The modified catheter has a thermal filament wrapped around the section where the PA catheter is sitting in the right ventricle of the heart. This thermal filament emits pulses of heat and a distal thermistor then detects these heat pulses. The cross-correlation of the input and output signal produces a time–temperature curve and the cardiac output can be calculated by using a Stewart–Hamilton equation. This process occurs every 30–60 s to give a semi-continuous cardiac output (Morgan 2003; Adam and Osborne 2005).

The pulmonary artery catheter

The PA catheter is inserted to obtain measurements of cardiac output (CO), pulmonary artery pressures, mixed venous oxygen saturation and to derive values for other indices of cardiovascular function such as systemic vascular resistance (SVR). The indications for a PA catheter include:

- patients with cardiogenic shock during supportive therapy
- patients with discordant right and left ventricular failure
- patients with severe chronic heart failure requiring inotropic, vasopressor and vasodilator therapy
- patients with suspected 'pseudo-sepsis' (high cardiac output, low systemic vascular resistance, elevated right atrial and pulmonary capillary wedge pressures)

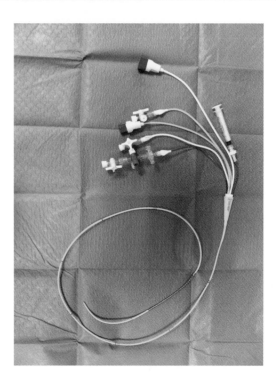

Figure 6.18 Pulmonary artery catheter (Dougherty and Lister 2011).

- patients with potentially reversible systolic heart failure such as fulminant myocarditis and peripartum cardiomyopathy
- to enable a haemodynamic differential diagnosis of pulmonary hypertension
- to assess response to therapy in patients with precapillary and mixed types of pulmonary hypertension
- during transplantation work-up.

(Morgan 2003; Chatterjee 2009)

The standard PA catheter is 110 cm long (marked in 10 cm increments) and has four lumens. This is shown in Figure 6.18. The functions of the various lumens are described below.

1 Proximal lumen: the 'proximal lumen' (that is, the lumen that has its opening closest to the external hub – sometimes referred to as the injectate port) opens 30 cm from the tip of the catheter. This lumen lies in the right atrium and is used to inject the cold 0.9% sodium chloride into the heart for the thermodilution cardiac output measurement. It is also connected to a transducer and monitoring system to measure the pressure in the right atrium. This lumen can also be used for drug and fluid administration.

2 Distal lumen: the distal lumen opens at the tip of the catheter and therefore the furthest opening from the external hub of the PA catheter. This is used to continuously measure the pressure in the pulmonary artery (PA).

Blood can be aspirated from this lumen to measure mixed venous blood saturation.

3 Balloon inflation lumen: this lumen is used to inflate a balloon that sits very close to the tip of the catheter. A specially designed 2 mL syringe, which limits the volume of air that can be injected into the balloon, is attached to the proximal end of this lumen. Once inflated in the right atrium the balloon assists flotation of the catheter into the PA. The inflated balloon is also necessary to measure the PA wedge pressure (Table 6.2). This is also known as the pulmonary occlusion pressure (PAOP) and the pulmonary artery catheter wedge pressure (PACWP).

4 Thermistor lumen: this lumen contains the thermistor, which is located 4 cm from the catheter tip. Its purpose is to measure blood temperature in the PA.

There are various modifications of the standard four-lumen catheter. This includes extra lumens for drug and fluid administration, and in some variations it can incorporate a lumen for connection to a SvO_2 monitor or pacing wires for connection to a pacing device (Adam and Osborne 2005; Morton and Fontaine 2009; Urden et al. 2010).

Prior to the insertion of a PA catheter, a wide-bore CVC called a PA introducer needs to be inserted into either the right or left internal jugular or subclavian vein in a similar manner to a narrow-bore CVC. At this stage, to make the monitoring of the waveform within the heart possible, a transducer set is connected to the distal port of the catheter. Once in place the PA catheter is advanced into the introducer then into the superior vena cava. Once the tip is inside the right atrium, the balloon sitting immediately proximal to the tip on the PA catheter is fully inflated. This allows the PA catheter to be floated slowly through to the right ventricle of the heart then into the PA. Once the catheter is in the PA it is advanced slowly until there is a 'wedged' appearance (flattened appearance demonstrated in Figure 6.19) and the balloon is then deflated and the monitor checked to ensure

the PA trace has returned to the monitor. As the PA catheter is floated through the chambers of the heart and into the PA, the position of the tip of the catheter is known, due to the characteristic waveform trace produced at each point on the monitor (Figure 6.19).

Once the PA catheter is inserted, a number of direct measurements can be obtained and from these a range of derived parameters can be calculated (Table 6.2).

Pulmonary artery wedge pressure

The PA wedge pressure (PAWP) is undertaken by inflating the balloon (see Procedure guideline 6.6). This causes the catheter to float into a smaller branch of the pulmonary artery and become wedged, resulting in an occlusion of blood flow through the vessel. As there are no valves between the catheter tip and the bicuspid valve in the left side of the heart, the pulmonary system is classed as 'open' to the left side of the heart. The pressure monitored therefore reflects left ventricular filling pressure or left ventricular end-diastolic pressure (normal 8–12 mmHg). This provides an indirect measurement of left ventricular preload. The normal PAWP waveform consists of an 'a' and 'v' wave, with the 'a' wave representing left atrial contraction and the 'v' wave representing right ventricular contraction. A high PAWP could indicate left-sided heart failure or pericardial tamponade, while a low pressure could indicate a reduced circulating volume (Adam and Osborne 2005; Jevon et al. 2007; Morton and Fontaine 2009; Urden et al. 2010).

The position of the catheter tip in the lungs is important for accurate PAWP recordings (Morgan 2003; Adam and Osborne 2005). As West (1990) identifies, there are three physiological zones where blood flow is dependent on PA pressure, pulmonary venous pressure (PVP) and the surrounding alveolar pressure. In zone one no blood flow occurs because the pulmonary capillaries are collapsed as alveolar pressure is greater than both the PA and PVP. In zone two some blood flow occurs because the PA pressure is greater than the alveolar pressure. In zone three PA pressure is higher than alveolar pressure, thus opening the capillaries resulting in blood flow. The catheter tip should be in this latter zone (Morgan 2003; Adam and Osborne 2005). Morgan (2003) suggests that this position can be checked at the bedside by a number of tests, including checking that the PAWP is less than the pulmonary artery diastolic pressure or checking that the respiratory swing in the PAWP during positive pressure ventilation does not exceed the respiratory swing in the pulmonary artery diastolic pressure. Another factor to consider when undertaking a PAWP measurement is the ventilatory status of the patient. Haemodynamic pressure measurements are more accurate when obtained at the end of expiration (Morton and Fontaine 2009). When a patient is breathing spontaneously, inspiration causes a negative intrathoracic pressure, which causes a negative deflection in the PAWP waveform. Therefore PAWP should be measured just before this deflection when the intrathoracic pressure influence is minimal (Morton and

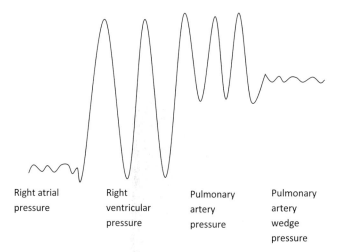

Right atrial
pressure

Right
ventricular
pressure

Pulmonary
artery
pressure

Pulmonary
artery
wedge
pressure

Figure 6.19 Waveforms on floating a pulmonary artery catheter.

Table 6.2 PA measurement parameters (Morgan 2003; Singer and Webb 2009)

Direct pressure measurements	Normal value	Indication
Right atrial (RA):	0–5 mmHg	Preload of the right ventricle
Right ventricular (RV)	20–25/0–5 mmHg	Systolic and diastolic pressure in the RV (measured during insertion)
Pulmonary artery pressure (PAP)	20–25/10–15 mmHg	Systolic and diastolic pressure in the PA
Pulmonary artery wedge pressure (PAWP)	6–12 mmHg	Reflects left ventricle end diastolic pressure (LVEDP) and LV preload
Cardiac output (CO) = HR × SV	4–6 L/min	Volume of blood ejected from the ventricle (primarily the left) per minute
Mixed venous oxygen saturation (SvO_2)	70–75%	SvO_2 is the percentage of saturated haemoglobin in blood returning to the PA

Derived parameters	Normal value	Indication
Stroke volume (SV)	70–100 mL	Volume of blood ejected from the ventricle (primarily the left) each beat
Cardiac index (CI) = CO × body surface area (BSA)	2.5–4.0 L/min/m^2	CO normalized (indexed) to the patient's body size
Systemic vascular resistance (SVR) $= \dfrac{(MAP - RAP) \times 79.9}{CO}$	960–1400 dynes·s/cm^5	SVR is the afterload that the left ventricle must overcome to eject its blood volume into the systemic circulation
Pulmonary vascular resistance (PVR) $= \dfrac{(MPA - PAW) \times 79.9}{CO}$	25–125 dynes·s/cm^5	PVR is the afterload that the right ventricle must overcome to eject its blood volume into the pulmonary circulation

Fontaine 2009; Urden et al. 2010). In a patient who is ventilated, inspiration causes a positive deflection in the PAWP waveform due to the corresponding increase in intrathoracic pressure. Therefore the PAWP should be measured just before the inspiratory rise (Morton and Fontaine 2009; Urden et al. 2010).

Mixed venous oxygen saturation

Another measurement that can be obtained directly either through continuous monitoring or intermittent sampling from the PA catheter is 'mixed venous oxygen saturation' (SvO_2). SvO_2 reflects the level of oxyhaemoglobin in desaturated blood returning to the PA. This is significantly lower (70–75%) than the level of oxyhaemoglobin (SaO_2) of blood returning from the lungs via the pulmonary vein, due to the extraction of oxygen during internal respiration (Morton and Fontaine 2009). Therefore measuring SvO_2 is an invaluable tool for monitoring the balance between oxygen delivery and consumption (Urden et al. 2010). A high SvO_2 could indicate increased oxygen supply or decreased oxygen demand, while a low SvO_2 could indicate increased oxygen consumption or low arterial saturation (SaO_2) (Urden et al. 2010).

Right atrial pressure and pulmonary artery pressure

Both RA and PA pressures fluctuate with the cardiac cycle and these variations can be displayed continuously in the shape of a waveform on the patient's monitor. The shape of these waveforms can then be analysed in relation to normal or abnormal function. The normal RA or CVP waveform consists of three peaks, which are an 'a', 'c' and 'v' wave (Pinnock et al. 2006) (see previous section 'Central Venous Pressure Monitoring'). A high RA pressure could indicate a number of clinical conditions, including right-sided heart failure, volume overload and pulmonary hypertension, while a low pressure could indicate a reduced circulating volume (Morton and Fontaine 2009).

The PA waveform is similar to an arterial waveform, consisting of systolic and diastolic components and a dicrotic notch on the downward slope of the waveform. This corresponds to the closure of the pulmonary valve (Morton and Fontaine 2009). The normal waveforms for the RA, RV, PA and PAWP during insertion can be can be seen in Figure 6.19. A high PA pressure (pulmonary hypertension) could be due to a number of clinical conditions, including pulmonary arterial hypertension, left-sided heart failure, chronic lung disease, thromboembolic disease and pericardial tamponade, while a low pressure could indicate a reduced circulating volume. A high PAWP could indicate left-sided heart failure.

Cardiac index

Derived parameters include cardiac index (CI), which indexes the CO measurement to the patient's body size thus providing a more precise assessment of cardiac function. CI is calculated by dividing the CO (L/min) by the patient's body surface area (BSA) (height [cm] × weight [kg]), e.g.

$$CI = \frac{CO}{BSA}$$

The normal CI is 2.5–4.0 L/min/m^2.

A high CI could indicate a high output state (septic shock), while a low pressure could indicate a number of clinical conditions including a reduced circulating volume (hypovolaemia) or reduced CO (cardiogenic shock).

Systemic vascular resistance

Systemic vascular resistance (SVR) can be calculated by measuring the difference between the MAP and the RA and multiplying this by a conversion factor of 79.9 to adjust the value into units of force (dynes·s/cm^5). This is then divided by the CO to give the afterload that the left ventricle must overcome to eject blood into the systemic circulation.

$$SVR = \frac{(MAP - RAP) \times 79.9}{CO}$$

The normal SVR is 960–100 dynes·s/cm^5.

A high SVR indicates peripheral vasoconstriction that could be caused by a number of clinical conditions including cardiogenic or hypovolaemic shock, while a low SVR indicates peripheral vasodilation caused by such conditions as septic shock.

Pulmonary vascular resistance

The pulmonary vascular resistance (PVR) can be calculated in a similar manner to the SVR, by measuring the difference between the mean pulmonary artery pressure (MPAP) and the PAWP and multiplying this by a conversion factor of 79.9 to adjust the value into units of force (dynes·s/cm^5). This is then divided by the CO to give the afterload that the right ventricle must overcome to eject blood into the pulmonary circulation:

$$PVR = \frac{(MPAP - PAWP) \times 79.9}{CO}$$

The normal PVR is 25–125 dynes·s/cm^5.

A high PVR indicates vasoconstriction in the pulmonary vasculature that could be caused by a number of clinical conditions including left ventricular failure, acute respiratory distress syndrome and pulmonary embolism. A low PVR can be found in patients receiving vasodilatory therapies.

Oxygen delivery (DO$_2$) and index (DO$_2$I) are the amount of oxygen transported to the tissues and depend on arterial oxygen content and CO (Morton and Fontaine 2009).

Complications of a PA catheter

Many complications exist with the insertion and use of a PA catheter (Morgan 2003; Adam and Osborne 2005; Jevon et al. 2007). These include:

- catheter insertion:
  - arrhythmias
  - heart block
  - knotting
  - malposition
- catheter:
  - balloon rupture
  - catheter disintegration
  - intracardiac trauma/perforation
  - PA rupture
  - catheter-related sepsis
  - PA thrombosis
  - pulmonary infarction
- in use:
  - arrhythmias
  - misinterpretation of data.

The management of a patient undergoing PA catheter monitoring is complex. Critical care practitioners must be able to interpret the various catheter waveforms and accurately collect and record data. They should also remain vigilant to potential complications and operator errors (Morton and Fontaine 2009). These are further described in the Procedure guideline 6.5.

199

Problem-solving table 6.5: Pulmonary artery catheter (Adam and Osborne 2005; Jevon et al. 2007)

Problem	Possible causes	Preventative measures	Suggested action
Spontaneous wedge[*1] (wedge trace on monitor even though balloon deflated)	Catheter migration further into pulmonary artery (PA)	Secure catheter, transducers and cables following local policy and manufacturer's guidelines Continuously monitor PA waveform and set alarm parameters	Check syringe for accidental inflation Urgently inform relevant senior practitioner(s) as the catheter will need repositioning

(Continued)

Right ventricular (RV) trace not PA	Catheter migration into RV	Secure catheter, transducers and cables following local policy and manufacturer's guidelines Continuously monitor PA waveform and set alarm parameters	Inform relevant senior practitioner(s) as the catheter will need repositioning
'Damped' trace on monitor	Loose connections Catheter tip against vessel wall	Set up pulmonary artery catheter components in line with manufacturer's guidelines	Check for loose connections – tighten Catheter tip against vessel wall – inform relevant senior practitioner(s) as the catheter will need repositioning
	Low pressure in pressure bag Air bubbles in transducer set Fibrin deposits on catheter tip	Continuously monitor PA waveform and set alarm parameters	Check pressure in pressure bag – reinflate (300 mmHg) as necessary. Air bubbles in transducer set – remove Fibrin deposits on tip – inform relevant senior practioner(s) as catheter needs aspirating/ flushing – follow local policy
Unable to obtain wedge when balloon inflated	Catheter tip not in the correct position	Set up pulmonary artery catheter components in line with manufacturer's guidelines Continuously monitor PA and PAWP waveform and set alarm parameters	Inform relevant senior practitioner as the catheter needs repositioning Balloon rupture – remove catheter
Trace rises steeply when balloon inflated ('over-wedged' trace)	Over inflation of balloon causes herniation over distal opening	Set up pulmonary artery catheter components in line with manufacturer's guidelines Continuously monitor PA and PAWP waveform and set alarm parameters	Inform relevant senior practitioner(s) as the catheter will need repositioning
Blood in syringe when air removed	Balloon rupture	Set up pulmonary artery catheter components in line with manufacturer's guidelines Continuously monitor PA and PAWP waveform and set alarm parameters Observe transducer set	Turn off tap and inform relevant senior practitioner(s) as the catheter needs replacing
Discrepancies in measurements of CO	Poor injection technique Cardiac arrhythmias Patient movement Incorrect injectate volume	Set up pulmonary artery catheter components in line with manufacturer's guidelines Continuously monitor ECG, PA and PAWP waveform and set alarm parameters Perform CO measurement in line with manufacturer's guidelines	Poor injection technique – repeat correct technique Patient movement – repeat when patient is not moving Incorrect injectate volume – use correct volume
Blood temperature not displayed	Faulty thermistor	Set up pulmonary artery catheter components in line with manufacturer's guidelines Continuously monitor temperature	Replace catheter if necessary
Injectate fluid temperature not displayed	Faulty temperature probe	Set up pulmonary artery catheter components in line with manufacturer's guidelines	Replace

*¹A 'wedged trace' is the terminology used to describe the change in the PA trace on the monitor when the balloon is inflated.

Transpulmonary dilution method

The transpulmonary dilution method encompasses a number of techniques that use either a known amount of cold fluid (transpulmonary thermodilution), or a chemical or dye (trans-pulmonary dilution) as indicators to calculate CO.

Transpulmonary thermodilution

The thermal method of transpulmonary dilution is similar to that of the PA catheter thermodilution technique in that the change in temperature of the indicator is plotted over a given period of time in the form of a time–temperature curve. An ice-cold fluid bolus (minimum of 15mL of 0.9% sodium chloride) acts as the thermal indicator and this is given via a central venous catheter. The fluid bolus rapidly disperses within the pulmonary and cardiac blood volumes. When the 0.9% sodium chloride indicator reaches an arterial thermistor, a temperature difference is detected and the time–temperature curve is plotted and CO is calculated using the Stewart–Hamilton equation (Tote and Grounds 2006; Jhanji et al. 2008). An example of the transpulmonary thermodilution technique is the Pulse Induced Continuous Cardiac Output System (PiCCO), which uses a specialized arterial catheter that has a temperature sensor built in to it (Singer and Webb 2009).

The PiCCO system

■ The PiCCO system (a transpulmonary thermodilution technique) can be utilized to monitor and calculate intermittent CO. Both a specialized arterial catheter that has a temperature sensor at its tip and a CVC for the administration of the thermal indicator are required. Temperature is measured as the indicator is injected into the CVC and the change in temperature is detected by the arterial catheter thermistor. The CO is then calculated. Three calibrations should be undertaken to achieve an accurate reading. A number of additional parameters are also determined from the time–temperature curve including global end-diastolic volume (GEDV). This is the total volume of all four chambers of the heart at the end of diastole and as a result is an indicator of preload (Cottis et al. 2003; Singer and Webb 2009). A high GEDV could indicate volume overload, while a low GEDV could indicate a reduced circulating volume. This can be indexed (GEDI) to the patient's body size thus providing a more precise assessment (normal values are shown in Table 6.3).

■ Intrathoracic blood volume (ITBV). This is the sum of the GEDV and the pulmonary thermal volume (or pulmonary blood volume). That is, the total volume of the blood in the four chambers of the heart plus the blood volume in the lungs, and like GEDV is an indicator of preload (Cottis et al. 2003; Morgan 2003). A high ITBV could indicate volume overload, while a low ITBV could indicate a reduced circulating volume. This can be indexed (ITBI) to the patient's body size thus providing a more precise assessment (normal values are shown in Table 6.3).

■ Extravascular lung water (EVLW). This is the volume of water in the lung tissue and provides a measure of the degree of pulmonary oedema (Singer and Webb 2009). This can indicate the severity of clinical conditions such as acute respiratory distress syndrome because EVLW would be raised in ARDS (Cottis et al. 2003). This can be indexed (EVLI) to the patient's body size thus providing a more precise assessment (normal values are shown in Table 6.3).

■ Cardiac function index (CFI). This is calculated from the ratio of CI to the GEDV and indicates the contractile state of the heart (Cottis et al. 2003; Ritter et al. 2009).

■ Global ejection fraction (GEF). This is the ratio of the stroke volume to the quarter of the global end-diastolic volume (Combes et al. 2004) and indicates cardiac performance (Ritter et al. 2009) (normal values are shown in Table 6.3).

■ Pulmonary vascular permeability index (PVPI). This gives a measure of how much pulmonary oedema there is in relation to the volume of preload. PVPI can be used

201

Table 6.3 Normal limits of haemodynamic status using PiCCO, LiDCO and ODM

	PiCCO	LiDCO	ODM
Heart rate	60–100 beats/min	60–100 beats/min	60–100 beats/min
CO (HR × SV)	4–8 L/min	4–8 L/min	4–8 L/min
Cardiac index (CO × BSA)	2.5–4.0 L/min/m²	2.5–4.0 L/min/m²	2.5–4.0 L/min/m²
Flow time corrected (FTc)			330–360 ms
Peak velocity (PV)			80–110 cm/s (40yrs)
Mean acceleration (MA)			Decreased MA: ■ decrease in contractility ■ increase in afterload Increased MA: ■ increase in contractility ■ decrease in afterload

(Continued)

Table 6.3 (*Continued*)

	PiCCO	LiDCO	ODM
Stroke distance (SD)			Dependent on patient's size and age A change of more than 10% − likely to be preload responsive A change of less than 10% − unlikely to be preload responsive
Cardiac function index (CFI = CI / GEDV)	4.5–6.5 L/min		
Global ejection fraction (GEF = SV / [GEDV/4])	25–35%		
Global end-diastolic volume index (the difference between intrathoracic thermal volume [ITTV] and pulmonary thermal volume [PTV indexed to the surface area])	680–800 mL/m²		
Intrathoracic blood volume index (GEDV × 1.25 indexed to the body surface area)	850–1000 mL/m²		
Extravascular lung water index (ELWI = intrathoracic thermal volume [ITTV] − intrathoracic blood volume [ITBV])	3–7 mL/kg		
Stroke volume	55–100 mL	55–100 mL	55–100 mL
Stroke volume variation (SVV %)	less than 10% − unlikely to be preload responsive greater than 13–15% − likely to be preload responsive	less than 10% − unlikely to be preload responsive greater than 13–15% − likely to be preload responsive	
Systolic pressure variation (SPV %)		less than 5 mmHg − unlikely to be preload responsive greater than 5 mmHg − likely to be preload responsive	
Pulse pressure variation (PPV %)	less than 10% − unlikely to be preload responsive greater than 13–15% − likely to be preload responsive	less than 10% − unlikely to be preload responsive greater than 13–15% − likely to be preload responsive	
Systemic vascular resistance (SVR) = (MAP − CVP) / (CO × 79.9)	960–1400 dynes·s/cm⁵	960–1400 dynes·s/cm⁵	
Systemic vascular resistance index (SVRI) (MAP − CVP) / (CI × 79.9)	1970–2390 dynes·s/cm⁵/m²	1970–2390 dynes·s/cm⁵/m²	
Oxygen delivery (DO₂) = (CaO₂ [arterial oxygen content] × CO × 10)	950–1150 mL/min (PiCCO₂)	950–1150 mL/min	
Oxygen delivery index (DO₂i) = (CaO₂ × CI × 10)	500–600 mL/min/m² (PiCCO₂)	500–600 mL/min/m²	

to determine if the cause of the pulmonary oedema is from a hydrostatic or a permeability problem (Monnet et al. 2007) (normal values are shown in Table 6.3).

- Oxygen delivery (DO_2), and index (DO_2I). This is the amount of oxygen transported to the tissues and depends on arterial oxygen content and CO (Morton and Fontaine 2009) (normal values are shown in Table 6.3).

Once the system has been calibrated using the transpulmonary thermodilution technique a continuous CO measurement can be obtained using pulse contour analysis. This method uses the arterial waveform to continuously analyse the curve and to calculate the CO. The calculation is based on the Wesseling algorithm, which is underpinned by the concept that the contour of the arterial pressure waveform is proportional to stroke volume (Singer and Webb 2009). Two other parameters can be calculated from the arterial pressure waveform (Figure 6.13) and these can be used as indicators of intravascular blood volume only in ventilated patients.

- Stroke volume variation (SVV%), which is the difference between the maximum and minimum stroke volume divided by the mean of the maximum and minimum stroke volumes over a given time period, described as a percentage.
- Pulse pressure variation (PPV%), which is the variation, as a percentage, of the pulse pressure (*see* Chapter 3).

This can give an indicator of how responsive the patient will be to fluid administration. For example, if a ventilated patient has more than 13–15% variation in these parameters they would be more likely to respond to fluid replacement (Parry-Jones and Pittman 2003; Ercole 2007). Like other advanced forms of monitoring, the management of a patient undergoing PiCCO monitoring is complex. Again critical care practitioners must be able to interpret various catheter waveforms and accurately collect and record data. They should also remain vigilant to potential complications and operator errors. These are further described in Procedure guideline 6.10.

Problem-solving table 6.6: Transpulmonary cardiac output monitoring using thermodilution (e.g. PiCCO) (Pulsion Medical Systems 2009)

PROBLEM	Possible causes	Preventative measures	Suggested action
Indicator injection was not detected	CVC malpositioned 3-way-stopcock incorrectly adjusted Temperature sensor housing pin clotted Temperature sensor housing/sensor not connected correctly Defective temperature sensor	Set up components in line with manufacturer's guidelines	CVC malpositioned – check position 3-way stopcock incorrectly adjusted – adjust Temperature sensor housing pin clotted – change Temperature sensor housing/sensor not connected correctly – check connection Defective temperature sensor – check and/or replace
Indicator injection error message	Incorrect technique/volume of injectate	Perform injection technique following manufacturer's guidelines	Repeat injection using correct technique/volume
Unstable temperature baseline measurement	Arterial connection cable broken or incorrectly connected Faulty thermistor on PiCCO catheter Thermistor lying against vessel wall	Set up components in line with manufacturer's guidelines	Arterial connection cable broken or incorrectly connected – check connection, replace if necessary Faulty thermistor on PiCCO catheter – replace catheter Thermistor lying against vessel wall – change patient position, replace catheter
Thermodilution curve is not displayed	Incorrect injection at central venous catheter Faulty thermistor on PiCCO catheter Poor connection on arterial cable	Set up components in line with manufacturer's guidelines Perform injection technique following manufacturer's guidelines	Incorrect injection at central venous catheter – repeat injection using correct technique Faulty thermistor on PiCCO catheter – replace catheter Poor connection on arterial cable – check and replace if necessary

(Continued)

Problem solving table 6.6: *(Continued)*

Thermodilution curve display is too late (time out limit)	Incorrect injection at central venous catheter Patient's CO very low or they have a very high EVLW	Perform injection technique following manufacturer's guidelines	Injection too slow – inject faster (less than 7 s) Very low CO or very high EVLW – use colder and/or more injectate
Thermodilution curve flattened	Inappropriate scale settings Injectate too warm Patient's CO very low or they have a very high EVLW	Set up components in line with manufacturer's guidelines Perform injection technique following manufacturer's guidelines	Inappropriate scale settings – adjust scale Injectate too warm – use colder injectate Very low CO or very high EVLW – use colder and/or more injectate

Transpulmonary dilution using dye or a chemical

In the transpulmonary dilution technique a chemical such as lithium is used as the indicator. This is given intravenously and disperses within the pulmonary and cardiac blood volumes. When the indicator reaches a specialized sensor attached to an arterial cannula, the dilution of the indicator is calculated and plotted on a time–plasma concentration curve. As with the other transpulmonary techniques the Stewart–Hamilton equation is then used to calculate CO (Adam and Osborne 2005: 514; Morton and Fontaine 2009: 313). An example of transpulmonary dilution technique is Lithium Dilution Cardiac Output system (LiDCO).

The LiDCO system

The LiDCO system uses lithium chloride as the transpulmonary indicator. This is injected into a CVC or a peripheral cannula usually in 0.3 mmol increments to a maximum of 3 mmol. A battery-powered peristaltic pump placed in the arterial tubing draws arterial blood through a disposable lithium-selective electrode sensor. The decreasing lithium dilution curve is then analysed in order to calculate the CO (Adam and Osborne 2005; Costa et al. 2008). The Nernst equation is used to calculate the plasma concentration of lithium in relation to the voltage across the sensor membrane (Jonas et al. 2002; Rhodes and Sunderland 2005). Cecconi et al. (2009) advise that three calibrations should be undertaken to obtain a high level of precision.

Once the system has been calibrated using the transpulmonary dilution technique, continuous CO measurements can be obtained using pulse contour analysis. This method uses the arterial catheter waveform and continuously analyses the curve to calculate the CO. The analysis is based on an autocorrelation algorithm (Jonas et al. 2002). Although calibration is generally advocated at least 8–12 hourly (Hamilton et al. 2002; Adam and Osborne 2005), a more recent study by Cecconi et al. (2008) advises that in order to maintain accuracy this should be undertaken every 4 hours. In addition to heart rate, BP, SV, CO and CI, a range of other haemodynamic parameters can be calculated, including the following.

- Systolic pressure variation (SPV). This is calculated from the minimum and maximum systolic pressure changes measured across a respiratory cycle.
- Stroke volume variation (SVV%). This is the difference between the maximum and minimum stroke volume divided by the mean of the maximum and minimum stroke volumes over a given time period, described as a percentage.
- Pulse pressure variation (PPV%). This is the variation, as a percentage, of the pulse pressure. This can give an indication of how responsive the patient will be to fluid administration.
- SPV, SVV and PPV. These can give an indicator of how responsive a ventilated patient will be to fluid administration (Parry-Jones and Pittman 2003; Ercole 2007).
- Systemic vascular resistance (SVR), and index (SVRI). This relates to the afterload that the left ventricle must overcome to eject its blood volume into the systemic circulation. A high SVR indicates peripheral vasoconstriction that could be caused by a number a number of clinical conditions including cardiogenic or hypovolaemic shock, whilst a low SVR indicates peripheral vasodilation caused by such conditions as septic shock.
- Oxygen delivery (DO_2) and index (DO_2I). This is the amount of oxygen transported to the tissues and depends on arterial oxygen content and CO (Parry-Jones and Pittman 2003; Ercole 2007; Morton and Fontaine 2009).

Like other forms of advanced monitoring, the management of a patient undergoing LiDCO monitoring is complex. Again critical care practitioners must be able to interpret the various catheter waveforms and accurately collect and record data. They should also remain vigilant to potential complications and operator errors. These are further described in the Procedure guidelines 6.7 and 6.8.

Oesophageal Doppler monitoring

Oesophageal Doppler monitoring (ODM) is an easy-to-use, accurate and minimally invasive method of monitoring haemodynamic parameters (Adam and Osborne 2005; Lowe et al. 2010). ODM involves the utilization of a single-use disposable probe that is inserted into the patient's oesophagus

Problem-solving table 6.7: Transpulmonary cardiac output monitoring using lithium dilution (e.g. LiDCOplus)

Problem	Possible causes	Preventative measures	Suggested action
Sensor voltage out of range	Incorrect set up Faulty sensor connections	Set up components in line with manufacturer's guidelines	Re-flush sensor Faulty sensor connections – check connections and replace if necessary
Unstable baseline	Incorrect calibration	Set up components in line with manufacturer's guidelines	Re-flush sensor Ensure calibration performed when there is no patient movement
Discrepancies in measurements of CO	Poor injection technique Cardiac arrhythmias	Perform injection technique following manufacturer's guidelines Observe for arrhythmias	Poor injection technique – repeat with correct technique

through either the mouth or nose. A low-frequency ultrasound signal is then directed through the descending aorta and is reflected back by the red blood cells as they travel down the aorta. The probe detects the reflected ultrasound signal and analysing the changes in the frequency (Doppler effect) determines the velocity of the travelling blood cells (Iregui et al. 2003). This produces real-time information about left ventricular flow by measuring the flow of blood down the descending aorta (Adam and Osborne 2005).

The ODM probe is inserted via the mouth or nose to a depth of approximately 25–40 cm. At this point the oesophagus lies close to the descending aorta in the region of T5 and T6 vertebrae. The probe is then positioned so that the ultrasound signal is directed towards the oesophagus and adjusted until a clear pulsatile triangular waveform appears (Morton and Fontaine 2009). The 'ideal' waveform should have a black central portion and a sharp outline in red, orange, yellow and white. The colours correspond to the proportion of blood cells moving at a given speed at that point in time. White indicates the speed at which most of the blood cells are moving, while red indicates the velocity at which few of the cells are moving. Black indicates no movement (Adam and Osborne 2005).

Interpretation of ODM waveform

The monitor uses a nomogram that includes the patient's height, weight and age to estimate the aortic cross-sectional area, which can then be used to calculate a number of derived and direct parameters (Gan et al. 2002; Morgan 2003). These include the following.

- Flow time corrected (FTc). This is the duration of blood flow during systole corrected for heart rate (adjusted to a heart rate of 60 bpm to give one cardiac cycle per second) and is an indicator of preload (Morgan 2003). When combined with peak velocity (PV), FTc can be a guide to afterload (Ott et al. 2001). Therefore a fall in FTc could indicate hypovolaemia or increased afterload, while a rise could indicate vasodilation (Singer and Webb 2009).

- Peak velocity (PV). This is the highest blood velocity detected during systole and gives an indication of left ventricular contraction (Singer and Webb 2009; Lowe et al. 2010). Therefore a fall in PV could indicate heart failure (Singer and Webb 2009).
- Mean acceleration. This is the average acceleration of blood from the start of systole to the PV and can be used as a marker of left ventricular contractility (Lowe et al. 2010).
- Stroke distance (SD). This is the distance in cm that a column of blood moves along the aorta and the SV is calculated from this measure (Lowe et al. 2010). A fall in SD and SV could indicate hypovolaemia (Lowe et al. 2010).

Again due to the complexity of ODM monitoring critical care practitioners when managing these patients must be able to interpret the various waveforms and also accurately collect and record data. They should also remain vigilant to potential complications and operator errors. These are further described in the Procedure guidelines 6.12.

Summary

The optimization of a patient's haemodynamic status is a key goal in the management of a critically ill patient. This requires the achievement of optimal cardiac output, oxygen delivery and adequate organ perfusion (Morton et al. 2009; Whiteley et al. 2010). Critical care practitioners need to possess the knowledge and skills to provide this care in a competent and effective manner. This chapter has outlined a range of advanced haemodynamic monitoring technologies that have been developed to support practitioners in monitoring the cardiovascular status of critically ill patients, to aid the diagnosis of disorders, and guide and evaluate treatments. These technologies include the pulmonary thermodilution approach, the transpulmonary thermodilution approach and the use of Doppler ultrasound.

Problem-solving table 6.8: Oesophageal Doppler monitoring (ODM) (e.g. CardioQ) (Deltex Medical 2009)

Problem	Possible causes	Preventative measures	Suggested action
Poor aortic velocity/time waveform	Poor probe position/focus	Reposition probe in line with manufacturer's guidelines	Check probe inserted to correct depth markers Re-focus probe Check NG tube not obstructing probe Reinsert probe
Waveform too large	Incorrect scale/range settings	Set up components in line with manufacturer's guidelines	Adjust the scale/range setting in the probe focus screen until the full waveform is visible
No probe connected message	Faulty connection	Set up components in line with manufacturer's guidelines	Check connections and replace if necessary

Procedure guideline 6.1: Application of continuous ECG monitoring (adapted with permission from the Royal Marsden Hospital Manual of Clinical Nursing Procedures)

Equipment

- Electrodes (3 or 5 depending on whether 3- or 5-lead monitoring is required)
- Appropriate cables to attach the electrodes to the monitor (3 or 5 wires depending on the monitoring required)

Procedure

Action	Rationale
1 Where possible, explain and discuss the procedure with the patient. If the patient lacks the capacity to make decisions the practitioner must act in the patient's best interests.	To ensure that the patient understands the procedure and gives their valid consent. To ensure the patient's best interests are maintained (Mental Capacity Act 2005).
2 Maintain good skin contact – clean and dry the skin and remove excess hair.	To prepare the skin for placement of electrodes in order to maximize the contact between electrode and skin.
3 Place the electrodes in the correct position, ensuring a good contact with skin.	To obtain an accurate and reliable ECG trace.
4 Attach a wire to each electrode and connect via a cable to the monitor.	To allow the ECG recording to be displayed on the monitor.
5 Ensure the alarm settings for upper and lower limits of heart rate are switched on the monitor.	To allow rapid detection of changes that may appear on the ECG trace and enable prompt intervention.
6 Document care.	To: ■ provide an accurate record ■ monitor effectiveness of procedure ■ reduce the risk of duplication of treatment ■ provide a point of reference or comparison in the event of later questions ■ acknowledge accountability for actions ■ facilitate communication and continuity of care. (NMC 2008; GMC 2013; HCPC 2012)

Procedure guideline 6.2: Setting up the arterial pressure monitoring system and insertion of an arterial cannula (adapted with permission from the Royal Marsden Hospital Manual of Clinical Nursing Procedures)

Equipment

- 500 mL pressure bag
- 500 mL bag of 0.9% sodium chloride
- 20G arterial cannula
- Sterile intravenous pack
- Sterile gloves
- 2% chlorhexidine gluconate in 70% isopropyl alcohol

- Sterile semi-permeable transparent polyurethane dressing
- 2 mL syringe
- Labels to identify infusion set as attached to an arterial cannula
- 1% lidocaine injection
- Pressure monitoring system equipment

Procedure

Action	Rationale
1 Where possible, explain and discuss the procedure with the patient. If the patient lacks the capacity to make decisions the practitioner must act in the patient's best interests. (Note: most arterial cannula are inserted when patients are anaesthetized.)	To ensure that the patient understands the procedure and gives their valid consent. To ensure the patient's best interests are maintained (Mental Capacity Act 2005).
2 Check that all Luer lock connections in the infusion set are secure.	To prevent disconnection.
3 Connect infusion set to 500 mL bag of 0.9% sodium chloride.	To prepare infusion.
4 Insert bag of 0.9% sodium chloride into pressure bag. Inflate to 300 mmHg.	To deliver 3 mL/h of 0.9% sodium chloride through the infusion set in order to prevent back flow of blood into the infusion set and maintain patency of the circuit, cannula and artery.
5 Open roller clamp fully.	To allow infusion to flow and to check the flow rate.
6 Squeeze the flush device-actuator (see instructions with set).	To prime the administration set and three-way tap ports with 0.9% sodium chloride.
7 Check thoroughly for air bubbles in the circuit and if any present continue to squeeze the flush device until they have been removed.	To reduce the risk of an air embolus and to prevent damping of the arterial pressure waveform.
8 Prepare trolley near the patient using an aseptic technique.	To reduce the risk of infection.
9 Wash hands and put on sterile gloves.	To reduce the risk of cross-infection. To prevent contamination of hands if blood spillage occurs.
10 Prepare the insertion site with 2% chlorhexidine gluconate in 70% isopropyl alcohol. Place a sterile drape around the insertion site.	To maintain asepsis. To provide a clean working area.

(Continued)

Procedure guideline 6.2: (Continued)

11 Inject local anaesthetic subcutaneously if cannulation is performed while the patient is conscious.	To minimize pain during the procedure.
12 If required, assistant to hold patient's hand in position requested by inserter.	To prevent movement and facilitate insertion.
13 Insert cannula using an aseptic technique.	To reduce the risk of infection.
14 Apply pressure to artery distal to the end of the cannula.	To reduce the risk of blood spillage.
15 Attach infusion set to cannula.	To allow pressure measurement.
16 Open roller clamp fully.	To allow infusion to flow and to prevent back flow of blood.
17 Check there is an arterial pressure waveform on the monitor.	To ensure the cannula is in the correct position.
18 Apply a semi-permeable transparent dressing over the cannula.	Leaving the site visible allows the observer to recognize immediately any dislodgement or disconnection or evidence of infection.
19 Clearly label the infusion set and cannula as 'arterial'.	Clear labelling prevents accidental injection of drugs into the artery rather than a vein.
20 Position the pressure transducer at the same level as the patient's right atrium.	To ensure an accurate recording of blood pressure can be obtained.
21 Calibrate (zero) the transducer by: ■ turning the tap at the transducer so it is 'off to the patient and open to air' ■ pushing button on the monitor to zero ■ returning the tap to 'on to patient and off to air'.	To enable accurate pressure measurements. To stop the fluid from the flush bag running down to the cannula and direct it to the opening in the tap to air. To calibrate the system to zero. To enable system to be continuous from patient to monitoring equipment to enable measurement of arterial pressure.
22 Set appropriate alarm limits for the arterial blood pressure on the monitor.	To detect significant changes in arterial blood pressure in a timely fashion.
23 Document care.	To: ■ provide an accurate record ■ monitor effectiveness of procedure ■ reduce the risk of duplication of treatment ■ provide a point of reference or comparison in the event of later questions ■ acknowledge accountability for actions ■ facilitate communication and continuity of care. (NMC 2008; GMC 2013; HCPC 2012)

Procedure guideline 6.3: Setting up the CVP monitoring system and insertion of a central venous catheter

Equipment

- 500 mL pressure bag
- 500 mL bag of 0.9% sodium chloride
- Central venous catheter with appropriate number of lumens
- Sterile intravenous pack
- Sterile gown and gloves
- Sterile drape
- 2% chlorhexidine gluconate in 70% isopropyl alcohol

- Sterile semi-permeable transparent polyurethane dressing
- 2 mL, 5 mL and 10 mL syringes
- 0.9% sodium chloride to flush the lumens of the catheter
- Labels to identify infusion set as attached to a CVC
- 1% lidocaine injection
- Appropriate suture material
- Pressure monitoring system equipment

Procedure

Action	Rationale
1 If possible, explain and discuss the procedure with the patient. If the patient lacks the capacity to make decisions the practitioner must act in the patient's best interests.	To ensure that the patient understands the procedure and gives their valid consent. To ensure the patient's best interests are maintained (Mental Capacity Act 2005).
2 Wash hands with antiseptic hand wash and alcohol gel, and wear appropriate personal protective equipment when handling equipment undertaking procedures.	To reduce the risk of microbial contamination (Pratt et al. 2007). To reduce risk of infection (Patient Safety First 2008).
3 Open infusion set and check that all Luer lock connections are tightly secure.	To prevent disconnection.
4 Connect infusion set to 500 mL bag of 0.9% sodium chloride.	To prepare infusion.
5 Insert bag of 0.9% sodium chloride into pressure bag. Inflate to 300 mmHg.	To deliver continuously 3 mL/h of 0.9% sodium chloride through the infusion set in order to prevent back flow of blood into the infusion set and maintain patency of the circuit, catheter and vein.
6 Open roller clamp fully.	To allow infusion to flow and to check the flow rate.
7 Squeeze the flush device actuator (see instructions with set).	To prime the administration set and three-way tap ports with 0.9% sodium chloride.
8 Check thoroughly for air bubbles in the circuit and if any present continue to squeeze the flush device until these are flushed out.	Reduces the risk of an air embolus entering the patient's circulation.
9 Attach the patient to a cardiac monitor as per unit protocol.	To assess and monitor patient for signs of arrhythmias during guide wire insertion.
10 Place the patient's bed in a head down position, as tolerated.	To reduce the risk of air embolism and aid insertion of the catheter.
11 Operator: put on sterile hat and mask, scrub up and put on sterile gown and gloves.	CVC insertion should be performed under strict asepsis (Pratt et al. 2007; Patient Safety First 2008).
12 Assistant: open the required equipment in a sterile manner and pass to the operator.	To maintain asepsis. To assist the operator.
13 Operator: clean skin with 2% chlorhexidine gluconate in 70% isopropyl alcohol and place a full sterile drape over the patient.	To maintain asepsis.

(Continued)

14	Assistant: for conscious patients ensure the patient is comfortable with the placement of the drapes. Reassure the patient.	To reduce anxiety of the patient. The drapes for internal jugular and subclavian vein placement are over the face and can cause anxiety.
15	Inject 1% lidocaine subcutaneously if CVC is inserted while the patient is conscious.	To prevent pain during insertion.
16	Operator: insert CVC using Seldinger technique (see below) under ultrasound guidance.	Use of ultrasound for the insertion of a CVC (NICE 2002).
17	Assistant: observe the cardiac monitor during insertion of the catheter.	To check for arrhythmias.
18	Operator: locate vein using ultrasound guidance.	To ensure the vein – not artery – is cannulated.
19	Operator: puncture vein using needle.	To access vein and provide route to vein for guide wire.
20	Operator: thread guide wire through needle.	To maintain access to vein when needle is removed.
21	Operator: remove needle from vein and guide wire.	To allow insertion of dilator.
22	Operator: pass dilator over guide wire into the vein.	To dilate vein to allow entry of the CVC.
23	Operator: remove dilator.	To allow insertion of CVC.
24	Operator: place CVC over guide wire to approximately 12 to 15 cm depending on site of insertion and size of the patient.	To enable CVC to be guided directly into vein and to correct position.
25	Operator: remove guide wire.	To allow blood and/or infusion to flow through the lumens.
26	Operator: aspirate all lumens of the CVC.	To check that blood is aspirated from all lumens to ensure the catheter is in the vein.
27	Operator: flush all lumens with 0.9% sodium chloride.	To prevent thrombosis.
28	Operator: suture catheter to the skin.	To prevent the catheter falling out.
29	Cover the insertion site with a semi-permeable transparent dressing.	To keep the area clean and aid inspection of the site for signs of infection.
30	Attach infusion set to the distal lumen while ensuring the lumen is closed to air.	To allow pressure measurement and prevent air embolism.
31	Open roller clamp fully.	To allow infusion to flow and to prevent back flow of blood.
32	Ensure the transducer is at the level of the patient's right atrium and calibrate (zero) the transducer by: ■ turning the tap at the transducer so it is 'off to the patient and open to air' ■ pushing button on the monitor to zero ■ returning the tap to 'on to patient and off to air'.	To enable accurate pressure measurements. To stop the fluid from the flush bag running down to the cannula and direct it to the opening in the tap to air. To calibrate the system to zero. To enable system to be continuous from patient to monitoring equipment to enable measurement of CVP.
33	Set appropriate alarm limits for the CVP on the monitor.	To detect significant changes in CVP in a timely fashion.
34	Document care.	To: ■ provide an accurate record ■ monitor effectiveness of procedure ■ reduce the risk of duplication of treatment ■ provide a point of reference or comparison in the event of later questions ■ acknowledge accountability for actions ■ facilitate communication and continuity of care. (NMC 2008; GMC 2013; HCPC 2012)

Procedure guideline 6.4: Insertion of a pulmonary artery catheter (PAC)

Equipment

- Central venous catheter insertion equipment
- PA catheter
- PAC introducer
- Cable to connect transducer to monitor
- Monitor with the ability to display pulmonary artery pressure, and measure CO and PAWP

- Bag of 0.9% sodium chloride and giving set attached to lumen of PAC to use as injectate to measure CO
- Connector to attach temperature sensor to lumen of PAC where 0.9% sodium chloride is injected for CO measurement
- Labels to identify infusion set as attached to a PA catheter

Procedure

Insertion of PAC introducer

Action	Rationale
1 If possible, explain and discuss the procedure with the patient. If the patient lacks the capacity to make decisions the practitioner must act in the patient's best interests.	To ensure that the patient understands the procedure and gives their valid consent. To ensure the patient's best interests are maintained (Mental Capacity Act 2005).
2 Wash hands with antiseptic hand wash and alcohol gel, and wear appropriate personal protective equipment when handling equipment and undertaking procedures.	To reduce the risk of microbial contamination (Pratt et al. 2007). To reduce risk of infection (Patient Safety First 2008).
3 Open infusion set and check that all Luer lock connections are tightly secure.	To prevent disconnection.
4 Connect infusion set to 500 mL bag of 0.9% sodium chloride.	To prepare infusion.
5 Insert bag of 0.9% sodium chloride into pressure bag. Inflate to 300 mmHg.	To continuously deliver 3 mL/h of 0.9% sodium chloride through the infusion set in order to prevent back flow of blood into the infusion set and maintain patency of the circuit, catheter and vein.
6 Open roller clamp fully.	To allow infusion to flow and to check the flow rate.
7 Squeeze the flush device-actuator (see instructions with set).	To prime the administration set and three-way tap ports with 0.9% sodium chloride.
8 Check thoroughly for air bubbles in the circuit and if any present continue to squeeze the flush device until these are flushed out.	To reduce the risk of an air embolus entering the patient's circulation.
9 Attach the patient to a cardiac monitor as per unit protocol.	To assess and monitor patient for signs of arrhythmias during guide wire insertion.
10 Place the patient's bed in a head down position, as tolerated.	To reduce the risk of air embolism and aid insertion of the catheter.
11 Operator: put on sterile hat and mask, scrub up and put on sterile gown and gloves.	PAC insertion should be performed under strict asepsis (Pratt et al. 2007; Patient Safety First 2008).
12 Assistant: open the required equipment in a sterile manner and pass to the operator.	To maintain asepsis. To assist the operator.
13 Operator: clean skin with 2% chlorhexidine gluconate in 70% isopropyl alcohol and place a full sterile drape over the patient.	To maintain asepsis.
14 Assistant: for conscious patients ensure the patient is comfortable with the placement of the drapes. Reassure the patient.	To reduce anxiety of the patient. The drapes for internal jugular and subclavian vein placement are over the face and can cause anxiety.

(Continued)

15 Inject 1% lidocaine subcutaneously if PAC is inserted while the patient is conscious.	To prevent pain during insertion.
16 Operator: insert PAC introducer using Seldinger technique (see below) under ultrasound guidance.	Use of ultrasound for the insertion of a PAC (NICE 2002).
17 Assistant: observe the cardiac monitor during insertion of the catheter.	To check for arrhythmias.
18 Operator: locate vein using ultrasound guidance.	To ensure the vein not artery is cannulated.
19 Operator: puncture vein using needle.	To access vein and provide route to vein for guide wire.
20 Operator: thread guide wire through needle.	To maintain access to vein when needle is removed.
21 Operator: remove needle from vein and guide wire.	To allow insertion of dilator and PAC introducer.
22 Operator: put dilator into PAC introducer and pass both over guide wire into the vein.	To dilate vein to allow entry of the PAC introducer into the vein.
23 Operator: remove dilator and guide wire.	To allow blood and or infusion to flow through the lumens.
24 Operator: aspirate the lumen of the PAC introducer.	To check that blood is aspirated from the lumen to ensure the catheter is in the vein.
25 Operator: flush the lumen with 0.9% sodium chloride.	To prevent thrombosis.
26 Operator: suture PAC introducer to the skin.	To prevent the catheter falling out.

Insertion of PAC

27 (a) Flush all lumens of the PA catheter and connect the infusion set attached to the pressure transducer to the distal lumen.	(a) To reduce the risk of an air embolus.
(b) Calibrate (zero) the transducer on the monitor.	(b) To avoid erroneous haemodynamic data being displayed.
(c) Check inflation syringe is connected to the lumen attached to the balloon.	(c) To prevent accidental disconnection and dislodging (Shoemaker et al. 2002; Adam and Osborne 2005; Morton et al. 2009; Urden et al. 2010).
(d) Perform a check inflation of the balloon.	(d) To observe for signs of rupture of the balloon and to prevent air embolus. To ensure the PAC is functioning correctly.
28 To insert PA catheter:	
(a) Attach sterile sheath over the PAC and insert PAC through the self-sealing diaphragm of the PAC introducer.	(a) To maintain catheter sterility.
(b) Observe both the PA pressure waveform for characteristic changes (Figure 6.20), and ECG for arrhythmias.	(b) To assess the position of the PAC and observe for arrhythmias as the catheter can cause arrhythmias as it floats through the chambers of the right side of the heart.
(c) Advance the catheter with the balloon deflated until a right atrial trace is obtained.	(c) To assess the position of the PAC.
(d) Inflate balloon and advance/float the catheter until a characteristic PAP trace is obtained. Slowly continue to advance until a wedged trace appears on the monitor.	(d) To aid insertion of the PAC.
(e) Stop advancing/floating the catheter and deflate the balloon (the PAP trace should return).	(e) To prevent rupture of the pulmonary artery and infarction of lung tissue.
(f) Cover the insertion site with a semi-permeable transparent dressing	(f) To keep the area clean and aid inspection of the site for signs of infection.
(g) Obtain a chest X-ray.	(g) To assess the position of the PAC (Shoemaker et al. 2002; Singer and Webb 2009).

29 Set up of the pulmonary artery catheter components in line with manufacturer's guidelines, including: ■ thermistor ■ cardiac output injectate components (If appropriate).	To allow CO measurements to be performed. To avoid erroneous haemodynamic data being displayed. To prevent accidental disconnection and dislodging (Shoemaker et al. 2002; Adam and Osborne 2005; Morton et al. 2009; Urden et al 2010).
30 Dispose of non-reusable components, sharps and waste following hospital guidelines.	To prevent accidental injury, contamination and maintain correct waste disposal process (Pratt et al. 2007).
31 Observe for potential problems including (see CVC insertion): ■ Catheter insertion: ○ arrhythmias ○ heart block ○ knotting ○ malposition.	To monitor for potential adverse affects of using a pulmonary artery catheter monitoring system (Morgan 2003; Adam and Osborne 2005; Jevon et al. 2007).
32 Document care.	To: ■ provide an accurate record ■ monitor effectiveness of procedure ■ reduce the risk of duplication of treatment ■ provide a point of reference or comparison in the event of later questions ■ acknowledge accountability for actions ■ facilitate communication and continuity of care. (NMC 2008; GMC 2013; HCPC 2012)

213

Procedure guideline 6.5: Pulmonary artery catheter monitoring

Equipment
As for Procedure guideline 6.4

Procedure	
Action	**Rationale**
1 Where possible, explain and discuss the procedure with the patient. If the patient lacks the capacity to make decisions the practitioner must act in the patient's best interests.	To ensure that the patient understands the procedure and gives their valid consent. To ensure the patient's best interests are maintained (Mental Capacity Act 2005).
2 Wash hands with antiseptic hand wash and alcohol gel, and wear appropriate personal protective equipment when handling equipment and undertaking procedures. Observe dressing for signs of infection, use visual infusion phlebitis (VIP) chart or local equivalent. Change dressing as required – follow local policy.	To reduce the risk of microbial contamination (Pratt et al. 2007) To reduce the risk of infection (Patient Safety First 2008).
3 Set up the pulmonary artery catheter components in line with manufacturer's guidelines, including: ■ proximal and distal port continuous flush transducer sets (follow local policy regarding heparinized saline for flush system) ■ balloon lumen and inflation syringe ■ thermistor lumen and cardiac output injectate components (if appropriate).	To avoid erroneous haemodynamic data being displayed. To prevent accidental disconnection and dislodging. To reduce adverse risk to patient (Shoemaker et al. 2002; Adam and Osborne 2005; Morton et al. 2009; Urden et al. 2010).

(Continued)

Procedure guideline 6.5: (Continued)

4 Calibrate (zero) catheter in line with manufacturer's guidelines (*see* arterial catheter insertion).	To calibrate the system to zero and enable accurate pressure measurements. To avoid erroneous haemodynamic data being displayed (Shoemaker et al. 2002; Adam and Osborne 2005; Morton et al. 2009; Urden et al. 2010).
5 Secure catheter, transducers and cables following local policy and manufacturer's guidelines.	To prevent accidental disconnection and dislodging (Shoemaker et al. 2002; Adam and Osborne 2005; Morton et al. 2009; Urden et al. 2010).
6 Continuously display pulmonary artery waveform and set alarms appropriately.	To monitor for any abnormal readings and initiate appropriate treatment in a timely manner (Shoemaker et al. 2002; Adam and Osborne 2005; Morton et al. 2009; Urden et al. 2010).
7 Observe for potential problems including (*see* Problem-solving table 6.5). **Catheter** ■ Balloon rupture ■ Catheter disintegration ■ Intra-cardiac trauma/perforation ■ Pulmonary artery rupture ■ Catheter related sepsis ■ Pulmonary artery thrombosis ■ Pulmonary infarction. **In use:** ■ Incorrect identification and labelling of tubing ■ Arrhythmias ■ Erroneous data ■ Misinterpretation of data.	To deliver clinical care while limiting adverse affects of using a pulmonary artery catheter monitoring system (Morgan 2003; Adam and Osborne 2005; Jevon et al. 2007).
8 Observe and document parameters, including: ■ right atrial pressure (RA) ■ right ventricular pressure (RV) – on insertion ■ pulmonary artery pressure (PAP) ■ pulmonary artery wedge pressure (PAWP) ■ cardiac output (CO) ■ cardiac index ■ systemic vascular resistance (SVR), and index (SVRI) ■ pulmonary vascular resistance (PVR), and index (PVRI) ■ mixed venous saturations (SvO_2).	To monitor for any abnormal readings and initiate appropriate treatment in a timely manner (Morgan 2003; Singer and Webb 2009). To: ■ provide an accurate record ■ monitor effectiveness of procedure ■ reduce the risk of duplication of treatment ■ provide a point of reference or comparison in the event of later questions ■ acknowledge accountability for actions ■ facilitate communication and continuity of care. (NMC 2008; GMC 2013; HCPC 2012)
9 Clearly identify and label tubing.	To reduce adverse risk to patient (Australian Commission on Safety and Quality in Health Care 2010).
10 Continuously monitor PA waveforms, and set audible alarms.	To monitor for any abnormal readings and initiate appropriate treatment in a timely manner. To detect accidental 'wedging' of catheter (Singer and Webb 2009). To ensure accountability and maintenance of patient records (GMC 2013; NMC 2008).

Procedure guideline 6.6: Undertaking pulmonary artery wedge pressure measurement

Equipment

As for Procedure guideline 6.4

Procedure

Action	Rationale
1 Where possible, explain and discuss the procedure with the patient. If the patient lacks the capacity to make decisions the practitioner must act in the patient's best interests.	To ensure that the patient understands the procedure and gives their valid consent. To ensure the patient's best interests are maintained (Mental Capacity Act 2005).
2 Wash hands with antiseptic hand wash and alcohol gel, and wear appropriate personal protective equipment when handling equipment and undertaking procedures.	To reduce the risk of microbial contamination (Pratt et al. 2007). To reduce the risk of infection (Patient Safety First 2008).
3 While observing the PA waveform slowly inflate balloon with no more than 1.5 mL of air. This should not be inflated for more than 15 seconds.	To 'wedge' balloon in the pulmonary artery. To prevent pulmonary ischaemia and/or infarction (Adam and Osborne 2005; Jevon et al. 2007; Singer and Webb 2009; Urden et al. 2010).
4 Stop inflating balloon once waveform changes and keep inflated for three respiratory cycles.	To prevent 'over wedging'. To inflate over three cycles to ensure an accurate reading (Adam and Osborne 2005; Jevon et al. 2007; Singer and Webb 2009).
5 Follow manufactory guidelines for calculating and recording a wedge pressure. Observe reading and align cursor to the end of expiration in the patient's respiratory cycle. The correct position depends on their respiratory support (that is, ventilated or breathing spontaneously).	To enable accurate assessment of pressures. To obtain a measurement at the end of expiration as this is closest to atmospheric pressure. If ventilated the recording should be taken prior to the inspired phase and the rise on the PA trace. If breathing spontaneously this should occur as the trace begins to fall (Adam and Osborne 2005; Jevon et al. 2007; Singer and Webb 2009).
6 Deflate balloon and ensure PA waveform present.	To ensure that the pulmonary artery is not occluded (Adam and Osborne 2005; Jevon et al. 2007; Singer and Webb 2009).
7 Document reading and care, and report findings.	To initiate appropriate treatment in a timely manner (Singer and Webb 2009). To: ■ provide an accurate record ■ monitor effectiveness of procedure ■ reduce the risk of duplication of treatment ■ provide a point of reference or comparison in the event of later questions ■ acknowledge accountability for actions ■ facilitate communication and continuity of care. (NMC 2008; GMC 2013; HCPC 2012)

Procedure guideline 6.7: Insertion of a transpulmonary cardiac output monitoring device using lithium dilution (e.g. LiDCO™plus)

Equipment

- Arterial cannula
- Central venous catheter
- LiDCO monitor
- Haemodynamic monitor with cables and adapters
- Lithium sensor
- Disposable blood collection bag and tube
- Lithium injectate pack and lithium chloride injection 0.15 mmol/mL
- Syringes: 2×20 mL, 1×2 mL
- Flow regulator pump

Procedure

Action	Rationale
1 Where possible, explain and discuss the procedure with the patient. If the patient lacks the capacity to make decisions the practitioner must act in the patient's best interests.	To ensure that the patient understands the procedure and gives their valid consent. To ensure the patient's best interests are maintained (Mental Capacity Act 2005).
2 Ensure arterial cannula inserted as described earlier in Procedure guideline 6.2.	To allow withdrawing of blood to determine lithium concentration. To produce arterial pressure waveform (Rhodes and Sunderland 2005).
3 Ensure central venous catheter inserted as described earlier in Procedure guideline 6.3.	To allow administration of lithium bolus (Rhodes and Sunderland 2005).
4 Wash hands with antiseptic hand wash and alcohol gel, and wear appropriate personal protective equipment when handling equipment and undertaking procedures.	To reduce the risk of microbial contamination (Pratt et al. 2007). To reduce the risk of infection (Patient Safety First 2008).
5 Set up the monitor components in line with manufacturer's guidelines. ■ Switch on LiDCO monitor and connect to patient bedside monitor via connection cable. ■ Enter patient details, height and weight.	To avoid erroneous haemodynamic data being displayed. To prevent accidental disconnection and dislodging. Reduce adverse risk to patient.
6 Set up the calibration components in line with manufacturer's guidelines. ■ Prime the wick of the sensor with 20 mL 0.9% sodium chloride and attach the manufacturer's waste bag. ■ Attach the sensor to the 3-way tap on the arterial tubing and flush the arterial set with 0.9% sodium chloride from the transducer system. ■ Attach the flow regulator. ■ Prime the 'park and ride' set (short infusion tubing) with 4–5 mL 0.9% sodium chloride. ■ Draw up of 2 mL of the lithium solution and inject into 'park and ride' set ■ Attach primed 'park and ride' set to venous access.	To avoid errors in the calibration of the monitor and prevent incorrect haemodynamic data being displayed. To prevent accidental disconnection and dislodging. Reduce adverse risk to patient.
7 Undertake calibration of the LiDCO monitor in line with manufacturer's guidelines. (a) Set monitor to calibration screen and follow instructions. (b) When 'ready to use' displayed press 'INJECT'. (c) Give a 20 mL 0.9% sodium chloride flush through 'park and ride' system. (d) Observe the 'dilution curve'. (e) Turn off flow regulator when 'switch flow regulator off and flush' message appears. (f) Flush tubing and detach 'park and ride' set, arterial set up and sensor.	(a) To avoid errors in the calibration of the monitor and prevent incorrect haemodynamic data being displayed. (b) and (c) To commence procedure and to flush the indicator solution through the CVC and into the circulation. (d) Observe for correct dilution curve. To ascertain results. (e) To prevent leakage should accidental disconnection and dislodging occur. (f) To reduce adverse risk to patient.

8 Clearly identify and label tubing.	To reduce the risk of tubing being used inappropriately and adverse risk to patient (Australian Commission on Safety and Quality in Health Care 2010).
9 Dispose of non-reusable components (e.g. 'park and ride' system, arterial set up and sensor), sharps and waste following hospital guidelines.	To prevent accidental injury, contamination and maintain correct waste disposal process (Pratt et al. 2007).
10 Accurately document reading and care, and report findings.	In order to initiate appropriate treatment in a timely manner. To: ■ provide an accurate record ■ monitor effectiveness of procedure ■ reduce the risk of duplication of treatment ■ provide a point of reference or comparison in the event of later questions ■ acknowledge accountability for actions ■ facilitate communication and continuity of care. (NMC 2008; GMC 2013; HCPC 2012)

Procedure guideline 6.8: Transpulmonary cardiac output monitoring using lithium dilution (e.g. LiDCOplus)

Equipment

- Haemodynamic monitor with cables and adapters
- Disposable blood collection bag and tube
- Lithium sensor
- Lithium chloride injectate and syringes
- Flow regulator pump

Procedure

Action	Rationale
1 Where possible, explain and discuss the procedure with the patient. If the patient lacks the capacity to make decisions the practitioner must act in the patient's best interests.	To ensure that the patient understands the procedure and gives their valid consent. To ensure the patient's best interests are maintained (Mental Capacity Act 2005).
2 Wash hands with antiseptic hand wash and alcohol gel, and wear appropriate personal protective equipment when handling equipment undertaking procedures.	To reduce the risk of microbial contamination (Pratt et al. 2007). To reduce the risk of infection (Patient Safety First 2008).
3 Observe dressing for signs of infection, use visual infusion phlebitis (VIP) chart or local equivalent. Change dressing as required – follow local policy.	To reduce the risk of microbial contamination (Pratt et al. 2007). To reduce the risk of infection (Patient Safety First 2008).

4 Set up components in line with manufacturer's guidelines:
 ■ cables
   ○ power
   ○ sensor interface and cable
   ○ bedside monitor connection cable
 ■ disposable blood collection bag and tube
 ■ lithium chloride injectate
 ■ flow regulator pump.
 	
 Secure catheter, transducers and cables following local policy and manufacturer's guidelines.
	To avoid erroneous haemodynamic data being displayed. To prevent accidental disconnection and dislodging. To reduce adverse events.

(Continued)

Procedure guideline 6.8: (Continued)

5 Clearly identify and label tubing.	To ensure that the correct tubing is used for the correct purpose. To reduce adverse risk to patient (Australian Commission on Safety and Quality in Health Care 2010).
6 (a) Input patient specific data. (b) Calibrate (zero) arterial catheter in line with manufacturer's guidelines. (c) Perform indicator dilution to calibrate the device in accordance with manufacturer's guidelines. (d) Administer the dilution indicator solution in line with manufacturer's guidelines and following local and national policies for medicine management.	To ensure accurate calibration of the monitor to avoid erroneous haemodynamic data being displayed.
7 Observe for potential complications. **Venous/arterial access** ■ Bleeding at site ■ Pneumo +/- haemothorax ■ Air embolism ■ Arterial puncture ■ Nerve injury ■ Venous thrombosis. **In use** ■ Incorrect calibration ■ Erroneous data ■ Misinterpretation of data.	To deliver clinical care while limiting adverse affects of using a transpulmonary cardiac output monitoring system (Morgan 2003; Adam and Osborne 2005; Singer and Webb 2009).
8 Observe and document parameters including: ■ Heart rate (HR) ■ Arterial blood pressure ■ Mean arterial blood pressure (MAP) ■ Systolic pressure variation (SPV) ■ Left ventricle stroke volume ■ Stroke volume variation (SVV %) ■ Pulse pressure variation (PPV %) ■ Cardiac output (CO) ■ Cardiac index (CI) ■ Systemic vascular resistance (SVR), and index (SVRI) ■ Pulmonary vascular resistance (PVR), and index (PVRI) ■ Oxygen delivery (DO_2), and index (DO_2I).	To monitor for any abnormal readings and communicate and initiate appropriate treatment in a timely manner. To: ■ provide an accurate record ■ monitor effectiveness of procedure ■ reduce the risk of duplication of treatment ■ provide a point of reference or comparison in the event of later questions ■ acknowledge accountability for actions ■ facilitate communication and continuity of care. (NMC 2008; GMC 2013; HCPC 2012)
9 Continuously monitor arterial waveform, and set audible alarms. Accurately record reading, report findings.	To monitor for any abnormal readings and initiate appropriate treatment in a timely manner. To ensure accountability and maintenance of patient records (GMC 2009 and NMC 2008).

218

Equipment

- Arterial cannula
- Central venous catheter
- Specific PiCCO 4 Fr femoral artery catheter
- PiCCO haemodynamic monitor with cables and adapters
- Injectate temperature sensor
- Injectate – 0.9% sodium chloride and 20mL syringe

Procedure

Action	Rationale
1 Where possible, explain and discuss the procedure with the patient. If the patient lacks the capacity to make decisions the practitioner must act in the patient's best interests.	To ensure that the patient understands the procedure and gives their valid consent. To ensure the patient's best interests are maintained (Mental Capacity Act 2005).
2 Specific PiCCO artery cannula insertion (as described in Procedure guideline 6.2).	To allow recording of an arterial pressure waveform for analysis. To allow temperature changes to be detected in the thermodilution method for measuring CO (Pulsion Medical Systems 2009).
3 Central venous catheter insertion (as described in Procedure guideline 6.3).	To allow boluses of cold 0.9% sodium chloride to be administered for the thermodilution method of measuring CO (Pulsion Medical Systems 2009).
4 Wash hands with antiseptic hand wash and alcohol gel, and wear appropriate personal protective equipment when handling equipment and undertaking procedures. Observe dressings for signs of infection, use visual infusion phlebitis (VIP) chart or local equivalent.	To reduce the risk of microbial contamination (Pratt et al. 2007). To reduce the risk of infection (Patient Safety First 2008).
5 Set up the monitor components in line with manufacturer's guidelines. (a) Prime transducer set. (b) Connect the thermistor cable to the PiCCO monitor and catheter. (c) Connect the injectate cable to the thermistor cable and injectate sensor housing. (d) Connect the pressure connection cable to the PiCCO monitor and the pressure transducer kit.	To avoid erroneous haemodynamic data being displayed. To prevent accidental disconnection and dislodging and reduce adverse risk to patient (Pulsion Medical Systems 2009).
6 Set up the monitor components in line with manufacturer's guidelines. (a) Switch the PiCCO monitor on and connect it to patient bedside monitor via connection cable. (b) Enter patient details, height and weight.	To avoid erroneous haemodynamic data being displayed. To reduce adverse risk to patient (Pulsion Medical Systems 2009).
7 Undertake calibration of the PiCCO monitor in line with manufacturer's guidelines. (a) Calibrate (zero) transducer to the PiCCO monitor and then to patient's bedside monitor. (b) Pressing the 'thermodilution' icon and follow instructions. (c) Give a 15mL bolus of iced 0.9% sodium chloride through the CVC system. (d) Observe the temperature dilution curve.	(a) To avoid errors in the calibration of the monitor and prevent incorrect haemodynamic data being displayed. To reduce adverse risk to patient. (b) and (c) To commence procedure and to flush the indicator solution through the CVC and into the circulation. (d) To observe for correct dilution curve. To ascertain results. (Pulsion Medical Systems 2009)

(Continued)

Procedure guideline 6.9: (Continued)

8 Clearly identify and label tubing.	To reduce the risk of tubing being used inappropriately and adverse risk to patient (Australian Commission on Safety and Quality in Health Care 2010).
9 Dispose of non-reusable components, sharps and waste following hospital guidelines.	To prevent accidental injury, contamination and maintain correct waste disposal process (Pratt et al. 2007).
10 Accurately document reading and care, and report findings.	In order to initiate appropriate treatment in a timely manner. To: ■ provide an accurate record ■ monitor effectiveness of procedure ■ reduce the risk of duplication of treatment ■ provide a point of reference or comparison in the event of later questions ■ acknowledge accountability for actions ■ facilitate communication and continuity of care. (NMC 2008; GMC 2013; HCPC 2012)

Procedure guideline 6.10: Transpulmonary cardiac output monitoring using thermodilution (e.g. PiCCO)

Equipment

- Arterial cannula
- Central venous catheter
- Haemodynamic monitor with cables and adapters
- Injectate temperature sensor
- Arterial catheter with thermistor
- Disposable pressure transducer
- Injectate and syringe

Procedure

Action	Rationale
1 Where possible, explain and discuss the procedure with the patient. If the patient lacks the capacity to make decisions the practitioner must act in the patient's best interests.	To ensure that the patient understands the procedure and gives their valid consent. To ensure the patient's best interests are maintained (Mental Capacity Act 2005).
2 Wash hands with antiseptic hand wash and alcohol gel, and wear appropriate personal protective equipment when handling equipment and undertaking procedures. Observe dressing for signs of infection, use visual infusion phlebitis (VIP) chart or local equivalent. Change dressing as required – follow local policy.	To reduce the risk of microbial contamination (Pratt et al. 2007). To reduce the risk of infection (Patient Safety First 2008).

3 Set up components in line with manufacturer's guidelines, including:
■ cables
  ○ power
  ○ injectate-temperature sensor cable
  ○ pressure
  ○ bedside monitor connection cable
■ injectate-temperature sensor housing
■ injectate
■ pressure transducer kit (primed and attached to a flush bag).
Correct securing of cathotor, transducers and cables following local policy and manufacturer's guidelines.
	To avoid erroneous haemodynamic data being displayed. To prevent accidental disconnection and dislodging. To reduce adverse risk to patient (Pulsion Medical Systems 2009).

4 Clearly identify and label tubing.	To reduce the risk of tubing being used inappropriately and adverse risk to patient (Australian Commission on Safety and Quality in Health Care 2010).
5 (a) Input patient specific data. (b) Calibrate (zero) arterial catheter in line with manufacturer's guidelines. (c) Perform three initial thermodilution measurements to calibrate the device in accordance with manufacturer's guidelines. (d) Administer the thermodilution indicator solution in line with manufacturer's guidelines and following local and national policies for medicine management.	(a), (b) and (c) To ensure accurate calibration of the monitor to avoid erroneous haemodynamic data being displayed. (d) To commence procedure and to flush the indicator solution through the CVC and into the circulation. (Pulsion Medical Systems 2009)
6 Observe for potential complications, including: **Venous/arterial access:** ■ bleeding at site ■ pneumo +/- haemothorax ■ air embolism ■ arterial puncture ■ nerve injury ■ venous thrombosis. **In use:** ■ incorrect calibration ■ erroneous data ■ misinterpretation of data.	To deliver clinical care while limiting adverse affects of using a thermodilution transpulmonary cardiac output monitoring system (Morgan 2003; Adam and Osborne 2005; Singer and Webb 2009).
7 Observe and document parameters, including: ■ arterial pressure (AP) ■ mean arterial blood pressure (MAP) ■ heart rate (HR) ■ stroke volume (SV) and index (SVI) ■ cardiac output (CO) ■ cardiac index (CI) ■ systemic vascular resistance (SVR) and index (SVRI) ■ global end-diastolic volume (GEDV) or index (GEDI) ■ intrathoracic blood volume (ITBV) or index (ITBI) ■ stroke volume variation (SVV %) ■ pulse pressure variation (PPV %) ■ extravascular lung water (EVLW), or index (ELWI) ■ pulmonary vascular permeability index (PVPI) ■ global ejection fraction (GEF %) ■ cardiac function index (CFI) ■ left ventricular contractility (dP/mx).	To monitor for any abnormal readings and communicate and initiate appropriate treatment in a timely manner (Pulsion Medical Systems 2009). To: ■ provide an accurate record ■ monitor effectiveness of procedure ■ reduce the risk of duplication of treatment ■ provide a point of reference or comparison in the event of later questions ■ acknowledge accountability for actions ■ facilitate communication and continuity of care. (NMC 2008; GMC 2013; HCPC 2012)
8 Continuously monitor arterial waveform, and set audible alarms. Accurately record reading, report findings.	To monitor for any abnormal readings and initiate appropriate treatment in a timely manner (Singer and Webb 2009). To ensure accountability and maintenance of patient records (NMC 2008; GMC 2013).

221

Procedure guideline 6.11: Insertion of the oesophageal Doppler probe (e.g. CardioQ™)

Equipment

- Oesophageal Doppler monitor
- Patient interface cable (PIC)
- Water-based lubricant
- Oesophageal Doppler probe

Procedure

Action	Rationale
1 Where possible, explain and discuss the procedure with the patient. If the patient lacks the capacity to make decisions the practitioner must act in the patient's best interests.	To ensure that the patient understands the procedure and gives their valid consent. To ensure the patient's best interests are maintained (Mental Capacity Act 2005).
2 Wash hands with antiseptic hand wash and alcohol gel, and wear appropriate personal protective equipment when handling equipment and undertaking procedures.	To reduce the risk of microbial contamination (Pratt et al. 2007).
3 Set up of components in line with manufacturer's guidelines. (a) Switch on the power. (b) Connect the probe to patient interface cable. (c) Enter the patient details, gender, height and weight. (d) Apply a water-based lubricant to probe.	(a) To commence procedure. (b) To prevent accidental disconnection and dislodging. (c) To ensure correct nomogram applied and to avoid erroneous haemodynamic data being displayed. (d) To ease insertion and reduce adverse risk to patient. (Deltex Medical 2009)
4 Insert oesophageal Doppler probe in line with manufacturer's guidelines. (a) Oral insertion – advance probe gently until incisors are between the distal marker (35 cm) on the probe and the middle marker (40 cm). (b) Nasal insertion – advance probe gently until nasal septum is between the middle marker (40 cm) and the proximal marker (45 cm) on the probe. (c) Locate the descending aortic signal by adjusting the probe depth. (d) Optimize the signal by rotating the probe to achieve the sharpest waveform and clearest audible sound.	(a) and (b) To ensure correct position of probe and reduce adverse risk to patient. (c) and (d) To ensure correct position of probe and avoid erroneous haemodynamic data being displayed. (Deltex Medical 2009)
5 Dispose of non-reusable components, sharps and waste following hospital guidelines.	To prevent accidental injury, contamination and maintain correct waste disposal process (Pratt et al. 2007).
6 Accurately document reading and care, and report findings.	In order to initiate appropriate treatment in a timely manner. To: - provide an accurate record - monitor effectiveness of procedure - reduce the risk of duplication of treatment - provide a point of reference or comparison in the event of later questions - acknowledge accountability for actions - facilitate communication and continuity of care. (NMC 2008; GMC 2013; HCPC 2012)

Procedure guideline 6.12: Oesophageal Doppler monitoring (ODM) (e.g. CardioQ)

Equipment

- Haemodynamic monitor with cables
- Oesophageal Doppler probe
- Water-based lubricant

Procedure

Action	Rationale
1 Where possible, explain and discuss the procedure with the patient. If the patient lacks the capacity to make decisions the practitioner must act in the patient's best interests.	To ensure that the patient understands the procedure and gives their valid consent. To ensure the patient's best interests are maintained (Mental Capacity Act 2005).
2 Wash hands with antiseptic hand wash and alcohol gel, and wear appropriate personal protective equipment when handling equipment and undertaking procedures.	To reduce the risk of microbial contamination (Pratt et al. 2007).

3 Set up of components in line with manufacturer's guidelines:
■ cables
  ○ power
  ○ patient interface cable
■ probe.
 	
Secure probe and cables following local policy and manufacturer's guidelines.
	To avoid erroneous haemodynamic data being displayed. To prevent accidental disconnection and dislodging. Reduce adverse risk to patient. (Deltex Medical 2009)

4 Input patient specific data.	To ensure accurate calibration of the monitor to avoid erroneous haemodynamic data being displayed (Deltex Medical 2009).
5 Observe for potential complications including: Insertion: ■ dislodgement of probe ■ damage to oesophageal mucosa and oesophageal bleeding ■ oesophagotracheal perforation ■ dysphagia. In use: ■ incorrect configuration ■ erroneous data ■ misinterpretation of data.	To deliver clinical care while limiting adverse affects of using an oesophageal Doppler monitoring (ODM) system (Deltex Medical 2009).
6 Observe and document parameters including: ■ heart rate (HR) ■ flow time corrected (FTc) ■ peak velocity (PV) ■ stroke distance ■ stroke volume (SV) and index (SVI) ■ cardiac output (CO) and index (CI).	To monitor for any abnormal readings and communicate and initiate appropriate treatment in a timely manner (Deltex Medical 2009).
7 Continuously monitor aortic waveform, and set audible alarms. Accurately record reading, report findings.	To monitor for any abnormal readings and initiate appropriate treatment in a timely manner. To: ■ provide an accurate record ■ monitor effectiveness of procedure ■ reduce the risk of duplication of treatment ■ provide a point of reference or comparison in the event of later questions ■ acknowledge accountability for actions ■ facilitate communication and continuity of care. (NMC 2008; GMC 2013; HCPC 2012)

Competency statement 6.1: Specific procedure competency statements for the application and use of continuous ECG monitoring

Complete assessment against relevant fundamental competency statements (*see* Chapter 2, pp. 20, 21)	Evidence
Specific procedure competency for the application and use of continuous ECG monitoring (3- and 5-lead)	**Evidence of competency for the application and use of continuous ECG monitoring (3- and 5-lead)**
Demonstrate ability to: ■ teach and assess or ■ learn from assessment.	Examples of evidence of teaching, assessing and learning.
Identify the indications for continuous ECG monitoring: ■ heart rate monitoring ■ detection of arrhythmias ■ detection of ischaemia ■ detection of conduction defects.	Discussion with supervisor/mentor on the indications for continuous ECG monitoring. Direct observation of clinical practice.
Identify risks, potential problems and complications of continuous ECG monitoring and how to prevent and manage them: ■ poor electrode contact ■ misinterpreting or missing information due to poor ECG trace ■ incorrect placement of electrodes giving inaccurate information ■ skin irritation from electrodes.	Discussion with supervisor/mentor. Direct observation of clinical practice.
Demonstrate knowledge and understanding of local and national policies, guidance and procedures in relation to the application and use of continuous ECG monitoring, including NICE guideline CG050 (2006).	Discussion with supervisor/mentor.
Demonstrate knowledge and understanding of evidence base in relation to the application and use of continuous ECG monitoring, including: ■ limited evidence ■ benefits of 5-lead compared to 3-lead ECG monitoring ■ benefits of 12-lead ECG.	Discussion with supervisor/mentor.
Demonstrate skills and correct technique that are required in relation to the application and use of continuous ECG monitoring, including: ■ adequate preparation of skin prior to electrode placement ■ correct positioning of electrodes ■ wires attached appropriately to electrodes and then to monitor ■ setting of appropriate alarm settings ■ recognition of common abnormalities on the ECG such as ischaemia and arrhythmias.	Direct observation of clinical practice. Discussion with supervisor/mentor.
Prepare equipment required in relation to applying and using continuous ECG monitoring.	Direct observation of clinical practice. Discussion with supervisor/mentor.

Competency statement 6.2: Specific procedure competency statements for insertion and use of invasive blood pressure monitoring

Complete assessment against relevant fundamental competency statements (*see* Chapter 2, pp. 20, 21)	Evidence
Specific procedure competency for insertion and use of invasive blood pressure monitoring	**Evidence for competency of insertion and use of invasive blood pressure monitoring**
Demonstrate ability to: ■ teach and assess or ■ learn from assessment.	Examples of evidence of teaching, assessing and learning.
Identify the reason(s) for insertion and use of invasive blood pressure monitoring, including: ■ continuous monitoring of arterial blood pressure in patients requiring inotropes or vasopressors or likely to have rapid changes in circulating blood volume ■ monitoring arterial blood gases.	Discussion with supervisor/mentor.
Identify risks, potential problems and complications of insertion and use of invasive blood pressure monitoring and to prevent and manage them, including: ■ air embolism ■ thrombosis ■ haemorrhage ■ inadvertent drug administration into the cannula ■ ischaemia ■ infection ■ arterial injury.	Direct observation of clinical practice. Discussion with supervisor/mentor.
Demonstrate knowledge and understanding of local and national policies, guidance and procedures in relation to insertion and use of invasive blood pressure monitoring, including the Department of Health guidelines on prevention of healthcare-associated infections.	Discussion with supervisor/mentor.
Demonstrate knowledge and understanding of evidence base in relation to insertion and use of invasive blood pressure monitoring, including: ■ comparison with non-invasive BP monitoring ■ use of systolic, or mean, blood pressure to guide treatment ■ omission of heparin from the flush bag.	Discussion with supervisor/mentor.
Demonstrate the skills and correct technique that are required in relation to insertion and use of invasive blood pressure monitoring, including: ■ aseptic technique ■ identification of appropriate site for insertion ■ use of local anaesthetic in awake patients ■ insertion of cannula ■ securing the cannula.	Discussion with supervisor/mentor. Direct observation of clinical practice.
Prepare equipment required in relation to insertion and use of invasive blood pressure monitoring, including: ■ preparing the flush bag and infusion set for the pressure monitoring system ■ preparing a sterile trolley containing equipment for insertion of the arterial cannula ■ calibrating the pressure monitoring system.	Direct observation of clinical practice. Discussion with supervisor/mentor.

Competency statement 6.3: Specific procedure competency statements for insertion and use of central venous pressure monitoring

Complete assessment against relevant fundamental competency statements (*see* Chapter 2, pp. 20, 21)	Evidence
Specific procedure competency for insertion and use of central venous pressure monitoring	**Evidence for competency of insertion and use of central venous pressure monitoring**
Demonstrate ability to: ■ teach and assess or ■ learn from assessment.	Examples of evidence of teaching, assessing and learning.
Identify the reason(s) for insertion and use of a central venous catheter: ■ to guide fluid administration ■ to administer drugs such as inotropes and vasopressors ■ for intravenous access.	Discussion with supervisor/mentor.
Identify risks, potential problems, and complications of insertion of a central venous catheter and to prevent and manage them, including: ■ pneumothorax/haemothorax ■ arrhythmias ■ air embolism ■ arterial puncture ■ nerve injury ■ infection ■ vein thrombosis.	Direct observation of clinical practice. Discussion with supervisor/mentor.
Demonstrate knowledge and understanding of local and national policies, guidance and procedures in relation to insertion and use of central venous catheters, including: ■ epic2 (Pratt et al. 2007) ■ NICE guidance on use of ultrasound during insertion (NICE 2002).	Discussion with supervisor/mentor.
Demonstrate knowledge and understanding of evidence base in relation to insertion and use of central venous pressure monitoring, including: ■ efficacy ■ insertion techniques (landmark or ultrasound guided) ■ reducing infection (epic2, Matching Michigan).	Discussion with supervisor/mentor.
Demonstrate skills and correct technique that are required in relation to insertion and use of central venous pressure monitoring, including: ■ aseptic technique ■ identification of appropriate site for insertion ■ use of local anaesthetic in awake patients ■ insertion of CVC ■ securing the CVC.	Discussion with supervisor/mentor. Direct observation of clinical practice.
Prepare equipment required in relation to insertion and use of central venous pressure monitoring, including: ■ preparing the flush bag and infusion set for the pressure monitoring system ■ preparing a sterile trolley containing equipment for insertion of a CVC.	Direct observation of clinical practice. Discussion with supervisor/mentor.

Competency statement 6.4: Specific procedure competency statements for insertion of a pulmonary artery catheter

Complete assessment against relevant fundamental competency statements (*see* Chapter 2, pp. 20, 21)

Evidence

Specific procedure competency statements for the insertion of a pulmonary artery catheter	Evidence of competency for the insertion of a pulmonary artery catheter
Demonstrate ability to: ■ teach and assess or ■ learn from assessment.	Examples of evidence of teaching, assessing and learning.
Identify indications for the insertion of a pulmonary artery catheter including: ■ patients with cardiogenic shock during supportive therapy ■ patients with discordant right and left ventricular failure ■ patients with severe chronic heart failure requiring inotropic, vasopressor and vasodilator therapy ■ patients with suspected 'pseudo-sepsis' (high cardiac output, low systemic vascular resistance, elevated right atrial and pulmonary capillary wedge pressures) ■ patients with potentially reversible systolic heart failure such as fulminant myocarditis and peripartum cardiomyopathy ■ to enable a haemodynamic differential diagnosis of pulmonary hypertension ■ to assess response to therapy in patients with precapillary and mixed types of pulmonary hypertension ■ during transplantation work-up. (Morgan 2003; Chatterjee 2009)	*May be demonstrated by:* ■ discussion with supervisor/mentor, providing an explanation of the indications for the insertion of a pulmonary artery catheter.
Identify the contraindications of inserting a pulmonary artery catheter, including: ■ recurrent sepsis ■ left bundle branch block ■ patients with tricuspid or pulmonary heart valve replacements ■ presence of endocardial pacing leads ■ hypercoagulable states ■ heparin-coated catheters where patients have a known sensitivity to heparin.	*May be demonstrated by:* ■ discussion with supervisor/mentor, providing an explanation of the contraindications of inserting a pulmonary artery catheter.

Demonstrate the skills that are required in relation to caring for a patient during the insertion of a pulmonary artery catheter.
■ The correct set up of the pressure transducer administration set in line with manufacturer's guidelines, including:
  ○ inserting intravenous administration set (single or bifurcated sets) into 0.9% sodium chloride bag. Following local policy/prescription regarding heparinized saline for flush system
  ○ opening roller clamp fully
  ○ priming the administration set and three-way tap ports by squeezing the flush device-actuator
  ○ checking thoroughly for air bubbles in the circuit
  ○ placing bag of 0.9% sodium chloride into pressure infuser cuff. Inflate to 300mmHg
  ○ checking that all Luer lock connections are secure.
■ The correct attachment of ECG monitoring with appropriately set alarms with the audible beat to beat sound set.
■ The correct positioning of the patient in the trendelenburg position as tolerated.
	May be demonstrated by:
	■ direct observation and discussion with supervisor/mentor of correct procedure for set up of:
	■ relevant components
	■ infusion preparation
	■ automatic flush preparation
	■ maintenance of circuit, and cannula.
	■ the waveform display
	■ alarms
	■ direct observation and discussion with supervisor/mentor of correct procedure for positioning a patient
	■ discussion with supervisor/mentor of the potential risks to patients
	■ discussion with supervisor/mentor of the rationale for the agreed haemodynamic parameter settings
	■ discussion with supervisor/mentor of relevant manufacturer, local and national guidelines and policies
	■ Where possible a testimonial from patient/client, and/or their carer.

(Continued)

Competency statement 6.4: (*Continued*)

Demonstrate skills that are required in relation to inserting (and/or assisting with insertion) the PAC introducer using a Seldinger technique, see CVC insertion.	*May be demonstrated by:* ■ direct observation and discussion with supervisor/mentor of the Seldinger technique ■ discussion with supervisor/mentor of relevant manufacturer, local and national guidelines and policies.
Demonstrate skills that are required in relation to inserting and/or assisting with insertion of the PAC under aseptic technique (*see* Competency statement 6.3), including: ■ the correct procedure for 'scrubbing up', including the wearing of a surgical hat, mask and sterile gown and gloves ■ the opening of all equipment in a sterile manner by the assistant and passed to the operator ■ skin preparation using 2% chlorhexidine ■ full barrier draping of the patient and ensuring their comfort. Demonstrate knowledge and understanding of local and national policies, guidance, in relation to infection control.	*May be demonstrated by:* ■ discussion with supervisor/mentor direct observation of the procedure, including: ○ acting to reduce risk with the multidisciplinary team.
Demonstrate skills that are required in preventing pain during the insertion of the pulmonary artery catheter, (*see* Competency statement 6.3), including: ■ the infiltration around the insertion site of 1% lidocaine if the patient is awake.	*May be demonstrated by:* ■ discussion with supervisor/mentor ■ direct observation of the procedure ■ discussion with supervisor/mentor of relevant manufacturer, local and national guidelines and policies. ■ acting to reduce risk with the multidisciplinary team.
Demonstrate skills that are required in relation to caring for a patient with a pulmonary artery catheter. ■ Safe and correct set up of pulmonary artery catheter components in line manufacturer's guidelines, including: ○ balloon lumen and inflation syringe ○ thermistor lumen ○ cardiac output injectate components (if appropriate). ■ Correct calibration/zeroing of catheter in line with manufacturer's guidelines. ■ Correct securing of catheter, transducers and cables following local policy and manufacturer's guidelines. ■ Clearly identify and label tubing. ■ Ensure pulmonary artery waveform is displayed at all times and alarms appropriately set.	*May be demonstrated by:* ■ direct observation and discussion with supervisor/mentor of correct procedure for set up of: ○ relevant components ○ calibration/zeroing ○ securing ○ monitor display ○ alarms. ■ discussion with supervisor/mentor of relevant manufacturer, local and national guidelines and policies ■ where possible a testimonial from patient/client and/or their carer ■ discussion with supervisor/mentor of the rationale for the agreed haemodynamic parameter settings.
Demonstrate skills that are required in relation to preventing potential pulmonary artery catheter introducer infection. ■ Observe dressing for signs of infection, use visual infusion phlebitis (VIP) chart or local equivalent. ■ Change dressing as required – follow local policy (Patient Safety First 2008). Demonstrate knowledge and understanding of local and national policies, guidance, in relation to infection prevention during invasive procedures.	*May be demonstrated by:* ■ discussion with supervisor/mentor ■ direct observation of the procedure ■ acting to reduce risk with the multidisciplinary team.

228

Demonstrate skills that are required in relation to inserting the PA catheter, including: ■ observation of both the PA pressure waveform for characteristic changes (*see* Figure 6.19) and ECG for arrhythmias ■ attaching the sterile sheath over the PAC and inserting catheter through the self-sealing diaphragm of the introducer sheath ■ advancing the catheter with the balloon deflated until a right atrial trace is obtained ■ inflating the balloon and advance/float the catheter until a characteristic PAWP trace is obtained ■ stopping the advancement/floatation of the catheter and deflate the balloon (the PA trace should return) ■ obtaining a chest X-ray.	*May be demonstrated by:* ■ direct observation and discussion with supervisor/mentor of the technique ■ discussion with supervisor/mentor of relevant manufacturer, local and national guidelines and policies.

Demonstrate skills that are required in relation to the safe and correct set-up of pulmonary artery catheter cardiac output components, in line with manufacturer's guidelines, including the:
■ thermistor lumen
■ cardiac output injectate components (If appropriate).
	May be demonstrated by:
	■ direct observation and discussion with supervisor/mentor of correct procedure for set up of:
	  ○ relevant components
	  ○ securing
	  ○ monitor display
	■ discussion with supervisor/mentor of relevant manufacturer, local and national guidelines and policies.

Demonstrate skills that are required in relation to the disposing of non-reusable components, sharps and waste following hospital guidelines. Demonstrate knowledge and understanding of local and national policies, guidance, in relation to infection control.	*May be demonstrated by:* ■ discussion with supervisor/mentor ■ direct observation of the procedure ■ discussion with supervisor/mentor of relevant manufacturer, local and national guidelines and policies ■ acting to reduce risk with the multidisciplinary team.
Identify the risks, potential problems and complications of pulmonary artery catheter monitoring and how to prevent or manage them (see CVC insertion), including: **Catheter insertion:** ■ arrhythmias ■ heart block ■ knotting ■ malposition.	*May be demonstrated by:* ■ acting to reduce risk with the multidisciplinary team ■ correctly assessing haemodynamic status following local guidelines ■ communicating in a timely and appropriate manner any changes or concerns regarding haemodynamic observations with the multidisciplinary team ■ able to deliver clinical care whilst limiting adverse affects on pulmonary artery catheter.
Demonstrate skills that are required in relation to the accurate documentation of readings and report findings.	*May be demonstrated by:* ■ direct observation by supervisor/mentor of documentation ■ communicating in a timely and appropriate manner any changes or concerns regarding haemodynamic observations with the multidisciplinary team ■ discussion with supervisor/mentor of relevant guidelines and policies ■ where possible a testimonial from patient/client and/or their carer.

Competency statement 6.5: Specific procedure competency statements for pulmonary artery catheter monitoring

Complete assessment against relevant fundamental competency statements (*see* Chapter 2, pp. 20, 21)	Evidence
Specific procedure competency statements for pulmonary artery catheter monitoring	**Evidence of competency for pulmonary artery catheter monitoring**
Demonstrate ability to: ■ teach and assess or ■ learn from assessment.	Examples of evidence of teaching, assessing and learning.
Identify indications for monitoring using a pulmonary artery catheter, including: ■ patients with cardiogenic shock during supportive therapy ■ patients with discordant right and left ventricular failure ■ patients with severe chronic heart failure requiring inotropic, vasopressor and vasodilator therapy ■ patients with suspected 'pseudo-sepsis' (high cardiac output, low systemic vascular resistance, elevated right atrial and pulmonary capillary wedge pressures) ■ patients with potentially reversible systolic heart failure such as fulminant myocarditis and peripartum cardiomyopathy ■ to enable a haemodynamic differential diagnosis of pulmonary hypertension ■ to assess response to therapy in patients with precapillary and mixed types of pulmonary hypertension ■ during transplantation work-up. (Morgan 2003; Chatterjee 2009)	*May be demonstrated by:* ■ discussion with supervisor/mentor, providing an explanation of the indications for monitoring using a pulmonary artery catheter.
Identify contraindications for monitoring using a pulmonary artery catheter, including: ■ recurrent sepsis ■ left bundle branch block ■ patients with tricuspid or pulmonary heart valve replacements ■ presence of endocardial pacing leads ■ hypercoagulable states ■ heparin-coated catheters where patients have a known sensitivity to heparin.	*May be demonstrated by:* ■ discussion with supervisor/mentor, providing an explanation of the indications for monitoring using a pulmonary artery catheter.

Demonstrate skills that are required in relation to caring for a patient with a pulmonary artery catheter.

- Safe and correct set up of pulmonary artery catheter components in line with manufacturer's guidelines, including:
  - distal (to the external hub) port continuous flush transducer set (discuss local policy regarding heparinized saline for flush system)
  - balloon lumen and inflation syringe
  - thermistor lumen
  - cardiac output injectate components (if appropriate).
- Correct calibration/zeroing of catheter in line with manufacturer's guidelines.
- Correct securing of catheter, transducers and cables following local policy and manufacturer's guidelines.
- Clearly identify and label tubing.
- Ensure pulmonary artery waveform is displayed at all times and alarms appropriately set.

May be demonstrated by:
- direct observation and discussion with supervisor/mentor of correct procedure for set up of:
  Relevant components.
  Calibration/zeroing
  Monitor display
  Alarms
- discussion with supervisor/mentor of relevant manufacturer, local and national guidelines and policies
- where possible a testimonial from patient/client, and or their carer
- discussion with supervisor/mentor of the rationale for the agreed haemodynamic parameter settings.

Demonstrate an understanding of:
- The rationale for the haemodynamic parameters agreed and set by the multidisciplinary team.

Demonstrate skills that are required in relation to preventing potential pulmonary artery catheter infection.

- Observe dressing for signs of infection, use visual infusion phlebitis (VIP) chart or local equivalent.
- Change dressing as required – follow local policy (Patient Safety First 2008).

May be demonstrated by:
- discussion with supervisor/mentor
- direct observation of the procedure
- acting to reduce risk with the multidisciplinary team.

Demonstrate knowledge and understanding of local and national policies, guidance, in relation to Infection prevention during invasive procedures.

Identify the risks, potential problems and complications of pulmonary artery catheter monitoring and how to prevent or manage them, including:

Catheter passage:
- arrhythmias
- haemorrhage
- damage to surrounding structures
- heart block
- knotting (catheter loops in the right ventricle causing a knot to form)
- malposition.

May be demonstrated by:
- acting to reduce risk with the multidisciplinary team
- correctly assessing haemodynamic status following local guidelines
- communicating in a timely and appropriate manner any changes or concerns regarding haemodynamic observations with the multidisciplinary team
- able to deliver clinical care whilst limiting adverse affects on pulmonary artery catheter
- direct observation of the procedure.

(Continued)

Competency statement 6.5: (*Continued*)

Catheter:
- balloon rupture
- catheter disintegration
- intracardiac trauma/perforation
- pulmonary artery rupture
- catheter-related sepsis
- pulmonary artery thrombosis
- pulmonary infarction.

In use:
- incorrect identification and labelling of tubing
- arrhythmias
- erroneous data
- misinterpretation of data.

232

Demonstrate knowledge and understanding of evidence base in relation to the impact of clinical interventions upon haemodynamic status.

Demonstrate knowledge and understanding of evidence base in relation to pulmonary artery catheter monitoring.
- Pulmonary artery catheter waveforms
- Pulmonary artery catheter parameters:
  1. right atrial pressure (RA)
  2. right ventricular pressure (RV) – on insertion
  3. right ventricular end-diastolic volume index (RVEDVI)
  4. pulmonary artery pressure (PAP)
  5. pulmonary artery wedge pressure (PAWP)
  6. stroke volume (SV), and index (SVI)
  7. cardiac output (CO)
  8. cardiac index
  9. systemic vascular resistance (SVR) and index (SVRI)
  10. pulmonary vascular resistance (PVR), and index (PVRI)
  11. left ventricular stroke work index (LVSWI)
  12. right ventricular stroke work index (RVSWI)
  13. mixed venous saturations (SvO_2).
- Implications of a 'dampened trace'.
	May be demonstrated by:
	- discussion with supervisor/mentor
	- direct observation of the procedure
	- correctly assessing haemodynamic status following local guidelines
	- communicating in a timely and appropriate manner any changes or concerns regarding the validity of the pulmonary artery catheter monitoring device observations with the multidisciplinary team.

Demonstrate how people benefit from records that promote communication and high quality care in relation to pulmonary artery catheter monitoring.	*May be demonstrated by:* - commencing and reviewing the pulmonary artery catheter monitoring management plan with respect to the agreed parameters identified by the multidisciplinary team.

Demonstrate knowledge and understanding of the potential problems that can occur during monitoring with a pulmonary artery catheter and how to troubleshoot these, including:
- catheter migration
- 'dampened' trace on monitor
- unable to obtain wedge pressure
- balloon rupture
- difficulty injecting solution
- inappropriate measurements.
	May be demonstrated by:
	- direct observation and discussion with supervisor/mentor of correct procedure for troubleshooting:
	  ○ catheter migration
	  ○ 'dampened' trace on monitor
	  ○ unable to obtain wedge pressure
	  ○ balloon rupture
	  ○ difficulty injecting solution
	  ○ inappropriate measurements
	- discussion with supervisor/mentor of relevant manufacturer, local and national guidelines and policies.

Competency statement 6.6: Specific procedure competency statements for undertaking pulmonary artery wedge pressure – measurement

Complete assessment against relevant fundamental competency statements (*see* Chapter 2, pp. 20, 21)	Evidence
Specific procedure competency statements for undertaking pulmonary artery wedge pressure measurement	**Evidence of competency for undertaking pulmonary artery wedge pressure measurement**
Demonstrate ability to: ■ teach and assess or ■ learn from assessment.	Examples of evidence of teaching, assessing and learning.
Identify indications for undertaking a pulmonary artery wedge pressure measurement. Explain and discuss the procedure if possible with the patient.	*May be demonstrated by:* ■ to ensure where possible that the patient understands the procedure and consent obtained.
Demonstrate skills that are required for undertaking pulmonary artery wedge pressure measurement, including: ■ correct inflation of the balloon following local and manufacturer guidelines ■ accurately document readings and report findings.	*May be demonstrated by:* ■ direct observation and discussion with supervisor/ mentor of correct procedure ■ discussion with supervisor/mentor of relevant manufacturer, local and national guidelines and policies ■ correctly assessing haemodynamic status following local guidelines ■ communicating in a timely and appropriate manner any changes or concerns regarding the validity of the pulmonary artery catheter monitoring device observations with the multidisciplinary team ■ discussion with supervisor/mentor of the rationale for the agreed haemodynamic parameter settings.
Demonstrate knowledge and understanding of evidence base in relation to pulmonary artery wedge pressure, including: ■ anatomy and physiology ■ PAWP technique ■ normal and abnormal measurements.	*May be demonstrated by:* ■ discussion with supervisor/mentor ■ direct observation of the procedure ■ correctly assessing haemodynamic status following local guidelines ■ communicating in a timely and appropriate manner any changes or concerns regarding the validity of the pulmonary artery catheter monitoring device observations with the multidisciplinary team.
Demonstrate knowledge and understanding of the potential problems that can occur during monitoring with a pulmonary artery catheter and how to troubleshoot these, including: ■ unable to obtain wedge pressure ■ over-inflation ■ prolonged inflation/pulmonary artery infarction ■ balloon rupture ■ pulmonary artery rupture ■ inappropriate measurements.	*May be demonstrated by:* ■ direct observation and discussion with supervisor/ mentor of correct procedure for troubleshooting: 　○ unable to obtain wedge pressure 　○ over-inflation 　○ prolonged inflation/pulmonary artery rupture 　○ balloon rupture 　○ pulmonary artery rupture 　○ inappropriate measurements ■ discussion with supervisor/mentor of relevant manufacturer, local and national guidelines and policies.

233

Competency statement 6.7: Specific procedure competency statements for undertaking CO studies with a pulmonary artery catheter

Complete assessment against relevant fundamental competency statements (*see* Chapter 2, pp. 20, 21)	Evidence
Specific procedure competency statements for undertaking CO studies with a pulmonary artery catheter	**Evidence of competency for undertaking CO studies with a pulmonary artery catheter**
Demonstrate ability to: ■ teach and assess or ■ learn from assessment.	Examples of evidence of teaching, assessing and learning.
Identify indications for undertaking CO studies. Explain and discuss the procedure if possible with the patient.	*May be demonstrated by:* ■ ensuring where possible that the patient understands the procedure and consent obtained.
Demonstrate skills that are required in undertaking cardiac output studies. ■ Safe and correct set up of cardiac output study components in line with manufacturer's guidelines. ■ Correct procedure for undertaking cardiac output studies in accordance with local and manufacturer's guidelines including measurements for a: 1. ventilated patient 2. non-ventilated patient. ■ Accurately document readings and report findings.	*May be demonstrated by:* ■ direct observation and discussion with supervisor/mentor of correct procedure for set-up ■ correct performance of procedure ■ discussion with supervisor/mentor of relevant manufacturer, local and national guidelines and policies ■ where possible a testimonial from patient/client and or their carer ■ discussion with supervisor/mentor of the rationale for the agreed haemodynamic parameter settings.
Demonstrate knowledge and understanding of evidence base in relation to cardiac output studies. ■ Pulmonary artery catheter parameters: 1. cardiac output (CO) 2. cardiac index (CI).	*May be demonstrated by:* ■ discussion with supervisor/mentor ■ direct observation of the procedure ■ correctly assessing haemodynamic status following local guidelines ■ communicating in a timely and appropriate manner any changes or concerns regarding the validity of the pulmonary artery catheter monitoring device observations with the multidisciplinary team.
Demonstrate knowledge and understanding of the potential problems that can occur during cardiac output studies including: ■ inappropriate measurements ■ inaccurate injectate temperature ■ inaccurate injectate volume ■ respiratory cycle influences.	*May be demonstrated by:* ■ direct observation and discussion with supervisor/mentor of correct procedure for troubleshooting: ○ inappropriate measurements ○ inaccurate injectate temperature ○ inaccurate injectate volume ○ respiratory cycle influences ■ discussion with supervisor/mentor of relevant manufacturer, local and national guidelines and policies.

234

Competency statement 6.8: Specific procedure competency statements for insertion of a transpulmonary cardiac output device using lithium dilution (e.g. LiDCOplus)

Complete assessment against relevant fundamental competency statements (*see* Chapter 2, pp. 20, 21)	Evidence
Specific Procedure Competency Statements for the insertion of a trans-pulmonary cardiac output device using lithium dilution (e.g. LiDCOplus)	**Evidence of competency for the insertion of a trans-pulmonary cardiac output device using lithium dilution (e.g. LiDCOplus)**
Demonstrate ability to: ■ teach and assess or ■ learn from assessment.	Examples of evidence of teaching, assessing and learning.
Identify indications for the insertion of a trans-pulmonary cardiac output device using lithium dilution (e.g. LiDCOplus), including: ■ high-risk surgical patients ■ acute heart failure ■ sepsis ■ severe hypovolaemia.	*May be demonstrated by:* ■ discussion with supervisor/mentor, providing an explanation of the indications for the insertion of a transpulmonary cardiac output device using lithium dilution (e.g. LiDCOplus).
Identify the contraindications of inserting a transpulmonary cardiac output device using lithium dilution (e.g. LiDCO plus), including: ■ patients with an IABP ■ patients with aortic regurgitation ■ patients with highly dampened peripheral arterial waveform ■ patients on oral lithium therapy ■ patients under 40 kg (paediatric patients) ■ patients during first trimester of pregnancy.	*May be demonstrated by:* ■ discussion with supervisor/mentor, providing an explanation of the contraindications of inserting a transpulmonary cardiac output device using lithium dilution (e.g. LiDCOplus).
Demonstrate the skills that are required in relation to caring for a patient during the insertion of a transpulmonary cardiac output device using lithium dilution (e.g. LiDCO™plus). The correct set-up of the monitor components in line with manufacturer's guidelines, including: ■ switching on LiDCO monitor and connect to patient bedside monitor via connection cable ■ entering patient details, height and weight ■ priming the wick of the sensor with 20 mL of 0.9% sodium chloride and attaching the waste bag ■ attaching the sensor to the three-way tap on the arterial tubing and flushing the arterial set with 0.9% sodium chloride from the transducer system ■ attaching the flow regulator ■ priming the park and ride system with 4–5 mL 0.9% sodium chloride ■ drawing up of 2 mL of the lithium chloride solution and inject into 'park and ride' ■ attaching primed 'park and ride' to venous access.	*May be demonstrated by:* ■ direct observation and discussion with supervisor/mentor of correct procedure for set up of: ○ relevant components ○ switching on LiDCO monitor and connect to patient bedside monitor via connection cable ○ entering patient details, height and weight ○ priming the wick ○ attaching the sensor ○ attaching the flow regulator ○ priming the 'park and ride' system ○ drawing up the lithium chloride solution (usually 2 mL) ○ attaching primed park and ride to venous access ○ the waveform display ○ alarms ■ discussion with supervisor/mentor of the potential risks to patients ■ discussion with supervisor/mentor of the rationale for the agreed haemodynamic parameter settings ■ discussion with supervisor/mentor of relevant manufacturer, local and national guidelines and policies. ■ where possible a testimonial from patient/client, and or their carer.

(Continued)

235

Competency statement 6.8: (*Continued*)

Demonstrate skills that are required in relation to undertaking the correct calibration procedure for the LiDCO monitor, in line with manufacturer's guidelines, including:

- Correct calibration/zeroing of the arterial catheter in line with manufacturer's guidelines.
- Correct calibration:
  - setting monitor to calibration screen and follow instructions
  - when 'ready to use' displayed press 'INJECT'
  - giving a 20 mL 0.9% sodium chloride flush through 'park and ride' system
  - observing the wash-out curve
  - turn off flow regulator when 'switch flow regulator off and flush' message appears
  - flushing tubing and detach 'park and ride' system, arterial set up and sensor.
- Correct securing of catheter, transducers and cables following local policy and manufacturer's guidelines.
- Clearly identify and label tubing.
- Ensure arterial waveform is displayed and alarms appropriately set.

May be demonstrated by:

- direct observation and discussion with supervisor/ mentor of correct procedure for set up of:
  - relevant components
  - calibration/zeroing
  - securing
  - displaying
  - alarms
- discussion with supervisor/mentor of relevant manufacturer, local and national guidelines and policies
- where possible a testimonial from patient/client and or their carer
- discussion with supervisor/mentor of the rationale for the agreed haemodynamic parameter settings.

Demonstrate skills that are required in relation to the disposing of non-reusable components, sharps and waste following hospital guidelines.

May be demonstrated by:

- discussion with supervisor/mentor
- direct observation of the procedure
- discussion with supervisor/mentor of relevant manufacturer, local and national guidelines and policies
- acting to reduce risk with the multidisciplinary team.

Demonstrate knowledge and understanding of local and national policies, guidance, in relation to infection control.

Demonstrate skills that are required in relation to the accurate documentation of readings and report findings.

May be demonstrated by:

- direct observation by supervisor/mentor of documentation
- communicating in a timely and appropriate manner any changes or concerns regarding haemodynamic observations with the multidisciplinary team
- discussion with supervisor/mentor of relevant guidelines and policies
- where possible a testimonial from patient/client and or their carer.

Competency statement 6.9: Specific procedure competency statements for transpulmonary cardiac output monitoring using lithium dilution (e.g. LiDCOplus)

Complete assessment against relevant fundamental competency statements (*see* Chapter 2, pp. 20, 21)	Evidence
Specific procedure competency statements for transpulmonary cardiac output monitoring using lithium dilution (e.g. LiDCOplus)	**Evidence of competency for transpulmonary cardiac output monitoring using lithium dilution (e.g. LiDCOplus)**
Demonstrate ability to: ■ teach and assess or ■ learn from assessment.	Examples of evidence of teaching, assessing and learning.
Identify indications for monitoring using the trans-pulmonary cardiac output monitoring using lithium dilution system, including: ■ high-risk surgical patients ■ acute heart failure ■ sepsis ■ severe hypovolaemia.	*May be demonstrated by:* ■ discussion with supervisor/mentor, providing an explanation of the indications for monitoring using the transpulmonary cardiac output monitoring using lithium dilution system.

Demonstrate skills that are required in relation to caring for a patient with this system.
■ Safe and correct set up of the system components in line with manufacturer's guidelines, including:
  ○ collection of correct components
  ○ correct connection to the transpulmonary monitoring device and patient monitor
  ○ correct input of patient data.
■ Correct calibration /zeroing of arterial catheter in accordance with manufacturer's guidelines.
■ Correct calibration of the system in line with manufacturer's guidelines, including:
  ○ correct set-up of calibration components
  ○ correct administration of the indicator dilution solution in line with manufacturer's guidelines and following local and national policies for medicine management.
■ Re-calibration in line with local and manufacturer's guidelines.
■ Correct securing of catheter, transducers and cables following local policy and manufacturer's guidelines.
■ Ensure that waveforms and parameters are displayed at all times and alarms appropriately set.
	May be demonstrated by:
	■ direct observation and discussion with supervisor/mentor of correct procedure for set-up of:
	  ○ relevant components
	  ○ calibration/zeroing
	  ○ securing
	  ○ displaying
	  ○ alarms
	■ discussion with supervisor/mentor of relevant manufacturer, local and national guidelines and policies
	■ discussion with supervisor/mentor of the rationale for the agreed haemodynamic parameter settings.

Demonstrate an understanding of: ■ The rationale for the haemodynamic parameters agreed and set by the multidisciplinary team.	
Demonstrate skills that are required in relation to preventing potential catheter infection. ■ Observe dressing for signs of infection, use visual infusion phlebitis (VIP) chart or local equivalent. ■ Change dressing as required – follow local policy.	*May be demonstrated by:* ■ discussion with supervisor/mentor ■ direct observation of the procedure ■ acting to reduce risk with the multidisciplinary team.
Demonstrate knowledge and understanding of local and national policies, guidance, in relation to infection control.	

(Continued)

Identify the contraindications, risks, potential problems and complications of using the lithium dilution transpulmonary cardiac output monitoring system, and how to prevent or manage them, including:

Contraindications:
- patients with an IABP
- patients with aortic regurgitation
- patients with highly dampened peripheral arterial waveform
- patients on oral lithium therapy
- patients under 40 kg (paediatric patient)
- patients during first trimester of pregnancy.

Complications:
- venous/arterial access
- bleeding at site
- pneumo +/- haemothorax
- air embolism
- arterial puncture
- nerve injury
- venous thrombosis.

In use:
- incorrect calibration
- erroneous data
- misinterpretation of data.

May be demonstrated by:
- acting to reduce risk with the multidisciplinary team
- correctly assessing haemodynamic status following local guidelines
- communicating in a timely and appropriate manner any changes or concerns regarding haemodynamic observations with the multidisciplinary team
- able to deliver clinical care whilst limiting adverse affects of using the lithium dilution trans-pulmonary cardiac output monitoring system.
- direct observation of the procedure.

Demonstrate knowledge and understanding of evidence base in relation to the impact of clinical interventions upon haemodynamic status.

Demonstrate knowledge and understanding of evidence base in relation to lithium dilution transpulmonary cardiac output monitoring.
- Waveforms
- Trend screen
- Chart screen
- Parameters:
    1. heart rate (HR)
    2. arterial blood pressure
    3. mean arterial blood pressure (MAP)
    4. systolic pressure variation (SPV)
    5. left ventricle stroke volume
    6. stroke volume variation (SVV %)
    7. pulse pressure variation (PPV %)
    8. cardiac output (CO)
    9. cardiac index (CI)
    10. systemic vascular resistance (SVR) and index (SVRI)
    11. pulmonary vascular resistance (PVR) and index (PVRI)
    12. oxygen delivery (DO_2) and index (DO_2I).

May be demonstrated by:
- discussion with supervisor/mentor
- direct observation of the procedure
- correctly assessing haemodynamic status following local guidelines
- communicating in a timely and appropriate manner any changes or concerns regarding the validity of the observations with the multidisciplinary team.

Demonstrate how people benefit from records that promote communication and high-quality care in relation to using the lithium dilution transpulmonary cardiac output monitoring system.

May be demonstrated by:
- commencing and reviewing the cardiac output monitoring management plan with respect to the agreed parameters identified by the multidisciplinary team.

Demonstrate knowledge and understanding of the potential problems that can occur during monitoring with the transpulmonary cardiac output monitoring using lithium dilution system and how to troubleshoot these, including:
- calibration problems
- inappropriate measurements.

May be demonstrated by:
- direct observation and discussion with supervisor/ mentor of correct procedure for troubleshooting:
    - calibration problems
    - inappropriate measurements
- discussion with supervisor/mentor of relevant manufacturer, local and national guidelines and policies.

Competency statement 6.10: Specific procedure competency statements for insertion of a transpulmonary cardiac output device using thermodilution (e.g. PiCCO)

Complete assessment against relevant fundamental competency statements (*see* Chapter 2, pp. 20, 21)	Evidence
Specific procedure competency statements for insertion of a transpulmonary cardiac output device using thermodilution (e.g. PiCCO)	**Evidence of competency for insertion of a transpulmonary cardiac output device using thermodilution (e.g. PiCCO)**
Demonstrate ability to: ■ teach and assess or ■ learn from assessment.	Examples of evidence of teaching, assessing and learning.
Identify indications for the insertion of a transpulmonary cardiac output device using thermodilution (e.g. PiCCO), including: ■ haemodynamic instability ■ shock ■ sepsis ■ lung injury ■ pulmonary oedema ■ organ failure ■ high-risk surgical patients.	*May be demonstrated by:* ■ Discussion with supervisor/mentor, providing an explanation of the indications for the insertion of a transpulmonary cardiac output device using thermodilution (e.g. PiCCO).
Identify the contraindications of inserting a transpulmonary cardiac output device using thermodilution (e.g. PiCCO), including: ■ peripheral arterial vasoconstriction ■ damped arterial trace ■ CVP in femoral vein (over-estimate) ■ intra-aortic balloon pumps ■ inaccurate readings: 　○ aortic aneurysm 　○ pneumonectomy 　○ aortic stenosis.	*May be demonstrated by:* ■ discussion with supervisor/mentor, providing an explanation of the contraindications of inserting a transpulmonary cardiac output device using thermodilution (e.g. PiCCO).
Demonstrate skills that are required in relation to caring for a patient with the specific PiCCO artery cannula insertion (*see* Procedure guideline 6.2).	*May be demonstrated by:* ■ direct observation and discussion with supervisor/mentor of correct management ■ discussion with supervisor/mentor of relevant manufacturer, local and national guidelines and policies ■ where possible a testimonial from patient/client and or their carer ■ discussion with supervisor/mentor of the rationale for the agreed haemodynamic parameter settings.

239

(*Continued*)

Competency statement 6.10: (*Continued*)

Demonstrate the skills that are required in relation to caring for a patient during the insertion of a transpulmonary cardiac output device using thermodilution (e.g. PiCCO), including:

- The correct set up of the monitor components in line with manufacturer's guidelines:
  - priming transducer set
  - connecting the thermistor cable to the PiCCO monitor and catheter
  - connecting the injectate cable to the thermistor cable and injectate sensor housing
  - connecting the pressure connection cable to the PiCCO monitor and the pressure transducer kit
  - switching the PiCCO monitor on and connecting it to patient bedside monitor via connection cable
  - entering patient details, height and weight.

May be demonstrated by:

- direct observation and discussion with supervisor/mentor of correct procedure for set up of:
  - relevant components
  - priming transducer set
  - the thermistor cable
  - the injectate cable
  - the pressure connection cable
  - switching the PiCCO monitor on and connecting it to patient bedside monitor
  - entering patient details, height and weight
  - the waveform display
  - alarms
- discussion with supervisor/mentor of the potential risks to patients
- discussion with supervisor/mentor of the rationale for the agreed haemodynamic parameter settings
- discussion with supervisor/mentor of relevant manufacturer, local and national guidelines and policies
- where possible a testimonial from patient/client and/or their carer.

Demonstrate skills that are required in relation to undertaking the correct calibration procedure for the PiCCO monitor, in line with manufacturer's guidelines, including:

- Correct calibration/zeroing of the arterial catheter in line with manufacturer's guidelines.
- Correct calibration:
  - 'zeroing' transducer to the PiCCO monitor and then to patient's bedside monitor
  - pressing the 'thermodilution' icon and following instructions
  - giving a 15 mL bolus of iced 0.9% sodium chloride through the CVC system.
  - observing the dilution curve.
- Correct securing of catheter, transducers and cables following local policy and manufacturer's guidelines.
- Clearly identify and label tubing.
- Ensure arterial pressure waveform is displayed and alarms appropriately set.

May be demonstrated by:

- direct observation and discussion with supervisor/mentor of correct procedure for set up of:
  - relevant components
  - calibration/zeroing
  - securing
  - displaying
  - alarms
- discussion with supervisor/mentor of relevant manufacturer, local and national guidelines and policies
- where possible a testimonial from patient/client and/or their carer
- discussion with supervisor/mentor of the rationale for the agreed haemodynamic parameter settings.

Demonstrate skills that are required in relation to the disposing of non-reusable components, sharps and waste following hospital guidelines.

May be demonstrated by:

- discussion with supervisor/mentor
- direct observation of the procedure
- discussion with supervisor/mentor of relevant manufacturer, local and national guidelines and policies
- acting to reduce risk with the multidisciplinary team.

Demonstrate knowledge and understanding of local and national policies, guidance, in relation to infection control.

Demonstrate skills that are required in relation to the accurate documentation of readings and report findings.

May be demonstrated by:

- direct observation by supervisor/mentor of documentation
- communicating in a timely and appropriate manner any changes or concerns regarding haemodynamic observations with the multidisciplinary team
- discussion with supervisor/mentor of relevant guidelines and policies
- where possible a testimonial from patient/client and/or their carer.

Competency statement 6.11: Specific procedure competency statements for transpulmonary cardiac output monitoring using thermodilution (e.g. PiCCO)

Complete assessment against relevant fundamental competency statements (*see* Chapter 2, pp. 20, 21)	Evidence
Specific procedure competency statements for transpulmonary cardiac output monitoring using thermodilution (e.g. PiCCO)	**Evidence of competency for transpulmonary cardiac output monitoring using thermodilution (e.g. PiCCO)**
Demonstrate ability to: ■ teach and assess or ■ learn from assessment.	Examples of evidence of teaching, assessing and learning.
Identify indications for monitoring using the transpulmonary cardiac output monitoring using a thermodilution system, including: ■ haemodynamic instability ■ shock ■ sepsis ■ lung injury ■ pulmonary oedema ■ organ failure ■ high-risk surgical patients.	*May be demonstrated by:* ■ discussion with supervisor/mentor, providing an explanation of the indications for monitoring using the transpulmonary cardiac output monitoring using a thermodilution system.
Demonstrate skills that are required in relation to caring for a patient with a thermodilution transpulmonary cardiac output monitoring system. ■ Safe and correct set up of the system components in line with manufacturer's guidelines, including: 1. collection of correct components 2. correct connection to the monitoring device and patient monitor 3. correct input of patient data. ■ Correct calibration/zeroing of catheter and arterial waveform in accordance with manufacturer's guidelines. ■ Correct configuration and calibration of system in line with manufacturer's guidelines, including: ■ correct set-up of calibration components ■ correct administration of the thermodilution indicator solution in line with manufacturer's guidelines and following local and national policies for medicine management. ■ Re-calibration in line with local and manufacturer's guidelines ■ Correct securing of catheter, transducers and cables following local policy and manufacturer's guidelines. ■ Ensure that waveforms and parameters are displayed at all times and alarms appropriately set.	*May be demonstrated by:* ■ direct observation and discussion with supervisor/mentor of correct procedure for set up of: ○ relevant components ○ calibration/zeroing ○ securing ○ monitor display ○ alarms ■ discussion with supervisor/mentor of relevant manufacturer, local and national guidelines and policies ■ discussion with supervisor/mentor of the rationale for the agreed haemodynamic parameter settings.
Demonstrate an understanding of: ■ the rationale for the haemodynamic parameters agreed and set by the multidisciplinary team.	
Demonstrate skills that are required in relation to preventing potential catheter infection. ■ Observe dressing for signs of infection, use visual infusion phlebitis (VIP) chart or local equivalent. ■ Change dressing as required – follow local policy.	*May be demonstrated by:* ■ discussion with supervisor/mentor ■ direct observation of the procedure ■ acting to reduce risk with the multidisciplinary team.
Demonstrate knowledge and understanding of local and national policies, guidance, in relation to infection control.	

241

(Continued)

Competency statement 6.11: *(Continued)*

Identify the contraindications, risks, potential problems and complications of the thermodilution transpulmonary cardiac output monitoring system, and how to prevent or manage them, including:

Contraindications:
- peripheral arterial vasoconstriction
- damped arterial trace
- CVP in femoral vein (over estimate)
- intra-aortic balloon pumps
- inaccurate readings:
  - aortic aneurysm
  - pneumonectomy
  - aortic stenosis.

Complications:
- venous/arterial access
- bleeding at site
- pneumo +/- haemothorax
- air embolism
- arterial puncture
- nerve injury
- venous thrombosis.

In use:
- incorrect calibration
- erroneous data
- misinterpretation of data.

May be demonstrated by:
- acting to reduce risk with the multidisciplinary team
- correctly assessing haemodynamic status following local guidelines
- communicating in a timely and appropriate manner any changes or concerns regarding haemodynamic observations with the multidisciplinary team
- able to deliver clinical care while limiting adverse affects of the thermodilution transpulmonary cardiac output monitoring system
- direct observation of the procedure.

Demonstrate knowledge and understanding of evidence base in relation to the impact of clinical interventions upon haemodynamic status.

Demonstrate knowledge and understanding of evidence base in relation to the transpulmonary cardiac output monitoring technique using a thermodilution system.
- Waveforms
- Parameters:
  1. arterial pressure (AP)
  2. mean arterial blood pressure (MAP)
  3. heart rate (HR)
  4. stroke volume (SV) and index (SVI)
  5. cardiac output (CO)
  6. cardiac index (CI)
  7. systemic vascular resistance (SVR) and index (SVRI)
  8. global end-diastolic volume (GEDV) or index (GEDI)
  9. intra-thoracic blood volume (ITBV) or index (ITBI)
  10. stroke volume variation (SVV%)
  11. pulse pressure variation (PPV%)
  12. extravascular lung water (EVLW) or index (ELWI)
  13. pulmonary vascular permeability index (PVPI)
  14. global ejection fraction (GEF%)
  15. cardiac function index (CFI)
  16. left ventricular contractility (dP/mx).

May be demonstrated by:
- discussion with supervisor/mentor
- direct observation of the procedure
- correctly assessing haemodynamic status following local guidelines
- communicating in a timely and appropriate manner any changes or concerns regarding the validity of observations with the multidisciplinary team.

242

Demonstrate knowledge and understanding of the potential problems that can occur during monitoring with the system and how to troubleshoot these, including:
- calibration problems
- inappropriate measurements.

May be demonstrated by:
- direct observation and discussion with supervisor/mentor of correct procedure for troubleshooting:
  - calibration problems
  - inappropriate measurements
- discussion with supervisor/mentor of relevant manufacturer, local and national guidelines and policies.

Competency statement 6.12: Specific procedure competency statements for insertion of an oesophageal Doppler probe (e.g. CardioQ)

Complete assessment against relevant fundamental competency statements (*see* Chapter 2, pp. 20, 21)	Evidence
Specific procedure competency statements for insertion of an oesophageal Doppler probe (e.g. CardioQ)	**Evidence of competency for insertion of an oesophageal Doppler probe (e.g. CardioQ)**
Demonstrate ability to: ■ teach and assess or ■ learn from assessment.	Examples of evidence of teaching, assessing and learning.
Identify indications for the use of an oesophageal Doppler monitor (ODM) (e.g. CardioQ), including: ■ moderate- to high-risk surgical patients ■ haemodynamically unstable patients ■ acute heart failure ■ sepsis ■ severe hypovolaemia.	*May be demonstrated by:* ■ discussion with supervisor/mentor, providing an explanation of the indications for the use of an oesophageal Doppler monitor (ODM) (e.g. CardioQ).
Identify the contraindications of inserting of an oesophageal Doppler probe (e.g. CardioQ), including: ■ facial trauma ■ nasal injuries or polyps ■ oesophageal varices and tears ■ severe coarctation of the aorta ■ known oesophageal tumours ■ severe bleeding diatheses ■ thoracic aorta aneurysms ■ intra-aortic balloon pumps.	*May be demonstrated by:* ■ discussion with supervisor/mentor, providing an explanation of the contraindications of inserting of an oesophageal Doppler probe (e.g. CardioQ).

(Continued)

Demonstrate the skills that are required in relation to caring for a patient during the use of an oesophageal Doppler monitor (ODM) (e.g. CardioQ), including:

- The correct set-up of the monitor components in line with manufacturer's guidelines:
  - switching on the power
  - connecting the probe to patient interface cable
  - entering the patient details, gender, height and weight
  - applying a water-based lubricant to the probe.

May be demonstrated by:

- direct observation and discussion with supervisor/ mentor of correct procedure for set up of:
  - relevant components
  - switching on the power
  - connecting the probe to patient interface cable
  - applying a water-based lubricant
  - entering patient details, height and weight
  - the waveform display
  - alarms
- discussion with supervisor/mentor of the potential risks to patients
- discussion with supervisor/mentor of the rationale for the agreed haemodynamic parameter settings
- discussion with supervisor/mentor of relevant manufacturer, local and national guidelines and policies.

Demonstrate skills that are required in relation to correctly inserting the oesophageal Doppler probe in line with manufacturer's guidelines.

- Orally – advancing probe gently until incisors are between the distal marker (Distal from connector), of the probe (depth of 35 cm) and the middle marker (depth of 40 cm).
- Nasally – advancing probe gently until nasal septum is between the middle marker (depth of 40 cm) and the proximal marker (proximal to the connector) of the probe (depth of 45 cm).
- Locating the descending aortic signal by adjusting the probe depth.
- Optimizing the signal by rotating the probe to achieve the sharpest waveform and clearest audible sound.

May be demonstrated by:

- discussion with supervisor/mentor
- direct observation of the procedure, including:
  - acting to reduce risk with the multidisciplinary team.

Demonstrate knowledge and understanding of local and national policies, guidance.

Demonstrate skills that are required in relation to the disposing of non reusable components, sharps and waste following hospital guidelines.

May be demonstrated by:

- discussion with supervisor/mentor
- direct observation of the procedure
- discussion with supervisor/mentor of relevant manufacturer, local and national guidelines and policies
- acting to reduce risk with the multidisciplinary team.

Demonstrate knowledge and understanding of local and national policies, guidance, in relation to infection control.

Demonstrate skills that are required in relation to the accurate documentation of readings and report findings.

May be demonstrated by:

- direct observation by supervisor/mentor of documentation
- communicating in a timely and appropriate manner any changes or concerns regarding haemodynamic observations with the multidisciplinary team
- discussion with supervisor/mentor of relevant guidelines and policies
- where possible a testimonial from patient/client and/ or their carer.

Competency statement 6.13: Specific procedure competency statements for oesophageal Doppler monitoring (ODM) (e.g. CardioQ)

Complete assessment against relevant fundamental competency statements (*see* Chapter 2, pp. 20, 21)	Evidence
Specific procedure competency statements for oesophageal Doppler monitoring (ODM)	**Evidence of competency for oesophageal Doppler monitoring (ODM)**
Demonstrate ability to: ■ teach and assess or ■ learn from assessment.	Examples of evidence of teaching, assessing and learning.
Identify indications for monitoring using an oesophageal Doppler monitor (ODM), including: ■ moderate- to high-risk surgical patients ■ haemodynamically unstable patients ■ acute heart failure ■ sepsis ■ severe hypovolaemia.	*May be demonstrated by:* ■ discussion with supervisor/mentor, providing an explanation of the indications for monitoring using an oesophageal Doppler monitor (ODM).

Demonstrate skills that are required in relation to caring for a patient with an oesophageal Doppler monitor (ODM).
■ Safe and correct set up of an oesophageal Doppler monitor (ODM) and components in line with manufacturer's guidelines, including:
  1. collection of correct components and appropriate probe
  2. correct connection to an ODM and patient monitor
  3. correct input of patient data.
■ Correct configuration an ODM in line with manufacturer's guidelines.
■ Correct securing of probe following local policy and manufacturer's guidelines.
■ Ensure that waveforms and parameters are displayed at all times and alarms appropriately set.
 	
Demonstrate an understanding of:
■ the rationale for the haemodynamic parameters agreed and set by the multidisciplinary team.
	May be demonstrated by:
	■ direct observation and discussion with supervisor/mentor of correct procedure for set up of:
	  ○ relevant components
	  ○ configuration
	  ○ securing
	  ○ displaying
	  ○ alarms
	■ discussion with supervisor/mentor of relevant manufacturer, local and national guidelines and policies
	■ discussion with supervisor/mentor of the rationale for the agreed haemodynamic parameter settings.

Demonstrate skills that are required in relation to preventing potential infection. Demonstrate knowledge and understanding of local and national policies, guidance, in relation to infection control.	*May be demonstrated by:* ■ discussion with supervisor/mentor ■ direct observation of the procedure ■ acting to reduce risk with the multidisciplinary team.
Identify the contraindications, risks, potential problems and complications of ODM and how to prevent or manage them, including: **Contraindications:** ■ facial trauma ■ nasal injuries or polyps ■ oesophageal varices and tears ■ severe coarctation of the aorta ■ known oesophageal tumours ■ severe bleeding diatheses ■ thoracic aorta aneurysms ■ intra-aortic balloon pumps.	*May be demonstrated by:* ■ acting to reduce risk with the multidisciplinary team ■ correctly assessing haemodynamic status following local guidelines ■ communicating in a timely and appropriate manner any changes or concerns regarding haemodynamic observations with the multidisciplinary team ■ able to deliver clinical care while limiting adverse affects of ODM ■ direct observation of the procedure.

(Continued)

Competency statement 6.13: (Continued)

Complications:
- dislodgement of probe
- damage to oesophageal mucosa and oesophageal bleeding
- oesophagotracheal perforation
- dysphagia.

In use:
- incorrect configuration
- erroneous data
- misinterpretation of data.

Demonstrate knowledge and understanding of evidence base in relation to the impact of clinical interventions on haemodynamic status.

Demonstrate knowledge and understanding of evidence base in relation to ODM:	*May be demonstrated by:*

- ODM waveforms
- ODM parameters:
  1. heart rate (HR)
  2. flow time corrected (FTc)
  3. peak velocity (PV)
  4. stroke distance
  5. stroke volume (SV) and index (SVI)
  6. cardiac output (CO) and index (CI).
	- discussion with supervisor/mentor
	- direct observation of the procedure
	- correctly assessing haemodynamic status following local guidelines
	- communicating in a timely and appropriate manner any changes or concerns regarding the validity of ODM device observations with the multidisciplinary team.

Demonstrate knowledge and understanding of the potential problems that can occur during monitoring with ODM and how to troubleshoot these, including:	*May be demonstrated by:*

- configuration problems
- inappropriate measurements.
	- direct observation and discussion with supervisor/mentor of correct procedure for troubleshooting:
	  ○ configuration problems
	  ○ inappropriate measurements
	- discussion with supervisor/mentor of relevant manufacturer, local and national guidelines and policies.

References

Abbas SM and Hill AG (2008) Systematic review of the literature for the use of oesophageal Doppler monitor for fluid replacement in major abdominal surgery. *Anaesthesia* **63**: 44–51.

Adam SK and Osborne S (2005) *Critical Care Nursing: Science and Practice*. Oxford: Oxford University Press.

Al-Shaikh B and Stacey S (2002) *Essentials of Anaesthetic Equipment* (2e). London: Churchill Livingstone.

Australian Commission on Safety and Quality in Health Care (2010) *National Recommendations for User-applied Labelling of Injectable Medicines, Fluids and Lines*. Darlinghurst: Australian Commission on Safety and Quality in Health Care.

Bersten AD, Soni N and Oh TE (2004) *Oh's Intensive Care Manual* (5e). Edinburgh: Butterworth-Heinemann.

Brzezinski M, Luisetti T and London MJ (2009) Radial artery cannulation: a comprehensive review of recent anatomic and physiologic investigations. *Anesthesia and Analgesia* **109**(6): 1763–1781.

Burtenshaw AJ and Isaac JL (2006) The role of trans-oesophageal echocardiography for perioperative cardiovascular monitoring during orthotopic liver transplantation. *Liver Transplant* **12**: 1577–1583.

Casey AL, Mermel LA, Nightingale P and Elliott TSJ (2008) Anti-microbial central venous catheters in adults: a systematic review and meta-analysis. *Lancet Infectious Diseases* **8**: 763–776.

Cecconi M, Fawcett J, Grounds RM and Rhodes A (2008) A prospective study to evaluate the accuracy of pulse power analysis to monitor cardiac output in critically ill patients. *BMC Anaesthesiology* **8**(3): 1–9.

Cecconi M, Dawson D, Grounds RM and Rhodes A (2009) Lithium dilution cardiac output measurement in the critically ill patient: determination of precision of the technique. *Intensive Care Medicine* **35**: 498–504.

Chatterjee K (2009) The Swan-Ganz catheters: past, present, and future a viewpoint. *Circulation* **119**: 147–152.

Combes A, Berneau J, Luyt C and Trouillet J (2004) Estimation of left ventricular systolic function by single trans-pulmonary thermodilution. *Intensive Care Medicine* **30**: 1377–1383.

Costa MG, Rocca GD, Chiarandini P et al. (2008) Continuous and intermittent cardiac output measurement in hyperdynamic conditions: pulmonary artery catheter vs. lithium dilution technique. *Intensive Care Medicine* **34**: 257–263.

Cottis R, Magee N and Higgins DJ (2003) Haemodynamic monitoring with pulse-induced contour cardiac output (PiCCO) in critical care. *Intensive and Critical Care Nursing* **19**: 301–307.

Deltex Medical (2009) *Oesophageal Doppler Monitoring using the CardioQ and CardioQ-ODM: Workbook for Nurses*. Chichester: Deltex Medical Great Britain.

Department of Health (2007) *Saving Lives: reducing infection, delivering clean and safe care*. High Impact Intervention No 1. Central venous catheter care bundle. http://www.clean-safe-care. nhs.uk/toolfiles/14_SL_HII_1_v2.pdf

Drew BJ, Califf RM, Funk M et al. (2004) Practice standards for electrocardiographic monitoring in hospital settings: an American Heart Association Scientific Statement from the Councils on Cardiovascular Nursing, Clinical Cardiology, and Cardiovascular Disease in the Young. Endorsed by the International Society of Computerized Electrocardiography and the American Society of Critical Care Nurses. *Circulation* **110**: 2721–2746.

Ercole A (2007) Assessing fluid responsiveness: the role of dynamic haemodynamic indices. *Trauma* **9**: 13–19.

Erdmann A (2004) *Concise Anatomy for Anaesthesia*. London: Greenwich Medical Media.

Gan TJ, Soppitt A, Maroof M et al. (2002) Goal-directed intra-operative fluid administration reduces length of hospital stay after major surgery. *Anaesthesiology* **97**(4): 820–826.

General Medical Council (2013) *Good Medical Practice*. London: GMC. http://www.gmc-uk.org/gmp2013 [accessed 25 March 2013].

Hadian M, Kim HK, Severyn DA and Pinsky MR (2010) Cross-comparison of cardiac output trending accuracy of LiDCO, PiCCO, FloTrac and pulmonary artery catheters. *Critical Care* **14**: 1–10.

Hamilton TT, Huber LM and Jessen ME (2002) Pulse CO: a less-invasive method to monitor cardiac output from arterial pressure after cardiac surgery. *Annals of Thoracic Surgery* **74**: 1408–1412.

Hampton JR (1998) *The ECG Made Easy* (5e). London: Churchill Livingstone.

Harvey S, Harrison D, Singer M et al. (2005) An assessment of the clinical effectiveness of pulmonary artery catheters in patient management in intensive care (PACMan): a randomised controlled trial. *Lancet* **366**(9484): 472–477.

Harvey S, Young D, Brampton W et al. (2006a) Pulmonary artery catheters for adult patients in intensive care. *Cochrane Database of Systematic Reviews* **3**: 1–35.

Harvey S, Stevens K, Harrison D et al. (2006b) An evaluation of the clinical and cost-effectiveness of pulmonary artery catheters in patient management in intensive care: a systematic review and a randomised controlled trial. *Health Technology Assessment* **10**(29): 1–6.

Health and Care Professions Council (2012) *Standard of Conduct, Performance and Ethics*. London: HCPC. http://www.hcpc-uk.org/ assets/documents/10003B6EStandardsofconduct,performance andethics.pdf [accessed January 2013].

Hutton P, Cooper GM, James III FM and Butterworth JF (2002) *Fundamental Principles and Practice of Anaesthesia* (1e). London: Martin Dunitz.

Iregui MG, Prentice D, Sherman G et al. (2003) Physicians' estimates of cardiac index and intravascular volume based on clinical assessment versus transoesopgageal Doppler measurements obtained by critical care nurses. *American Journal of Critical Care* **12**(4): 336–342.

Jevon P, Ewens B and Pooni JS (2007) *Monitoring the Critically Ill Patient* (2e). Oxford: Blackwell Publishing.

Jhanji S, Dawson J and Pearse RM (2008) Cardiac output monitoring: basic science and clinical application. *Anaesthesia* **63**: 172–181.

Jonas M, Hett D and Morgan J (2002) Real-time, continuous monitoring of cardiac output and oxygen delivery. *International Journal of Intensive Care* **9**(1): 33–42.

Kannan A (2008) Heparinised saline or normal saline? *Journal of Perioperative Practice* **18**: 440–441.

Kemps HMC, Thijssen EJM, Schep G et al. (2008) Evaluation of two methods for continuous cardiac output assessment during exercise in chronic heart failure patients. *Journal of Applied Physiology* **105**: 1822–1829.

Kumar A, Anel R, Bunnell E et al. (2004) Pulmonary artery occlusion pressure and central venous pressure fail to predict ventricular filling volume, cardiac performance, or the response to volume infusion in normal subjects. *Critical Care Medicine* **32**:691–699.

LiDCO. *Normal Hemodynamic Parameters*. LiDCO Ltd. http://www. lidco.com/html/clinical/nhp.asp [accessed 10 November 2010].

LiDCO. *LiDCOplus set-up procedure* [DVD-ROM]. LiDCO Ltd.

Lowe GD, Chamberlain BM, Philpot EJ and Willshire RJ (2010) Oesophageal Doppler monitor (ODM) guided individualised goal directed fluid management (iGDFM) in surgery – a technical review. *Deltex Medical Technical Review* **4**: 1–12.

Marieb EN and Hoehn K (2007) *Human Anatomy and Physiology* (7e). San Francisco: Pearson Benjamin Cummings.

Marik PE, Baram M and Vahid B (2008) Does central venous pressure predict fluid responsiveness? *Chest* **134**: 172–178.

Mental Capacity Act (2005) http://www.legislation.gov.uk/ukpga/ 2005/9/pdfs/ukpga_20050009_en.pdf [accessed 9 February 2012].

Mireles SA, Jaffe RA, Drover DR and Brock-Utne JG (2009) A poor correlation exists between oscillometric and radial arterial blood pressure as measured by the Philips MP90 monitor. *Journal of Clinical Monitoring and Computing*; **23**:169-174.

Monnet X, Anguel N, Osman D et al. (2007) Assessing pulmonary permeability by trans-pulmonary thermodilution allows differentiation of hydrostatic pulmonary edema from ALI/ARDS. *Intensive Care Medicine* **33**: 448–453.

Moore KL (1985) *Clinically Orientated Anatomy* (2e). Baltimore, MD: Williams and Wilkins,

Morgan A (2003) Haemodynamic monitoring. In: Bersten A, Soni N and Oh TE (eds) *Oh's Intensive Care Manual* (5e). London: Butterworth-Heinemann.

Morton PG and Fontaine DK (eds) (2008) *Critical Care Nursing: a holistic approach* (9e). Philadelphia: Lippincott Williams and Wilkins.

Morton PG, Reck K, Tucker T et al. (2009) Patient assessment: cardiovascular system. In: Morton PG and Fontaine DK (eds) *Critical Care Nursing: a holistic approach* (9e). Philadelphia: Wolters Klumer Health.

National Institute for Health and Clinical Excellence (2002) *Technology Appraisal Guidance No.49: Guidance on the use of ultrasound locating devices for placing central venous catheters*. London: NICE.

National Institute for Health and Clinical Excellence Short Clinical Guidelines Technical Team (2006) *Acutely Ill Patients in Hospital: recognition of and response to acute illness in adults in hospital*. London: NICE. www.nice.org.uk/CG050

National Institute for Health and Clinical Excellence (2011) *NICE Medical Technologies Guidance 3, CardioQ-ODM oesophageal Doppler monitor*. London: NICE.

Nursing and Midwifery Council (2008) *The Code: standards of conduct, performance and ethics for nurses and midwives*. London: NMC.

Ott K, Johnson K and Ahrens T (2001) New technologies in the assessment of haemodynamic parameters. *Journal of Cardiovascular Nursing* **15**(2): 41–55.

Parry-Jones AJD and Pittman JAL (2003) Arterial pressure and stroke volume variability as measurements for cardiovascular optimization. *International Journal of Intensive care* **10**(2): 67–72.

Patient Safety First (2008) *The 'How to Guide' for Reducing Harm in Critical Care*. Patient Safety First Campaign. NHS Institute for Innovation and Improvement.

Pinnock C, Lin T and Smith T (2006) *Fundamentals of Anaesthesia* (2e). Cambridge: Cambridge University Press.

Power I and Kam P (2008) *Principles of Physiology for the Anaesthetist* (2e). London: Hodder Arnold.

Pratt RJ, Pellowe CM, Wilson JA et al. (2007) epic2: National Evidence-Based Guidelines for Preventing Healthcare-Associated Infections in NHS Hospitals in England. *Journal of Hospital Infection* 65S: S1–S64.

Pronovost P, Needham D, Berenholtz S et al. (2006) An intervention to decrease catheter-related bloodstream infections in the ICU. *New England Journal Of Medicine* 335: 2725–2732.

Pulsion Medical Systems (2009) *Train the Trainer Folder Advanced Hemodynamic Monitoring PiCCO-Technology: Theory and Practice*. Irving: Pulsion Medical Systems. http://www.pulsion.com/fileadmin/pulsion_share/Education/Training/TraintheTrainer/TtT_US_MPI851405US_R00_101008_Complete.pdf [accessed 26 April 2011].

Rhodes A and Sunderland R (2005) Arterial pulse contour analysis: the LiDCOplus system. In: Pinsky MR and Payen D (eds) *Functional haemodynamic monitoring update*. *Intensive Care and Emergency Medicine* 42: 183–192.

Ritter S, Rudiger A and Maggiorini M (2009) Trans-pulmonary thermodilution-derived cardiac function index identifies cardiac dysfunction in acute heart failure and septic patients: an observational study. *Critical Care* 13: 1–10.

Rivers E, Nguyen B, Havestad S et al. (2001) Early goal-directed therapy in the treatment of severe sepsis and septic shock. *New England Journal of Medicine* 345: 1368–1377.

Roizen MF, Berger DL, Gabel RA et al. (2003) Practice guidelines for pulmonary artery catheterization: an updated report by the American Society of Anesthesiologists Task Force on Pulmonary Artery Catheterization. *Anesthesiology* 99: 988–1014.

Selleng K, Warkentin T and Creinacher A (2007) Heparin-induced thrombocytopenia in intensive care patients. *Critical Care Medicine* 35(4): 1165–1176.

Shoemaker WC, Velmahos GC and Demetriades D (2002) *Procedures and Monitoring for the Critically Ill*. Pennsylvania: WB Saunders.

Singer M and Webb AR (2009) *Oxford Handbook of Critical Care* (3e). Oxford: Oxford University Press.

Thibodeau GA and Patton KT (2007) *Anatomy and Physiology* (6e). St Louis, MO: Mosby Elsevier.

Timsit J-F, Schwebel C, Bouadma L et al. (2009) Chlorhexidine-impregnated sponges and less frequent dressing changes for prevention of catheter-related infections in critically ill adults: a randomized controlled trial. *Journal of the American Medical Association* 301(12): 1231–1241.

Tortora GJ and Derrickson BH (2011) *Principles of Anatomy and Physiology* (13e). New Jersey: John Wiley and Sons.

Tote SP and Grounds RM (2006) Performing perioperative optimization of the high-risk surgical patient. *British Journal of Anaesthesia* 97(1): 4–11.

Tuncali BE, Kuvaki B, Tuncali B and Capar E (2005) A comparison of the efficacy of heparinized and nonheparinized solutions for the maintenance of perioperative radial artery catheter patency and subsequent occlusion. *Anesthesia and Analgesia* 100(4): 1117–1121.

Urden LD, Stacy KM and Lough ME (2010) *Critical Care Nursing: Diagnosis and Management* (6e). St Louis, MO: Mosby Elsevier.

Walsh SR, Tang T, Bass S and Gaunt ME (2008) Doppler-guided intra-operative fluid management during major abdominal surgery: systematic review and meta-analysis. *International Journal of Clinical Practice* 62(3): 466–470.

West IB (1990) *Respiratory Physiology – the essentials* (4e). Baltimore, MD: Williams and Wilkins.

Whiteley SM, Bodenham A and Bellamy MC (2010) *Churchill's Pocketbooks: intensive care* (3e). London: Churchill Livingstone.

248

Chapter 7

Titration of inotropes and vasopressors

Kirsty Rutledge

Newcastle upon Tyne Hospitals NHS Foundation Trust, Newcastle upon Tyne, UK

Critical Care Manual of Clinical Procedures and Competencies, First Edition.
Edited by Jane Mallett, John W. Albarran, and Annette Richardson.
© 2013 John Wiley & Sons, Ltd. Published 2013 by John Wiley & Sons, Ltd.

Definition

Inotropes are drugs that improve the performance of heart muscle fibres, thereby improving cardiac output. They have either an inotropic effect, altering heart contractility, or a chronotropic effect, altering heart rate. Vasopressors are drugs that increase blood pressure through vasoconstriction (Ellender and Skinner 2008). Some drugs can have both inotropic and vasopressor actions depending on the dose delivered; however, they are distinguished by their main actions (Hollenberg 2007).

Aims and indications

Inotropes and vasopressors are used to support or enhance blood flow and organ perfusion in haemodynamically unstable patients. Throughout their delivery the dose of these drugs is titrated to achieve a desired response, through increasing and decreasing the infusion rate.

Background

Circulatory failure is a common, life-threatening problem in patients who are critically ill, which results in poor organ and tissue perfusion and reduced oxygen delivery. Persistent hypotension leads to irreversible tissue damage and organ failure, and can ultimately end in death (Mitchell 2005). However, if circulatory failure is promptly recognized, patients effectively resuscitated and the underlying cause corrected, then the consequences may be reversible (Ellender and Skinner 2008). The aim of titration of inotropes and vasopressors is, therefore, to support cardiac function and improve blood pressure while correcting the underlying cause.

The first line of treatment for hypotension is the administration of intravenous fluids to increase circulatory blood flow (Mullner et al. 2008), with volume status and responsiveness to fluid boluses being regularly measured (Sturgess et al. 2007).

Blood pressure is often the first measurement taken; however, while this is important, it should not be utilized solely as a reliable parameter for resuscitation (Dellinger et al. 2008) or to determine perfusion. One sign of adequate perfusion is adequate urine output, as the renal circulation is known to respond sensitively to perfusion pressure (Hollenberg 2007); other signs can be normal blood lactate levels, consciousness, adequate capillary refill time and skin that is pink and warm (see Table 7.1 for normal values). When these measurements indicate that the patient's circulating blood flow is adequate but blood pressure remains low, the administration of inotropes and vasopressors is often required to support adequate organ and tissue perfusion (Holmes 2005). Administration of vasopressors prior to correcting circulatory blood flow may be detrimental to pre-existing inadequate organ perfusion because vasoconstriction further reduces blood flow to the extremities and organs. Inotropes and vasopressors can, however, be used

Table 7.1 Normal values that guide intervention

Clinical indicators	Normal values (Carpenito-Moyet 2009)
Systolic blood pressure	above 90 mmHg
Mean arterial blood pressure	above 70 mmHg
Central venous pressure	0–8 cm H_2O
Urine output	above 0.5 mL/kg/h
Lactate	below 2 mmol/L

Table 7.2 Terminology

Term	Definition (Klabunde 2005)
Cardiac output	The amount of blood ejected from the heart each minute
Heart rate	The number of heart beats per minute
Stroke volume	The amount of blood ejected from the heart with each contraction
Contractility	The force of cardiac contraction
Preload	The amount of stretch in the cardiac muscles prior to contraction
Afterload	The force against which the left ventricle must contract to eject blood from the heart
Systemic vascular resistance	The resistance in the blood vessels of the systemic circulation

in emergency situations prior to adequate fluid replacement in order to restore a dangerously low blood pressure quickly (Beale et al. 2004), but should be titrated as response to fluid replacement occurs (Dellinger et al. 2008).

Anatomy and physiology

In order to administer the appropriate treatment to improve a patient's blood pressure, it is important that the determinants of blood pressure and how they can be influenced are understood (see Table 7.2). Blood pressure is ultimately determined by cardiac output and systemic vascular resistance (SVR). Cardiac output is, in turn, influenced by heart rate and stroke volume, with stroke volume being determined by preload, afterload and contractility. All of these determinants can be manipulated pharmacologically through the administration of selected fluids and drugs. The administration of fluids, for example, will increase the volume of blood returning to the heart, optimizing preload, which increases cardiac contractility and stroke volume, improving cardiac output. This follows Frank–Starling's Law of the Heart (Marieb 2004). Administering inotropes affects heart rate and contractility. Administering vasopressors increases SVR, reducing the diameter of blood vessels, and hence the amount of blood required to fill them to achieve an acceptable blood pressure (Ellender and Skinner 2008) (Figure 7.1). See also Chapter 6.

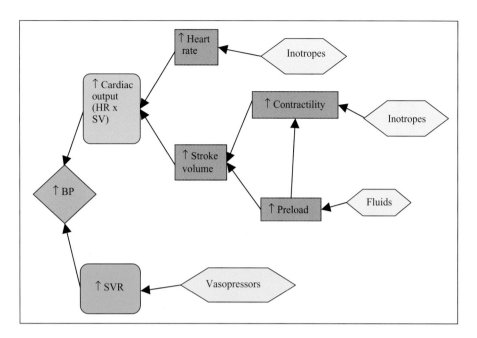

Figure 7.1 How blood pressure can be improved.

Choice of inotrope or vasopressor

Inotropes and vasopressors act in different ways, having excitatory and/or inhibitory effects on the heart and blood vessels as well as important effects on the central nervous system, autonomic nervous system and metabolism (Overgaard and Dzavik 2008). Inotropes mainly activate β-receptors in the cardiac muscle with minimal effects on α-receptors; however, some inotropes, e.g. phosphodiesterase inhibitors, do not depend on receptors to elicit their effect on the cardiac muscle. Vasopressors mainly activate α-receptors with minimal effect on β-receptors. Adrenaline is unique in that it acts equally on both receptors, making it a vital drug in emergency situations (Resuscitation Council UK 2010). In order to select the appropriate drug and exert the required response it is vital to understand how each of them works, what their side effects are and how different combinations will affect patients (*see* Table 7.3).

Components of titration of inotropic drug therapies

Administration of inotropic drugs via syringe pumps

Inotropes and vasopressors can cause irritation to peripheral vasculature and should therefore be administered via a central venous catheter (CVC) (Miller 2007). A CVC is a venous access system used to access the large veins in the

neck, chest, or groin. It has a varying number of lumens used for the administration of drugs and fluids, to withdraw blood samples and to obtain diagnostic information such as the central venous pressure. Inotropes and vasopressors should be administered via a designated lumen of the CVC, with no other drugs on that lumen, to avoid drug compatibility issues and bolus delivery, and to allow accurate titration. To allow safe changeover, the lumen used to administer inotropes and vasopressors should have a device attached to it which allows multiple infusions to run together on the same lumen. Depending on local hospital policy this will be either an 'octopus' device with bionectors, a three-way tap with bionectors, or a three-way tap with bungs. When accessing CVCs it is vital to adhere to infection control policies to minimize the risk of potential infection (Trim and Roe 2004). The Department of Health (DH 2007) has devised a 'care bundle' for CVCs – a set of research-based guidelines that inform healthcare practitioners of best practice for the insertion and ongoing care of CVCs (see Chapter 6 for further guidance). Once connected to the lumen, drug administration tubing should be labelled to enable staff to quickly identify, change, or discontinue infusions in an emergency (Miller 2007).

Delivery of inotropes and vasopressors should occur through a syringe fitted in to a syringe pump, rather than a bag of fluid dripping through a volumetric pump. This is because inotropes and vasopressors are often delivered at rates of less than 10 mL/h and syringe pumps are able to deliver a more constant, accurate flow at these low rates (MHRA 2010).

Syringe pumps are specifically designed to deliver high-risk drugs with greater accuracy and the shortest time delay

Table 7.3 Actions of inotropes and vasopressors

	Activation of α1 receptors Smooth muscle contraction, leading to increased SVR	Activation of β1 receptors Enhanced myocardial contractility	Activation of β2 receptors Vasodilatation	Activation of dopaminergic receptors Renal and mesenteric vasodilatation	Activation of vasopressin receptors Vasoconstriction of the systemic, splanchnic, renal and coronary arteries (Cooper 2008). May reduce the need for the use of catecholamines (Russel et al. 2008)
Inotropes					
Dopamine (Fischer and Bland 2007)	Active in high doses only (greater than 6 micrograms/kg/min)	**Increases contractility*** (3–6 micrograms/kg/min)	x	Active in low doses only (1–3 micrograms/kg/min)	x
Dobutamine	x	**Increases contractility**	Encourages vasodilatation	x	x
Dopexamine	x	**Increases contractility**	**Encourages vasodilatation in cardiac muscle**	x	x
Phosphodiesterase inhibitors (PDIs) – milrinone, amrinone, and levosimendan	x	**Increases contractility** (although this is through the activation of calcium channels rather than through activation of receptors)	**Causes venous and arterial dilation** (although this is through the activation of calcium channels rather than through activation of receptors)	x	x
Vasopressors					
Noradrenaline	**Potent vasoconstrictor**	Very mild inotropic results	x	x	x
Phenylephrine	**Potent vasoconstrictor**	x	x	x	x
Vasopressin	x	x	x	x	**Potent vasoconstrictor**
Adrenaline (Fischer and Bland 2007)	Active in high doses (greater than 1 micrograms/kg/min)	Active in low doses (0.01–1 micrograms/kg/min)	Active in low doses (0.01–1 micrograms/kg/min)	x	x

*Main mode of action of drug is indicated in bold.

possible prior to delivery of the medication. They also have a sensitive alarm to indicate any occlusion that is preventing the administration of the medication (Trim and Roe 2004). Neff et al. (2007) studied syringe size and accuracy and found that larger syringes deliver less accurately at very low rates, i.e. 0.1 mL/h, when compared with smaller syringes. However, a small reduction in accuracy becomes less significant with higher rates. It may, however, be necessary to reduce the concentration of medication in the syringe, using larger volumes to improve accuracy.

When commencing a syringe pump there is a period of time between the start of the infusion and the medication being delivered to the patient, before the syringe pump engages with the plunger. This is known as mechanical slack. Inotropes and vasopressors are usually required immediately and at a steady rate (Neff et al. 2007), but infusion at low rates could result in the mechanical slack time prior to administration being as long as 40–60 minutes (Amoore et al. 2001). A delay in delivery of inotropes and vasopressors can result in adverse effects such as a drop in blood pressure (Llewellyn 2007; De Barbieri et al. 2009), therefore it is vital that start-up time is as short as possible (Neff et al. 2007). Mechanical slack is avoided by purging the infusion in the pump prior to connecting the line to the patient (Morrice et al. 2004). This allows the mechanical slack to be taken up by the pump and avoids delay in the administration of the drug, hence maintaining haemodynamic stability and patient safety as much as possible (Trim and Roe 2004).

Titration of inotropic drugs to meet patient requirements

Selection and titration of inotropes and vasopressors should be performed in keeping with set targets (Ellender and Skinner 2008), and the dose of inotropes and vasopressors should be increased or decreased until the target is achieved or until the maximum dose is reached (Sheppard 2001 cited in Trim and Roe 2004). The aim of inotropic and vasopressor therapy is to maintain an adequate blood pressure and ensure organ perfusion, with the general aim of a mean arterial blood pressure of 65–70 mmHg (Rossinen et al. 2007) (see Table 7.1). However, it is vital to understand that a normal blood pressure in one patient may signify inadequate perfusion in another, therefore aims should be individualized (Hollenberg 2007). Juarez (2005) highlights the importance of knowing:

- how each drug affects the body
- the correct starting and maximum dose
- appropriate intervals for titration
- appropriate methods for reduction and withdrawing of the medication.

Knowledge of the acceptable patient parameters in terms of blood pressure, cardiac output, etc., allows practitioners to determine starting doses (Juarez 2005) and titrate medications safely and appropriately (Miller 2007). Titration should occur in accordance with patient response and within the prescribed range; however, where assessment of the patient indicates the therapy is no longer achieving the desired response the prescriber should be informed and they should consider further treatment options (GMC 2013; NMC 2007). For ease and accuracy, and to ensure haemodynamic stability, titration of inotropes and vasopressors should occur in 0.5–1 mL volumes, and syringe changes should be infrequent, therefore concentrations of these drugs may need to be changed to facilitate this. That is, concentrations may need to be increased if a patient is receiving high volumes of medication and requiring frequent syringe changes, or they may need to be decreased if a patient is receiving very small volumes of medication, difficult to titrate in 0.5–1 mL increments.

Dosages

Inotropes and vasopressors are mainly prescribed as micrograms per kilogram per minute and this should be documented on patients' charts, alongside the rate of infusion. Exceptions to this are vasopressin, which is calculated in pressor units per minute, and glyceryltrinitrate (GTN), which is calculated in micrograms per minute. Maximum dosages are also usually specified for both inotropes and vasopressors, allowing practitioners to titrate medications within the prescribed range and introduce additional drugs when one does not attain its goal (Juarez 2005). Documenting dosages requires the ability to perform accurate calculations. Examples of how to do this are given below (see Tables 7.4 and 7.5), further calculations can be found in the guidelines section. It is important to refer to local policy, however, as different organizations may have different approaches to dosages.

Side effects

The effect of inotropes and vasopressors varies depending on the dose administered, producing a dose-response curve. Resulting side effects can be counteractive to the desired response, therefore titration and combination of these drugs can be problematic (Ellender and Skinner 2008). However, most inotropes and vasopressors have a very short half-life of approximately 2–3 minutes (Arino et al. 2004), enabling them to be titrated quickly to achieve the desired response while avoiding side effects (Cooper 2008). The minimum dose possible to achieve target blood pressure and perfusion should be used. High dosages of vasopressors can lead to peripheral ischaemia as a result of decreased blood flow to the peripheral circulation (Cooper 2008). Afterload is also increased, which can lead to an unsustainable increase in left ventricular effort, ultimately worsening cardiac output and hence organ perfusion (Beale et al. 2004). Excessive vasoconstriction leads to decreased blood flow to the kidneys and gastrointestinal tract, resulting in decreased urine

253

Table 7.4 Converting the infusion of inotropes and vasopressors from millilitres per hour (mL/h) to micrograms per kilogram per minute (micrograms/kg/min)

Procedure	Example Noradrenaline 4 mg in 50 mL administered at 10 mL/h; patient weight = 70 kg
1. Convert the dose of the inotrope or vasopressor in the infusion to micrograms	4 mg × 1000 = 4000 μg
2. Divide the dose of the drug in micrograms by total volume of diluted drug to calculate micrograms/mL	4000 μg/50 mL = 80 μg/mL
3. Multiply micrograms/mL by current infusion rate to calculate micrograms/h	(80 μg/mL) × (10 mL/h) = 800 μg/h
4. Divide micrograms/h by 60 to calculate micrograms/min	(800 μg/h)/60 = 13.33 μg/min
5. Divide micrograms/min by patient's weight in kilograms to calculate micrograms/kg/min	13.33/70 kg = 0.19047619047 (0.19 μg/kg/min)

Table 7.5 Converting the infusion of inotropes and vasopressors from micrograms per kilogram per minute (micrograms/kg/min) to millilitres per hour (mL/h)

Procedure	Example Noradrenaline 4 mg in 50 mL to be infused at 0.1 micrograms/kg/min; patient weight = 70 kg
1. Convert the dose of the inotrope or vasopressor in the infusion to micrograms	4 mg × 1000 = 4000 μg
2. Divide the dose of the drug in micrograms by total volume of diluted drug to calculate micrograms/mL	4000 μg/50 mL = 80 μg/mL
3. Multiply required micrograms/kg/min by 60 to calculate micrograms/kg/h	0.1 μg/kg/min × 60 = 6 μg/kg/h
4. Multiply micrograms/kg/h by patient's weight in kilograms to calculate micrograms/h	6 μg/kg/h × 70 kg = 420 μg/h
5. Divide required micrograms/h by calculated micrograms/mL to calculate required rate in mL/h	(420 μg/h) / (80 μg/mL) = 5.25 mL/h

output, lactic acidosis and translocation of bacteria from the gastrointestinal tract to the bloodstream (Cooper 2008). Inotropes can lead to thrombocytopenia, dyspnoea and arrhythmias (BNF 2012), and increased oxygen consumption (Rossinen 2007). Despite the risks involved with inotrope and vasopressor use, it is recognized that the benefits outweigh the risks when they are used temporarily until underlying causes of hypotension are treated (Overgaard and Dzavik 2008).

Monitoring

Patients' response to any medical intervention should be monitored throughout its duration (GMC 2013; NMC 2007). Arterial blood pressure should be continuously monitored via an arterial cannula, as this is more reliable than using a sphygmomanometer (Beale et al. 2004) (*see* Chapters 6). This also enables practitioners to see the immediate effects of therapy, which is especially important given the potential for life-threatening hypotension or hypertension (Overgaard and Dzavik 2008). Cardiac output monitoring is also advised to help guide appropriate therapy (Dellinger et al. 2008) (*see* Chapter 6).

Withdrawing

When weaning (withdrawing drugs in a manner that allows the patient's physiology to compensate for the reduction) a patient off a combination of inotropes and vasopressors a specific decision should be made regarding which drug to reduce first. The desired effects of each individual inotrope or vasopressor should be considered separately and each infusion titrated to separate goals. That is, vasopressors should be titrated to a specific and agreed mean arterial blood pressure (MAP) while inotropes should be titrated to achieve the desired cardiac output (Cooper 2008). Additionally, documenting dosages (micrograms/kg/min, units/min and micrograms/min) rather than rates (mL/h) gives a clearer indication of patient requirements and allows more accurate titration of medications in individual patients (Juarez 2005) (*see also* Table 7.4 and 7.5).

Changeover of inotrope and vasopressor infusions

Inotropes and vasopressors are seen as high-risk drugs due to their rapid effect on the cardiovascular system and their short duration of action (Crisp 2002), both of which could have serious consequences if the drugs are administered incorrectly. Continuous infusions of these drugs are necessary to ensure a constant plasma drug concentration. However, this can be problematic if infusions need to be changed regularly (Arino et al. 2004), resulting in interrupted drug flow and potential haemodynamic instability (Argaud et al. 2007). Safe inotrope and vasopressor administration will reduce the number of adverse effects associated with the changeover procedure, hence improving patient care (Morrice et al. 2004). This is a major responsibility of practitioners (Crisp 2002); however, many staff are relatively new to critical care and lack some specialist skills. In order to deliver continuous inotropic and vasopressor therapy, practitioners require additional and specialist training to develop necessary competencies. This should be completed under supervision in their probationary period (Crisp 2002). It is essential that practitioners are competent to change inotropic and vasopressor medications in order to minimize the number of adverse events associated with each stage of changeover and respond appropriately to those that occur (Trim and Roe 2004). The patient should be observed and monitored during the changeover of inotropes and vasopressors to ascertain any adverse effects and ensure appropriate treatment and care is given (Crisp 2002; NMC 2008). It is essential that practitioners are updated regularly to maintain their knowledge and skills, not only in their use of medical devices but also on the use of medications, side effects and correct dosages (GMC 2013; NMC 2008).

Changeover method

A review of the literature reveals no definitive evidence as to how infusion changeovers should be carried out, but shows many different techniques used among critical care practitioners (Llewellyn 2007). A lack of guidance or protocol for changeover of inotropes and vasopressors reflects the lack of evidence available. It is reported that only 21% of critical care units have specific guidance (Crisp 2002), with most nurses adopting methods based on how they were taught and their previous experience (Llewellyn 2007). One study compared the volume of drug infused while changing just the syringe and using the same syringe pump, with changing both the syringe and syringe pump. Results indicated that using two pumps provide better consistency. It should be noted, however, that haemodynamic stability was not assessed (Powell and Carnevale 2004). Morrice et al. (2004) also suggest that two syringe pumps are necessary when changing inotrope and vasopressor drug syringes. These should be located next to each other to prevent complications.

Crisp (2002) acknowledges that two infusions running concurrently are necessary during changeover, and the two main methods of changing inotropes and vasopressors are the 'piggybacking' technique and the 'quick change' technique (Table 7.6) (Llewellyn 2007).

Although both methods allow a continuous delivery of drug to the patient they are not without complications (Arino et al. 2004). Haemodynamic instability is the major complication during syringe changeover, and the administration of a bolus in times of severe blood pressure loss is debated in the literature. It has been suggested that administering a bolus may lead to further haemodynamic instability, therefore instead, infusion rates should be increased until blood pressure stabilizes (Morrice et al. 2004) However, it has also been acknowledged that on rare occasions it is necessary to give the patient a rescue bolus of inotrope if there is a greater than 20% drop in MAP during changeover of infusion (Arino et al. 2004).

A direct comparison between the two methods has indicated no statistical difference in haemodyamic stability (Arino et al. 2004; De Barbieri et al. 2009). The most frequently utilized technique is piggybacking; however, the techniques used for this are inconsistent (Crisp 2002). There is no evidence to support either method, but it has been concluded that the quick change method should be utilized as it is the quickest, easiest and most cost-effective (De Barbieri et al. 2009) while also maintaining haemodynamic stability. In addition, the quick change method does not risk tolerance to higher levels of inotropes (Arino et al. 2004).

However, where a change of concentration of medication is required the situation is different, as there will still be some of the original drug concentration in the CVC. To avoid an abrupt change of concentration or medication, and the possibility of haemodynamic instability, the piggybacking method should be used in this instance, although there is currently no research describing how this should be undertaken (Crisp 2002).

Troubleshooting

The practitioner administering and titrating inotropes and vasopressors must be competent and have knowledge of the pharmacology of these drugs, their effects and adverse reactions. They must also be aware of other potential problems that may occur during administration and how to solve them. The problems associated with the administration of inotropic and vasopressor drugs can be split into two categories: those associated with the infusion device and those associated with the medication being delivered.

Table 7.6 'Piggybacking' technique compared with 'quick change' technique when keeping the drug and its concentration constant

Technique name	Technique	Evidence for	Evidence against
Piggybacking	Two infusions are administered together while titrating in opposing rates, i.e. gradually decrease the rate of the original infusion while at the same rate gradually increase the new infusion, until only one infusion is running	Less haemodynamic instability (Morrice et al, 2004) The volume of drug infused increases during the changeover period. This results in less potential for hypotensive episodes (Powell and Carnevale 2004)	Infusing higher volumes of drugs during switchover results in patients becoming tolerant to a higher level of inotrope. This is particularly so if the switchover lasts longer than 10 minutes (Karch 2003) Greater practitioner workload due to the length of time required for monitoring and titration of the medications (Powell and Carnevale 2004) The greatest rises in blood pressure are seen in the piggybacking method (Llewellyn 2007) as a result of syringe pump mechanics and practitioner inexperience and technique, i.e. practitioners fail to effectively adjust the rates according to patient response (Crisp 2002)
Quick change	A new infusion is started at the same rate as the original infusion. The new infusion is then connected to the patient's CVC and commenced as the original infusion is turned off (Arino et al. 2004; Argaud et al. 2007; Llewellyn 2007)	Maintains haemodynamic stability and does not risk patient becoming tolerant to higher levels of inotropes (Arino et al. 2004) Less frequent rises in blood pressure occur (Llewellyn 2007) Quicker, easier and more cost-effective (De Barbieri et al. 2009) Following training and guidance the occurrence of haemodynamic instability can be reduced by approximately 67% (Argaud et al. 2007)	Hypotension and hypertension can occur (Llewellyn 2007)

Problem-solving table 7.1: Syringe pumps

Problem	Possible causes	Preventative measures	Suggested action
Drive disengaged	Incorrect fitting of syringe	Ensure syringe is correctly fitted in the syringe pump	Reposition the syringe
Low battery	Pump not plugged into mains and losing battery charge	Ensure pumps are plugged in whenever possible	If possible plug the syringe driver into mains to enable battery to charge
		Ensure power lead is securely inserted in the pump	If no mains electricity available change pump
Occlusion alarm	Kinked syringe infusion administration set	Ensure the syringe infusion administration set is positioned in a way that will prevent kinking. Ensure tubing is kept free from moving bed parts	Reposition syringe infusion administration set
	Kinked central venous catheter	Ensure central venous catheter dressing is secure and maintains the position of the catheter	Redress central venous catheter if necessary
		Try to maintain the patient's position so it does not affect the central venous catheter position	Reposition the patient while ensuring the central venous catheter is not kinked
	Three-way tap off to infusion	Ensure three-way tap is open to current infusion	Open three-way tap to infusion
	High pressure detected by syringe pump	Ensure pressure alarms in the syringe pump are appropriate, particularly if infusing two drugs on the same port	Check for all other potential occlusions and eliminate these. If the syringe pump continues detecting high pressure and all other potential factors for occlusion are eliminated consider increasing pressure alarm limit
Other error messages	Technical fault with pump	Ensure pumps are maintained and serviced regularly	Change syringe pumps, label faulty pump and send to be serviced. Complete incident form
Under-/ over-infusion	Technical fault	Ensure pumps are serviced regularly	Change syringe pumps and immediately remove faulty pump from use, label and send to be serviced and repaired. Complete incident form
	Incorrect rate setting	Ensure the correct rate is calculated and programmed accurately. Check rate at least hourly and at change over of the practitioner looking after patient	Correct infusion rate. Check patient's condition. Inform prescriber and practitioner managing the unit at that time. Complete incident form

257

Problem-solving table 7.2: **Medication**

Problem	Possible causes	Preventative measures	Suggested action
Heart rate, blood pressure, or urine output outside required parameters	Under-/over-infusion of drugs	Constantly monitor patient response to therapy and titrate medications as required	Titrate medications to achieve desired effect
Maximum prescribed drug dose almost reached without heart rate, blood pressure, or urine output being within required parameters	Patient not responding to treatment	Monitor infusion dose at least hourly, and on titration, and discuss with prescriber regarding the need for additional fluid and or medications	Discuss the next necessary intervention with senior practitioners
No response to newly connected infusion	Syringe infusion administration set not correctly connected	Ensure infusion administration set is connected correctly at changeover	Connect infusion administration set
	Three-way tap between infusion and patient turned off	Ensure three-way tap is open to new infusion and closed to original infusion at changeover	Open three-way tap to new infusion
	Syringe pump on hold or not turned on	Ensure syringe pump is turned on and start button is pressed prior to attaching new infusion to three-way tap	Switch on syringe pump, disconnect infusion administration set from the three-way tap, press purge to take up mechanical slack, start infusion, and reconnect to three-way tap
	Unknown cause		In all cases where problems occur at changeover of syringes consider switching off the new infusion and restarting the original infusion until problems are solved. It may be necessary to increase the rate of the infusion if the patient's blood pressure/heart rate have decreased
Dose requirement and infusion rate high, requiring numerous syringe changes	Lower-concentration solutions can result in high volumes to achieve the required dose	Change concentrations of drug when possible and appropriate	Increase drug concentrations, limiting the volume of drug infused and frequency of syringe change
Dose requirement and infusion rate reducing, making titration difficult	Higher-concentration solutions need lower volumes to achieve the required dose, and titration can be difficult as well as less accurate	Change concentrations of drug when possible and appropriate	Reduce drug concentrations, increasing the volume of drug infused, making dosage more accurate and titration easier

Procedure guideline 7.1: **Preparation of inotropes and vasopressors for administration via a syringe pump**

Equipment

- Patient's drug chart
- Ampoules of drug to be administered
- Container of prescribed dilutent
- Drug additive label
- Protective clothing as per hospital policy
- Swab saturated with 2% chlorhexidine in 70% alcohol
- 50 mL syringe in which to draw up dilutent
- 25 G needle for drawing up dilutent
- Sterile bung
- Sterile topical swab
- Needle for drawing up the drug, 21 G or smaller
- Syringe of appropriate size in which to draw up the amount of drug to be administered
- Syringe infusion administration set
- Clinically clean receiver or tray in which to place the prepared syringe of drug

Procedure

Action	Rationale
1. Where possible, explain and discuss the procedure with the patient. If the patient lacks the capacity to make decisions the practitioner must act in the patient's best interests.	To ensure that the patient understands the procedure and gives their valid consent. To ensure the patient's best interests are maintained (Mental Capacity Act 2005).
2. Collect and check all equipment.	To prevent delays and enable full concentration on the procedure.
3. If continuing an infusion of the same medication, dilutent, concentration and volume, inspect the infusion in progress and compare with the new infusion to be commenced.	To ensure the infusion being delivered is replaced with an infusion of the same medication, dilutent, concentration and volume.
4. If changing an infusion concentration or starting an infusion of a new medication, check the current infusion rate and concentration.	To ensure the dose is correctly calculated and administered at an appropriate rate and concentration to maintain required parameters.
5. Check that the packaging of all equipment is sealed, complete and dry.	To ensure sterility. Discard if seals are broken or packaging damaged.
6. Select the appropriate volume or dosage of drug and dilutent and, with a second qualified practitioner, consult the patient's drug chart and check the following: ■ drug ■ dose ■ dilutent and compatibility with drug ■ date and time of administration ■ route and method of administration ■ validity and legibility of prescription ■ prescriber's signature ■ expiry dates of drug and dilutent.	Two practitioners reduces the risk of error. For nurses to comply with NMC (2007) guidelines for the administration of medicines. To ensure the patient is given the correct drug at the correct dosage in the correct dilutent via the correct route. To reduce wastage by using the appropriate volume. Expiry dates indicate when the drug is no longer pharmacologically efficacious. To use beyond this date is dangerous. To ensure safe and effective administration of the drug.
7. Both practitioners sign the drug additive label.	Two practitioners reduces the risk of error. For nurses to comply with NMC (2007) guidelines for the administration of medicines. To comply with local intravenous drug administration policy.
8. Wash hands with bactericidal soap and water or bactericidal hand rub.	To reduce risk of contamination of medication or equipment.

259

(Continued)

Procedure guideline 7.1: (Continued)

9. Apply protective clothing, gloves and apron.	To reduce risk of contamination of medication or equipment.
10. Inspect the drug and dilutent for discolouration, particles or cloudiness.	To prevent foreign objects or degraded drug being delivered to the patient.
11. Place the bag containing the dilutent on a flat surface.	To make the injection site more easily accessible, and leave two hands free to undertake the process, thus minimizing the risk of puncturing the bag.
12. Remove the seal and swab the injection site of the bag containing the dilutent with the swab saturated with 2% chlorhexidol in 70% alcohol. Allow to dry.	To remove any bacteria present on the injection site and, therefore, to minimize the risk of contamination.
13. Using a 50 mL syringe and 25 G needle draw up the volume of dilutent required.	Drugs are usually prescribed in 50 mL of fluid, and a syringe pump is used to administer inotropes and vasopressors, therefore 50 mL syringes should be used. 25 G needles have a large enough bore to allow easy withdrawal of fluids.
14. Tap the syringe to dislodge any air bubbles. Discard the needle, expel any air and place a bung on the syringe.	To ensure correct volume in the syringe. To avoid needlestick injury. To reduce the risk of contact of the dilutent with equipment and maintain sterility of the dilutent.
15. Cover the neck of the ampoule with sterile topical swab and snap open.	To minimize the risk of contamination of the drug with foreign particles. To minimize the risk of injury to the practitioner.
16. Inspect the ampoule for glass particles and discard if present.	To ensure glass particles are not infused into the patient.
17. Draw up the required volume of drug to be infused using a 21 G or smaller needle and appropriate-sized syringe.	Using a 21 G or smaller needle reduces the risk of drawing up large shards of glass (Shaw and Lyall 1985).
18. Tap the syringe to dislodge air bubbles and expel air.	To ensure the correct volume of drug in the syringe.
19. Remove the bung from the syringe of dilutent and pull back plunger to at least double the volume of the drug to be added.	To make enough space for the drug and prevent overflow of the drug out of the syringe.
20. Inject the drug into the 50 mL syringe of dilutent, place a bung on the syringe and agitate gently.	To instil the medication into the dilutent. To maintain sterility of the infusion. To ensure adequate mixing of the drug.
21. Tap the syringe to dislodge air bubbles, expel any air.	To prevent infusion of air.
22. Attach syringe infusion administration set and prime the infusion administration set by applying gentle pressure to the plunger until fluid is noted at the end of the set.	To ensure all air is expelled from the administration set and prevent infusion of air.
23. Apply the completed additive label to the syringe and place in a clean receiver ready to be administered.	All syringes containing injectable medicines should be labelled (NPSA, 2007). To ensure the correct drug is administered to the patient. To ensure safe storage of the prepared drug prior to administration.

24. Document care provided.	To: ■ provide an accurate record ■ monitor effectiveness of procedure ■ reduce the risk of duplication of treatment ■ provide a point of reference or comparison in the event of later questions ■ acknowledge accountability for actions ■ facilitate communication and continuity of care. (NMC 2008; GMC 2013; HCPC 2012)
25. Dispose of all waste as per hospital policy.	To ensure the safe disposal of domestic waste, clinical waste and sharps. To prevent harm to all users of healthcare premises (NPSA 2009).

Procedure guideline 7.2: Calculating dosages for the administration of inotropes and vasopressors

Equipment
■ Patient's drug chart
■ Calculator

■ Knowledge of the patient's weight in kilograms (*see also* Table 7.4 and Table 7.5)

Converting the infusion of inotropes and vasopressors from millilitres per hour (mL/h) to units per minute (units/min)

Procedure	Example: Vasopressin 20 units in 50 mL infused at 6 mL/h
1. Divide the total units in the syringe by the total volume to calculate units/mL	20 units/50 mL = 0.4 units/mL
2. Multiply units/mL by current rate to calculate units/h	(0.4 units/mL) × (6 mL/h) = 2.4 units/h
3. Divide units per hour by 60 to calculate units/min	(2.4 units/h)/60 = 0.04 units/min

Converting the infusion of inotropes and vasopressors from units per minute (units/min) to millilitres per hour (mL/h)

Procedure	Example: Vasopressin 20 units in 50 mL infused at 0.02 units/min
1. Divide the total units in the syringe by the total volume to calculate units/mL	20 units/50mL = 0.4 units/mL
2. Multiply the required units/min by 60 to calculate the required units/h	(0.02 units/min) × 60 = 1.2 units/h
3. Divide required units/h by the number of units/mL to calculate required mL/h	(1.2 units/h)/(0.4 units/mL) = 3 mL/h

(Continued)

Procedure guideline 7.2: (Continued)

Converting the infusion of inotropes and vasopressors from millilitres per hour (mL/h) to micrograms per minute (μg/min)

Procedure	Example: GTN 50 mg in 50 mL infused at 5 mL/h
1. Convert the dose of the inotrope or vasopressor in the infusion to micrograms	50 mg × 1000 = 50 000 μg
2. Divide the dose of the drug in micrograms by total volume of diluted drug to calculate micrograms/mL	50 000 μg/50 mL = 1000 μg/mL
3. Multiply micrograms/mL by current infusion rate to calculate micrograms/h	(1000 μg/mL) × (5 mL/h) = 5000 μg/h
4. Divide micrograms/h by 60 to calculate micrograms/min	5000/60 = 83.33 μg/min

Converting the infusion of inotropes and vasopressors from micrograms per minute (μg/min) to millilitres per hour (mL/h)

Procedure	Example: GTN 50 mg in 50 mL infused at 100 μg/min
1. Convert the dose of the inotrope or vasopressor in the infusion to micrograms	50 mg × 1000 = 50 000 μg
2. Divide the dose of the drug in micrograms by total volume of diluted drug to calculate micrograms/mL	50 000 μg/50 mL = 1000 μg/mL
3. Multiply the required micrograms/min by 60 to calculate the required micrograms/h	(100 μg/min) × 60 = 6000 μg/h
4. Divide required micrograms/h by calculated micrograms/mL to calculate required rate in mL/h	(6000 μg/h)/(1000 μg/mL) = 6 mL/h

Procedure guideline 7.3: Administration of inotropic and vasopressor drugs via a syringe pump (commencing a new infusion)

Equipment

- Protective clothing as per hospital policy
- Clean dressing trolley
- 10 mL syringe
- 5 mL syringe
- 10 mL 0.9% sodium chloride
- Swab saturated with 2% chlorhexidine in 70% alcohol
- Sterile dressing pack
- Prepared inotrope or vasopressor syringe and syringe infusion administration set
- Patient's drug chart
- Syringe pump

Procedure

Action	Rationale
1. Follow steps 1–23 in Procedure guideline 7.1.	
2. Wash hands with bactericidal soap and water or bactericidal hand rub.	To reduce the risk of contamination of medication or equipment.
3. Where possible, explain and discuss the procedure with the patient. If the patient lacks the capacity to make decisions the practitioner must act in the patient's best interests.	To ensure that the patient understands the procedure and gives their valid consent. To ensure the patient's best interests are maintained (Mental Capacity Act 2005).

4. On the bottom of the dressing trolley place 10 mL syringe, 5 mL syringe, 10 mL 0.9% sodium chloride; swab saturated with 2% chlorhexidine in 70% alcohol and sterile dressing pack.	To ensure all required equipment is together, to prevent delays and enable full concentration on the procedure.
5. With a second qualified practitioner take the syringe and connected syringe infusion administration set containing the prepared inotrope or vasopressor and the drug chart to the patient. Check the patient's identity against that on the drug chart and drug additive label. Ask the patient to confirm details if possible or use the patient's identification band.	To ensure the correct drug is given to the correct patient.
6. With the other qualified practitioner use the starting dosage on the prescription to calculate the starting rate of the infusion (*see* section on Dosages and Procedure guideline 7.2).	To minimize error and ensure drugs are given at the prescribed dose.
7. Load the syringe into a syringe pump designed for the delivery of high-risk drugs, ensuring correct fitting of the syringe.	To prevent any delivery problems and/or delays. Syringe pumps designed for high-risk medications deliver the most accurate and constant flow pressures, have the shortest time delay at start-up, and have the most accurate occlusion alarms (MDA 1998; Trim and Roe 2004).
8. Wash hands with bactericidal soap and water or bactericidal hand rub.	To reduce the risk of contamination of medication or equipment with any bacteria that may be present on the hands.
9. Open the sterile dressing pack on to the top of the dressing trolley.	To create a sterile field on which to open the sterile equipment.
10. Wash hands with bactericidal soap and water or bactericidal hand rub.	To reduce the risk of contamination of medication or equipment.
11. On to sterile field open 5 mL syringe, 10 mL syringe and swab saturated with 2% chlorhexidine in 70% alcohol.	To maintain sterility of the equipment needed for the procedure.
12. Wash hands with bactericidal soap and water or bactericidal hand rub.	To reduce the risk of infection and prevent contamination.
13. Apply sterile gloves and apron and any other protective clothing as appropriate, e.g. visor if the patient has any blood-borne viruses.	To reduce the risk of contamination of practitioner, medication or equipment.
14. Draw up a 10 mL flush of 0.9% sodium chloride.	To ensure the flush is ready for when it is needed.
15. Identify a lumen on the patient's central venous catheter which has no other medications infusing through it and which has a three-way tap.*	To ensure that inotropes and vasopressors are not administered on the same port as other drugs. This is to avoid giving boluses when administering other drugs, and to enable titration. To allow uninterrupted infusion of medication when the syringe needs to be changed.
16. Place a sterile towel under the lumen to be used for inotropes and vasopressors.	To create a sterile field on which to work, in order to minimize the risk of contamination.
17. Remove one bung from the three-way tap, clean the port with the swab saturated with 2% chlorhexidine in 70% alcohol and allow to air dry.	To minimize the risk of contamination and infection.
18. Aspirate 5 mL from the designated lumen into the 5 mL syringe and discard.	To assess patency and clear the line of any previously administered medications.
19. Flush the lumen with the 10 mL of 0.9% sodium chloride.	To ensure patency, thus enabling the drug to be delivered to the patient.

(*Continued*)

20. Switch on the syringe pump containing the previously loaded syringe and press the button for purging or priming the infusion until the fluid is at the end of the infusion administration set (this can be seen when two or three drops of fluid exit the infusion administration set).	To take up mechanical slack and ensure prompt delivery of the drug (Morrice et al. 2004).
21. Set the calculated infusion rate and press start.	To commence the infusion at the correct rate and allow any remaining mechanical slack to be taken up, ensuring prompt delivery of the drug to the patient.
22. Attach the infusion administration set to the exposed port on the three-way tap and turn the three-way tap to 'on' for the infusion.	To commence the infusion of the drug to the patient.
23. Continuously monitor the patient's blood pressure and heart rate and cardiac output if available, in response to the infusion.	To determine any change and the effects of the infusion and to enable prompt adjustment of the infusion as necessary.
24. Dispose of all waste as per hospital/national policy.	To ensure the safe disposal of domestic waste, clinical waste and sharps. To prevent harm to all users of healthcare premises (NPSA 2009).
25. Document care provided including documenting on patient's chart when the infusion commenced.	To: ■ provide an accurate record ■ monitor effectiveness of procedure ■ reduce the risk of duplication of treatment ■ provide a point of reference or comparison in the event of later questions ■ acknowledge accountability for actions ■ facilitate communication and continuity of care. (NMC 2008; GMC 2013; HCPC 2012)

*For the purposes of this guideline, it is assumed that three-way taps with bungs are used; however, bionectors and octopus devices may be used – refer to local hospital policy.

Procedure guideline 7.4: Titration of inotropic and vasopressor drugs up and down to meet patient requirements

In order to titrate any medication it is necessary to know the intended outcome of the use of the medication, i.e. the intended blood pressure, cardiac output and heart rate. Different medications act differently and have differing duration of action and time of onset of action, therefore the practitioner titrating the drugs must have a full understanding of these actions in order to titrate safely and effectively. Practitioners must also be aware of the side effects of infusion that may counteract the desired response.

Equipment

■ Patient's drug chart
■ Calculator

■ Parameters for heart rate/blood pressure/urine output

Action	Rationale
1. Calculate the maximum and minimum rate for current inotrope or vasopressor infusion from prescribed dose on patient's drug chart.	To ensure drugs are given within the prescribed dosages.
2. Monitor the patient's blood pressure and heart rate constantly, ensuring these are kept within pre-determined limits.	To ensure therapy is adequate and detect problems early.

3. When the patient's blood pressure/heart rate deviates from the pre-determined value, decide which drug will have the desired response and titrate an increased or decreased amount in 0.5–1 mL increments.	To ascertain which inotrope or vasopressor has the desired effect. Inotropes and vasopressors have varying effects so it is important to know which one needs to be altered to maintain parameters and by how much they should be titrated. The volume is titrated at a known concentration of the drug. The concentration of the drug has been calculated to be suitable for titration in 0.5–1.0 mL volumes for ease and accuracy. The increment will depend on the drug concentration, how sensitive the patient is to rate change and the level of deviation from the desired outcomes.
4. Constantly monitor the patient's blood pressure/heart rate, continuing to titrate the infusion up or down every 2–3 minutes as required until blood pressure/cardiac output/heart rate returns to within the pre-determined limits.	To determine the effects of titration and ensure adequate amounts of inotrope and/or vasopressor are being infused.
5. If the maximum prescribed dose is nearly reached without therapeutic parameters being attained or maintained, discuss with clinical prescriber as additional inotropes or an increase in dose may be required.	Adding further inotropes and vasopressors may enable a reduction of the current inotrope or vasopressor infusion or return to specified clinical parameters (such as the predetermined limits of blood pressure and or heart rate).
6. If the medication is titrated down to a rate where it is safe to be switched off, turn the infusion off at the pump, turn the three-way tap* of the CVC off to the infusion, but leave the infusion connected.	Turning the three-way tap off at the CVC prevents inadvertent bolus delivery of the drug when disconnecting later. Leaving the infusion connected, rather than disconnecting and disposing of it ensures it is available if the patient's condition deteriorates to the point where the medication is required again.
7. Document care and rate/dose change, and care on patient's charts.	To: ■ provide an accurate record ■ monitor effectiveness of procedure ■ reduce the risk of duplication of treatment ■ provide a point of reference or comparison in the event of later questions ■ acknowledge accountability for actions ■ facilitate communication and continuity of care. (NMC 2008; GMC 2013; HCPC 2012)

*For the purposes of this guideline, it is assumed that three-way taps with bungs are used; however, bionectors and octopus devices may be used – refer to local hospital policy.

Procedure guideline 7.5: Changeover of inotrope and vasopressor infusions

There is no definitive evidence as to how infusion changeovers should be carried out. The most popular choice seems to be the 'quick change' method when changing infusions of the same drug and concentration (Arino et al. 2004; Argaud et al. 2007; Llewellyn 2007; De Barbieri et al. 2009). However, 'piggybacking' is necessary when changing concentrations. There is no evidence to describe piggybacking for changing concentrations, so the guideline included here is simply the best technique from personal experience; however, local guidelines and policies should be referred to wherever possible.

(a) Quick change for the same concentration of drugs via a syringe pump

Equipment

- Protective clothing as per hospital policy
- Clean dressing trolley
- Swab saturated with 2% chlorhexidine in 70% alcohol
- Sterile dressing pack
- Prepared inotrope or vasopressor syringe and syringe infusion administration set
- Patient's drug chart
- Syringe pump designed for delivering high-risk infusions

Procedure

Action	Rationale
1. Wash hands with bactericidal soap and water or bactericidal hand rub.	To reduce the risk of contamination of medication or equipment.

(Continued)

Procedure guideline 7.5: *(Continued)*

2. Where possible, explain and discuss the procedure with the patient. If the patient lacks the capacity to make decisions the practitioner must act in the patient's best interests.	To ensure that the patient understands the procedure and gives their valid consent. To ensure the patient's best interests are maintained (Mental Capacity Act 2005).
3. Place on the bottom of the dressing trolley swab saturated with 2% chlorhexidine in 70% alcohol and sterile dressing pack.	To ensure all required equipment is together, to prevent delays and enable full concentration on the procedure.
4. With a second qualified practitioner take the syringe and connected syringe infusion administration set containing the prepared inotrope or vasopressor and the drug chart to the patient. Check the patient's identity against that on the drug chart and drug additive label. Ask the patient to confirm details if possible or use the patient's identification band.	To ensure the correct drug is given to the correct patient.
5. Load the syringe into a syringe pump designed for the delivery of high-risk drugs, ensuring correct fitting of the syringe.	To prevent any delivery problems and/or delays. Syringe pumps designed for high-risk medications deliver the most accurate and constant flow pressures, have the shortest time delay at start-up and have the most accurate occlusion alarms.
6. Wash hands with bactericidal soap and water or bactericidal hand rub.	To reduce the risk of contamination of medication or equipment with any bacteria that may be present on the hands.
7. Open the sterile dressing pack on to the top of the dressing trolley.	To create a sterile field on which to open the sterile equipment.
8. Wash hands with bactericidal soap and water or bactericidal hand rub.	To reduce the risk of contamination of medication or equipment.
9. On to sterile field open swab saturated with 2% chlorhexidine in 70% alcohol.	To maintain sterility of the equipment needed for the procedure.
10. Wash hands with bactericidal soap and water or bactericidal hand rub.	To reduce the risk of infection and prevent contamination.
11. Apply sterile gloves and apron and any other protective clothing as appropriate, e.g. visor if the patient has any blood-borne viruses.	To reduce the risk of contamination of practitioner, medication or equipment.
12. Identify the designated inotrope lumen on the patient's central venous catheter.	To ensure that inotropes and vasopressors are not administered on the same port as other drugs. This is to avoid giving boluses when administering other drugs, and to enable titration. To allow uninterrupted infusion of medication when the syringe needs to be changed.
13. Place a sterile towel under the lumen to be used for inotropes and vasopressors.	To create a sterile field on which to work, in order to minimize the risk of contamination.
14. Remove the bung from the spare port of the three-way tap*, clean the port with the swab saturated with 2% chlorhexidine in 70% alcohol and allow to dry.	To minimize the risk of contamination and infection.
15. Switch on the syringe pump containing the previously loaded new syringe and press the button for purging or priming the infusion until the fluid is at the end of the infusion administration set.	To take up mechanical slack and ensure prompt delivery of the drug.

16. With the original infusion still running set the new infusion rate the same as that of the current infusion and press start.	To commence the infusion at the correct rate, and allow any remaining mechanical slack to be taken up, ensuring prompt delivery of the drug to the patient.
17. Attach the syringe infusion administration set to the exposed port on the three-way tap and turn the three-way tap to 'on' for the new infusion and to 'off' for the old infusion.	To prevent the infusion of double the amount of drug.
18. Continuously monitor the patient's blood pressure and heart rate and cardiac output if available, in response to the infusion.	To determine any change and the effects of the infusion and to enable prompt adjustment of the infusion as necessary.
19. If no signs of problems, switch off the old infusion.	Keeping the current infusion connected and running enables prompt conversion back to the original infusion should any problems occur with the new infusion.
20. Dispose of all waste as per hospital/national policy.	To ensure the safe disposal of domestic waste, clinical waste and sharps. To prevent harm to all users of healthcare premises (NPSA 2009).
21. Document care, and when infusion is changed on patient's charts.	To: ■ provide an accurate record ■ monitor effectiveness of procedure ■ reduce the risk of duplication of treatment ■ provide a point of reference or comparison in the event of later questions ■ acknowledge accountability for actions ■ facilitate communication and continuity of care. (NMC 2008; GMC 2013; HCPC 2012)

*For the purposes of this guideline it is assumed that three-way taps with bungs are used; however, bionectors and octopus devices may be used – refer to local hospital policy.

(b) Piggybacking for changing the concentration of infusions via a syringe pump

(e.g. from 6 mL/h single concentration to 3 mL/h double concentration or vice versa)

Equipment

- Protective clothing as per hospital policy
- Clean dressing trolley
- Swab saturated with 2% chlorhexidine in 70% alcohol
- Sterile dressing pack
- Prepared inotrope or vasopressor syringe containing double or half the concentration of drug of the current infusion and syringe infusion administration set
- Patient's drug chart
- Syringe pump designed for delivering high-risk infusions

Procedure

Action	Rationale
1. Wash hands with bactericidal soap and water or bactericidal hand rub.	To reduce the risk of contamination of medication or equipment.

(*Continued*)

267

Procedure guideline 7.5: (*Continued*)

2. Where possible, explain and discuss the procedure with the patient. If the patient lacks the capacity to make decisions the practitioner must act in the patient's best interests.	To ensure that the patient understands the procedure and gives their valid consent. To ensure the patient's best interests are maintained (Mental Capacity Act 2005).
3. On the bottom of the dressing trolley place swab saturated with 2% chlorhexidine in 70% alcohol and sterile dressing pack.	To ensure all required equipment is together, to prevent delays and enable full concentration on the procedure.
4. With a second qualified practitioner take the syringe and connected syringe infusion administration set containing the prepared inotrope or vasopressor and the drug chart to the patient. Check the patient's identity against that on the drug chart and drug additive label. Ask the patient to confirm details if possible or use the patient's identification band.	To ensure the correct drug is given to the correct patient.
5. Load the syringe into a syringe pump designed for the delivery of high-risk drugs, ensuring correct fitting of the syringe.	To prevent any delivery problems and/or delays. Syringe pumps designed for high-risk medications deliver the most accurate and constant flow pressures, have the shortest time delay at start-up and have the most accurate occlusion alarms.
6. Wash hands with bactericidal soap and water or bactericidal hand rub.	To reduce the risk of contamination of medication or equipment with any bacteria that may be present on the hands.
7. Open the sterile dressing pack on to the top of the dressing trolley.	To create a sterile field on which to open the sterile equipment.
8. Wash hands with bactericidal soap and water or bactericidal hand rub.	To reduce the risk of contamination of medication or equipment.
9. On to sterile field open swab saturated with 2% chlorhexidine in 70% alcohol and three-way tap.	To maintain sterility of the equipment needed for the procedure.
10. Wash hands with bactericidal soap and water or bactericidal hand rub.	To reduce the risk of infection and prevent contamination.
11. Apply sterile gloves and apron and any other protective clothing as appropriate, e.g. visor if the patient has any blood-borne viruses.	To reduce the risk of contamination of practitioner, medication or equipment.
12. Identify the designated inotrope or vassopressor lumen on the patient's central venous catheter.	To ensure that inotropes and vasopressors are not administered on the same port as other drugs. This is to avoid giving boluses when administering other drugs, and to enable titration. To allow uninterrupted infusion of medication when the syringe needs to be changed.
13. Place a sterile towel under the lumen to be used for inotropes and vasopressors.	To create a sterile field on which to work, in order to minimize the risk of contamination.
14. Remove the bung from the spare port of the three-way tap, clean the port with the swab saturated with 2% chlorhexidine in 70% alcohol and allow to dry.	To minimize the risk of contamination and infection.
15. While the original infusion continues to run, switch on the syringe pump containing the previously loaded new syringe and press the button for purging or priming the infusion until the fluid is at the end of the infusion administration set.	To take up mechanical slack and ensure prompt delivery of the drug.

268

If doubling the concentration of the drug follow 15a–19a **15a.** Set the new infusion rate at half the rate of the original infusion and press start.	To allow any remaining mechanical slack to be taken up, ensuring prompt delivery of the drug to the patient. To ensure the same dose of drug is administered to the patient. Half of the rate of the original infusion is still the same dosage of drug, e.g. 6 mL/h single concentration = 3 mL/h double concentration.
16a. With both original and new syringe pumps administering together, attach the infusion administration set to the exposed port on the three-way tap on the central venous catheter and turn the three-way tap to 'on' for both infusions.	To allow the infusion of both drugs.
17a. Halve the rate of the original infusion.	The drug already in the CVC is still the original infusion. This must be delivered at the same rate as before the change, e.g. 6 mL/h original = 3 mL/h original + 3 mL/h new.
18a. Continuously monitor the patient's blood pressure and heart rate and cardiac output if available, in response to the infusion.	To determine any change and the effects of the infusion and to enable prompt adjustment of the infusion as necessary.
19a. When an increase in the patient's blood pressure is seen, gradually reduce the original infusion until only the new infusion is running.	To ensure that the new, correct dose is gradually being delivered to the patient. There will still be a mixture of concentrations of drug in the central venous catheter so this needs to be gradually altered to support haemodynamic stability until only the new concentration drug is infusing.
If halving the concentration of the drug follow 15b–19b **15b.** Set the new infusion rate at 1 mL/h and press start.	To allow any remaining mechanical slack to be taken up, ensuring prompt delivery of the drug to the patient. Commencing the infusion at 1 mL/h allows a slow, gradual changeover, with the least haemodynamic instability.
16b. With both original and new syringe pumps administering together, attach the new three-way tap to the exposed port on the three-way tap on the central venous catheter and turn the three-way tap to 'on' for both infusions.	To allow the infusion of both drugs.
17b. Reduce the rate of the original infusion by 1 mL/h.	To ensure the drug already in the CVC is delivered at the same rate as before the change, e.g. 4 mL/h original = 3 mL/h original +1 mL/h new.
18b. Continuously monitor the patient's blood pressure and heart rate and cardiac output if available, in response to the infusion.	To determine any change and the effects of the infusion and to enable prompt adjustment of the infusion as necessary.
19b. When a decrease in the patient's blood pressure is seen gradually reduce the original infusion while increasing the new infusion until only the new infusion is running.	To ensure that the new, correct dose is gradually being delivered to the patient. There will still be a mixture of concentrations of drug in the central venous catheter so this needs to be gradually altered to support haemodynamic stability until only the new concentration drug is infusing.
20. If no signs of severe haemodynamic instability are noted switch off the original infusion.	To ensure the patient is receiving the correct dose. Keeping the original infusion connected enables prompt conversion back to the original infusion (and concentration) should any problems occur with the new infusion.

(Continued)

Procedure guideline 7.5: *(Continued)*

21. Dispose of all waste as per hospital/national policy.	To ensure the safe disposal of domestic waste, clinical waste and sharps. To prevent harm to all users of healthcare premises (NPSA 2009).
22. Document care, and when infusion is changed on patient's charts.	To: ■ provide an accurate record ■ monitor effectiveness of procedure ■ reduce the risk of duplication of treatment ■ provide a point of reference or comparison in the event of later questions ■ acknowledge accountability for actions ■ facilitate communication and continuity of care. (NMC 2008; GMC 2013; HCPC 2012)

*For the purposes of this guideline, it is assumed that three-way taps with bungs are used; however, bionectors and octopus devices may be used – refer to local hospital policy.

Competency statement 7.1: Specific procedure competency statements for preparation of inotropes and vasopressors for clinical use

Complete assessment against relevant fundamental competency statements (*see* Chapter 2, pp. 20, 21)	Evidence
Specific procedure competency statements for preparation of inotropes and vasopressors for clinical use	**Evidence of competency for preparation of inotropes and vasopressors for clinical use**
Demonstrate ability to: ■ teach and assess or ■ learn from assessment.	Examples of evidence of teaching, assessing and learning.
Identify reasons for the use of inotropes and vasopressors.	There are a number of ways in which competency can be judged. These include: ■ direct observation of the preparation of inotropes and vasopressors ■ testimonial from staff members ■ teaching sessions from peers ■ completion of a reflective text, workbook or educational package ■ examination/test ■ discussion with supervisor/mentor in relation to the preparation of inotropes and vasopressors for clinical use.
Identify risks, potential problems and complications for the preparation of inotropes and vasopressors and how they can be avoided or managed, including: ■ maintaining the sterility of the equipment ■ avoiding contamination of the infusion ■ ensuring the correct drug is prepared for the correct patient ■ ensuring the correct concentration of the drug is prepared.	
Demonstrate knowledge and understanding of local and national policy, procedures and guidelines relating to the preparation of intravenous medications, including: ■ hospital IV policy ■ NMC guidelines ■ DH guidelines.	
Demonstrate knowledge and understanding of the evidence base in relation to the preparation of inotropes and vasopressors.	

Demonstrate the skills and correct procedure required in preparing inotropes and vasopressors, including:
- gathering the appropriate equipment
- checking the drug and dilutent against the prescription
- avoiding contamination of the infusion
- drawing up the drug and dilutent accurately
- labelling the prepared infusion.

Prepare and check the equipment and drugs required for drawing up inotropes and vasopressors.

Competency statement 7.2: Specific procedure competency statements for calculating dosages for the administration of inotropes and vasopressors

Complete assessment against relevant fundamental competency statements (see Chapter 2, pp. 20, 21)	Evidence
Specific procedure competency statements for calculating dosages for the administration of inotropes and vasopressors	**Evidence of competency for calculating dosages for the administration of inotropes and vasopressors**
Demonstrate ability to: - teach and assess or - learn from assessment.	Examples of evidence of teaching, assessing and learning.
Identify reasons for knowing the correct dosages, including: - appropriate starting dosages - patient safety - accurate titration - awareness of complications/necessity for further intervention.	There are a number of ways in which competency can be judged. These include: - direct observation of the preparation of inotropes and vasopressors - testimonial from staff members - teaching sessions from peers - completion of a reflective text, workbook, or educational package - examination/test - discussion with supervisor/mentor in relation to the preparation of inotropes and vasopressors for clinical use.
Identify potential problems and errors in calculating dosages and how they can be avoided or managed, including: - too much/little drug given to patient - hypotension - hypertension.	
Demonstrate knowledge and understanding of local and national policy, procedures and guidelines relating to the delivering medications at the correct dosage, including: - hospital IV policy - NMC guidelines - DH guidelines.	

(Continued)

Competency statement 7.2: (*Continued*)

Demonstrate knowledge and understanding of the evidence base in relation to the dosages of inotropes and vasopressors including:
- identify which drug dosages should be calculated in micrograms/kg/min, micrograms/kg/h and micrograms/min.

Demonstrate the skills and correct procedure required in calculating dosages, including:
- converting rates to dosages
- converting dosages to rates
- calculating maximum and minimum dosages and rates.

Competency statement 7.3: Specific procedure competency statements for administration of inotropic and vasopressor drugs via syringe pumps

Complete assessment against relevant fundamental competency statements (*see* Chapter 2, pp. 20, 21)	Evidence
Specific procedure competency statements for administration of inotropic and vasopressor drugs via syringe pumps	**Evidence of competency for administration of inotropic and vasopressor drugs via syringe pumps**
Demonstrate ability to: ■ teach and assess or ■ learn from assessment.	Examples of evidence of teaching, assessing and learning.
Identify reasons for administering inotropes and vasopressors via syringe pumps, including: ■ the difference between syringe pumps and volumetric pumps ■ the safety devices of syringe pumps that enable quick detection of problems/prevent delay in infusion delivery.	There are a number of ways in which competency can be judged. These include: ■ direct observation of the preparation of inotropes and vasopressors ■ testimonial from staff members ■ teaching sessions from peers ■ completion of a reflective text, workbook, or educational package ■ examination/test ■ discussion with supervisor/mentor in relation to the preparation of inotropes and vasopressors for clinical use.
Identify risks, potential problems and complications for the administration of inotropes and vasopressors via syringe pumps and how they can be avoided or managed, including: ■ low battery power ■ incorrect syringe loading ■ mechanical slack.	
Demonstrate knowledge and understanding of local and national policy, procedures and guidelines relating to the use of syringe pumps, including: ■ hospital IV policy ■ medicines and healthcare products regulatory agency (MHRA) guidelines.	

Demonstrate knowledge and understanding of the evidence base in relation to the use of syringe pumps.

Demonstrate the skills and correct procedure required in administering inotropes and vasopressors via syringe pumps, including:
- correct syringe loading
- purging the syringe to take up mechanical slack
- commencing the infusion prior to attaching to the patient.

Prepare and check the equipment required.

Competency statement 7.4: Specific procedure competency statements for titration of inotropic and vasopressor drugs to meet patient requirements

Complete assessment against relevant fundamental competency statements (*see* Chapter 2, pp. 20, 21)	Evidence
Specific procedure competency statements for titration of inotropic and vasopressor drugs to meet patient requirements	**Evidence of competency for titration of inotropic and vasopressor drugs to meet patient requirements**
Demonstrate ability to: - teach and assess or - learn from assessment.	Examples of evidence of teaching, assessing and learning.
Identify reasons for the titration of inotropes and vasopressors to meet patient requirements, including: - accurate maintenance of patient blood pressure, etc. - avoiding unnecessary side effects.	There are a number of ways in which competency can be judged. These include: - direct observation of the preparation of inotropes and vasopressors - testimonial from staff members - teaching sessions from peers - completion of a reflective text, workbook, or educational package - examination/test - discussion with supervisor/mentor in relation to the preparation of inotropes and vasopressors for clinical use.
Identify risks, potential problems and complications for the titration of inotropes and vasopressors and how they can be avoided or managed, including: - hypotension - hypertension.	
Demonstrate knowledge and understanding of local and national policy, procedures and guidelines relating to the titration of IV medications, including: - hospital IV policy - NMC guidelines.	
Demonstrate knowledge and understanding of the evidence base in relation to the titration of inotropes and vasopressors, including: - comparative advantages and disadvantages of 'piggybacking' and 'quick change' techniques - ability to correctly calculate dosages in different concentrations, at different rates.	

(Continued)

Demonstrate the skills and correct procedure required in titrating inotropes and vasopressors to meet patient requirements, including:
- adjusting infusion rates
- monitoring the effects of adjustments
- documenting changes
- informing senior practitioners when necessary.

Prepare and check the equipment and drugs required.

Competency statement 7.5: Specific procedure competency statements for changeover of inotrope and vasopressor infusions

Complete assessment against relevant fundamental competency statements (*see* Chapter 2, pp. 20, 21)	Evidence
Specific procedure competency statements for changeover of inotrope and vasopressor infusions	**Evidence of competency for changeover of inotrope and vasopressor infusions**
Demonstrate ability to: ■ teach and assess or ■ learn from assessment.	Examples of evidence of teaching, assessing and learning.
Identify reasons for safe and effective changeover of inotropic and vasopressor infusions, including: ■ continuity of infusion ■ maintenance of adequate blood pressure ■ avoidance of complications ■ continued patient safety.	There are a number of ways in which competency can be judged. These include: ■ direct observation of the preparation of inotropes and vasopressors ■ testimonial from staff members ■ teaching sessions from peers ■ completion of a reflective text, workbook, or educational package ■ examination/test ■ discussion with supervisor/mentor in relation to the preparation of inotropes and vasopressors for clinical use.
Identify risks, potential problems and complications for the changeover of inotropic and vasopressor infusions and how they can be avoided or managed, including: ■ hypotension ■ hypertension.	
Demonstrate knowledge and understanding of local and national policy, procedures and guidelines relating to the changeover of inotropic and vasopressor infusions, including: ■ hospital IV policy ■ unit guidelines.	
Demonstrate knowledge and understanding of the evidence base in relation to the changeover of inotropic and vasopressor infusions.	
Demonstrate the skills and correct procedure required in the changeover of inotropic and vasopressor infusions, including: ■ loading the syringe into the pump ■ purging the infusion to take up mechanical slack ■ commencing the infusion prior to connecting to the patient ■ switching off original infusion once new infusion is connected ■ monitoring the patient for any adverse effects.	
Prepare and check the equipment and drugs required.	

274

References and further reading

Amoore J, Dewar D, Ingram P and Lowe D (2001) Syringe pumps and start-up time: ensuring safe practice. *Nursing Standard* **15**: 43–45.

Annane D, Vignon P, Renault A et al. (2007) Norepinephrine plus dobutamine versus epinephrine alone for the management of septic shock: a randomised trial. *Lancet* **370**: 676–684.

Argaud L, Cour M, Martin O et al. (2007) Changeovers of vasoactive drug infusion pumps: impact of a quality improvement program. *Critical Care* **11**(6): R133–R138.

Arino M, Barrington JP, Morrison AL and Gillies D (2004) Management of the changeover of inotrope infusions in children. *Intensive and Critical Care Nursing* **20**: 275–280.

Barochia AV, Cui X, Vitberg D et al. (2010) Bundled care for septic shock: an analysis of clinical trials. *Critical Care Medicine* **38**(2): 668–678.

Beale RJ, Hollenberg SM, Vincent JL and Parrillo JE (2004) Vasopressor and inotropic support in septic shock: An evidence based review. *Critical Care Medicine* **32**(11): S455–S465.

De Barbieri I, Frigo AC and Zampieron A (2009) Quick change versus double pump while changing the infusion of inotropes: an experimental study. *Nursing in Critical Care* **14**(4): 200–206.

Carpenito-Moyet LJ (2009) *Nursing Care Plans and Documentation: nursing diagnoses and collaborative problems* (5e). Philadelphia: Lippincott Williams & Wilkins.

Cooper BE (2008) Review and update on inotropes and vasopressors. *AACN Advanced Critical Care* **19**(1): 5–15.

Crisp H (2002) Minimising the risks: safe administration of inotropic drug infusions in intensive care. *Nursing in Critical Care* **7**(6): 283–289.

Deckert D, Buerkle C, Neurauter A et al. (2009) The effects of multiple infusion line extensions on occlusion alarm function of an infusion pump. *Anesthesia & Analgesia* **108**(2): 518–520.

Dellinger RP, Levy MM, Carlet JM et al. for the International Surviving Sepsis Campaign Guidelines Committee (2008) Surviving Sepsis Campaign: International guidelines for management of severe sepsis and septic shock: 2008. *Critical Care Medicine* **36**(1): 296–327.

Department of Health (2007) *Saving Lives: reducing infection, delivering clean and safe care*. London: Department of Health.

Ellender TJ and Skinner JC (2008) The use of vasopressors and inotropes in the emergency medical treatment of shock. *Emergency Medical Clinics Of North America* **26**: 759–786.

Fischer JE and Bland KI (2007) *Mastery of Surgery, Volume 1* (5e). Philadelphia: Lippincott Williams & Wilkins.

General Medical Council (2013) *Good Medical Practice*. London: GMC. http://www.gmc-uk.org/gmp2013 [accessed 25 March 2013].

Health and Care Professions Council (2012) *Standard of Conduct, Performance and Ethics*. London: HCPC. http://www.hcpc-uk.org/assets/documents/10003B6EStandardsofconduct,performance andethics.pdf [accessed January 2013].

Hollenberg SM (2007) Vasopressor support in septic shock. *Chest* **132**: 1678–1687.

Hollenberg SM, Ahrens TS, Annane D et al. (2004) Practice parameters for hemodynamic support of sepsis in adult patients: 2004 update. *Critical Care Medicine* **32**(9): 1928–1948.

Holmes CL (2005) Vasoactive drugs in the intensive care unit. *Current Opinion in Critical Care* **11**: 413–417.

Jerath N, Frndova H, McCrindle BW et al. (2008) Clinical impact of vasopressin infusion on hemodynamics, liver and renal function in pediatric patients. *Intensive Care Medicine* **34**: 1274–1280.

Juarez P (2005) Safe administration of IV infusions: Part 1. Vasopressors. *American Journal of Nursing* **105**(9): 72AA–72FF.

Karch AM (2003) *Lippincott's Nursing Drug Guide*. Springhouse: Lippincott Williams and Wilkins.

Klabunde RE (2005) *Cardiovascular Physiological Concepts*. Philadelphia: Lippincott Williams & Wilkins.

Llewellyn L (2007) Changing inotrope infusions: which technique is best? *Nursing Times* **103**(8): 30–31.

Marieb E (2004) *Human Anatomy and Physiology* (6e). San Francisco: Pearson Benjamin Cummings.

McIntyre LA, Hebert PC, Fergusson D et al. (2007) A survey of Canadian intensivists' resuscitation practices in early septic shock. *Critical Care* **11**: R74–R82.

Medicines and Healthcare products Regulatory Agency (2010) *Infusion Systems DB 2003(02)*. London: MHRA.

Mental Capacity Act (2005) http://www.legislation.gov.uk/ukpga/2005/9/pdfs/ukpga_20050009_en.pdf [accessed 9 February 2012].

Miller J (2007) Keeping your patient hemodynamically stable. *Nursing 2007* **37**(5): 36–41.

Mitchell RN (2005) Shock. In: Kumar V (ed.) *Robins and Cotran: pathologic basis of disease* (6e), pp. 134–138. Philadelphia: Saunders.

Morrice A, Jackson E and Farnell S (2004) Practical considerations in the administration of intravenous vasoactive drugs in the critical care setting part two – how safe is our practice. *Intensive and Critical Care Nursing* **20**: 183–189.

Mullner M, Urbanek B, Havel C, Losert H, Gamper G and Herkner H for The Cochrane Collaboration (2008) *Vasopressors for Shock (Review)*. London: John Wiley & Sons

National Patient Safety Agency (2007) *Risk Assessment Tool for Injectable Medicines*. London: NPSA.

National Patient Safety Agency (2009) *The Revised Healthcare Cleaning Manual*. London: NPSA.

Neff SB, Neff TA, Gerber S and Weiss MM (2007) Flow rate, syringe size and architecture are critical to start-up performance of syringe pumps. *European Journal of Anaesthesiology* **24**: 602–608.

Nursing and Midwifery Council (2007) *Standards for Medicine Management*. London: NMC.

Nursing and Midwifery Council (2008) *The Code – standards of conduct, performance and ethics for nurses and midwives*. London: NMC.

Overgaard CB and Dzavik V (2008) Inotropes and vasopressors – review of physiology and clinical use in cardiovascular disease. *Circulation* **118**: 1047–1056.

Patel BM, Chittock DR, Russel JA and Walley KR (2002) Beneficial effects of short term vasopressin infusion during septic shock. *Anaesthesiology*: **96**, 576–582.

Powell ML and Carnevale FA (2004) A comparison between single and double-pump syringe changes of intravenous inotropic medications in children. *Canadian Association of Critical Care Nurses* **15**(4): 10–14.

Resuscitation Council (UK) (2010) *Resuscitation Guidelines*. London: Resuscitation Council (UK).

Rokyta R, Tesarova J, Pechman V et al. (2010) The effects of short-term norepinephrine up-titration on hemodynamics in cardiogenic shock. *Physiological Research* **59**: 373–378.

Rossinen J, Harjola VP, Siirila-Waris K et al. (2007) The use of more than one inotrope in acute heart failure is associated with increased mortality: a multi-centre observational study. *Acute Cardiac Care* **10**: 209–213.

Royal Pharmaceutical Society of Great Britain & British Medical Association (2012) *BNF 64*. London: BMJ Publishing Group Ltd and Royal Pharmaceutical Society.

Russel JA, Walley KR, Singer J and Gordon AC (2008) Vasopressin versus norepinephrine infusion in patients with septic shock. *New England Journal of Medicine* **358**(9): 877–884.

275

Shaw NJ and Lyall EGH (1985) Hazards of glass ampoules. *British Medical Journal* **291**: 1390.

Sturgess DJ, Joyce C, Marwick TH and Venkatesh B (2007) A clinician's guide to predicting fluid responsiveness in critical illness: applied physiology and research methodology. *Anaesthesia and Intensive Care* **35**(5): 669–678.

Trim JC and Roe J (2004) Practical considerations in the administration of intravenous vasoactivedrugs in the critical care setting: the double pumping or piggyback technique – part one. *Intensive and Critical Care Nursing* **20**: 153–160.

Chapter 8

Assessment and support of hydration and nutrition status and care

Kirsty Rutledge[1] and Ian Nesbitt[2]

[1]Newcastle upon Tyne Hospitals NHS Foundation Trust, Newcastle upon Tyne, UK
[2]Freeman Hospital, Newcastle upon Tyne, UK

Critical Care Manual of Clinical Procedures and Competencies, First Edition.
Edited by Jane Mallett, John W. Albarran, and Annette Richardson.
© 2013 John Wiley & Sons, Ltd. Published 2013 by John Wiley & Sons, Ltd.

Definition

Hydration and nutrition status is the condition of the body resulting from the intake, absorption and utilization of fluids and food, and the influence of disease-related factors (Academisch Ziekenhuls Maastricht 2012).

Aims and indications

The aim of assessment and support of a patient's hydration and nutritional status is to:

- evaluate pre-existing hydration and nutritional conditions
- identify any hydration and nutrition related complications that could affect outcome
- establish an individualized plan of care for specialized hydration and nutrition support
- maintain the optimum level of intake and promote adequate utilization of hydration and food in order to promote growth, healing and recovery.

(Cresci 2005)

Approximately 30% of patients in hospital are malnourished; many present in this condition on admission to hospital and remain in this state throughout their stay (Kondrup et al. 2003a). All patients should therefore have their hydration and nutritional status assessed as soon as possible, and regularly throughout their hospital stay, to ensure their individual needs are identified and catered for. Given the importance of hydration and nutrition for health and recovery, this assessment and the resulting actions should form part of the daily care and management of critically ill patients.

Background

Anatomy and physiology
Organs of the digestive system

The digestive system consists of the gastrointestinal tract (also known as the alimentary canal) and the accessory digestive organs (Figure 8.1). The gastrointestinal tract includes:

- mouth
- some of the pharynx
- oesophagus
- stomach
- small and large intestines.

The digestive organs include:

- teeth
- tongue
- salivary glands
- liver
- gall bladder
- pancreas.

The gastrointestinal tract (GI) is 5–7 metres in length (Tortora and Derrickson 2011).

Layers of the GI tract

The GI tract generally has four main layers (*see* Figure 8.2) (there are some variations along its length). Generally the tract is composed of:

- mucosa (inner lining)
- submucosa
- muscularis
- serosa (outer layer).

Mucosa

The mucosa is further divided into three layers:

- epithelium (inner layer) – mainly non-keratinized stratified squamous epithelium in the mouth, pharynx, oesophagus and anal canal, which have a protective role. In the stomach and intestines the layer consists of simple columnar epithelium, which have secretory and absorption functions. The epithelium also includes exocrine and endocrine cells, which secrete mucus and fluid, and hormones respectively
- lamina propria (middle layer) – contains connective tissue, and blood and lymphatic vessels, which support the epithelium and transport nutrients to other parts of the body. Lymphatic nodules (also known as mucosa-associated lymphatic tissue [MALT]) – which have an immune function – are also within this layer
- muscularis mucosae (outer layer) – consists of muscle fibres, which cause folding and increase the surface area of the muscosa in contact with food and fluid in order to promote absorption (Tortora and Derrickson 2011).

Submucosa

The submucosa contains:

- connective tissue, which attaches the mucosa to the muscularis
- blood vessels, to transport food molecules
- lymphatic vessels, to transport food molecules
- network of neurons (submucosal plexus), to control movement of the GI tract and secretions from digestive organs
- glands
- lymphatic tissue (Tortora and Derrickson 2011).

Muscularis

The longitudinal and circular smooth muscle fibres in this layer are found in most of the GI tract. They contract in order to help break down and mix food, and to move it along the tract towards the anus. However, skeletal muscle

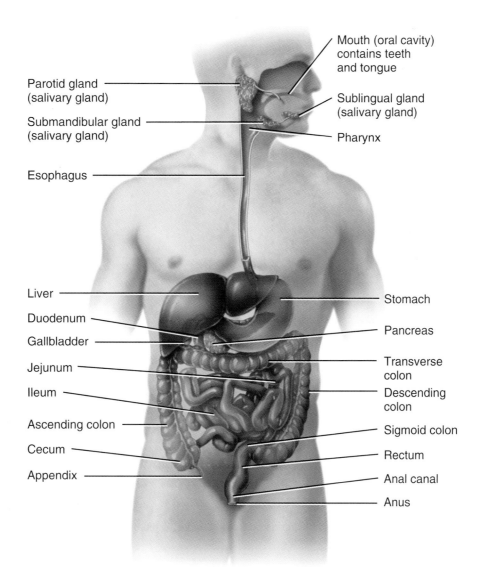

Mouth (oral cavity) contains teeth and tongue

Parotid gland (salivary gland)

Sublingual gland (salivary gland)

Submandibular gland (salivary gland)

Pharynx

Esophagus

Liver

Stomach

Duodenum

Pancreas

Gallbladder

Jejunum

Transverse colon

Ileum

Descending colon

Ascending colon

Sigmoid colon

Cecum

Rectum

Appendix

Anal canal

Anus

279

Figure 8.1 Right lateral view of the head and neck and anterior view of the trunk (from Tortora and Derrickson 2011, reproduced with permission from Wiley).

is found in the mouth, pharynx and parts of the oesophagus, which enables swallowing (Tortora and Derrickson 2011).

Serosa

The serosa consists of connective tissue and mesothelium, and forms part of the visceral peritoneum. It surrounds part of the GI tract, but not all (for example, the oesophagus is not surrounded by serosa) (Tortora and Derrickson 2011).

Functions of the digestive system

The functions of the digestive system are to utilize food and fluids to provide energy, maintain the integrity of the tissues (by building and repair) and to contribute to immunity. It does this by:

- ingestion (taking food into the digestive system)
- secretion (releasing substances, particularly enzymes, into the GI tract, either by cells lining the tract, or by glands [salivary, pancreas, liver] directly connected to it. This is in order to lubricate the tract, protect it from gastric acid and aid in the breakdown of food)
- propulsion (mixing food and moving it through the GI tract by peristalsis)
- digestion (mechanically breaking down food – for example, chewing, churning by the stomach – and chemically breaking down food by enzymes into small molecules)
- absorption (the passage of digested food products through the walls of the GI tract into the blood or lymph)

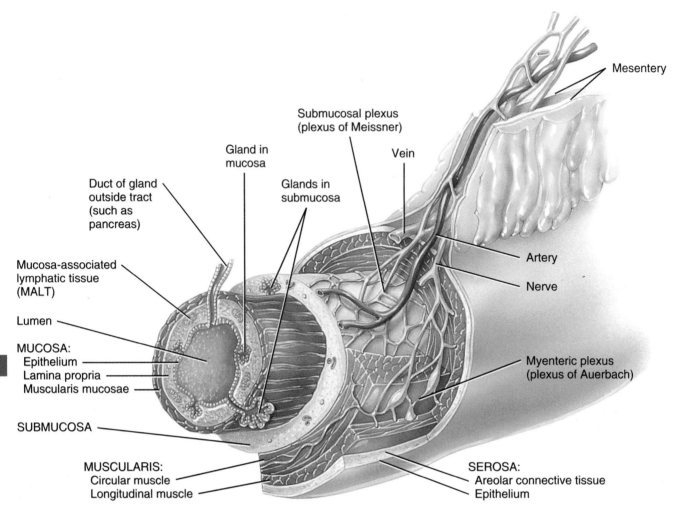

Figure 8.2 Layers of the gastrointestinal tract (from Tortora and Derrickson 2011, reproduced with permission from Wiley).

■ mounting an immune response (Tortora and Derrickson 2011).

Immune function

The lymphatic system is divided into branches (or trunks) and capillaries. The intestinal branch receives lymph from the stomach, intestines, pancreas, spleen and part of the liver. This then drains into the left lymphatic (or thoracic) duct and into the venous blood (Tortora and Derrickson 2011).

The role of the lymphatic system is to:

■ transport lipids, and vitamins that are lipid soluble (A, D, E and K), which have been absorbed by the GI tract
■ initiate highly specific immune responses against particular microbes and abnormal cells
■ drain excess fluid from interstitial areas and return it to the blood circulation (Tortora and Derrickson 2011).

MALT (mucosal-associated lymphatic tissues) are found in the GI tract (and also the urinary tract, reproductive tract and respiratory airways), and form part of the lymphatic system. MALT occur in large numbers in areas such as the tonsils, ileum (Peyer's patches) and appendix. These assist in defending the body against toxins and pathogens.

Other means of assisting in the immune function of the digestive system is by the:

■ acidity of the gastric juice (pH 1.2 to 3.0), which kills many bacteria and bacterial toxins
■ presence of IgA antibodies in saliva and other GI secretions. IgA protects local mucous membrane against bacteria and viruses (Tortora and Derrickson 2011).

Body fluid

The human body is largely (65% or more) composed of water (Chappell et al. 2008), although the exact proportion

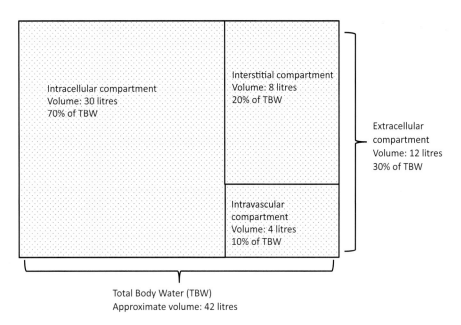

Figure 8.3 Traditional conceptual model of body fluid compartments.

varies with age, gender and obesity. The traditional view, based largely on the work of Starling in the 19th century (Starling 1896), dividing the body into several compartments (Figures 8.3 and 8.4), provides a useful conceptual background to current understanding of the importance of hydration in patient care and the effect of treatments on clinically measureable outcomes. However, Starling's model is probably too simplistic for clinical practice and has been recently challenged.

The 'intracellular fluid compartment' pertains to fluid within cells, and comprises around two-thirds of total body water. As the cell membrane is relatively impermeable, any change in the composition of intracellular fluid depends largely on active transport of water, ions, or other chemicals through pores, ion channels, or similar. This is a relatively slow and controlled process, with the result that the concentration of ions, proteins, etc., is very different between intracellular fluid and extracellular fluid (Table 8.1) (Pain 1977).

Extracellular fluid is fluid outside cells, and is divided into two parts – a relatively small amount within the vascular system (intravascular fluid) and the larger part contained by the spaces between blood vessels and cells (interstitial or 'third space' fluid).

Separating the intravascular and interstitial compartments is a capillary wall, containing the endothelial membrane system. Like the cell membrane, this is relatively impermeable to larger molecules (proteins and cellular components), but is much more permeable to small molecules (water and ions). This allows water and ions to move freely between intra- and extracellular compartments, but, under normal circumstances, allows only minimal movement of proteins and cells between the two compartments. Movement across this membrane is regulated by a variety of complex, inter-related factors such as hydrostatic pressure, ionic forces, molecular size and active transport (Ellis 2000).

This means that blood has a cellular component (red cells, white cells and platelets) and a fluid component (plasma), while interstitial fluid has a similar composition to plasma, but without the protein.

Turnover of water (input/output) is finely balanced. A loss of as little as 1% of total body water causes hyperosmolarity of plasma, the sensation of thirst, and triggers homeostatic mechanisms (for example antidiuretic hormone, renin-aldosterone). These act to restore equilibrium by causing oliguria, peripheral vasoconstriction, shunting of blood from skin and muscle to core organs, and increasing fluid intake (*see also* Chapter 9 for more anatomy and physiology).

The effect of critical illness on hydration and nutrition

Critical illness is a form of stress on the body, stimulating a metabolic response, which the body uses in an attempt to protect and heal itself (Scott et al. 1998). Stressors can include arterial and venous pressure and volume, pH, osmolality, pain, anxiety, arterial oxygen content, toxic mediators from infection and tissue injury (Cresci 2005), septic shock, inflammation and necrotic tissue (Scott et al, 1998).

The metabolic response to injury can be separated into an 'ebb' phase and a 'flow' phase. The 'ebb' phase occurs immediately after the initial insult, and is portrayed by hypoperfusion of the tissues, reduced metabolic activity, hyperglycaemia, and the release of catecholamines to increase heart rate, contractility and vasoconstriction to improve cardiac performance and venous return, restoring an adequate blood pressure. This phase may last between

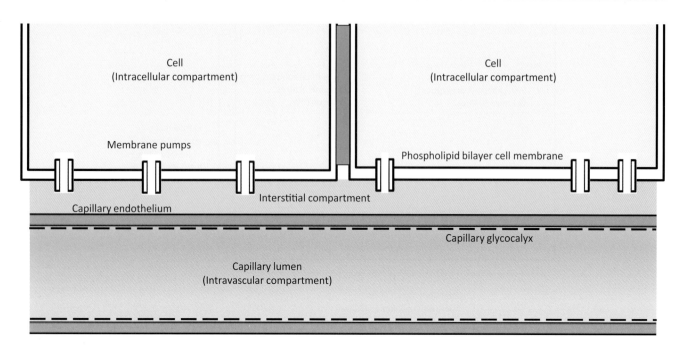

Figure 8.4 Detail of three compartment model.

Table 8.1 Composition of different fluid compartments

Content	Intracellular	Interstitial	Intravascular
Sodium (mmol/L)	10	140	140
Potassium (mmol/L)	150	5	5
Chloride (mmol/L)	10	105	105
Protein (g/L)	25	0	60–80
Albumin(g/L)	0	20	30–40
Cells	N/A	Minimal	Red cells, white cells, platelets

12 and 24 hours, depending on the severity of the insult and how well the patient is resuscitated.

The 'flow' phase is portrayed by a restoration of blood flow to the tissues, delivering oxygen and metabolic substrates. Increased levels of hormones, such as catecholamines, glucagon and cortisol, lead to catabolism of the peripheral muscles and adipose tissues to provide energy. Insulin release is increased during this phase; however, most of its effects are counteracted by the increased levels of circulating glucagon. The consequence of the flow phase is a considerable loss of muscle, resulting in an overall change in the composition of the body. Carbohydrate and fat stores are also reduced and there is an increase in the fluid in the extracellular and intracellular compartments (Cresci 2005).

To maintain hydration, the composition of the different fluid compartments depends to a great degree on the integrity and proper functioning of the capillary endothelium and cell membrane (Chappell et al. 2008). One common consequence of the inflammatory cascades involved in critical illness is a breakdown of this function, with capillary leak syndrome and cellular dysfunction. Often, the increased permeability leads to movement of fluid, solute and also some osmotically active molecules (such as albumin) from the intravascular to interstitial compartment, sometimes called 'third space losses'. Along with vasodilation, the consequent intravascular hypovolaemia due to third space losses results in hypoperfusion of cells, oedema in the lungs and end organ damage (Chappell et al. 2008).

The critically ill patient may also undergo substantial fluid loss. The rate of fluid loss may be so rapid (for example exsanguination of the intravascular component, massive gastrointestinal losses from infective diarrhoea) that the body's normal compensatory responses are inadequate. The resulting hypoperfusion and cellular hypoxia disrupts the workings of the cell membranes and intracellular organelles, causing organ dysfunction or death (Dutton 2006).

Injudicious administration of fluids resulting in fluid overload, long understood to worsen heart failure and acute lung injury, is now shown to be independently associated with worse outcome following major abdominal surgery (Brandstrup et al. 2003); in cases of acute kidney injury requiring renal replacement therapy (Payen et al 2008); and sepsis (Vincent et al 2006).

Thus the balance between hydration and haemodynamic stability must be carefully managed and the administration of routine hydration fluids regularly reviewed.

In addition, many patients admitted to critical care units are already malnourished due to the decline in their condition, and this is compounded by the fact that many of them are also undergoing a metabolic stress response to their critical illness. Malnutrition takes a very long time to overcome and therefore evidence-based interventions should take place early, allowing the GI system to return to its normal functions (Galley 2001).

Hydration and nutrition status declines in critically ill patients for a number of reasons:

- patients may be unable to drink and eat
- patients may be catabolic and nutritional replacements may not be adequate to replace metabolic losses
- patients may have impaired ingestion due to neurological or other conditions
- patients may have impaired absorption (Galley 2001).

Table 8.2 Fluid input and output sources

Input	Output
Oral (drinks and food)	Faeces (bowel management systems)
Enteral (continuous gastric/jejostomy feed or infusions, drugs and fluid used to flush tubing)	Gastric secretions (gastric drainage, gastric aspirations, vomit)
Intravenous fluids (parenteral, infusions and drugs)	Urine
	Insensible losses (estimated and therefore often not recorded)
	Wounds and drains
	Net losses during renal replacement therapy

Optimizing hydration and nutrition

Therapy to maintain hydration and nutrition status

Hydration and nutrition in the critically ill patient have evolved from being seen as adjunctive or part of supportive care to being understood as fundamental therapeutic interventions with a major influence on outcomes (McClave et al. 2009). In particular, the importance of:

- maintaining gut integrity in order to provide adequate hydration and nutrition, and to preserve the immune function of the gut
- the role of nutrients in tissue integrity and healing
- the adverse effects of hyper- or hypovolaemia (see also Chapter 6).

have highlighted the requirement for detailed monitoring and care to achieve the best outcomes.

Maintaining fluid balance in the critically ill

Fluid replacement

There are several important issues regarding appropriate fluid maintenance and replacement. These include the need for:

- accurate measurement of hydration status
- choice of appropriate fluid

- appropriate volume and timing of fluid administration
- choice of appropriate physiological endpoints.

Assessment of hydration status

Assessment of the patient's fluid status is important on a continuous basis, and many input and output sources should be included (Table 8.2). These inputs and outputs are usually recorded on a fluid balance chart every hour, with a calculated running hourly fluid balance. Then once a day, an overall 24-hour daily balance is calculated and recorded.

However, fluid balance is only one way to asses a patient's hydration status, and there are many other signs and symptoms that indicate fluid deficit or overload (Table 8.3 displays details of other ways to assess hydration [Dougherty and Lister 2011]).

The clinical assessment of whether or not a patient is adequately hydrated is difficult, particularly in the critically ill. This is because hypotension, tachycardia, oliguria, poor skin turgor, dry tongue and other signs may be poor indicators of dehydration, and can also accompany a myriad of other situations. For example, a large 'swing' or pulse pressure variation on the arterial pressure waveform may indicate hypovolaemia, but is inaccurate for patients breathing spontaneously (Heenen et al. 2006). Central venous pressure is dependent on intravascular volume, but also on cardiovascular function and ventilator settings, so may bear little relation to volume state in many conditions (Marik et al. 2008). Minimally invasive cardiac output monitors, for example oesophageal Doppler monitors (ODM), have limitations for many patient groups, such as those who are awake, or patients with arrhythmias.

An assessment of hydration status therefore relies on using multiple imprecise measures to build up a clinical impression, but even for experienced staff, this is often an

Table 8.3 Assessment of fluid status (adapted with permission from The Royal Marsden Hospital Manual of Clinical Nursing Procedures)

Assessment	Usual findings	Indications	
Signs and symptoms		**Fluid deficit**	**Fluid overload**
History To establish any condition, medication or lifestyle that may contribute to or predispose the patient to a fluid imbalance	Differs for each patient	For example, chronic or acute diarrhoea, medication such as diuretics, poor oral fluid intake	Ingestion of too much water/ fluid, renal failure/dysfunction
Thirst Ask the patient	Occasional; resolved by taking an oral drink	Unusually thirsty	No thirst
Mucosa and conjunctiva Inspect	Usually moist and pink	Dry and whitened mucosa, dry conjunctiva and 'sunken' eyeballs	Very moist, pink
Clinical signs			
Heart rate	Usual resting 60–100 beats per minute	Raised	Normal or raised
Peripheral pulse character	Radial pulse is normal volume and can be easily palpated	Thready, difficult to palpate	Bounding, easy to palpate
Blood pressure	Patient's own normal should be used as a guide	BP will fall if blood volume falls beyond compensatory mechanisms. Patient may experience postural hypotension	Rise in blood pressure, or may remain normal
Pulse pressure variation (PPV) or stroke volume variation (SVV)	Less than 10% variation with respiration	Greater than 10% variation in PPV or SVV with respiration with fluid challenge	No change, or decrease in PPV/SVV with respiration following fluid challenge
Central venous pressure	0–5 mmHg non-ventilated patients. 5–10 mmHg ventilated patients (*see* Chapter 6)	Low	Raised
Passive straight leg raising (SLR)	Minimal increase in cardiac output with SLR	Increased cardiac output with SLR	Little change in cardiac output with SLR
Echocardiography	'Normal' appearances	Dynamic, 'empty' heart, collapsed inferior vena cava	Dilated heart with possible impaired function. Distended inferior vena cava
Respiratory rate	12–20 breaths/min	High, to meet increased oxygen demands of compensatory mechanisms	High
Capillary refill	Within 3 seconds	Slower	Faster
Urine output	0.5 to 1 mL/kg	Low	Increase, if good renal function
Lung sounds, auscultation	Vesicular breath sounds, 'rustling' heard mainly on inspiration	Normal	Abnormal adventitious (additional) course crackles *may* indicate pulmonary oedema (*see* Chapter 5)
Skin turgor	Following a gentle pinch, the fold of skin should return to normal	Skin will take much longer to 'bounce' back to normal. Unreliable in elderly who may have lost some elasticity of their skin	May be normal; however, may be oedematous, therefore skin remains dented/pinched
Serum electrolyte levels			
Sodium	135–145 mmol/L	Raised	Lowered
Potassium	3.5–5 mmol/L	May be lowered if cause of fluid deficit is GI losses	Normal
Urea	2.5–6.4 mmol/L	Decreased	Normal
Creatinine	Male: 63–116 micromol/L Female: 54–98 micromol/L	Normal, but eventually rises with prolonged poor renal perfusion	Normal

Table 8.3 (*Continued*)

Assessment	Usual findings	Indications	
		Fluid deficit	Fluid overload
Serum osmolarity	275–295 mosmol/kg	Increased	Decreased
Urine osmolarity	50–1400 mosmol/kg	Increased	Decreased
Daily weight	A person's daily weight should be fairly stable; large losses or gain in weight may indicate fluid imbalance	Reduced each day	Increased each day
Temperature	36.5–37.5°C	May be elevated and this may also contribute to the fluid deficit (increased insensible losses)	Normal

Table 8.4 Composition of intravenous fluids

Fluid	Sodium (mmol/L)	Ppotassium (mmol/L)	Chloride (mmol/L)	Dextrose (g/L)	Lactate (mmol/L)	Typical molecular size (kDa)
5% dextrose	0	0	0	50	0	0.18
0.9% sodium chloride	154	0	154	0	0	0.06
0.4% dextrose, 0.18% sodium chloride 'dextrose-saline'	30	0	30	40	0	0.18
Hartmann's solution	131	5	111	0	29	0.06
Gelatin	145	5	145	0	0	30
Starch	154	0	154	0	0	130–200
Albumin	155	1	135	0	0	67

inaccurate process (Shippy et al. 1984; Iregui et al. 2003). Consulting fluid balance and observation charts, and cross-referencing these with the response to interventions such as fluid challenges or passive straight leg raising (Cavallaro et al. 2010) may help in decision making.

Choice of fluid

Intravenous fluids may be classified as crystalloid or colloid. A crystalloid is essentially water with small molecules (ions such as sodium, potassium and chloride). A colloid is water containing larger molecules (e.g. proteins, gelatins and starches). Table 8.4 shows the composition of various intravenous fluids.

Distribution of administered fluid

Traditionally, it was viewed that a colloid would remain in the intravascular compartment, while an ionic fluid (crystalloid) would distribute uniformly into the extracellular compartment. Water would distribute throughout all three compartments (Figure 8.5). Although experiments in normal, healthy subjects tend to support this, studies in critically ill patients have shown this model to be of limited relevance.

For example, differences in vascular expansion for various fluids are less than predicted. This difference may be explained by our increased understanding of the complexities of the endothelial glycocalyx (a 1 micron thick layer on the luminal side of normal vessels) (Weinbaum et al. 2007).

Intravenous fluid replacement is one of the most commonly prescribed medical interventions, but it is only recently that adequate studies to inform rational use of this therapy have been designed and carried out (*see* Table 8.6). At present, which fluid, and how much of that fluid a particular patient receives, depends almost entirely on geography, practitioner beliefs and marketing, rather than physiology (Miletin et al. 2002).

Dextrose

Dextrose is a fluid containing a variable amount of dextrose dissolved in water. A 5% solution contains 50 g dextrose in 1000 mL water. Other available solutions are 10%, 20% and 50%. Although there is a small amount of energy available from a solution of 5% dextrose, the main use for this is to provide water. Water should not be administered intravenously in large quantities, partly because it may damage red blood cells, and partly because it may cause acute

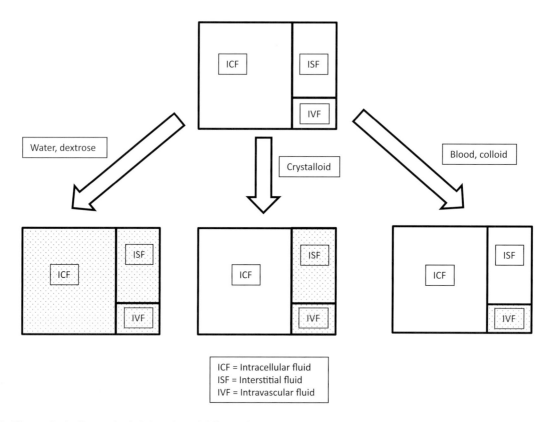

ICF = Intracellular fluid
ISF = Interstitial fluid
IVF = Intravascular fluid

Figure 8.5 Theoretical effects of administration of different fluids.

disturbances in serum electrolyte concentrations. Dextrose, therefore, is a way to deliver water: the dextrose is slowly metabolized by cells, leaving the carrier water to distribute throughout the body. Thus, in theory, for every litre of dextrose administered intravenously only around 100 mL will remain within the intravascular compartment (Figure 8.5) (Powell-Tuck et al. 2011).

0.9% Sodium chloride ('normal' saline)

This crystalloid contains equal amounts of sodium and chloride. This provides an electrically neutral solution. However, although the sodium concentration (154 mmol/L) is similar to that in plasma, the chloride concentration (154 mmol/lL is significantly higher than plasma concentrations (97–105 mmol/L). Thus, administration of large volumes of 0.9% sodium chloride results in hyperchloraemia. This causes a metabolic acidosis, and may impair renal function, cytokine release, immune function and ultimately patient survival (Shaw et al. 2012). Theoretically, for every litre administered intravenously, around 350 mL of 0.9% sodium chloride will remain in the intravascular compartment (Powell-Tuck et al. 2011).

Hartmann's solution

This is a solution containing a more physiological, or balanced, concentration of ions than 0.9% sodium chloride

(White and Goldhill 1997). The sodium concentration is lower in Hartmann's solution (131 mmol/L), and the chloride concentration in particular is much lower (98 mmol/L). Electrical neutrality is maintained with lactate, hence the alternative name, compound sodium lactate. As with 0.9% sodium chloride, around 350 mL should remain in the intravascular compartment for every litre given intravenously, with the remainder passing into the interstitial compartment.

Albumin

This is a colloid, containing the protein albumin (which typically has a molecular weight 67 kDa). These molecules are too large to cross from intravascular to extracellular compartments, leading to the presumption that the interstitial concentration of albumin would be zero. The actual concentration is higher because some capillary beds are more permeable to albumin-sized molecules (e.g. fenestrated and sinusoidal capillaries in the glomeruli, spleen, bone marrow and intestines).

It could be expected that human albumin solution would be an ideal replacement fluid for intravascular losses, especially in the critically ill, who often have a moderate or severe degree of hypoalbuminaemia. Unfortunately, studies have demonstrated that, outside the setting of hepatorenal failure, there currently seems a limited role for intravenous albumin in critically ill patients (Ortega et al. 2002; SAFE 2004; Boldt 2010).

Table 8.5 Daily requirements for fluid replacement, and possible regimens

	Approximate daily requirement	Actual amount (typical 70 kg adult)	Possible prescription	Alternative prescription
Sodium	2–3 mmol/kg	200 mmol	1.5 L 0.9% sodium chloride	1.5 L dextrose-sodium chloride
Potassium	1–2 mmol/kg	100 mmol	1 L 5% dextrose	1 L 0.9% sodium chloride
Water	1.5 mL/kg/h	2500 mL	Each 500 mL bag has 20 mmol potassium added	Each 500 mL bag has 20 mmol potassium added

Starch solutions

There are a range of starch solutions, typically differing by the size of molecules (typically 130–200 kDa, although a proportion of molecules in each infusion bag will be outside this range). Despite theoretical benefits, clinical experience has demonstrated that starch use is associated with increased renal dysfunction. In addition, concerns about sequestration in the reticuloendothelial system with potentially long-term adverse effects have been raised.

Requirements for fluid replacement

Fluid replacement has two components – normal daily requirements and replacement of lost fluid. Daily requirements may be relatively standardized, while replacement fluids will vary dependent on the composition of lost fluid. For example, high gastric aspirates may cause a large loss of hydrogen and chloride, while pancreatic and small bowel losses may cause large amounts of bicarbonate loss. Replacement regimens may need to be tailored to the individual's clinical condition circumstances (Powell-Tuck et al. 2011).

In theory, if fluid output is measured, then the input required can be calculated, and an appropriate fluid, or combination of fluids, used to replace losses. Using this approach would typically predict daily requirements as shown in Table 8.5. Various ways to provide fluid requirements for individual patients are also shown. In reality, adjustments must be made for insensible and unmeasured losses, so any estimate is inaccurate, and the effects of fluid and electrolyte replacement must be checked by clinical and biochemical measurement at appropriate intervals. Patients with capillary leak syndrome, vasomotor paresis or very high insensible losses (for example in patients with burns) may require much higher replacement rates of both fluid and electrolytes.

For the critically ill patient, a common sequence of events following clinical assessment is that of high fluid requirements for immediate resuscitation on initial admission to critical care. As the patient stabilizes, the requirements reduce and the daily cumulative fluid balance becomes less positive. As the patient recovers, fluid in the third space is mobilized and returned to the intravascular compartment, from where it is excreted. Thus, polyuria and a negative net fluid balance often form part of recovery from critical illness.

Thus, not only is the amount and type of fluid required important, but also the timing of fluid replacement.

Choice of physiological endpoints

In former years, physiological measurements were principally based on pressure measurements (e.g. central venous pressure, arterial blood pressure). Recognition of serious shortcomings in this approach have led to a more dynamic, flow-based approach to managing fluid therapy (for example oesophageal Doppler, stroke volume variation models). The use of the Frank–Starling theory to assess cardiac function remains the underlying principle of estimating a patient's response to fluid boluses (*see* Chapter 6 for more information regarding the Frank–Starling mechanism and the administration of a fluid challenge).

Ultimately, patient-centred outcomes such as time to eat, drink, mobilize and be discharged from hospital are the most relevant outcome measures, rather than secondary, proxy indicators of adequate tissue perfusion and oxygen delivery. However, these are of limited utility in the acute and critical care environment, so secondary indicators are most commonly used.

For elective, fast-track surgery, an individualized, pre-emptive approach to maintaining adequate hydration is recommended (Mythen et al. 2012). For the critically ill, the situation is less clear, in part due to the difficulties in conducting any study in critical care, and in part to the additional complexity of critically ill patients compared with elective surgical groups.

Several studies have addressed important questions (Table 8.6), but this is a rapidly changing field, so at present, only broad conclusions can be drawn for day-to-day management, although national expert opinion (Powell-Tuck et al. 2011) has attempted (with limited success) to produce evidence-based recommendations (Soni 2009).

General conclusions would suggest that albumin should rarely be used, that colloids have minimal advantages over crystalloids (and starches in particular may cause harm), and that 'normal' saline is perhaps more harmful than balanced solutions.

Maintenance of patent vascular access

Delivery of intravenous fluid therapy relies on the insertion of an intravascular access catheter. Insertion of an intravascular catheter will cause a break in the skin and bypass normal defence mechanisms, therefore posing a constant risk to patients. This risk may be due to:

Table 8.6 Key studies of fluid therapy

Study, authors, journal and date	Question	Main results
SAFE study, SAFE study investigators NEJM, 2004	Albumin v 0.9% sodium chloride in adult critical care patients	No benefit from albumin
FEAST study, Maitland et al., NEJM, 2011	Albumin bolus v 0.9% sodium chloride bolus v nil in children	No benefit from aggressive fluid replacement
6S study, Perner et al., NEJM, 2012	HES (starch) 130/0.4 v Hartmann's in adults with sepsis	Harm from HES
CHEST study, Myburgh et al., NEJM, 2012	HES (starch) 130/0.4 v 0.9% sodium chloride in adult critical care patients	Not yet known

- poor insertion technique
- infection at the insertion site
- thrombophlebitis due to drug administration or irritation
- another reason, such as disconnection leading to blood loss or air embolus.

No vascular device should be left in place for longer than its recommended indwelling life. This can vary from, for example, 48–96 hours for peripheral cannulae to perhaps several weeks or months for peripherally inserted central catheters, depending on need and type (Dougherty and Lister 2011). While in place, vascular devices should be cared for appropriately (see Chapter 18 in *The Royal Marsden Hospital Manual of Clinical Nursing Procedures* [Dougherty and Lister 2011] for further information on this topic).

Summary

Superficially, intravenous fluid management appears straightforward. However, there is still uncertainty concerning how best to measure hydration status; how much and which type of fluid is best in different clinical situations; and what are appropriate endpoints in treatment. Many long-held beliefs have recently been challenged or overturned by high-quality studies, but much work remains to be done in this area.

Maintaining nutrition

Assessment of nutrition status

The National Institute of Health and Clinical Excellence (NICE 2006) recommended that all patients should undergo nutritional screening on admission to hospital. All healthcare organizations should, therefore, have policies and protocols in place to identify patients at nutritional risk. This should be followed by the development of appropriate care plans through estimation of energy and protein requirements followed by the prescription of food, oral supplements, tube feeding or parenteral nutrition, or a combination of these (Kondrup et al. 2003a).

The steps for appropriate management of care for a patient group are:

- screening
- assessment
- monitoring and outcome
- communication
- audit.

1 Screening

All patients should be screened on admission to healthcare settings. This process categorizes patients into the following groups:

(a) 'not at risk', but re-screening should be carried out at specified intervals, for example weekly during hospital stay
(b) 'at risk' and a nutritional care plan can be developed by practitioners
(c) 'at risk, but metabolic or functional problems prevent a standard care plan being carried out'
(d) 'doubt as whether the patient is at risk'.

In the two latter cases, referral should be made to an expert for more detailed assessment (Kondrup et al. 2003a).

2 Assessment

A detailed examination of metabolic, nutritional or functional variables should be conducted by an expert practitioner (for example, a dietician or nutrition nurse). Consideration should be paid to patient history, laboratory investigations, current medication and gastrointestinal assessment (including ability to swallow [see below] and bowel function), etc. The assessment should provide information leading to an appropriate care plan, which takes into account indications, possible side effects and, in some cases, special feeding techniques.

3 Monitoring and outcome

The effectiveness of the nutritional intervention should be monitored, leading to alterations in treatment as necessary throughout the patient's stay.

288

4 Communication

Screening and assessment results and the developed nutritional care plans should be communicated to other practitioners when the patient is transferred elsewhere.

5 Audit

If steps 1 to 4 are carried out systematically, this will allow audit of outcomes which can inform future policy decisions.

Components of nutritional screening

The purpose of screening tools is to detect protein and energy malnutrition, and predict whether malnutrition is likely to develop or worsen.

Screening tools should therefore contain four main areas.

1   An assessment of the patient's present condition. This can be partly determined using the Body Mass Index (BMI = weight (kg)/height (m)^2). If it is not possible to measure weight and height, then a general indication of BMI can be obtained from a measurement of mid-upper arm circumference. This is achieved by measuring the distance between the shoulder and elbow, identifying the mid-point and, with the arm hanging loose, measuring the circumference of arm at the mid-point. If mid-upper arm circumference is less than 23.5 cm, BMI is likely to be less than 20 kg/m^2. If mid-upper arm circumference is greater than 32.0 cm, BMI is likely to be greater than 30 kg/m^2 (Malnutrition Advisory Group 2004).

2   An assessment of whether the condition is stable. For example, an estimate of the amount of involuntary weight loss or gain.

3   An assessment of whether the condition will get worse. For instance, determine whether intake has reduced prior to screening. If intake has been less than the patient's normal requirements then further weight loss is likely.

4   An assessment of whether the disease process will accelerate nutritional deterioration. Nutritional requirements may be increased due to the stress metabolism associated with severe disease (for example major surgery, sepsis, trauma), leading to worsening nutritional status, even where 1 to 3 above are normal.

(Kondrup et al. 2003a)

The most widely used tool in hospital settings is the Malnutrition Universal Screening Tool (MUST; Russell and Elia 2011). The European Society for Clinical Nutrition and Metabolism (ESPEN) for screening recommends three main tools.

1   **Malnutrition Universal Screening Tool (MUST)** – This is a five-step screening tool for use in hospitals, community and other care settings. It analyses BMI, recent weight loss and acute disease to identify adults who are malnourished, at risk of malnutrition, or obese. Management guidelines that can be used to develop care plans are included in the tool (Malnutrition Advisory Group 2004). Assessment of malnutrition using MUST will normally score every critically ill patient as requiring dietician review.

2   **Nutritional Risk Screening (NRS-2002)** – The purpose of the NRS-2002 system is to analyse BMI, weight loss, recent dietary intake and severity of illness to detect the presence, and risk, of developing malnutrition in the hospital setting (Kondrup et al. 2003b).

3   **Mini Nutritional Assessment (MNA)** – The objective of the MNA is to detect malnutrition and the risk of malnutrition developing in the elderly in home-care programmes, nursing homes and hospitals. The MNA includes physical and mental aspects that frequently affect the nutritional status of the elderly, as well as a dietary questionnaire. Therefore it is more likely to identify those at risk of developing malnutrition, and malnutrition at an early stage.

These tools are available in the ESPEN Guidelines for Nutrition Screening 2002 (Kondrup et al. 2003a), available at http://www.espen.org/documents/Screening.pdf

Components of assessment for choice of route for nutrition

In addition to a nutritional status assessment there is a requirement to assess the best route of administration of nutrition for the patient. Oral nutrition is generally considered the first-line method, followed by enteral, then parenteral routes. This is because enteral and parenteral feeding have more associated risks. However, this is dependent on various factors, such as whether the patient is conscious and able to swallow, the presence of a tracheostomy tube, whether the gut needs to be rested, etc. If there are no contraindications prior to oral feeding, the patient's ability to receive safely oral nutrition and hydration needs to be assessed. This involves a swallowing assessment.

Swallowing assessment of patient with tracheal tube

An initial assessment can be carried out at the bedside by a practitioner so long as the following are not present:

- neurological involvement
- head and neck surgery
- evidence of aspiration of food, fluid and/or oral secretions on tracheal suctioning
- persistent wet or weak voice when speaking valve or decannulation cap in place
- coughing occurs in relation to oral intake
- oxygen desaturation in conjunction with oral intake
- patient anxiety or distress during oral intake.

(St George's Healthcare NHS Trust 2012)

In all of the above situations a speech and language therapist's expertise is required for more detailed assessment.

Bedside assessment of swallowing should only be considered when the tracheostomy cuff is deflated. Cuff deflation should be checked prior to testing swallowing ability.

Assessment of ability to swallow begins with a trial of sips of water. If this is successful, the patient may progress to small amounts of smooth yogurt, followed by larger amounts of fluid and food (see Box 8.1). Traditionally blue dye has been added to the water (and yogurt) as it is possible to see the dye on suctioning if aspiration occurs. However, this may produce false negative results (that is, no detection of blue dye but patient still aspirating) (Peruzzi et al. 2001). As long as it is recognized that this test is only one of the factors to consider when observing for aspiration, then blue dye may

still be used. See the guidelines section for a flowchart on swallowing assessment of patients with a tracheostomy.

Any patient who fails the initial bedside swallow test should be referred to a speech and language therapist (St George's Healthcare NHS Trust 2012).

Therapy

Enhanced recovery programmes

Recent developments in the care of patients undergoing major abdominal and pelvic surgery have led to 'enhanced recovery' or 'fast-track' programmes that ameliorate the metabolic response to illness and challenge established practices of minimal monitoring, preoperative fasting and failure of early mobilization. In particular, there are three areas relating to nutrition and hydration that might be of clinical use in critically ill patients.

1 *Optimizing preoperative nutrition and hydration*: it has been demonstrated that, following 7–10 days of preoperative parenteral nutrition, postoperative outcome improves in severely malnourished patients who cannot be adequately orally or enterally fed. However, its use in well-nourished or mildly undernourished patients is associated with either no benefit or with increased morbidity (Braga et al. 2009). A 400 mL carbohydrate-rich drink ingested 2–3 hours before surgery has been shown to reduce preoperative thirst, hunger and anxiety In addition, this significantly reduced postoperative insulin resistance, leaving patients more likely to benefit from postoperative nutrition (commenced within 3 hours of surgery) (Hausel et al. 2001; Soop et al 2001). However, the complexity of the critically ill patient's condition and their subsequent management does not always allow for preoperative optimization due to multiple physiological imbalances and competing clinical priorities. For example, in emergency procedures maintenance of airway may take precedence over obtaining fluid balance. This makes research in this area difficult.

2 *Intra- and or postoperative goal-directed fluid therapy to optimize hydration status* (that is, without causing overload or dehydration): fluid therapy can reduce the incidence of ileus, complications and hospital stay (Lobo et al. 2002; Grocott et al. 2005; Pearse et al. 2005; Bundgaard-Neilsen et al. 2007).

3 *Avoidance of nasogastric intubation as routine* (for example, to decompress the stomach): this leads to lower incidence of fever, atelectasis and pneumonia (Cheatham et al. 1995).

Therefore using the above strategies the metabolic insult of surgery can be attenuated, the length of stay and complications reduced, and recovery enhanced. Nevertheless, further research is required in patients who are critically ill to establish whether outcomes are improved.

Box 8.1 Swallowing assessment of patients with tracheal tube

Equipment for 'swallow screen'

- Individual vial/ampoule sterile blue dye
- Drinking water
- Smooth yoghurt
- 'Normal' cup/glass, not spouted beaker with lid (no straws)
- Teaspoon

General principles

- Prior to commencing the assessment the patient should be assessed for:
  - level of alertness and cognitive awareness
  - laryngeal competency and voicing ability
  - strength of reflexive and spontaneous cough
  - strength of voice
  - ability to swallow sputum
  - risk of aspiration
- Universal precautions should be adhered to throughout the assessment and eye protection should be worn
- The patient should be sat upright
- The tracheal cuff should be deflated for all oral intake, if the patient can tolerate this
- Regular suctioning should be available throughout the assessment
- Assessment should begin with small sips of water
- The assessment can proceed to thicker fluids and then solids, following success at prior levels
- The assessment should end if:
  - the patient's condition deteriorates
  - the patient becomes tired or distressed
  - the patient's voice sounds consistently wet/gurgling
  - persistent coughing is evident
  - there are signs of aspiration on tracheal suction
  - there are signs of respiratory distress (e.g. increased respiratory rate, decreased SpO_2)

Refer to the speech and language team if any of the above signs are noted.

Feeding critically ill patients

Critically ill patients who cannot tolerate oral feeding can be fed enterally or parenterally, the route of choice being enteral (see below). The route used will depend on:

- if the patient has a functioning GI system
- which route is appropriate
- how long feeding will be required.

All key decision makers should be involved in this decision to ensure patients receive the appropriate route, type and volume of nutrition.

Enteral feeding

Enteral feeding (feeding patients liquid feed via a tube placed either in the stomach or post-pyloric) is the route of choice for critically ill patients where oral feeding is not possible. It is vital in counteracting the catabolic state induced by critical illness (Kreymann et al. 2006). This method is used when patients are malnourished or at risk of malnourishment; have inadequate oral intake or are unsafe and/or unable to have oral intake; and have a functional, accessible GI tract (NICE 2006). The benefits of enteral feeding include:

- the preservation of GI tract morphology and function
- support of the immune function of the GI tract
- nutritional delivery is more closely matched to normal physiology
- enteral nutrition is less expensive than parenteral nutrition
- enteral nutrition leads to fewer complications than parenteral nutrition.

(Scott 1998)

Studies concerning whether early enteral feeding reduces length of stay, rates of infection and mortality demonstrate varied findings. However, it is recommended that all patients who are expected to be without a full oral diet within 3 days of admission to critical care should receive enteral nutrition (Kreymann et al. 2006). Nevertheless, it is accepted that metabolic requirements of the critically ill cannot be met in full in this way. Kreymann et al. (2006) suggest that supplementary parenteral nutrition should be used in patients who cannot tolerate sufficient enteral intake; however, this should be avoided where enteral intake is approximately at target values.

Enteral feeding in critical care should be administered continuously, 24 hours a day unless contraindicated. Continuous pump feeding can reduce gastrointestinal discomfort, may maximize levels of nutrition support when absorptive capacity is diminished (Stroud et al. 2003) and may reduce the risk of aspiration (Pearce and Duncan 2002). Specific volumes of enteral nutrition can be adjusted depending on the progression/course of the illness and to gut tolerance (Kreymann et al. 2006). ESPEN guidelines indicate that:

- during the acute and initial phase of critical illness, in excess of 20–25 kcal/kg body weight (BW)/day may be associated with a less favourable outcome
- during the anabolic recovery phase, the aim should be to provide 25–30 kcal/kg BW/day
- patients with a severe malnutrition should receive enteral nutrition up to 25–30 total kcal/kg BW/day. If these target values are not reached supplementary parenteral nutrition should be given
- intravenous administration of a GI motility stimulant, for example metoclopramide or erythromycin, should be considered in patients with intolerance to enteral feeding (e.g. with high gastric residuals).

See Procedures guideline 8.3 at the end of this chapter for a suggested enteral feeding regimen (see Box 8.2).

The choice of enteral feed may vary depending on the patient's clinical condition. Further advice from ESPEN (Kreymann et al. 2006) indicates the following.

- Whole protein formulae are appropriate in most patients because no clinical advantage of peptide-based formulae can be shown.
- Immune-modulating formulae (formulae enriched with arginine, nucleotides and omega-3 fatty acids) have been demonstrated to improve patient outcomes and reduce length of stay compared to standard enteral formulae, although their exact method of action in different critical illness varies (Worthington and Cresci 2011). They can be used:
  - in elective upper GI surgical patients
  - in patients with mild sepsis

291

Box 8.2 Enteral feeding

General principles for enteral feeding

- Assess the patient's requirements for feeding on admission. Involve the dietician to ensure patient's needs are being met
- Feeding should commence as soon as possible
- Nutritional support should be provided by the enteral route where possible
- Feeding should be continuous for 24 hours a day
- Change the feed and administration set every 24 hours using a clean technique
- Commence feed at prescribed rates usually between 25 and 50 mL/h
- Aspirate every 6 hours and follow the prescribed feeding regimen
- Consider the administration of GI motility stimulants to reduce high aspirates of over 500 mL
- Increase feed as prescribed and tolerated
- Reassess daily regarding possible oral feeding

- in patients with severe sepsis; however, immune-modulating formulae may be harmful and are therefore not recommended
- in patients with trauma
- in patients with acute respiratory distress syndrome (ARDS) (formulae containing omega-3 fatty acids and antioxidants).

- Patients with very severe illness who do not tolerate more than 70 mL of enteral formulae per day should not receive an immune-modulating formula enriched with arginine, nucleotides and omega-3 fatty acids, as these formulae have been linked to higher mortality among this patient group (Heyland et al. 2001).

- Glutamine has been found to improve wound healing, reduce mortality and reduce rates of bacteraemia, pneumonia and sepsis in burns and trauma patients, therefore it is recommended that this is added to standard enteral formula in these patients.

- There are not sufficient data to support glutamine supplementation in surgical or heterogeneous critically ill patients groups.

(Kreymann et al. 2006)

Glycaemic control

'Glycaemic control' (controlling the level of glucose in the blood) is an essential part of critical care. Hyperglycaemia is more common than hypoglycaemia as the release of cortisol, catecholamines and glucagon during the metabolic stress response stimulates the breakdown of fat and glycogen, causing a rise in blood glucose levels. If untreated, hyperglycaemia leads to polyuria, dehydration, hypotension and electrolyte imbalance, abdominal pains, nausea and vomiting, cardiac irregularities, lipidaemia, weight loss, ketoacidosis, coma and death. Hypoglycaemia may be caused by hepatic or renal impairment, salicylate poisoning, insulin-secreting tumours and insufficient clearing of insulin, or with insufficient dietary intake (Marini & Wheeler 1997). Early symptoms of hypoglycaemia are hypertension, tachycardia and sweating. If left untreated seizures and reduced levels of consciousness may develop (Dougherty and Lister 2011).

To avoid these extremes and maintain normoglycaemia, all patients should have their blood glucose level checked (at least 4-hourly), and further action should be taken depending on the result of this measurement. Blood glucose levels can be obtained from an arterial (*see* Chapter 5, Arterial blood gas sampling) or central venous catheter blood sample, or from a finger prick, and can be measured either through a blood gas machine or a blood glucose monitor.

There has been much debate around what blood sugar measurements are considered to be necessary in critical care. Following Van den Berghe et al.'s 2001 publication suggesting that intensive insulin therapy was associated with better outcomes, many have tried to replicate the results but with sparse success. In 2009, the NICE-SUGAR Study Investigators reported on a large, multicentre trial that showed that

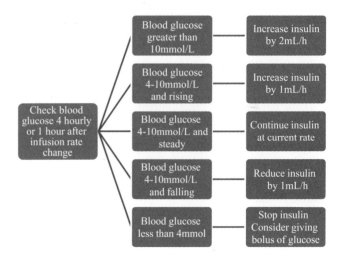

Figure 8.6 Insulin titration to blood glucose 4–10 mmol/L.

patients receiving intensive insulin for 'tight' glycaemic control (4.5–6.0 mmol/L) had a significantly higher 90-day mortality than those treated less intensively (blood sugar kept below 10 mmol/L) and suffered more than 15 times as many episodes of severe hypoglycaemia (blood sugar less than 2.2 mmol/L). Deaths during the NICE-SUGAR study were predominantly caused by cardiovascular events, although the investigators acknowledge that further research is required to determine the mechanisms of this (NICE-SUGAR Study Investigators 2009). Practices are therefore changing to the NICE-SUGAR recommendation of maintaining blood glucose levels below 10 mmol/L. This can be achieved using the algorithm of insulin titration (Figure 8.6).

Insulin titration

The following algorithm can be used as an example of insulin titration when using an insulin infusion of 1 unit/mL (Figure 8.6).

Problems with providing hydration and nutrition

Overfeeding

Providing effective nutritional support in critical care can help to maintain existing energy stores and avoid catabolism (Beer et al. 2012), however, excess energy provision should be avoided. For example, giving too large an amount of:

- calories supplied as glucose results in increased CO_2 production and retention
- carbohydrate results in steatosis of the liver, increased CO_2 production and hyperglycaemia
- fat results in lipid deposits in the lungs impairing gas exchange, and impairs the reticular endothelial system

- protein increases the rate of protein synthesis and breakdown with no net effect on nutritional balance.

(from Klein et al. 1998)

Refeeding syndrome

Refeeding syndrome is a constellation of metabolic disturbances resulting from the provision of nutrition to patients who are starved or severely malnourished (Mehanna et al. 2008). Reduced carbohydrate intake in malnourished patients leads to a decreased secretion of insulin. Fat and protein stores are catabolized to produce energy, leading to intracellular loss of phosphate and other electrolytes. When regular nutrition is re-established, carbohydrate metabolism recommences, resulting in increased insulin secretion. This then stimulates cellular uptake of phosphate, leading to profound hypophosphataemia (Hearing 2004).

Patients are determined to be at risk of refeeding when the patient has one or more of the following:

- BMI less than $16 \, kg/m^2$
- unintentional weight loss greater than 15% within the past 3–6 months
- little or no nutritional intake for more than 10 days
- low levels of potassium, phosphate, or magnesium prior to feeding

or two or more of the following:

- BMI less than $18.5 \, kg/m^2$
- unintentional weight loss greater than 10% within the past 3–6 months
- little or no nutritional intake for more than 5 days
- a history of alcohol abuse or drugs, including insulin, chemotherapy, antacids, or diuretics.

(NICE 2006)

In patients at risk, no more than 50% of their daily requirements should be provided for the first two days of feeding. Feeding should be started at a low rate, vitamins are recommended, and close monitoring and replacement of electrolyte levels are essential as follows:

- start nutrition support at a maximum of 10 kcal/kg/day, increasing levels slowly to meet full needs by 4–7 days
- use 5 kcal/kg/day in extreme cases of malnutrition (for example, BMI less than $14 \, kg/m^2$ or negligible intake for more than 15 days) and monitor cardiac rhythm
- restore circulatory volume and monitor fluid balance closely
- provide immediately before and during the first 10 days of feeding: oral thiamin 200–300 mg daily, vitamin B co strong 1 or 2 tablets, three times a day (or full dose daily intravenous vitamin B preparation, if necessary) and a balanced multivitamin/trace element supplement once daily

- provide oral, enteral, or intravenous supplements of potassium, phosphate and magnesium where necessary to prevent refeeding syndrome.

(NICE 2006)

Enteral feeding access in an intubated patient

Enteral feeding can be carried out in an intubated patient using the following.

- *Nasogastric (NG) tube* (fine bore or wider diameter). However, these tubes are absolutely contraindicated for patients with severe mid-face trauma or recent nasal surgery, and should be used with caution for patients with abnormal coagulation, oesophageal varices or stricture, recent banding or cauterization of varices or alkaline ingestion (Shlamovitz and Shah 2011). The NG tube should be inserted post intubation, using a laryngoscope and Magills forceps (a specific type of angled forceps) to give an adequate view.
- *Orogastric tube.* This type of tube is used to overcome some of the above contraindications of nasogatric tubes. For example, it can be used following nasal surgery and where there is abnormal coagulation. It is inserted post intubation using a laryngoscope and Magills forceps to give an adequate view. These are not appropriate for conscious patients as they stimulate the gag reflex.
- *Post-pyloric* (for example nasoduodenal and nasojejunal) tube. These tubes are effective when patients have upper GI dysfunction or an inaccessible upper GI tract (NICE 2006). They can be blindly inserted; however, successful placement using this method is difficult. It is therefore preferable that post-pyloric tubes are either inserted when a laparotomy is being performed, or endoscopically (Galley 2001).
- *Percutaneous endoscopic gastrostomy (PEG) tube.* NICE (2006) suggests that PEG tubes should be considered when enteral tube feeding is necessary long term (4 weeks or more). As the name indicates, tubes are placed endoscopically (Galley 2001).

Advantages of fine-bore and wide-bore enteral tubes

Wide-bore tubes are useful in gastric decompression and feeding as they can be aspirated easily. This allows practitioners to measure how much enteral feed is being absorbed, thus determining a patient's tolerance to feeding (Stroud et al. 2003). Complications associated with wide-bore tubes include mucosal irritation, oesophageal ulceration, oesophageal perforation, sinusitis and tracheo-oesophageal fistula (Scott et al. 1998). Therefore where patients are able to tolerate adequate volumes of enteral feed, a tube of the smallest diameter which allows delivery of the optimal volume of feed should be utilized, as these are more comfortable for patients and lead to fewer complications (Cresci 2005). Securing feeding tubes so that they are not accidentally removed is vital to ensure sufficient volumes of feed are administered, and to avoid further trauma to patients when new tubes need to be administered. Oral and nasal tubes can be secured safely using tape applied to the patient's cheek or nose and wrapped around the tube. However, if the patient is at risk of pulling out a nasal tube then a bridle system (a securing device passed behind the nasal septum and tied around the nasal tube) may be used to prevent this (*see* Figure 8.7a and 8.7b).

(a)

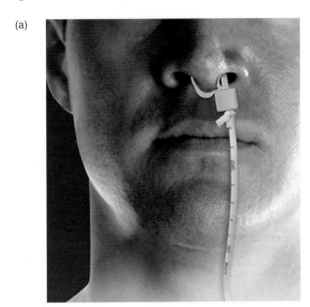

(b)

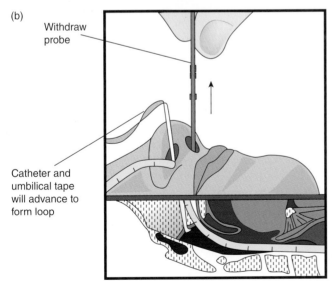

Withdraw probe

Catheter and umbilical tape will advance to form loop

Figure 8.7 AMT Bridle™ Nasal Tube Retaining System. (a) Nasogastric bridle in situ. (b) Nasogastric bridle position. Images supplied with compliments of Applied Medical Technology, Inc.

Risks and complications of nasogastric tube insertion (Durai et al. 2009)

Following correct insertion techniques and guidelines should help to avoid risks and complications associated with NG tube insertion. The most common complications relate to poor placement and include the following.

- Inadvertent insertion into the lungs. Due to the anatomy of the larynx and oesophagus it is possible that the nasogastric tube will pass into the trachea (Lo et al. 2008), which could result in a pneumothorax (Zausig et al. 2008). If this is not readily identified and the correct procedure is not followed for checking the tube position, it is possible that the feed will enter the patient's lungs. This can lead to pneumonia and severe sepsis, which could be fatal.
- Inadvertent insertion into the brain. There are numerous reports of NG tubes entering the brain through perforations in the base of the skull, for example caused by basal skull fractures (Elliott and Jones 2003).
- Coiling in the patient's throat. Refrigerating tubes prior to use may help to keep the tube stiff and less likely to coil. The use of a tube with a guide wire will also help.
- Perforation of the oesophagus. Although rare (Hutchinson et al. 2008), it is possible this may occur in pre-existing oesophageal disease.
- Retropharyngeal abscess. This may develop following perforation of a piriform sinus (Makay et al. 2008; Obon Azuara et al. 2007).
- Damage to the ciliary epithelium, and infection and sinusitis if in position for an extended period of time.
- Reflux of stomach contents into the oesophagus and risk of aspiration. The performance of the lower oesophageal sphincter can be disrupted, causing reflux of stomach contents, which may lead to aspiration pneumonitis. The risk is increased when patients are fed when lying down flat.

Checking NG tube position

Nasogastric and orogastric tubes should not be flushed, nor any liquid/feed administered through the tube until the position of the tube tip is confirmed (NPSA 2011). The NPSA (2011) has issued guidelines on how NG tube position should and should not be checked. This includes the following.

- All practitioners involved in checking the position of the NG tube have been assessed as competent in this task.
- All NG tubes used for feeding should be radio-opaque and have externally visible length markings.

- pH testing of aspirate from NG tube should be the first-line test method, with pH between 1 and 5.5 as the safe range indicating that the aspirate is acidic and from the stomach. pH indicator paper should be CE marked and intended by the manufacturer to test human gastric aspirate. Each test result should be documented on a chart kept at the patient's bedside.
- An X-ray should be used only as a second-line test when no aspirate can be obtained or pH indicator paper has failed to confirm a pH of 1 to 5.5.
- Once the position of the tube has been confirmed the documentation should include how placement was interpreted, confirm that any X-ray viewed was the most current X-ray for the correct patient, and include clear instructions as to further actions. Any tubes identified as being incorrectly placed should be removed immediately.

Only the above methods for checking tube position should be used, the following methods **must not** be used:

- the 'whoosh' test (auscultation of air injected through the NG tube)
- acidity/alkalinity testing of aspirate using blue litmus paper
- the absence of respiratory distress
- bubbling at the end of the NG tube
- appearance of feeding aspirate in the NG tube (NPSA 2005).

(*See also* Table 8.7)

Parenteral nutrition

Parenteral nutrition is liquid nutrition administered via a single dedicated lumen on either a central or peripheral vascular access device. This route is used when oral and/or enteral nutrition is unable to fully meet the patient's nutritional requirements. The aim of parenteral nutrition is to provide sufficient calories, nutrients and amino acids to match energy expenditure, hence avoiding negative energy balance. Critically ill patients should generally initially receive 25 kcal/kg/day, increasing to full requirements over the next 2–3 days. The main element of parenteral nutrition is carbohydrates, with minimal glucose requirements of approximately 2 g/kg/day. Other constituents include lipids, essential for fatty acid provision, amino acids, multivitamins and trace elements. Parental nutrition can be categorized as:

- low osmolarity, which includes only a proportion of nutritional needs and is generally delivered peripherally
- high osmolarity, which is designed to meet fully nutritional needs and which should be administered via a central venous catheter (Singer et al. 2009).

There is some debate concerning the optimal timing for starting total parenteral nutrition (TPN). European guidance indicates that TPN should be commenced within 24–48 hours for all patients in whom normal nutrition is not expected within 3 days, or where enteral nutrition is contraindicated or not tolerated (Singer et al. 2009). However, contemporaneous US recommendations state that it should be started relatively late – after 7 days of hospitalization where enteral feeding is not possible (McClave et al. 2009). The latter position is supported by more recent research, which compared early (at day 2) and late (day 8) initiation of TPN to supplement insufficient enteral feeding and found that the late initiation group had faster recovery and fewer complications (Casaer et al. 2011).

The debate about TPN composition and delivery, as well as its role in feeding the critically ill, will continue as different formulations are studied in relevant populations.

Table 8.7 Aspiration of stomach contents following enteral feeding and subsequent care

Step 1	Insert enteral feeding tube and confirm position				
Step 2	Commence feeding at 25–50 mL/h				
Step 3	Aspirate stomach contents after 6 hours of feeding				
Step 4					
Amount of aspirate	Aspirate less than 300 mL	Aspirate 300–400 mL	Aspirate 400–500 mL	Aspirate greater than 500 mL	Vomiting
Replacement/Discard plan	Replace aspirate Increase feed as tolerated	Replace 300 mL Discard balance	Replace 300 mL Discard balance	Replace 300 mL Discard balance	Stop feed Aspirate and discard stomach contents
Amended rate		Continue at the same rate	Reduce rate to 15–30 mL/h	Reduce rate to 10–20 mL/h	Restart feed after 1 hour at half the original rate

Complications

The main complications of TPN are:

- catheter-related sepsis (in about 50% of patients)
- glucose abnormalities (hyperglycaemia or hypoglycaemia)
- liver dysfunction (in more than 90% of patients)
- serum electrolyte and mineral disturbances
- volume overload.

Less common complications include:

- adverse reactions to lipid emulsions – hyperlipidemia
- hepatomegaly
- mild elevation of liver enzymes
- splenomegaly
- thrombocytopenia and leukopenia
- gallbladder complications – cholelithiasis, gallbladder sludge and cholecystitis caused or worsened by prolonged gallbladder stasis.

TPN should be administered in the same way as other intravenous infusions (see Dougherty and Lister 2011 for further information).

Ethical considerations

There are ethical challenges that arise in critical care hydration and nutrition. These focus primarily on negotiating nutrition with the conscious, but confused and agitated, patient deemed incompetent to make a decision, and also in respect of withdrawing or withholding nutrition and hydration at the end of life (*see* Chapter 17). In the former case, issues around truth-telling, restraint, manipulation and even bribery may undermine the dignity of the patient, and any trust between practitioners and the patient. In the case of end of life care, there is an understanding that loss of appetite and a diminished need for fluid are normal parts of the dying process (Marie Curie Palliative Care Institute 2009). However, while tools such as integrated care pathways for the dying in critical care may aid with directing cessation of feed and hydration during palliation, there may be staff and family members who feel uncomfortable with this aspect of care.

Procedure guideline 8.1: **Blood glucose monitoring**

Essential equipment

- Blood glucose monitor
- Test strips
- Control solution
- Single-use safety lancets

- Gloves
- Cotton wool/gauze
- Sharps box

Procedure

Action	Rationale
1 Before taking the device to the patient, the equipment needs to be checked for the following: ▪ testing trips are in date and have not been left exposed to air ▪ the monitor and test strips have been calibrated together ▪ if a new pack of strips is required, the monitor is recalibrated ▪ internal quality control carried out in accordance to hospital guidelines ▪ result of internal quality control is recorded in equipment log book and signed.	To ensure accuracy of the result and ensure patient safety (Roche Diagnostics 2004).
2 Where possible, explain and discuss the procedure with the patient. If the patient lacks the capacity to make decisions the practitioner must act in the patient's best interests.	To ensure that the patient understands the procedure and gives their valid consent. To ensure the patient's best interests are maintained (Mental Capacity Act 2005).

3 If appropriate, ask patient to sit or lie down.	To ensure the patient's safety and minimize the risks if they feel faint when blood is taken (Roche Diagnostics 2004).
4 Wash hands and put on gloves.	To minimize the risk of cross-infection and contamination (Fraise and Bradley 2009).
5 Take a single-use lancet and if it has depth settings, ensure the correct setting is used (most commonly middle one).	To minimize the risk of cross-infection and accidental needlestick injury (Fraise and Bradley 2009).
6 Take a blood sample from the side of the finger using the lancet, ensuring that the site of piercing is rotated. Avoid frequent use of index finger and thumb. Other areas may be used if finger or palm of hand is unusable. The fingertip may need 'milking' from palm of hand towards the finger to gain a large enough droplet of blood.	The side of the finger is less painful and easier to obtain a hanging droplet of blood. Sites are rotated to avoid infection from multiple stabbings, area becoming toughened and to reduce pain (Roche Diagnostics 2004).
7 Insert testing strip into blood glucose monitor and apply the blood to the testing strip. Some strips are hydrophilic and are dosed/filled from the side instead of dropping blood directly on to the strip. Ensure that the window on the test strip is entirely covered with blood.	The window on the test strip allows verification of a correctly dosed strip which needs to be covered to ensure accurate results (Blake and Nathan 2004; Roche Diagnostics 2004).
8 Dispose of lancet in a sharps container.	To reduce the risk of needlestick injury (Roche Diagnostics 2004).
9 Place gauze over puncture site and monitor for excess bleeding.	To ensure patient safety (Wallymahmed 2007).
10 Once result is obtained, document and sign.	To ensure accuracy (NMC 2009; Roche Diagnostics 2004).
11 Report any abnormal results.	To ensure appropriate treatment and obtain optimal blood glucose range (Wallymahmed 2007).
12 Document care.	To: ■ provide an accurate record ■ monitor effectiveness of procedure ■ reduce the risk of duplication of treatment ■ provide a point of reference or comparison in the event of later questions ■ acknowledge accountability for actions ■ facilitate communication and continuity of care. (NMC 2008; HCPC 2012; GMC 2013)

Procedure guideline 8.2: Insertion of a nasogastric tube in a sedated and intubated patient (adapted from The Royal Marsden Hospital Manual of Clinical Nursing Procedures 2011)

Essential equipment

- Clinically clean tray
- Fine-bore nasogastric tube with introducer OR wide bore nasogastric tube that has been stored in a deep freeze for at least half an hour before the procedure is to begin, to ensure a rigid tube that will allow for easy passage
- Receiver
- Sterile water

- Laryngoscope and blade
- Magills forceps (a specific type of angled forceps)
- 50 mL enteral syringe
- Hypoallergenic tape
- Adhesive patch if available
- Lubricating jelly
- CE marked-indicator strips with pH range of 0–6 or 1–11 with gradations of 0.5

Preprocedure

Action	Rationale
1 Where possible, explain and discuss the procedure with the patient. If the patient lacks the capacity to make decisions the practitioner must act in the patient's best interests.	To ensure that the patient understands the procedure and gives their valid consent. To ensure the patient's best interests are maintained (Mental Capacity Act 2005).
2 Position the patient supine in the bed.	To allow for easy passage of the NG tube.
3 Select the appropriate distance mark on the tube by measuring the distance on the tube from the patient's earlobe to the bridge of the nose plus the distance from the earlobe to the bottom of the xiphisternum (the NEX measurement).	To ensure that the appropriate length of tube is passed into the stomach NPSA 2011.
4 Wash hands with bactericidal soap and water or bactericidal alcohol hand rub, and assemble the equipment required. Put on gloves, apron and visor.	To minimize cross-infection (Fraise and Bradley 2009).
5 Follow manufacturer's instructions to prepare the NG tube, for example injecting sterile water down the tube and lubricating the proximal end of the tube with lubricating jelly.	Contact with water activates the coating inside the tube and on the tip. This lubricates the tube, assisting its passage through the nasopharynx and allowing easy withdrawal of the introducer.
6 Check that the nostrils are clear.	To identify any obstructions liable to prevent passage of the tube.
7 Using a laryngoscope, open the patient's mouth to visualize the back of the throat.	To enable the NG tube to be seen as it passes into the oropharynx.
8 Insert the proximal end of the tube into the clearer nostril and slide it backwards and inwards along the floor of the nose to the nasopharynx. If any obstruction is felt, withdraw the tube and try again in a slightly different direction or use the other nostril.	To facilitate the passage of the tube by following the natural anatomy of the nose.
9 As the tube passes down into the nasopharynx, look into the mouth and visualize the NG tube.	To ensure the NG tube is following the correct route.

10 Advance the tube through the pharynx using the Magills forceps until the predetermined mark has been reached (NEX measurement). If the patient shows signs of distress, for example coughing or ventilation problems, remove the tube immediately.	The tube may have accidentally been passed down the trachea instead of the pharynx. Distress may indicate that the tube is in the bronchus. However, absence of distress is not sufficient to assume the tube is not misplaced (NPSA 2005, 2011).
11 Secure the tape to the nostril with adherent dressing tape, for example Elastoplast, or an adhesive nasogastric stabilization/securing device (Burns et al 1995.). Alternatively Tegaderm/Deoderm can be applied to the cheek and then covered in Mepore to secure the nasogastric tube; this can help to prevent skin irritation. A hypoallergenic tape should be used if an allergy is present.	To hold the tube in place. To ensure patient comfort.
12 Measure the part of the visible tube from tip of nose and record this and the NEX measurement in care plan. Mark the tube at the exit site (nares) with a permanent marker pen.	To provide a record to assist in detecting movement of the tube (Metheny and Titler 2001; NPSA 2011).
13 Check the position of the tube to confirm that it is in the stomach by using the following methods.	To ensure that the tube is in the correct position. Feeding via the tube must not begin until the correct position of the tube has been confirmed (NPSA 2011) as this may lead, inter alia, to aspiration of stomach contents. To confirm placement of NG tube.

First-line test method: pH paper

(a) Aspirate 0.5–1 mL of stomach contents and test pH on indicator strips (NPSA 2011; Rollins 1997).	(a) Indicator strips should have gradations of 0.5 or paper with a range of 0–6 or 1–11 to distinguish between gastric acid and bronchial secretions (NPSA 2011).
(b) When aspirating fluid for pH testing, wait at least 1 hour after a feed or medication has been administered (either orally or via the tube). Before aspirating, flush the tube with 20 mL of air to clear other substances (Metheny et al. 1993).	(b) To prove an accurate test result because the feed or medication may raise the pH of the stomach.
(c) Assess pH of aspirate.	(c) A pH level of between 1 and 5.5 is unlikely to be pulmonary aspirates and it is considered appropriate to proceed to feed through the tube (Metheny and Meert 2004; NPSA 2011). If a pH falls within the range 5–6, it is recommended that a second competent practitioner checks the reading to ascertain whether the reading indicates it is safe (pH 1–5.5) to commence feeding. If a pH of 6.0 or above is obtained then feeding **must not** commence. This is because there is a risk of the nasogastric tube being incorrectly placed (NPSA 2011).
	The nasogastric tube may need to be repositioned or checked with an X-ray.
Second-line test method: X-ray confirmation. Organize an X-ray of chest and upper abdomen.	X-ray of radio-opaque tubes is the most accurate confirmation of position and is the method of choice in patients with altered anatomy, those who are aspirating or are unconscious with no gag reflex (NPSA 2011).

299

(Continued)

Procedure guideline 8.2: (Continued)

Action	Rationale
14 The following methods **must not** be used to test the position of a nasogastric feeding tube: auscultation (introducing air into the nasogastric tube and checking for a bubbling sound via a stethoscope, also known as the 'whoosh test'), use of litmus paper or absence of respiratory distress.	These tests are not accurate or reliable as a method of checking the position of a nasogastric tube as they have been shown to give false-positive results (Metheny and Meert 2004; NPSA 2011).
15 When the position is confirmed as correct, (a) remove the introducer by using (b) gentle traction. If appropriate, secure nasogastric tube with a bridle system.	(a) The introducer is no longer required. (b) To avoid damaging the mucosa. Using a bridle will help to prevent accidental nasogastric tube removal in agitated patients.
16 Document the tip position in the patient's notes.	To record the position (NMC 2009).
17 Document care.	To: ■ provide an accurate record ■ monitor effectiveness of procedure ■ reduce the risk of duplication of treatment ■ provide a point of reference or comparison in the event of later questions ■ acknowledge accountability for actions ■ facilitate communication and continuity of care. (NMC 2008; HCPC 2012; GMC 2013)

Procedure guideline 8.3: Administration of enteral feed (adapted from The Royal Marsden Hospital Manual of Clinical Nursing Procedures 2011)

Essential equipment

■ 50 mL enteral or catheter-tipped syringe
■ Administration set
■ Administration pump

■ Prescribed feed (for example, commercially available 'ready-to-hang' feed)

Optional equipment

■ Sterile water. Water should be fresh and kept covered

Procedure

Action	Rationale
1 Where possible, explain and discuss the procedure with the patient. If the patient lacks the capacity to make decisions the practitioner must act in the patient''s best interests.	To ensure that the patient understands the procedure and gives their valid consent. To ensure the patient's best interests are maintained (Mental Capacity Act 2005).
2 Check the date on the feed container.	To ensure that the feed has not passed its expiry date.
3 Shake the feed container gently.	To ensure the feed is evenly dispersed therefore reducing the risk of blocking the administration set.

4	Take a new administration set from sealed package and ensure that the roller clamp/tap is closed.	To avoid accidental spillage of feed from end of administration set.
5	Screw the giving set tightly on to the feed container.	In order to pierce the seal on the container and maintain a sealed system (Matlow *et al.* 2006).
6	Hang the container upside down from the hook on a stand.	To avoid backflow of intestinal contents into the feed container (Matlow *et al.* 2006).
7	Open the roller clamp/tap and prime the feed to the end of the administration set (follow instructions for individual pump).	This ensures that air is not fed into the stomach when feeding commences.
8	Position the tubing of the administration set into the pump as directed by the manufacturer's instructions.	To connect the administration set to the pump device.
9	Set the rate of the feed as directed by the manufacturer's instructions and according to the patient's feeding regimen.	To ensure the correct rate of feed is administered.
10	Flush the feeding tube slowly with a minimum of 30 mL of sterile water using an enteral syringe attached to the end of the feeding tube.	To ensure the patency of the feeding tube; 30 mL will ensure the full tube is thoroughly flushed and doing this slowly enables the practitioner to identify any blockages and safely unblock the tube without causing harm to the patient or splash-back to the practitioner. The use of sterile water helps to avoid the introduction of bacteria and infection. All enteral administration should take place using dedicated enteral syringes with special connectors to avoid IV administration.
11	Remove the end cover from the administration set and connect to the feeding tube.	To ensure that the feed is delivered via the enteral feeding tube.
12	Set the rate of the feeding pump and commence administration of feed.	To ensure that the feed is delivered via the enteral feeding tube.
13	Document care and the time that the feed commenced and the rate of administration.	To ensure accurate documentation of nutritional and fluid intake (NMC 2008). To: ■ provide an accurate record ■ monitor effectiveness of procedure ■ reduce the risk of duplication of treatment ■ provide a point of reference or comparison in the event of later questions ■ acknowledge accountability for actions ■ facilitate communication and continuity of care. (NMC 2008; HCPC 2012; GMC 2013)
14	Dispose of any equipment that is no longer required.	To reduce the chance of equipment being re-used and to reduce cross-contamination with new equipment.

Competency statement 8.1: Specific procedure competency statements for blood glucose monitoring

Complete assessment against relevant fundamental competency statements (*see* Chapter 2, pp. 20, 21)	Evidence
Specific procedure competency statements for blood glucose monitoring	**Evidence of competency for specific procedures blood glucose monitoring**
Demonstrate ability to: ■ teach and assess or ■ learn from assessment.	Examples of evidence of teaching, assessing and learning.
Identify reason(s) for blood glucose monitoring, including: ■ patient is diabetic ■ patient is known to have unstable blood glucose levels ■ patient has had surgery which may affect blood glucose levels ■ patient is on enteral or parenteral feed ■ patient is on insulin infusion.	There are a number of ways in which competency can be judged. These include: ■ direct observation of procedure ■ testimonial from *people*, carer and or staff members ■ teaching session for peers ■ completion of a reflective text, workbook, or educational package ■ examination ■ test ■ discussion with supervisor/mentor.
Identify risks, potential problems and complications of blood glucose monitoring and how to prevent or manage them, including: ■ introduction of infection at sample site ■ bleeding at sample site ■ inaccurate results ■ needle stick injury.	
Demonstrate knowledge and understanding of local and national policies, guidance and procedures in relation to blood glucose monitoring.	
Demonstrate knowledge and understanding of evidence base in relation to blood glucose monitoring.	
Demonstrate skills that are required in relation to blood glucose monitoring, including: ■ ability to take sample effectively ■ use of blood glucose monitor ■ use of blood gas machine ■ adjustment of insulin infusion ■ administration of glucose where necessary.	
Prepare equipment required in relation to blood glucose monitoring.	
Demonstrate the correct technique for the procedure in relation to blood glucose monitoring: ■ take a blood sample from the side of the finger using the lancet or from arterial/central line ■ insert testing strip into blood glucose monitor and apply the blood to the testing strip ■ once result is obtained, document and sign ■ dispose of materials as per local infection control guidelines ■ report any abnormal results.	

Competency statement 8.2: Specific procedure competency statements for insertion of a nasogastric tube in an intubated patient

Complete assessment against relevant fundamental competency statements (*see* Chapter 2, pp. 20, 21)	Evidence
Specific procedure competency statements for Insertion of a nasogastric tube in an intubated patient	**Evidence of competency for insertion of a nasogastric tube in an intubated patient**
Demonstrate ability to: ■ teach and assess or ■ learn from assessment.	Examples of evidence of teaching, assessing and learning.
Identify reason(s) for insertion of a nasogastric tube in an intubated patient, including: ■ malnourishment or risk of malnourishment ■ patient unable to swallow ■ patient has a functioning GI system.	There are a number of ways in which competency can be judged. These include: ■ direct observation of procedure ■ testimonial from people, carer and/or staff members
Identify risks, potential problems and complications of insertion of a nasogastric tube in an intubated patient and how to prevent or manage them, including: ■ inadvertent insertion into the lungs ■ inadvertent insertion into the brain ■ coiling in the patient's throat ■ perforation of the oesophagus ■ retropharyngeal abscess ■ damage to the ciliary epithelium.	■ teaching session for peers ■ completion of a reflective text, workbook, or educational package ■ examination ■ test ■ discussion with supervisor/mentor.
Demonstrate knowledge and understanding of local and national policies, guidance, and procedures in relation to insertion of a nasogastric tube in an intubated patient, including: ■ NICE (2006) ■ Kreymann et al. (2006).	
Demonstrate knowledge and understanding of evidence base in relation to insertion of a nasogastric tube in an intubated patient: ■ why a nasogastric tube is required ■ wide bore tube versus fine bore tube and when to change ■ contraindications of nasogastric tube insertion.	
Demonstrate skills that are required in relation to insertion of a nasogastric tube in an intubated patient: ■ measuring the NEX measurement ■ preparing the tube ■ using a laryngoscope and Magills forceps to insert the tube ■ securing the tube to the nostril ■ checking the position of the tube.	
Prepare equipment required in relation to insertion of a nasogastric tube in an intubated patient, including: ■ nasogastric tube ■ laryngoscope and blade ■ Magills forceps ■ lubrucating jelly ■ pH paper.	

303

(Continued)

Competency statement 8.2: (*Continued*)

Demonstrate the correct technique for the procedure in relation to insertion of a nasogastric tube in an intubated patient:

- ensure the patient is adequately sedated
- ensure the patient has no contraindications to nasogastric tube insertion, e.g. skull fractures, varices, abnormal coagulation
- select the appropriate distance mark on the tube by measuring the distance on the tube from the patient's earlobe to the bridge of the nose plus the distance from the earlobe to the bottom of the xiphisternum
- prepare the NG tube, for example inject sterile water down the tube and lubricate the proximal end of the tube with lubricating jelly
- using a laryngoscope open the patient's mouth to visualize the back of the throat
- insert the proximal end of the tube into the nostril and advance the tube through the pharynx using the Magills forceps until the predetermined mark has been reached
- secure the tube to the nostril
- measure the part of the visible tube from tip of nose and record this and the NEX measurement in care plan
- check the position of the tube.

Competency statement 8.3: Specific procedure competency statements for administration of enteral feed

Complete assessment against relevant fundamental competency statements (*see* Chapter 2, pp. 20, 21)	Evidence
Specific procedure competency statements for administration of enteral feed	**Evidence of competency for administration of enteral feed**
Demonstrate ability to: ■ teach and assess or ■ learn from assessment.	Examples of evidence of teaching, assessing and learning.
Identify reason(s) for administration of enteral feed including: ■ patient is sedated and ventilated ■ patient is unable to tolerate oral nutrition ■ patient is unable to fulfil nutritional requirements with oral nutrition alone.	There are a number of ways in which competency can be judged. These include: ■ direct observation of procedure ■ testimonial from people, carer and or staff members ■ teaching session for peers
Identify risks, potential problems and complications of administration of enteral feed and how to prevent or manage them, including: ■ re-feeding syndrome ■ over-feeding ■ nausea and vomiting ■ aspiration.	■ completion of a reflective text, workbook, or educational package ■ examination ■ test ■ discussion with supervisor/mentor.
Demonstrate knowledge and understanding of local and national policies, guidance and procedures in relation to administration of enteral feed: ■ NICE (2006).	

Demonstrate knowledge and understanding of evidence base in relation to administration of enteral feed:
■ Kreymann et al. (2006).

Demonstrate skills that are required in relation to administration of enteral feed, including:
■ clean technique
■ setting up administration set and pump.

Prepare equipment required in relation to administration of enteral feed, including:
■ appropriate syringe
■ administration set
■ administration pump
■ correct enteral feed.

Demonstrate the correct technique for the procedure in relation to administration of enteral feed:
■ check the date on the feed container
■ shake the feed container gently
■ connect new administration set to the feed container and prime
■ position the tubing of the administration set into the pump and set the rate of the feed according to the patient's feeding regimen
■ flush the feeding tube and connect the administration set to the tube.

References and further reading

Alexander JW, MacMillan BG, Stinnett JD et al. (1980) Beneficial effects of aggressive protein feeding in severely burned children. *Annals of Surgery* **192**(4): 505–517.

Academisch Ziekenhuls Maastricht (AZM) (2012) *What is Nutritional Assessment?* http://www.nutritionalassessment.english.azm.nl/wat+is+na.htm [accessd 2 October 2012].

Beer R, Fischer M, Dietmann A et al. (2012) Hypothermia and nutrition: at present more questions than answers? *Critical Care* **16**(Suppl 2): A28.

Blake DR and Nathan DM (2004) Point-of-care testing for diabetes. *Critical Care Nurse* **27**(2): 150–161.

Boldt J (2010) Use of albumin: an update. *British Journal of Anaesthesia* **104**(3): 276–284.

Braga M, Ljungqvist O, Soeters P et al. (2009) ESPEN guidelines on parenteral nutrition: surgery. *Clinical Nutrition* **28**: 378–386.

Brandstrup B, Tonnesen H, Beier-Holgersen R et al. (2003) Effects of intravenous fluid restriction on postoperative complications: comparison of two perioperative fluid regimens: a randomized assessor-blinded multicentre trial. *Annals of Surgery* **238**(5): 641–648.

Bundgaard-Neilsen M, Holte K and Secher NH (2007) Monitoring of peri-operative fluid administration by individualized goal-directed therapy. *Acta Anaesthesiologica Scandinavica* **105**: 465–474.

Burns SM, Martin M, Robbins V et al (1995) Comparison of nasogastric tube securing method and tube types in medical intensive care patients. *American Journal of Critical Care* **4**(3): 198–203.

Casaer MP, Mesotten D, Hermans G et al. (2011) Early versus late parenteral nutrition in critically ill adults. *New England Journal of Medicine* **365**: 506–517.

Cavallaro F, Sandroni C, Marano C et al. (2010) Diagnostic accuracy of passive leg raising for prediction of fluid responsiveness in adults: systematic review and meta-analysis of clinical studies. *Intensive Care Medicine* **36**(9): 1475–1483.

Chappell D, Jacob M, Hofmann-Keifer K et al. (2008) A rational approach to perioperative fluid management. *Anesthesiology* **109**: 723–740.

Cheatham ML, Chapman WC, Key SP and Sawyers JL (1995) A meta-analysis of selective versus routine nasogastric decompression after elective laparotomy. *Annals of Surgery* **221**(5): 469–476.

Cresci G (2005) *Nutrition Support for the Critically Ill Patient.* Boca Raton: Taylor & Francis.

Dougherty L and Lister S (2011) *The Royal Marsden Manual of Clinical Nursing Procedures* (8e). Oxford: Wiley-Blackwell.

Durai R, Venkatraman R andPhilip CH (2009) Nasogastric tubes 2: risks and guidance on avoiding and dealing with complications. *Nursing Times* **105**: 17. http://www.nursingtimes.net/nursing-practice/clinical-specialisms/gastroenterology/nasogastric-tubes-2-risks-and-guidance-on-avoiding-and-dealing-with-complications/5000684.article [accessed 29 June 2012].

Dutton RP (2006) Fluid management for trauma; where are we now? *Continuing Education in Anaesthesia, Critical Care & Pain* **6**(4): 144–147.

Elliott M and Jones L (2003) Inadvertent intracranial insertion of nasogastric tubes: an overview and nursing implications. *Australian Emergency Nursing Journal* **6**(1): 10–14.

Ellis KJ (2000) Human body composition: in vivo methods. *Physiological Reviews* **80**(2): 649–680.

Fraise AP and Bradley T (eds) (2009) *Ayliffe's Control of Healthcare-associated Infection: a practical handbook* (5e). London: Hodder Arnold.

Galley H (2001) *Critical Care Focus 7: Nutritional issues*. London: BMJ Books.

General Medical Council (2013) *Good Medical Practice*. London: GMC. http://www.gmc-uk.org/gmp2013 [accessed 25 March 2013].

Grocott MP, Mythen MG and Gan TJ (2005) Perioperative fluid management and clinical outcomes in adults. *Anesthia & Analgesia* **100**: 1093–1106.

Hausel J, Nygren J, Lagerkranser M et al. (2001) A carbohydrate-rich drink reduces preoperative discomfort in elective surgery patients. *Anesthesia & Analgesia* **93**(5): 1344–1350.

Health and Care Professions Council (2012) *Standard of Conduct, Performance and Ethics*. London: HCPC. http://www.hcpc-uk.org/assets/documents/10003B6EStandardsofconduct,performanceandethics.pdf [accessed January 2013]

Hearing S (2004) Refeeding syndrome is underdiagnosed and under-treated, but treatable. *British Medical Journal* **328**: 908–909.

Heenen S, De Backer D and Vincent J-L (2006) How can the response to volume expansion in patients with spontaneous respiratory movements be predicted? *Critical Care* **10**: R102.

Heyland D, Cook D, Winder B et al. (1995) Enteral nutrition in the critically ill patient: a prospective study. *Critical Care Medicine* **23**: 1055–1060.

Heyland DK, Novak F, Drover JW et al. (2001) Should immunonutrition become routine in critically ill patients? A systematic review of the evidence. *Journal of the American Medical Association* **286**: 944–953.

Hutchinson R, Ahmed A and Menzies D (2008) A case of intramural oesophageal dissection secondary to nasogastric tube insertion. *Annals of the Royal College of Surgeons of England* **90**(7): W4–W7.

Iregui MG, Prentice D, Sherman G et al. (2003) Physicians' estimates of cardiac index and intravascular volume based on clinical assessment versus transesophageal Doppler measurements obtained by critical care nurses. *American Journal of Critical Care* **12**(4): 336–342.

Klein CJ, Stanek GS and Wiles CE (1998) Overfeeding macronutrients to critically ill adults: metabolic complications. *Journal of the American Dietetic Association* **98**: 795–806.

Kondrup J, Allison SP, Elia M et al. (2003a) ESPEN guidelines for nutrition screening 2002. *Clinical Nutrition* **22**(4): 415–421.

Kondrup J, Rasmussen HH, Hamberg O et al. (2003b) Nutritional risk screening (NRS 2002): a new method based on an analysis of controlled clinical trials. *Clinical Nutrition* **22**: 321–336.

Kreymann KG, Berger MM, Deutz NE et al. (2006) ESPEN guidelines on enteral nutrition: intensive care. *Clinical Nutrition* **25**(2): 210–223.

Lo JO, Wu V, Reh D et al (2008) Diagnosis and management of a misplaced nasogastric tube into the pulmonary pleura. *Archives of Otolaryngology, Head and Neck Surgery* **134**(5): 547–550.

Lobo DN, Bostock KA, Neal KR et al. (2002) Effect of salt and water balance on recovery of gastrointestinal function after elective colonic resection: a randomised controlled trial. *Lancet* **359**(9320): 1812–1818.

Long CL, Schaffel BS, Geiger JW et al. (1979) Metabolic response to injury and illness: estimation of energy and protein needs from indirect calorimetry and nitrogen balance. *Journal of Parenteral and Enteral Nutrition* **3**: 452–456.

Maitland K, Kiguli S, Opoka RO et al. (2011) Mortality after fluid bolus in African children with severe infection. *New England Journal of Medicine* **364**: 2483–2495.

Makay O, Icoz G, Akyildiz S et al. (2008) Pyriform sinus perforation secondary to nasogastric tube insertion. *ANZ Journal of Surgery* **78**(7): 624.

Malnutrition Advisory Group (2004) *Malnutrition Universal Screening Tool*. Redditch: BAPEN.

Marie Curie Palliative Care Institute Liverpool (2009) *The Liverpool Care Pathway for the Dying Patient (LCP) version 12 core documentation*. http://www.mcpcil.org.uk/liverpool-care-pathway/documentation-lcp.htm#core

Marik PE and Zagola GP (2001)Early enteral nutrition in acutely ill patients: a systematic review. *Critical Care Medecine* **29**(12): 2264–2270.

Marik PE, Baram M and Vahid B (2008) Does central venous pressure predict fluid responsiveness? A systematic review of the literature and the tale of seven mares. *Chest* **134**: 172–178.

Marini J and Wheeler A (1997) *Critical Care Medicine: the essentials* (2e). Baltimore: Williams & Wilkins.

Matlow A, Jacobson M, Wray R et al. (2006) Enteral tube hub as a reservoir for transmissible enteric bacteria. *American Journal of Infection Control* **34**(3): 131–133.

Mehanna H, Moledina J and Travis J (2008) Refeeding syndrome: what it is, and how to prevent and treat it. *British Medical Journal* **336**: 1495.

Mental Capacity Act (2005) http://www.legislation.gov.uk/ukpga/2005/9/pdfs/ukpga_20050009_en.pdf [accessed 9 February 2012].

McClave SA, Martindale RG, Vanek VW et al., ASPEN board of directors (2009) Guidelines for the provision and assessment of nutrition support therapy in the adult critically ill patient: Society of Critical Care Medicine (SCCM) and American Society for Parenteral and Enteral Nutrition (ASPEN). *Journal of Parenteral and Enteral Nutrition* **33**: 277–316.

Metheny NA and Meert KL (2004) Monitoring feeding tube placement. *Nutrition in Clinical Practice* **19**(5): 487–495.

Metheny NA and Titler MG (2001) Assessing placement of feeding tubes. *American Journal of Nursing* **101**(5): 36–45; quiz 45–46.

Metheny N, Reed L, Wiersema L et al. (1993) Effectiveness of pH measurements in predicting feeding tube placement: an update. *Nursing Research* **42**(6): 324–331.

Miletin MS, Stewart TE and Norton PG (2002) Influences on physicians' choices of intravenous colloids. *Intensive Care Medicine* **28**(7): 917–924.

Moore EE and Jones TN (1986) Benefits of immediate jejunostomy feeding after major abdominal trauma: a prospective randomized study. *Journal of Trauma* **26**: 874–881.

Myburgh JA, Finfer S, Bellomo R, et al. for the CHEST (Crystalloid versus Hydroxy-Ethyl Starch Trial) Investigators and the Australian and New Zealand Intensive Care Society Clinical Trials Group (2012) Hydroxyethyl starch or saline for fluid resuscitation in intensive care. *New England Journal of Medicine* 2012DOI: 10.1056/NEJMoa1209759.

Mythen M, Swart M, Acheson N et al. (2012) Perioperative fluid management: consensus statement from the enhanced recovery partnership. *Perioperative Medicine* **1**: 2–4.

NICE (2006) *Nutrition Support in Adults* CG32. www.nice.org.uk/nutrition-support-in-adults-cg32

NICE-SUGAR Study Investigators (2009) Intensive versus conventional glucose control in critically ill patients. *New England Journal of Medicine* **360**: 1283–1297.

Nursing and Midwifery Council (2008) *The Code: standards of conduct, performance and ethics for nurses and midwives*. London: NMC. http://www.nmc-uk.org/Documents/Standards/The-code-A4-20100406.pdf [accessed 15 February 2012].

Nursing and Midwifery Council (2009) Record Keeping. Guidance for nurses and midwives. London: NMC. http://www.nmc-uk.org/Documents/NMC-Publications/NMC-Record-Keeping-Guidance.pdf [accessed 12 February 2013].

National Patient Safety Agency (2005) *Reducing the harm caused by misplaced nasogastric feeding tubes*. Patient Safety Alert 05. London: NPSA.

National Patient Safety Agency (2011) *Reducing the harm caused by misplaced nasogastric feeding tubes in adults, children and infants*. Patient Safety Alert NPSA/2011/PSA002. London: NPSA.

Obon Azu, Gutiérrez Cía I and Montoiro Allué R (2007) Adverse events by nasogastric tube placement. *Anales de Medicina Interna* 24(9): 461–462.

Ortega R, Gines P, Uriz J et al. (2002) Terlipressin therapy with and without albumin for patients with hepatorenal syndrome: results of a prospective, nonrandomized study. *Hepatology* 36(4): 941–948.

Pain RW (1977) Body fluid compartments. *Anaesthesia & Intensive Care* 5(4): 284–294.

Payen D, de Pont AJM, Sakr Y et al. (2008) A positive fluid balance is associated with a worse outcome in patients with acute renal failure. *Critical Care* 12: R74.

Pearce CB and Duncan HD (2002) Enteral feeding. Nasogastric, nasojejunal, percutaneous endoscopic gastrostomy, or jejunostomy: its indications and limitations. *Postgraduate Medical Journal* 78: 198–204.

Pearse R, Dawson D, Fawcett J et al. (2005) Early goal-directed therapy after major surgery reduces complications and duration of hospital stay. A randomised controlled trial. *Critical Care* 9(6): R687–693.

Perner A, Haase N, Guttormsen AB et al. for the 6S Trial Group and the Scandinavian Critical Care Trials Group (2012) Hydroxyethyl starch 130/0.4 versus Ringer's acetate in severe sepsis. *New England Journal of Medicine* 367: 124–134.

Peruzzi WT, Logemann JA, Currie D and Moen SG (2001) Assessment of aspiration in patients with tracheostomies: comparison of the bedside colored dye assessment with videofluoroscopic examination. *Respiratory Care* 46: 243–247.

Powell-Tuck J, Gosling P, Lobo DN et al. (2011) *British Consensus Guidelines on Intravenous Fluid Therapy for Adult Surgical Patients (GIFTASUP)*. London: NHS National Library of Health. http://www.bapen.org.uk/pdfs/bapen_pubs/giftasup.pdf [accessed 1 October 2012].

Roche Diagnostics (2004) Accu-Chem Safe T-Pro Plus: information leaflet. East Sussex: Roche.

Rollins H (1997) A nose for trouble. *Nursing Times* 93(49): 66–67.

Russell CA and Elia M (2011) *Nutrition screening survey in the UK and Republic of Ireland in 2010*. Redditch: BAPEN.

SAFE Study Investigators (2004) A comparison of albumin and saline for fluid resuscitation in the intensive care unit. *New England Journal of Medicine* 350(22): 2247–2256.

St George's Healthcare NHS Trust (2012) *Tracheostomy guidelines: swallowing*. http://www.stgeorges.nhs.uk/trachswallowing.asp [accessed 6 July 2012].

Scott A, Skerratt S and Adam S (1998) *Nutrition for the Critically Ill: a practical handbook*. London: Arnold.

Shaw AD, Bagshaw SM, Goldstein SL et al. (2012) Major complications, mortality and resource utilization after open abdominal surgery. *Annals of Surgery* 255: 821–829.

Shippy CR, Appel PL and Shoemaker WC (1984) Reliability of clinical monitoring to assess blood volume in critically ill patients. *Critical Care Medicine* 12(2): 107–112.

Shlamovitz G and Shah N (2011) *Nasogastric tube*. http://emedicine.medscape.com/article/80925-overview#a01 [accessed 29 June 2012].

Singer P, Berger M, Van den Berghe G et al. (2009) ESPEN Guidelines on parenteral nutrition: intensive care. *Clinical Nutrition* 28: 387–400.

Soni N (2009) British consensus guidelines on intravenous fluid therapy for adult surgical patients (GIFTASUP) – Cassandra's view. *Anaesthesia* 64: 235–238.

Soop M, Nygren J, Myrenfors P et al. (2001) Perioperative oral carbohydrate treatment attenuates immediate postoperative insulin resistance *American Journal of Physiology – Endocrinology & Metabolism* 280(4): E576–E583.

Starling E (1896) On the absorption of fluid from the connective tissue spaces. *Journal of Physiology (Lond)* 19: 312–326.

Stroud M, Duncan H and Nightingale J (2003) Guidelines for enteral feeding in adult hospital patients. *Gut* 52(Suppl VII): vii1–vii12.

Tortora B and Derrickson GJ (2011) *Principles of Anatomy and Physiology* (13e). New Jersey: John Wiley and Sons.

Van den Berghe G, Wouters P, Weekers F et al. (2001) Intensive insulin therapy in critically ill patients. *New England Journal of Medicine* 345: 1359–1367.

Van der Riet P, Brooks D and Ashby M (2006) Nutrition and hydration at the end of life: pilot study of a palliative care experience. *Journal of Law & Medicine* 14: 182–198.

Vincent JL, Sakr Y, Sprung CL et al. (2006) Sepsis in European intensive care units: results of the SOAP study. *Critical Care Medicine* 34(2): 344–353.

Wallymahmed M (2007) Capillary blood glucose monitoring. *Nursing Standard* 21(38): 35–38.

Weinbaum S, Tarbell JM and Damiano ER (2007) The structure and function of the endothelial glycocalyx layer. *Annual Review of Biomedical Engineering* 9: 121–167.

White SA and Goldhill DR (1997) Is Hartmann's the solution? *Anaesthesia* 52(5): 422–427.

Worthington ML and Cresci G (2011) Immune-modulating formulas: who wins the meta-analysis race? *Nutrition in Clinical Practice* 26(6): 650–655.

Zausig YA, Graf BM and Gust R (2008) Occurrence of a pneumothorax secondary to malpositioned nasogastric tube: a case report. *Minerva Anestesiologica* 74(12): 735–738.

Chapter 9

Continuous renal replacement therapies: assessment, monitoring and care

Annette Richardson and Jayne Whatmore

Newcastle upon Tyne Hospitals NHS Foundation Trust, Newcastle upon Tyne, UK

Critical Care Manual of Clinical Procedures and Competencies, First Edition.
Edited by Jane Mallett, John W. Albarran, and Annette Richardson.
© 2013 John Wiley & Sons, Ltd. Published 2013 by John Wiley & Sons, Ltd.

Definition

Continuous renal replacement therapy (CRRT) is an extra-corporeal process in which blood is circulated outside the body and through an artificial filter (haemofilter) to remove excess fluid and waste products of metabolism from the patient.

Blood is removed from and returned to the patient through a double-lumen central venous catheter (CVC) continuously using a pump. Waste products are removed into a collection bag and other tubing delivers dialystate and/or substitution fluid. All tubing and the haemofilter are generally referred to as the CRRT circuit (Figure 9.1).

Aims and indications

Continuous renal replacement therapy (CRRT) acts in place of failing kidneys by withdrawing excess fluid and waste

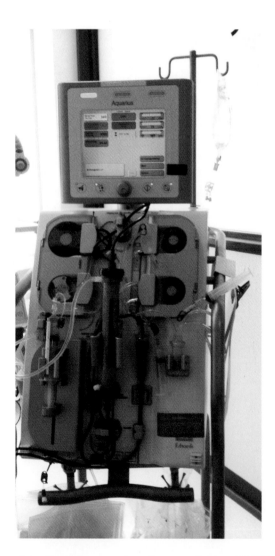

Figure 9.1 Continuous renal replacement therapy (CCRT) circuit.

from the body. CRRT allows slow continuous removal of fluid and waste from the blood to regulate its volume, chemical composition and pH. This minimizes dangerous electrolyte imbalance, the risk of hypotension and arrhythmias (Levy et al. 2004), making this therapy particularly suitable for patients who are critically ill. CRRT is a common supportive renal replacement therapy for critically ill patients with acute kidney injury (AKI).

Anatomy and physiology of the kidney

The kidney consists of the cortex, medulla and renal pelvis (Figure 9.2) (Tortora and Derrickson 2011). The cortex (outer layer) and the medulla (inner layer) are referred to as the functioning part of the kidney. The renal pelvis is a funnel-shaped structure which connects to the ureter, allowing urine to pass from the kidney into the bladder. Each kidney has about 1 million nephrons, each of which is situated in both the cortex and medulla (Figure 9.3). A nephron is made up of a glomerulus (a collection of capillaries) and a renal tubule. The renal tubule consists of a Bowman's capsule (also known as the glomerular capsule), the proximal convoluted tube, the loop of Henle, followed by the distal convoluted tubule. The first part of the nephron is the glomerulus.

Blood enters the kidney through the renal artery. The renal artery divides into branches of arteries until it becomes the afferent arteriole, which carries blood to the glomerulus. Blood then leaves the glomerulus through the efferent arteriole and is returned to the venous system and leaves the kidneys via the renal vein. As the diameter of the efferent arteriole is smaller than that of the afferent arteriole, a pressure gradient is built up in the glomerulus, which pushes out small molecules (salts, glucose and urea) and water – a process known as ultrafiltration. However, larger molecules (proteins and glycogen) stay within the capillary network. The particles that are pushed out with water enter the renal tubule via Bowman's capsule, which surrounds the glomerulus. The filtrate then passes down the proximal convoluted tubule and the loop of Henle to the distal convoluted tubule, allowing the removal of waste products and water, and the reabsorption of beneficial solutes and water to enable the concentration of urine to be adjusted according to fluid balance status. The process is complicated and is carried out by the specialized cells within each part of the nephron. Much of the salt and water, glucose and amino acids are reabsorbed into the capillaries surrounding the proximal convoluted tubule. The ascending loop of Henle concentrates the salt in the surrounding renal tissue, causing water to be reabsorped by osmosis in the descending loop. The distal convoluted tubule regulates pH via secretion or reabsorption of hydrogen ions and bicarbonate. Active transport of ions (for example sodium and calcium) also occurs in this tubule, much of which is regulated by the endocrine system via, for example, the hormone aldosterone. The distal convoluted tubules from several nephrons empty into a system of urine-collecting ducts (which are normally impermeable

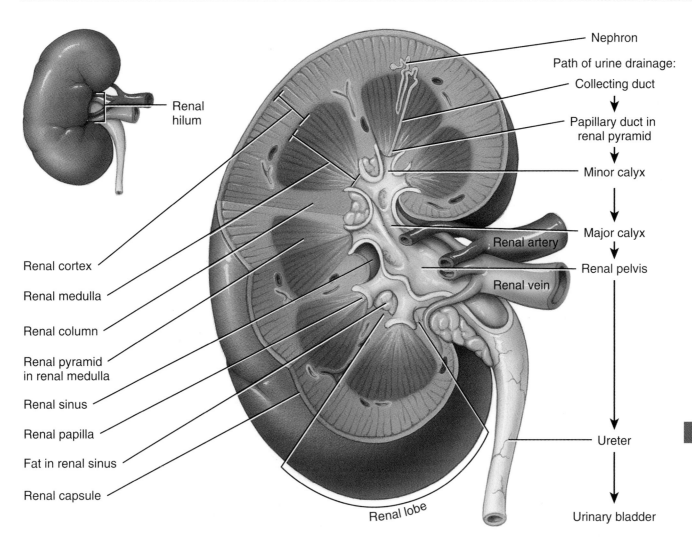

Figure 9.2 Anterior view of dissection of right kidney (from Tortora and Derrickson 2011, reproduced with permission from Wiley).

311

to water) and from here the urine drains into large papillary ducts in the renal pelvis. The juxtaglomerular apparatus (near the glomerular) regulates the nephron and is responsible for production and secretion of rennin.

Kidney functions

The main functions of the kidney include the following.

- Secretion of hormones:
  - erythropoietin (which is also synthesized in the kidney), which stimulates the bone marrow to produce red blood cells
  - renin, which controls the production of angiotensin and aldosterone. These cause, respectively, systemic vasoconstriction and renal salt and water retention to maintain effective circulating volume. This contributes to the regulation of blood pressure and fluid balance.

- Regulation and maintenance of:
  - fluid balance
  - electrolyte balance
  - acid-base balance.
- Excretion of drugs and byproducts of metabolism, nitrogen, urea, creatinine.
- Maintenance of calcium and phosphorus balance and activation of vitamin D.

(Tortora and Derrickson 2011)

Acute kidney injury

Acute kidney injury (AKI) formally known as acute renal failure is a common complication of critical illness, occurring in up to 25% of critically ill patients. It is associated with a high mortality rate when AKI worsens (Griffiths and Kanagasundaram 2011). The causes of AKI can be split into three main types (Griffiths and Kanagasundaram 2011):

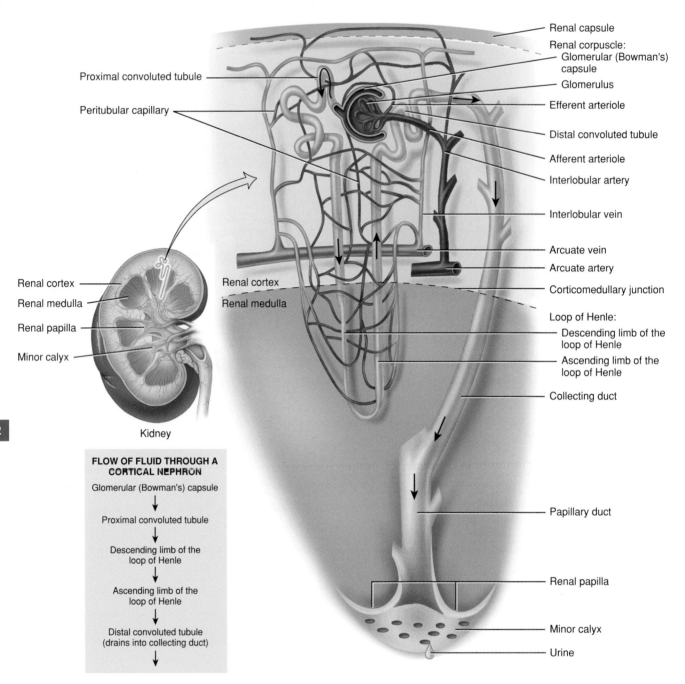

Proximal convoluted tubule

Peritubular capillary

Renal cortex
Renal medulla
Renal papilla
Minor calyx

Kidney

Renal cortex
Renal medulla

Renal capsule
Renal corpuscle:
  Glomerular (Bowman's) capsule
  Glomerulus
Efferent arteriole
Distal convoluted tubule
Afferent arteriole
Interlobular artery

Interlobular vein

Arcuate vein
Arcuate artery
Corticomedullary junction

Loop of Henle:
  Descending limb of the loop of Henle
  Ascending limb of the loop of Henle

Collecting duct

Papillary duct

Renal papilla

Minor calyx

Urine

FLOW OF FLUID THROUGH A CORTICAL NEPHRON

Glomerular (Bowman's) capsule
↓
Proximal convoluted tubule
↓
Descending limb of the loop of Henle
↓
Ascending limb of the loop of Henle
↓
Distal convoluted tubule (drains into collecting duct)
↓

Figure 9.3 Cortical nephron and vascular supply (from Tortora and Derrickson 2011, reproduced with permission from Wiley).

- pre-renal uraemia (azotaemia)
- intrinsic AKI uraemia
- post-renal uraemia (obstructive).

Pre-renal uraemia (azotaemia)

This is a response to reduced renal perfusion sometimes referred to as azotaemia. The kidney attempts to retain sodium and water, resulting in an impaired excretory capacity. No renal cellular injury occurs so the terms 'azotaemia' refers to a build-up of uraemic waste products, such as urea

and creatinine. Causes of pre-renal uraemia include anything that reduces cardiac output, such as haemorrhage and sepsis.

Intrinsic AKI uraemia

This is tubular in aetiology and usually takes the form of acute tubular necrosis, which is the death of tubular cells due to lack of oxygen. The causes of acute tubular necrosis are ischaemia, hypotension, nephrotoxins (drugs and chemical agents that damage the renal tubule epithelium) and some systemic vascular diseases, such as lupus erythematosus (Hilton 2006). Intrinsic AKI is principally due to all the causes of severe pre-renal disease, particularly hypotension, and nephrotoxins (Åhlström 2006).

Post-renal (obstructive) uraemia

The underlying cause of post-renal uraemia is often a bilateral obstruction below the level of the renal pelvis and may be due to tumour development, thrombi, urinary tract obstruction, or enlarged prostate (Hilton 2006). The obstruction causes increased pressure within the renal collecting system and renal blood flow is reduced.

Classification and staging system for acute kidney injury

The Kidney Disease: Improving Global Outcomes (KDIGO) *Clinical Practice Guideline for AKI* sets out to assist practitioners caring for patients with AKI (KDIGO 2012) and provides guidance on definition and staging of AKI. The guidance is based on an earlier classification system called RIFLE – an acronym indicating:

- Risk of renal dysfunction
- Injury to the kidney
- Failure of kidney function
- Loss of kidney function
- End stage kidney disease.

(Bellomo et al. 2004)

Early detection and treatment of AKI may improve outcomes, so definitions on serum creatinine and urine output have been defined as any of the following (KDIGO 2012):

- increase in serum creatinine by greater than or equal to 26.5 micrograms/mol/L within 48h *or*
- increase in serum creatinine to greater than or equal to 1.5 times baseline, which is known or presumed to have occurred within the prior 7 days *or*
- urine output is less than 0.5 mL/kg/h for 6h.

Once AKI is diagnosed its severity can be determined using a staging system. The staging system uses levels of serum creatinine or urine output (Table 9.1) as indicators (KDIGO 2012). As the stage increases so does mortality (Lewington and Kanagasundaram 2011).

Indications for CCRT in acute kidney injury

The indications for CRRT in AKI are:

- *To control circulating volume of fluid or to maintain control of circulating volume of fluid.* Critically ill patients often require large amounts of fluid and CRRT is adaptable giving continuous control of intravascular and extravascular volume (Bellomo and Ronco 2000), avoiding fluid overload.

Table 9.1 Staging of AKI (KDIGO 2012)

Stage	Serum creatinine	Urine output
1	1.5 to 1.9 times baseline OR greater than or equal to 0.3mg/dL (greater than or equal to 26.5micromol/L) increase	less than 0.5mL/kg/h for 6–12h
2	2.0 to 2.9 times baseline	less than 0.5mL/kg/h for greater than or equal to 12h
3	3.0 times baseline OR increase in serum creatinine to greater than or equal to 4.0mg/dL (greater than or equal to 353.6micromol/L) OR initiation of renal replacement therapy OR in patients less than 18 years, decrease in eGFR to less than 35mL/min per 1.73m²	less than 0.3mL/kg/h for greater than or equal to 24h OR anuria for greater than or equal to 12h

- *To control cardiovascular instability.* CRRT avoids rapid changes in fluid levels, thus preventing multiple hypotensive episodes which could further damage the kidney (Bellomo and Ronco 2000). It may also remove inflammatory mediators which can cause haemodynamic instability (Sarkar 2009).
- *For uraemic and electrolyte control.* CRRT can maintain homeostatic (a stable and constant) urea and electrolyte levels (Levy et al. 2009).
- *For metabolic control.* CRRT can correct blood acidosis (Levy et al. 2009).
- *For nutritional support.* Protein rich nutrition can be administered to maintain nitrogen balance and prevent protein malnutrition (Levy et al. 2009).
- *To treat raised intracranial pressure.* CRRT helps to improve cardiovascular stability in patients with raised ICP, therefore preventing hypotension and avoiding decreases in cerebral perfusion (Bellomo and Ronco 2000).
- *To remove intoxications*, such as lithium, toxic alcohols and salicylates (Pannu and Gibney 2005). CRRT will remove these from the blood.
- *To treat severe sepsis.* Severe sepsis and septic shock with acute renal failure carries a high mortality in those who are critically ill. Sepsis represents a systemic response to infection and excessive inflammatory mediators are released, it is therefore hypothesized that patients with sepsis may benefit from CRRT as it has the ability to remove or absorb many of the soluble inflammatory mediators of sepsis (Bellomo and Ronco 2000).

Aims of CRRT

The aims of CRRT therefore include:

- removal of waste products
- restoration of acid-base balance
- correction of electrolyte abnormalities
- stabilization of the cardiovascular system
- maintenance of fluid balance.

How CRRT works

Principles of renal replacement therapy

There are three mechanisms used with CRRT: ultrafiltration, convection and diffusion. Ultrafiltration and convection work in a similar way so are often grouped together providing two core physical processes (Kanagasundaram 2007). The mechanisms, how these are used in CRRT and the effects on the blood and patient are detailed in Table 9.2.

Continuous versus intermittent renal replacement therapy

AKI was traditionally treated with intermittent renal replacement therapy (IRRT) in the ICU setting; however, CRRT therapy has emerged as an alternative therapy (Mehta et al. 2001). Table 9.3 shows the differences between IRRT and CRRT.

Types of CRRT

There are four types of CRRT (*see* Table 9.4). These include:

- slow continuous ultrafiltration (SCUF)
- continuous veno-venous haemofiltration (CVVH)

- continuous veno-venous haemodialysis (CVVHD)
- continuous veno-venous haemodiafiltration (CVVHDF).

The main differences between the different types of CRRTs are the ability to remove and replace fluid, with varying degrees of solute elimination.

Slow continuous ultrafiltration (SCUF) (Figure 9.4)

- Patient is attached to the CRRT machine and their blood is pumped through the haemofilter.
- Principle used: ultrafiltration. Primarily removes water from the bloodstream, taking small amounts of solutes, but usually not enough to be clinically significant.
- The amount of fluid in the effluent bag represents the volume of fluid removed from the patient.
- Primary indication: fluid overload without uraemia or significant electrolyte imbalance, e.g. cardiac failure.

Continuous veno-venous haemofiltration (CVVH) (Figure 9.5)

- Patient is attached to the CRRT machine and their blood is pumped through the haemofilter with replacement fluid (balanced physiological electrolyte fluid) added either before or after the filter.
- Principle used: ultrafiltration and convection.
- Replacement fluids are used to replace the high electrolyte and fluid loss in the ultrafiltrate.
- Extremely effective method for removing large molecules and a wider range of solute due to the convection mechanism.
- Indicated for uraemia or severe acid-base or electrolyte imbalance with or without fluid overload (Dirkes and Hodge 2007).

314

Table 9.2 Mechanisms and effects of CRRT

Mechanism	Definition of mechanism	How mechanism is used in CRRT	Effects on the blood and patient
Ultrafiltration	Movement of fluid through a semi-permeable membrane along a pressure gradient	The blood side of the membrane generates a positive pressure and the negative pressure is created on the fluid side	Results in a net fluid removal from the patient Minimal solutes cleared from blood
Convection	One-way movement of solutes through a semi-permeable membrane	The pressure (hydrostatic) in the blood is higher than the pressure in the ultrafiltrate, causing plasma water to be removed; this also causes solute removal, often known as 'solvent drag' Solutes of high molecular weight are retained, while water and low molecular weight solutes pass through the membrane	Efficient at removal of both large and small molecules The faster the flow rate the higher the clearance
Diffusion	Movement of particles from higher concentration to regions of lower concentration	Solutes move across from the blood (high concentration) across the membrane to the dialysate (low concentration) The dialysate flows counter-current to the blood flow to facilitate this process	Removes small to medium molecules efficiently but not large molecules

Table 9.3 Characteristics of IRRT and CRRT

	IRRT	CRRT
Duration of therapy	3–4 hours every 2–3 days	Continuous
Haemodynamic stability	■ Haemodynamic compromise common ■ Hypotensive episodes common	■ Haemodynamic stability easier to maintain ■ Hypotensive episodes comparatively fewer. This reduces the risk of further ischemia to the nephrons (Dirkes and Hodge 2007)
Fluids, electrolyte and toxin removal	■ Large amounts of fluids removed quickly ■ Peaks and troughs in uraemia level ■ Difficulties with volume control when fluids required	■ Gradual removal of fluids circulating volume ■ Maintains a steady uraemia level maintaining lower levels of blood urea and creatinine, may have improved survival rates (Bellomo and Ronco 2000) ■ Large amounts of fluids can be administered and volume control maintained
Protein intake	■ Fluid restricted so difficulties administering adequate protein in lower fluid volumes	■ Unlimited fluid intake so protein can be administered in volumes large enough to achieve optimal nutrition (Bellomo and Ronco 2000)
Patient mobility	■ Patient able to be fully mobile when therapy not in progress	■ Patient's mobility restricted as continuously attached to the therapy
Anticoagulation	■ Patient exposure to anticoagulation limited to short periods	■ Patient exposure to anticoagulation is continuous

Continuous veno-henous haemodialysis (CVVHD) (Figure 9.6)

■ Patient is attached to the CRRT machine and their blood is pumped through the filter with dialysate running in a countercurrent flow (opposite direction to the blood flow), in the outside compartment of the haemofilter.

■ Principles used: ultrafiltration and diffusion.

■ Indicated for removal of fluid and small to medium-sized molecules, in patients with severe uraemia, acid-base and electrolyte imbalance.

Continuous veno-venous haemodiafiltration (CVVHDF) (Figure 9.7)

■ Patient is attached to the CRRT machine and their blood is pumped through the filter with dialysate running in a countercurrent flow, in the outside compartment of the haemofilter and replacement fluid is pumped in after the filter.

■ Principles used: ultrafiltration, diffusion and convection.

■ It is an effective way of enhancing metabolic control if this is not being achieved with CVVH, as it combines the benefits of all principles, but it is not always necessary to use this therapy to achieve the desired renal replacement.

Slow extended daily dialysis (SLEDD)

An alternative, but not continuous, renal replacement therapy is slow extended daily dialysis (SLEDD). This can be conducted using any of the first four types of CRRT but is completed in a shorter time – usually 8–12 hours. The advantage of SLEDD over CRRT, therefore, is that it can be performed overnight and allows time for patient rehabilitation during the day. The therapy time is reduced, so increased amounts of fluid may need to be removed in a shorter period. Consequently it is indicated for patients with a more stable haemodynamic and fluid status (Dirkes and Hodge 2007).

CRRT priming and treatment choices

Consensus is lacking on precisely when to start CRRT, probably due to limited evidence available to guide recommendations (Kanagasundaram 2007). Despite the uncertainty, early intervention with CRRT is advised when AKI is established (Bellomo and Ronco 2000, Kanagasundaram 2007). CRRT should be started when conventional indications (such as hyperkalaemia, fluid overload and severe metabolic acidosis) are present (Kanagasundaram 2007).

Priming the CRRT machine

Before starting CRRT, the CRRT circuit (tubing and haemofilter) must be primed. This is usually with 1 L of 0.9% sodium chloride with or without heparin (dependent on the patient's requirements (see below)). The purpose of the priming is to remove all air from the circuit; it also allows detection of leaks before connecting the patient and commencing treatment (Faber and Klein 2009).

The rate of filtration

Research by Ronco et al. (2000) recommended a standard starting ultrafiltrate rate of 35 mL/kg using CRRT as this was found to improve outcomes for critically ill patients.

315

Table 9.4 Types of CRRT

Type	Method	Principle action	Other clinical information	Indications
Slow continuous ultrafiltration (SCUF) (Figure 9.4)	■ Patient is attached to the CRRT machine and their blood is pumped through the haemofilter	■ Ultrafiltration	■ Primarily removes water from the bloodstream, taking small amounts of solutes, but usually not enough to be clinically significant (Dirkes and Hodge 2007) ■ The amount of fluid in the effluent bag represents the volume of fluid removed from the patient	■ Fluid overload without uraemia or significant electrolyte imbalance, e.g. cardiac failure
Continuous veno-venous haemofiltration (CVVH) (Figure 9.5)	Patient is attached to the CRRT machine and their blood is pumped through the haemofilter with replacement fluid (balanced physiological electrolyte fluid) added either before or after the filter	■ Ultrafiltration and convection	■ Replacement fluids are used to replace the high electrolyte and fluid loss in the ultra filtrate ■ Extremely effective method for removing large molecules and a wider range of solute due to the convection mechanism	■ Uraemia ■ Severe acid-base or electrolyte imbalance with or without fluid overload
Continuous veno-venous haemodialysis (CVVHD) (Figure 9.6)	Patient is attached to the CRRT machine and their blood is pumped through the filter with dialysate running in a counter current flow, in the outside compartment of the haemofilter	■ Ultrafiltration and diffusion		■ Removal of fluid and small to medium-sized molecules in patients with severe uraemia, acid-base and electrolyte imbalance
Continuous veno-venous haemodiafiltration (CVVHDF) (Figure 9.7)	Patient is attached to the CRRT machine and their blood is pumped through the filter with dialysate running in a countercurrent flow, in the outside compartment of the haemofilter and replacement fluid is pumped in after the filter	■ Ultrafiltration, Diffusion and convection	Combines the benefits of ultrafiltration, diffusion and convection principles but it is not always necessary to use this therapy to achieve the desired renal replacement	■ Enhancing metabolic control if this is not being achieved with CVVH

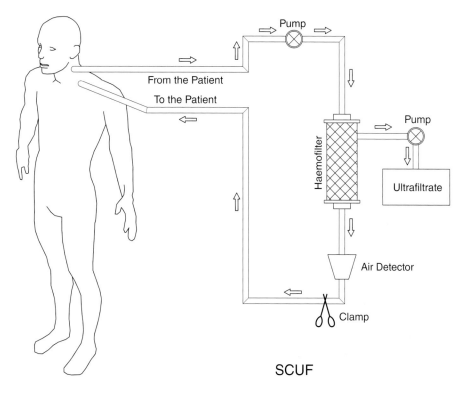

Figure 9.4 Slow continuous ultrafiltration (SCUF).

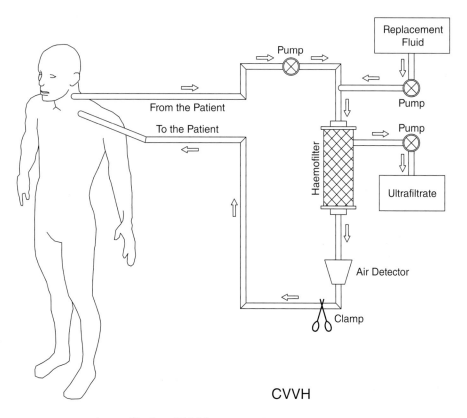

Figure 9.5 Continuous veno-venous haemofiltration (CVVH).

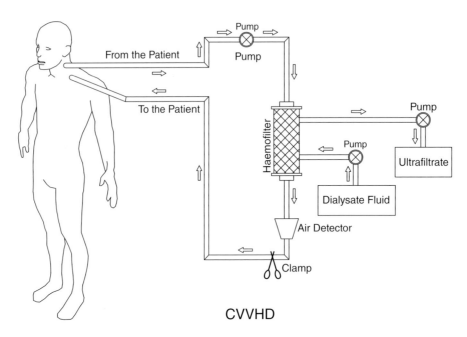

Figure 9.6 Continuous veno-venous haemodialysis (CVVHD).

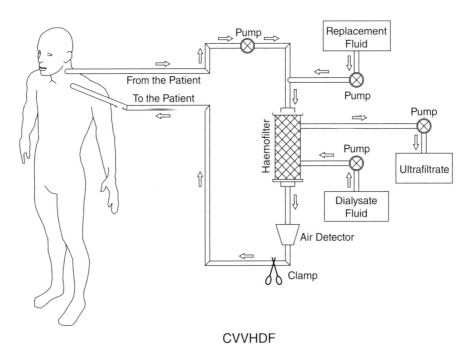

Figure 9.7 Continuous veno-venous haemodiafiltration (CVVHDF).

Type of haemofilter

The haemofilter (Figure 9.8) is often referred to as the artificial kidney. It consists of thousands of hollow narrow fibres with semipermeable walls within a tubular casing. Blood flows through the fibres and the effluent/dialysate flows on the outside of the fibres. Water and solutes from the blood move through the walls of the fibres into the effluent/dialysate fluid (Teo et al. 2007). There are various types of haemofilter, which differ in the permeability of their membrane and the thickness and pore size, factors that determine their utility (Kanagasundaram 2007). Guidance on use should be sought from local policies/manufacturer's guidelines.

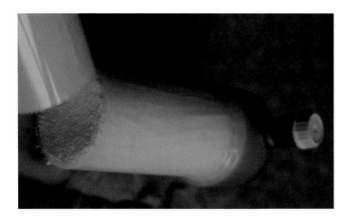

Figure 9.8 A haemofilter.

Replacement fluid

All CRRT, except SCUF, requires sterile replacement fluid or dialysate fluid (Dirkes and Hodge 2007). The optimal replacement solution should be similar to normal plasma composition, in order to replace electrolytes and minerals (Pannu and Mehta 2006).

During ultrafiltration bicarbonate is moved from the blood, therefore it must be replaced to avoid causing or worsening any acidosis. Some replacement fluids substitute lactate for bicarbonate, as lactate improves the shelf-life of replacement fluid and is cheaper. As long as the patient is able to metabolize lactate to carbon dioxide and water, which generates new bicarbonate ions, it can be a suitable substitute (Hilton et al. 1998). However, the capacity to convert lactate to bicarbonate is limited in critically ill patients with multiple organ failure, liver failure and lactate acidosis (Pannu and Mehta 2006). This situation can then lead to a worsening of the acidosis when undergoing CRRT (Hilton et al. 1998). In these cases, Faber and Klein (2009) suggest that lactate-free solutions are used with a separate bicarbonate infusion. More recently bicarbonate-based solutions have become available, particularly for use with patients in liver failure (Kanagasundaram 2007). These are better tolerated, often resulting in fewer cardiovascular events and hypotensive episodes (Barenbrock et al. 2000; Pannu and Gibney 2005).

Double-lumen access

For CRRT in critical care, temporary veno-venous access is generally achieved with a large-bore (for example 12 Fr) double-lumen CVC in a large central vein (Sarkar 2009). Common sites include internal jugular, femoral or subclavian veins.

Drug adjustments

Correct dosage of drugs is important, particularly in patients who are critically ill (Levy et al. 2009). One unwanted effect of CRRT is the concurrent removal of some drugs, such as antimicrobials. This leads to reduced levels of drugs in the blood and tissues, and poses a real problem in relation to providing the correct dose for the patient (Schetz 2007). Drugs removed by CRRT will vary according to the type of CRRT, and the rate of clearance will depend on the ultrafiltration rate (Levy et al. 2009). Therefore prescriptions and administration of medication must be completed on an individual basis according to the needs of the patient and the levels of specific drugs within their body (Schetz 2007). Drug clearance is continuous during CRRT, so if this is stopped the prescribers should be made aware so that adjustments can be made to drug doses (Levy et al. 2009). The renal drug handbook (Ashley and Currie 2009) provides individual drug adjustment requirements.

Nutritional adjustments

Nutritional input may need adjusting before and after CRRT. CRRT results in significant losses of glucose, amino acids, proteins, trace elements and water-soluble vitamins, and this loss should be compensated. Therefore individual nutritional assessment is essential before and after CRRT in order to design optimal nutrition (Wooley et al. 2005).

Maintaining the CRRT circuit

The aim is to safely administer CRRT for as long as clinically indicated, therefore preserving the life of a CRRT circuit is important to avoid unnecessary interruptions to the patient's therapy. The provision of good vascular access is essential (Davies and Leslie 2007) for lengthening the life of the circuit, as is using a wide-bore CVC (Dirkes and Hodge 2007). This helps to maintain a high blood flow, which reduces the possibility of thrombus forming in the circuit as it is more likely to clot if blood flow is allowed to drop below 100 mL/min (Davies and Leslie 2006). If clots occur in the circuit, CRRT will not function and it will not be possible to return the blood to the patient. A rise in circuit pressures is an early indication that thrombi are within the system (Dirkes and Hodge 2007), but it is crucial also to observe the circuit for the presence of clots.

The use of anticoagulation

The clotting cascade is a complex cascade of enzymatic reactions in which each clotting factor initiates the release of the next clotting factor, and finally insoluble protein fibrin is formed (Tortora and Derrickson 2011). Anticoagulants are used to prevent the blood from clotting within the extracorporeal circuit and to maximize the circuit life. The choice of anticoagulant is dependent on the patient's condition and whether or not they require systemic anticoagulation medication (Bellomo and Ronco 2000). Anticoagulation may not be required in patients who have a high risk of bleeding, as in the case of coagulopathy, severe sepsis or hepatic failure (Dirkes and Hodge 2007), where the likelihood of clotting in the circuit is reduced.

All types of anticoagulation have risks and benefits, so it is important to consider the attendant risks (such as bleeding) against the risk of filter clotting. Types of anticoagulation used for CRRT include the following:

- heparin
- prostacycline
- regional citrate
- thrombin inhibitors.

Heparin

Heparin is the most often-used anticoagulant (Kanagasundaram 2007), and the least expensive (Dirkes and Hodge 2007). Heparin affects the clotting cascade by binding to antithrombin III to inhibit thrombin and factor Xa to prevent clot formation (Davies and Leslie 2007). Heparin is commonly used in the priming solution as it is thought to adhere to the plastic of the circuit lines (Davies and Leslie 2007). It is delivered through an infusion pump on a continuous basis and is administered prior to the filter in the circuit. On occasions heparin can be administered systemically due to a pre-existing requirement for anticoagulation – such as in patients undergoing treatment for a pulmonary embolism. The disadvantages of heparin include risks of haemorrhage, heparin resistance (patients requiring greater than 35 000 units of heparin/day to achieve the therapeutic range [Anderson and Saenko 2002]) and heparin-induced thrombocytopenia. Heparin-induced thrombocytopenia occurs when antibodies to heparin bind to coagulation factor IV on platelets, causing platelet activation and aggregation, which generates thrombi. If a patient has heparin-induced thrombocytopenia the heparin must be stopped (Dirkes and Hodge 2007).

It is important that the efficacy of anticoagulation achieved with heparin should be assessed on a regular basis. This can be undertaken by measuring the 'activated partial thromboplastin time' (the time taken in seconds for a clot to form) (Chacko 2008). Activated partial thromboplastin ratio is also sometimes calculated, this is the ratio of activated partial thromboplastin time to the normal coagulation time. Both tests will need to be repeated regularly, followed by the titration of heparin dosage. The testing and titration should be undertaken according to local protocols to maintain the prescribed limits.

Prostacycline

Prostacycline prevents platelet aggregation by reducing the formation of fibrin, leukocyte and platelet-based microaggregates (Davies and Leslie 2006). It is a suitable alternative to heparin in patients with increased risk of bleeding (Kanagasundaram 2007) and/or with acute liver failure, as it does not affect the clotting cascade (Davies and Leslie 2007). Possible alternatives should be sought when patients have a platelet count of less than 80 units and/or are hypotensive. This is because prostacycline is a potent vasodilator, often reducing the mean arterial pressure by 15 mmHg (Hall and Fox 2006).

Prostacycline can be used in combination with heparin to prolong the life of the CRRT filter. The combination also reduces the haemodynamic instability associated with using prostacycline alone (Davies and Leslie 2007). The main disadvantages of prostacycline are its high cost and its unwanted systemic vasodilatory effects (Kanagasundaram 2007).

Regional citrate

Calcium plays an important role in the clotting cascade (Dirkes and Hodge 2007). Regional citrate binds to calcium in blood within the CRRT circuit and prevents clotting. It is infused into the extracorporeal circuit before the filter by separate infusion or in replacement fluid (Dirkes and Hodge 2007). The administration of citrate induces hypocalcaemia in the filter, preventing clotting of the CRRT, but it also reduces calcium levels within the patient's blood, resulting in a requirement to replace calcium. This can be achieved by administering calcium via different intravenous tubing directly to the patient (Dirkes and Hodge 2007).

The indications for its use are active bleeding or a high risk of bleeding and heparin-induced thrombocytopenia. Citrate is contraindicated in severe liver failure as it is metabolized in the liver (Davies and Leslie 2007). Regional citrate requires monitoring for potential complications, including metabolic alkalosis, hyponatreamia and hyocalcaemia. In summary, it is effective but is technically complex (Kanagasundaram 2007) as it requires preparation of specific replacement fluids and close monitoring of calcium, sodium and acid-base status (Davies and Leslie 2007).

Thrombin inhibitors

Thrombin inhibitors are used as an alternative means of anticoagulation for patients diagnosed with heparin-induced thrombocytopenia (Dirkes and Hodge 2007). The use of a thrombin inhibitor is associated with a higher risk of bleeding (Davies and Leslie 2007), it has no reversal agent (Pannu and Gibney 2005) and it is also considered to be considerably expensive (Dirkes and Hodge 2007). It is administered before the haemofilter (Dirkes and Hodge 2007).

No anticoagulation

In some cases no anticoagulation medication may be warranted. This is because the patient's blood is unlikely to clot. This occurs particularly in cases of severe coagulopathy, hepatic failure and recent haemorrhage, and in patients who have low platelets (Davies and Leslie 2007).

The use of pre-dilution and post-dilution

For CVVH and CVVHDF, the replacement fluid can be added before the haemofilter (often referred to as 'pre-dilution') or after the haemofilter (often referred to as 'post-dilution'). Pre-dilution prolongs the life of the filter by diluting the blood haematocrit (concentration of red blood cells). A consequence of diluting the blood before the filter is the dilution of all solutes within the blood, which reduces the clearance (Faber and Klein 2009). Post-dilution replacement fluid can result in a higher chance of filter blockage due to the haemoconcentration effect (Faber and Klein 2009). This indicates that combining both pre- and post-dilution methods by administering a proportion of replacement fluid before the filter and a proportion post filter (usually slightly more post filter) has the advantage of extending filter life and maintaining adequate clearance.

Assessment and monitoring of the patient on CRRT

An accurate patient history, physical examination, review of medication, allergies and laboratory tests should be undertaken prior to commencement of CRRT. In addition, the need to rule out any renal obstruction should be assessed for all patients. A renal ultrasound can be undertaken for patients suspected of obstruction from possible causes such as stones or a tumour (Raggio and Umans 2006).

There are a number of major complications of CRRT so continuous assessment and monitoring of the patient is important to detect and treat complications of CRRT. The main complications of CRRT include:

- haemodynamic instability
- bleeding
- hypothermia
- electrolyte and acid- base imbalance
- inappropriate drug dosing
- infection.

Cardiovascular status and fluid management

Current research suggests that CRRT is more effective than IRRT for fluid and cardiovascular control. However, major complications can result if appropriate care and actions are not implemented (Mehta 2001). CRRT patients must have a full assessment of their fluid status, including their intake and output, baseline observations of blood pressure, heart rate, cardiac rhythm, central venous pressure, cardiac output (if being measured) and dosages of any vasopressor drugs being administered prior to commencing CRRT. An assessment of weight and an agreed fluid balance goal should be set (Dirkes and Hodge 2007).

Fluid management requires the calculation of the patient's fluid balance, taking into account the patient's intake (for example infusions, medications and nutritional input) plus any fluid output (for example urine, sweating, nasogastric/

bowel loss and drain/wound loss) on an hourly basis. The patient's fluid balance and the ordered fluid loss need to be considered so the CRRT machine can be programmed for the desired hourly volume removal (Dirkes and Hodge 2007). An accurate measurement/assessment of fluid balance is important as inaccuracies can result in either under- or over-hydration of the patient (Mehta 2001). This can lead to a significant decrease in blood pressure, which could have an impact on vasopressor requirements (Dirkes and Hodge 2007). Errors in calculating the rate of fluid removal can easily occur when frequent readjustments are required to maintain the desired CRRT prescription (Langford et al. 2008).

Ongoing assessment of the cardiovascular status and fluid balance must continue throughout the therapy, with continual measurement of blood pressure, pulse, heart rate, central venous pressure and cardiac output/pulmonary artery pressures as available. Some patients will not tolerate the predetermined fluid removal and the prescriber will need to be notified of any adverse effects due to fluid loss (Dirkes and Hodge 2007). The achievement of fluid goals should be compared with prescribed goals, with adjustments in machine programming when necessary (Mehta 2001). Most CRRT machines have a scales system, balancing the weight of the replacement fluid and the weight of the fluid lost (Dirkes and Hodge 2007).

Intravenous access and infection control

Bacteraemia can be caused by entry of bacteria via the temporary CVC. Therefore, it is important that the intravenous access for CRRT is dedicated for this single use (Faber and Klein 2009) and only used for other purposes in life-threatening situations (Sarkar 2009). See Chapter 6.

Maintaining patency of intravenous access

Monitoring the blood flow of the CVC is important, as poor patency will affect treatment, especially if poor patency results in the circuit stopping intermittently. Therefore prior to commencement of CRRT the double-lumen CVC should be checked to ensure good blood flow. This is achieved by the withdrawal of blood from the CVC. Good patency is indicated if blood easily fills the syringe (Dirkes and Hodge 2007).

Once CRRT has commenced, assessing the blood flow within the CVC can be carried out by monitoring and documenting the access and return pressures on the CRRT machines on an hourly basis. The trend of pressures over time will enable the detection of access problems (Dirkes and Hodge, 2007).

The double-lumen CVC has two lumens:

- a red lumen, which is generally used to pull blood out of the patient. This opens into the vein proximal to the line tip

321

■ a blue lumen for blood to be returned to the patient, distal to or at the line tip.

If adequate flow to the machine cannot be achieved then it may be necessary to reverse the use of the lines. Reversal of the lines can give a small reduction in clearance due to a small amount of internal recirculation; however, maintaining the circuit life should be the priority (Sarkar 2009).

Maintaining a patent double-lumen catheter when it is not in use is important, to enable immediate connection to the CRRT machine once indicated. A catheter blocked with blood clot will require a new CVC insertion before CRRT can commence. Therefore following the disconnection of CRRT, the double-lumen catheter should be flushed with 10 mL of 0.9% sodium chloride and then anticoagulant administered as prescribed. This procedure is to prevent thrombi forming within the lumen when not in use (Sarkar 2009).

Monitoring electrolytes and metabolic status

CRRT removes electrolytes in an unselected way, so it is important to replace the necessary electrolytes lost in the ultrafiltrate (Culley et al. 2006). This is done by providing a replacement solution that is physiologically similar to plasma composition, which enables electrolytes and minerals to be administered (Pannu and Mehta 2006). A wide range of replacement fluids are available commercially but most require the addition of electrolytes (for example potassium in the form of potassium chloride) to correct the patient's electrolyte imbalance (Pannu and Mehta 2006). It is important to test the patient's systemic blood regularly for electrolyte balance. Generally this should be done 4- to 6-hourly, although the frequency should be escalated if patient electrolyte levels are outside normal ranges. It is also beneficial to ascertain electrolyte levels prior to changing bags of replacement fluid, so that the correct dosage of additional electrolytes can be added and administered.

A major part of the management of the patient on CRRT is the control of serum potassium. The use of a potassium 'sliding scale' (where dose is dependent on concentration in the blood) is a good method of giving clear step-by-step instructions for all practitioners to avoid the risk of therapy-induced arrhythmias associated with hypokaleamia (Brooks 2006). Hypophosphataemia (low phosphate levels) is another recognized problem during CRRT, so monitoring of phosphate levels and, where appropriate, administering replacement is essential (Bellomo and Ronco 2000).

Metabolic acidosis occurs with AKI, due to the failure to excrete hydrogen ions and waste product accumulation. This leads to increased muscle breakdown (Levy et al. 2009). Arterial blood gases should be monitored for any deterioration or improvement in pH balance, base excess and increase in lactate (where possible). CRRT can then be altered as appropriate by increasing or decreasing the ultrafiltrate rates or changing the mode of therapy (Dirkes and Hodge 2007).

Hypothermia

Hypothermia is a complication of CRRT (Levy et al. 2009). A typical extracorporeal circuit contains 110–200 mL of blood that is outside the body and this contributes significantly to cooling the patient (Dirkes and Hodge 2007). The patient's temperature must be monitored at least 4-hourly and the replacement and/or dialysate fluids warmed prior to entering the CRRT circuit to help prevent hypothermia (Lee et al. 2008). Most CRRT machines allow adjustments in temperature of replacement and/or dialysate fluid; however, if this is not sufficient, warming blankets can be used on the patient and/or the temperature of the room increased (Dirkes and Hodge 2007).

Nutritional support

Patients in AKI often have problems with electrolyte balance due to restrictions on their diet and fluid intake. Patients with AKI on CRRT do not need a limit on their fluid intake (Levy et al. 2009) and the electrolyte intake can become less restricted. This enables patients to receive full nutritional support.

Nutritional status in AKI is influenced by the underlying disease and severely catabolic patients require nutritional support. Malnutrition in patients with AKI can develop as a result of protein breakdown and negative nitrogen balance, so treatment should involve delivering appropriate nutritional supplements (Brady and Kieran 2006). Where the gastrointestinal tract is functioning, enteral feeding is recommended (Levy et al. 2009), as Lewington and Kanagasundaram (2011) suggest it helps maintain gut integrity and reduces the risk of bacterial translocation (the passage of bacteria from the gastrointestinal tract to normally sterile tissues and other internal organs).

Respiratory management

One of the goals of CRRT in patients with fluid overload and pulmonary oedema is to reduce fluid overload and treat pulmonary oedema. Therefore continuous assessment of respiratory status is necessary, which includes respiratory rate, arterial blood gas levels, oxygen saturation and presence of chest secretions. Following assessment, any changes to the respiratory observations must be considered and modifications made to CRRT as required, particularly with potential adjustments to volume removal. Further adjustments maybe considered with the respiratory ventilation parameters, such as oxygen concentration and level of respiratory support (Dirkes and Hodge 2007).

322

Neurological care

Patients in AKI often become confused as their urea levels increase. Their conscious level can be assessed using the Glasgow Coma Scale (*see* Chapter 11).

Using CRRT for patients with cerebral oedema and in AKI (typically found in patients with acute liver failure) has been found to help maintain fluid status and prevent brainstem herniation (Davenport 1999). However, the patient should also be monitored for increased intracranial pressure. That is, the pupils should be assessed and intracranial pressures and waveforms (if available) should be observed for elevations and fluctuations (Arbour 2004).

Monitoring and problem solving on the CRRT circuit

Continuous monitoring and assessment of the CRRT circuit is important to ensure the prescribed treatment can be delivered and for early recognition of CRRT circuit failure. The following should be monitored on a continuous basis and recorded hourly (Dirkes and Hodge 2007) (Table 9.5).

CRRT machine alarms

The CRRT machine has a number of alarms to alert practitioners to changes within the CRRT circuit and/or the patient's CVC. The alarms indicate various problems which require action to safely resolve and maintain the CRRT circuit. A variety of manufacturers make CRRT machines resulting in some differences with alarms and ways of resolving problems. However, despite this, most of the alarms are similar on all machines (Edwards 2004; Levy et al.).

Table 9.5 Continuous CRRT monitoring requirements

Blood pump speed (mL/min)	Speed of blood removal from the patient
Access pressure (mmHg)	Pressure generated to remove blood from the patient
Return pressure (mmHg)	Pressure generated to return blood to the patient
Transmembrane pressure (TMP) (mmHg)	Pressure gradient exerted across the semipermeable membrane of the fibres in the haemofilter. TMP needs to be sufficient to enable ultrafiltration. It can be used as an indicator of filter fibre clogging across the membrane
Prefilter pressure (mmHg)	Positive pressure generated in the circuit immediately before the blood enters the haemofilter

323

Problem solving table 9.1 **Continuous renal replacement therapy**

Alarm	Possible causes	Preventative measures	Suggested action
Low access pressure (negative pressure generated to remove blood from the patient)	■ CVC is sucking against a vessel wall ■ CVC lumen is partially clotted or fully clotted ■ Lumen is kinked or clamped	Make sure both lumens and all tubing are straight and unclamped	1. Reposition the patient and/or CVC with a little external manipulation to maintain alignment 2. Swap the access and return tubing 3. Temporarily reduce the blood pump speed 4. Clamp off tubing and access lumen, and attempt to aspirate lumen with a syringe to remove clot. If clot is removed and good flow is restored, flush access lumen with 0.9% sodium chloride, reconnect tubing and release clamps. If clot is not removed and blood cannot be withdrawn, consider stopping the CRRT by returning the blood, followed by re-siting the CVC

(Continued)

Problem solving table 9.1 (Continued)

High return pressure (pressure generated to return the blood back to the patient)	■ CVC lumen is clotted or occluded ■ Lumen or line is kinked, clamped ■ Circuit clotting	Make sure all the lumens and tubing are straight and unclamped	1. Reposition the patient and/or CVC 2. Clamp off tubing and CVC return lumen and attempt to aspirate lumen with a syringe to remove clot. If clot is removed and good flow is restored, flush return lumen with 0.9% sodium chloride, reconnect tubing and release clamps. If clot is not removed and blood cannot be withdrawn, consider stopping the CRRT by returning the blood, followed by re-siting the CVC 3. If circuit clotting, prepare to discontinue treatment
Low return pressure (pressure generated to return the blood)	■ Low blood pump speed ■ Return tubing disconnected	Ensure tubing is securely connected	1. Increase blood flow rate to prescribed rate 2. If disconnected reattach tubing to CVC
High transmembrane pressures (TMP) (reflects the positive pressure inside the fibres and negative pressure outside the filter)	Rapid rise in TMP: ■ Filtrate tubing or bags occluded by a clamp or kink Slow rise in TMP: ■ Filter clotting slowly High TMP from beginning of treatment: ■ Ratio of pressure between the blood flow and replacement fluid is too high	Ensure all tubing is straight and unclamped Consider increasing pre-dilution rate on commencing of next treatment (particularly if CRRT circuit prematurely clotted on previous treatments)	1. Remove the kink or unclamp the tubing or bag 2. Consider increasing pre-dilution rates and decreasing post-dilution rate. Then, if the TMP decreases, continue treatment. If TMP continues to rise, discontinue CRRT (to return blood to patient to prevent blood loss). Consider more pre dilution on commencement of next CRRT 3. Increase the blood flow speed or decrease the exchange rate
High pre-filter (positive pressure generated in the circuit immediately before the blood enters the haemofilter)	■ Tubing kinked ■ 'Return chamber' clotting ■ Filter clotting	Ensure tubing is straight Consider more pre-dilution on next CRRT	1. Prepare to end treatment 2. Prepare to end treatment and consider more pre-dilution on next treatment
Air detected (air or microfoam in CRRT tubing prior to returning blood to patient)	■ Air in the tubing returning to the patient ■ Blood level is too low in 'return chamber' ■ Return tubing is not in the air detector clamp correctly	When setting up circuit ensure air detector is securely fitted When priming, ensure that all air is cleared from the circuit	1. Remove air with syringe 2. Using a syringe manually raise the blood level in the return chamber. This will remove excess air 3. Place the tubing correctly within the air detector
Blood leak (traces of blood in the ultrafiltrate this is sometimes discoloured [usually rose])	■ Filter membrane ruptured causing a leak of blood into the ultrafilrate ■ Blood leak detection chamber not correctly in housing ■ Sensor in housing is unclean	When setting up circuit, ensure blood leak detection chamber is housed in correct position and machine sensor cleaned	1. Cease treatment and change filter and circuit 2. Replace chamber in housing 3. Clean the sensor in housing and replace the chamber

324

| Fluid balance* (deviation in weight from the values set by the operator) | ■ Fluid bags moving or swinging below machine ■ Fluid bags not connected properly ■ Fluid tubing are kinked or clamped ■ As above | Ensure tubing is straight and free from obstruction Ensure fluid replacement bags and ultrafiltrate bags unclamped | 1. Stop replacement bags and ultrafiltrate bags from moving 2. Check all connections are secure between the fluid bags and the tubing 3. Ensure all clamps are undone and tubing is not kinked 4. Do not override the balance alarm, always identify the cause |

Procedure guideline 9.1: Preparation and priming of the CRRT machine

Equipment

- CRRT machine
- Machine lines and haemofilter
- Priming solution: 1 L 0.9% sodium chloride with or without heparin (dependent on individual need)
- Replacement and or dialysate fluid with or without potassium (dependent on patient's electrolyte balance)
- Prescribed anticoagulant (if required)

Procedure

Action	Rationale
1 Where possible, explain and discuss the procedure with the patient. If the patient lacks the capacity to make decisions the practitioner must act in the patient's best interests.	To ensure that the patient understands the procedure and gives their valid consent. To ensure the patient's best interests are maintained (Mental Capacity Act 2005).
2 Ensure Chest X-ray is assessed for correct position (except femoral CVCs).	To ensure the CVC is in the correct place (Gladwin et al. 1999).
3 Obtain prescription for CRRT.	To ensure that a CRRT can be set up, primed programmed and ready for commencement (Dirkes and Hodge 2007) according to the individual needs of the patient.
4 Obtain CRRT equipment required.	To ensure that all the equipment is available and treatment commenced as required (Kanagasundaram 2007).
5 Prime the circuit using the prescribed solution, following the manufacturer instructions on the CRRT machine.	To ensure all air is expelled from the system (Faber and Klein 2009).
6 Assess the patient's fluid status, blood pressure, heart rate, cardiac rhythm, central venous pressure, cardiac output (if being measured) and dosages of any vasopressor drugs being administered.	To detect patient's potential risk of haemodynamic instability on commencement of CRRT (Dirkes and Hodge 2007).
7 Observe vascular access site for signs of infection.	To detect early recognition of infection (DH 2007).
8 Check vascular access for patency and blood flow.	To ensure that the vascular access will allow adequate blood flow to achieve the prescribed CRRT (Levy et al. 2009).

Procedure guideline 9.2: Commencement of CRRT

Equipment

- Primed CRRT machine
- Sterile dressing pack
- 2% chlorhexidine gluconate in 70% isopropyl alcohol solution
- Sterile gloves
- Apron and personal protective equipment
- Syringes × 5 mL

Procedure

Action	Rationale
1 Prior to connecting the CRRT lines, program the primed CRRT machine (according to manufacturer's guidelines) and attach anticoagulation infusion as prescribed.	To ensure that once the tubing is connected to the patient, the CRRT can be commenced as prescribed. Anticoagulation programmed to prevent circuit clotting (Kanagasundaram 2007).
2 Check correct patient against CRRT prescription.	To ensure correct patient receives correct CRRT (NMC 2012).
3 Measure the patient's temperature and set the fluid warmer to an appropriate temperature.	To warm the replacement fluid or dialysate to prevent hypothermia (Dirkes and Hodge 2007).
4 Put on apron, use personal protective equipment, wash hands, apply sterile gloves and open sterile dressing pack.	To reduce the risk of microbial contamination (Pratt et al. 2007).
5 Remove caps from the two hubs at the end of the double-lumen CVC and using an aseptic non-touch technique swab ports with 2% chlorhexidine gluconate in 70% isopropyl alcohol and allow to air dry.	To open up access to the CVC for connection and to reduce the risk of microbial contamination (Pratt et al. 2007).
6 Apply a 5 mL syringe to each lumen and one at a time release the CVC clamp and withdraw 5 mL of blood. Then re-clamp and remove syringe.	To remove all the solution contained in the lumen and to check patency of CVC (Baxter and Edwards 2007; Sarkar 2009).
7 Connect the renal replacement tubing: red tubing to the red lumen on the double-lumen access CVC; blue tubing to the blue lumen on the double-lumen access CVC.	To ensure the double-lumen CVC is safely connected to prevent accidental disconnection and subsequent blood loss (Baxter and Edwards 2007).
8 Ensure double-lumen CVC clamps and tubing clamps are open.	To ensure blood flows from the patient into the CRRT circuit (Baxter and Edwards 2007).
9 Start CRRT machine blood pump, increasing speed slowly. Aim to increase the blood pump speed to the prescribed level, usually 200 mL/min (Levy et al. 2009).	To slowly assess patient's cardiovascular response to commencing CRRT (Dirkes and Hodge 2007). A blood pump speed of 200 mL/min will maximize CRRT (Baxter and Edwards 2007).
10 If blood flow is inadequate consider swapping the access tubing (that is red tubing) to the blue lumen and blue return tubing to the red lumen. (Note: a 3–10% recirculation could occur [Levy et al. 2009].)	To maintain good blood flow (Pannu and Mehta 2006).
11 Once prescribed blood pump speed is established start prescribed replacement fluid and/or dialysate.	To fully commence CRRT and maintain fluid balance (Baxter and Edwards 2007).
12 Observe the patient's fluid status, blood pressure, heart rate, cardiac rhythm, central venous pressure and cardiac output (if being measured).	To detect any adverse reactions or cardiovascular instability, report to appropriate clinicians and treat accordingly (Dirkes and Hodge 2007).

13 Document date and time CRRT commenced plus any adverse reactions.	To: ■ provide an accurate record ■ monitor effectiveness of procedure ■ reduce the risk of duplication of treatment ■ provide a point of reference or comparison in the event of later questions ■ acknowledge accountability for actions ■ facilitate communication and continuity of care. (NMC 2008; HCPC 2012; GMC 2013)

Procedure guideline 9.3: Managing the patient on CRRT

Procedure

Action	Rationale
1 Continuously observe and monitor of the patient's vital signs and fluid status, e.g. blood pressure, heart rate, cardiac rhythm, central venous pressure, cardiac output (if being measured), fluid input and output.	To detect any changes and take action to maintain stability. This may necessitate alterations in fluid calculations or alterations in inotropic drugs (*see* Chapter 7) (Dirkes and Hodge 2007).
2 Monitor blood urea, creatinine and electrolytes. Consider the need to change potassium levels in replacement fluids and alter doses of replacement phosphate.	To detect changes with essential electrolyes during CRRT (Brooks 2006). To prevent hypokalaemia (Brooks 2006) and hypophosphateamia (Bellomo and Ronco 2000) and possibly arrhythmias.
3 Monitor blood clotting and titrate anticoagulation.	To prevent risk of bleeding (Levy et al. 2009) and reduce risk of clotting to maintain circuit life (Davies and Leslie 2007).
4 Observe access entry site.	To monitor for signs of infection (DH 2007).
5 Monitor CRRT circuit. Keep circuit free from obstruction, kinks and accidental clamping.	To maintain CRRT and prolong circuit life (Baxter and Edwards 2007).
6 Observe circuit for the presence of air in the circuit.	To prevent air embolism entering the patient (Dirkes and Hodge 2007).
7 Ensure the tubing remains securely connected.	To ensure the double-lumen CVC is safely connected to prevent accidental disconnection and subsequent blood loss (Baxter and Edwards 2007).
8 Monitor and document CRRT machine pressures, such as access and return pressures, TMP (transmembrane pressures) and prefilter pressures.	To provide an indication or a trend of the life of the filter (Baxter and Edwards 2007).
9 Monitor and respond to all CRRT alarms.	To provide early detection of potential circuit problems such as clotting, inadequate blood flow, disconnection and air in the circuit (Dirkes and Hodge 2007).
10 Calculate and document hourly fluid totals.	To ensure that the prescribed fluid balance target is reached (Dirkes and Hodge 2007).

327

Procedure guideline 9.4: Disconnection of CRRT

Equipment

- Sterile dressing pack
- 2% chlorhexidine gluconate in 70% isopropyl alcohol solution
- Sterile gloves
- Apron and personal protective equipment
- 500 mL 0.9% sodium chloride

- 10 mL amps of 0.9% sodium chloride × 2
- 2 mL syringes with required locking-off solution × 2
- 5 mL syringes × 2
- 10 mL syringes × 2
- Sterile caps × 2

Procedure

Action	Rationale
1 Collect all necessary equipment.	To ensure CRRT machine is disconnected correctly (Baxter and Edwards 2007).
2 Put on apron, use personal protective equipment, wash hands, apply sterile gloves and open sterile dressing pack.	To reduce the risk of microbial contamination (Pratt et al. 2007).
3 Clamp access lumen (red lumen) on CVC.	To prevent blood loss directly from patient (Baxter and Edwards 2007).
4 Disconnect access tubing (red tubing) from the double-lumen CVC and using an aseptic non-touch technique connect access tubing to 0.9% sodium chloride.	To enable blood to be returned from the circuit to the patient. To reduce the risk of microbial contamination (Pratt et al. 2007).
5 Commence disconnection according to manufacturer's guidelines, following the CRRT machine on-screen instructions.	To ensure CRRT machine is disconnected safely and blood returned to patient (Dirkes and Hodge 2007). To minimize blood loss (Levy et al. 2009).
6 Swab access hub with 2% chlorhexidine gluconate in 70% isopropyl alcohol and allow to air dry.	To reduce the risk of microbial contamination (Pratt et al. 2007).
7 Attach 5 mL syringe and withdraw blood from access lumen of the CVC.	The withdrawal of a small volume of blood from within the CVC allows thrombi to be removed prior to flushing the lumen with 0.9% sodium chloride (Levy et al. 2009).
8 Flush access lumen with 10 mL of 0.9% sodium chloride and then administer prescribed anticoagulant.	To prevent thrombi forming within the lumen when not in use (Sarkar 2009).
9 Apply sterile cap to access hub.	To reduce the risk of microbial contamination (Pratt et al. 2007).
10 Once all blood returned to patient and CRRT blood pump stopped, clamp return lumen (blue lumen) on CVC.	To prevent blood loss directly from the patient (Baxter and Edwards 2007).
11 Disconnect return tubing (blue tubing) from the double-lumen CVC and swab access hub with 2% chlorhexidine gluconate in 70% isopropyl alcohol and allow to air dry.	To reduce the risk of microbial contamination (Pratt et al. 2007).
12 Attach 5 mL syringe and withdraw blood from return lumen of the CVC.	The withdrawal of a small volume of blood from within the CVC allows thrombi to be removed prior to flushing the lumen with 0.9% sodium chloride (Levy et al. 2009).
13 Flush access lumen with 10 mL of 0.9% sodium chloride and then administer prescribed anticoagulant.	To prevent thrombi forming within the lumen when not in use (Sarkar 2009).

14 Apply sterile cap to return hub.	To reduce the risk of microbial contamination (Pratt et al. 2007).
15 Ensure CVC clamps are on securely.	To prevent haemorrhage from CVC (Baxter and Edwards 2007).
16 Discard used circuit appropriately in line with national and local waste disposal guidelines.	To prevent contamination and maintain correct waste disposal process.
17 Document, sign, date and time the CRRT discontinued.	To: ■ provide an accurate record ■ monitor effectiveness of procedure ■ reduce the risk of duplication of treatment ■ provide a point of reference or comparison in the event of later questions ■ acknowledge accountability for actions ■ facilitate communication and continuity of care. (NMC 2008; HCPC 2012; GMC 2013)

Competency statement 9.1: Specific procedure competency statements for CRRT

Complete assessment against relevant fundamental competency statements (*see* Chapter 2, pp. 20, 21)	Evidence
Specific procedure competency statements for CRRT	**Evidence of competency for CRRT**
Demonstrate ability to: ■ teach and assess or ■ learn from assessment.	Examples of evidence of teaching, assessing and learning.
Demonstrate an understanding of the anatomy and physiology of the kidney.	*May be demonstrated by:* ■ discussion with supervisor/mentor ■ teaching session for peers.
Identify the causes and phases of acute renal failure (AKI), including: ■ pre-renal uraemia (azotaemia) ■ intrinsic AKI uraemia ■ post-renal uraemia (obstructive).	*May be demonstrated by:* ■ discussion of causes with supervisor/mentor and correctly identifying reason for AKI with individual patients ■ teaching session for peers.
Demonstrate an understanding of the principles of renal replacement therapy, including: ■ mechanisms and effects of CRRT ■ characteristics of IRRT and CRRT ■ indications for CRRT ■ types of CRRT: 　■ SCUF 　■ CVVH 　■ CVVHD 　■ CVVHDF.	*May be demonstrated by:* ■ discussion of mechanisms, characteristics and indications for each type of CRRT and IRRT with supervisor/mentor ■ teaching session for peers.

(Continued)

Competency statement 9.1: (*Continued*)

Identify complications associated with CRRT, including: ■ bleeding ■ hypothermia ■ infection ■ electrolyte and acid-base imbalance ■ haemodynamic instability ■ inappropriate drug dosing.	*May be demonstrated by:* ■ discussion of the complications associated with CRRT with supervisor/mentor. ■ teaching session for peers.
Demonstrate skills to prepare equipment and solutions for setting up and priming CRRT: ■ CRRT machine ■ machine lines and haemofilter ■ priming solution: 1 L 0.9% sodium chloride with or without heparin (dependent on individual need) ■ replacement and or dialysate fluid with or without potassium (dependent on patients electrolyte balance) ■ prescribed anticoagulant (if required) ■ prime machine as per manufacturer's instructions.	*May be demonstrated by:* ■ discussion with supervisor/mentor. ■ teaching session for peers ■ observation of setting up and preparation of CRRT in practice by supervisor/mentor.
Demonstrate an understanding of the importance of good vascular access and skills in maintenance and monitoring of vascular access.	*May be demonstrated by:* ■ discussion with supervisor/mentor ■ teaching session for peers.
Demonstrate knowledge and skills of the correct procedure for CRRT connection and disconnection, including: ■ aseptic non-touch technique ■ hub preparation ■ unlocking and locking of the double-lumen CVC ■ following manufacturer's instructions ■ following procedure for disposal of CRRT circuit.	*May be demonstrated by:* ■ discussion with supervisor/mentor ■ teaching session for peers ■ observation of correct connection and disconnection in practice by supervisor/mentor.
Demonstrate knowledge and understanding of continuous monitoring, including: ■ anticoagulation ■ cardiovascular status and fluid management ■ IV access and infection control ■ monitoring electrolytes and metabolic status ■ hypothermia ■ nutritional support ■ respiratory management ■ neurological care ■ monitoring the CRRT circuit.	*May be demonstrated by:* ■ discussion of the monitoring requirements of individual patients with supervisor/mentor ■ teaching session for peers.
Demonstrate knowledge and skills to safely problem solve on CRRT: ■ CRRT problems and alarms ■ causes ■ preventative measures ■ actions.	*May be demonstrated by:* ■ discussion of problems and causes with supervisor/mentor ■ teaching session for peers ■ observation of actions to prevent and solve problems associated with CRRT in practice by supervisor/mentor.
Demonstrate understanding and skill to correctly document CRRT, including: ■ commencement of CRRT as per prescription ■ assessment and monitoring the patient ■ recording and monitoring of alarms ■ discontinuation or CRRT.	*May be demonstrated by:* ■ discussion with supervisor/mentor ■ teaching session for peers ■ observation of documentation by supervisor/mentor.

References

Anderson JAM and Saenko EL (2002) Editorial 1, Heparin resistance. *British Journal of Anaesthesia* 88(4): 467–469.

Åhlström A (2006) Acute renal failure in critically ill patients. Academic dissertation for the Medical Faculty of the University of Helsinki. ISBN (PDF): 952-10-3394-0.

Arbour R (2004) Intracranial hypertension. Monitoring and nursing assessment. *Critical Care Nurse* 24: 19–32.

Ashley C and Currie A (2009) *The Renal Drug Handbook* (3e). Oxford: Radcliffe Publishing.

Barenbrock M, Hausberg M, Matzkies F et al. (2000) Effects of bicarbonate and lactate – buffered replacement fluids on cardiovascular outcome in CVVH patients. *Kidney International* 58: 1751–1757.

Baxter & Edwards (2007) *Module 1 CRRT Overview* (CD:ROM). Berkshire: Edwards Lifesciences Ltd.

Bellomo R and Ronco C (2000) Continuous haemofiltration in the intensive care unit. *Critical Care* 4: 339–345.

Bellomo R, Ronco C, Kellum JA, Mehta RL, Palevsky P and the ADQI (2004) Acute renal failure – definition, outcome measures, animal models, fluid therapy and information technology needs: the Second International Consensus Conference of the Acute Dialysis Quality Initiative (ADQI) Group. *Critical Care* 8(4): 204–212.

Brady HR and Kieran N (2006) Acute renal failure. In: Murray P, Brady H and Hall J (eds) *Intensive Care in Nephrology*, pp. 125–136. Oxon: Taylor & Francis.

Brooks G (2006) Potassium additive algorithm for use in continuous renal replacement therapy. *Nursing in Critical Care* 11(6): 273–280.

Chacko J (2008) Renal replacement therapy in the intensive care unit. *Indian Journal of Critical Care Medicine* 12: 174–180.

Culley CM, Bernardo JF, Gross PR et al. (2006) Implementing a standard safety procedure for continuous renal replacement therapy solutions. *American Journal Health-system Pharmacy* 63(8): 756–763.

Davenport A (1999) Is there a role for continuous renal replacement therapies in patients with liver and renal failure? *Kidney International* 56(72): S62–S66.

Davies H and Leslie G (2006) Maintaining the CRRT circuit: non-anticoagulant alternatives. *Australian Critical Care* 19(4): 133–138.

Davies H and Leslie G (2007). Anticoagulation in CRRT: agents and strategies in Australian ICUs. *Australian Critical Care* 20: 15–26.

Department of Health (2007) *High Impact Intervention No 1 central venous catheter care bundle*. London: DH.

Dirkes S and Hodge K (2007) Continuous renal replacement therapy in the adult intensive care unit: history and current trends. *Critical Care Nurse* 27: 61–80.

Edwards (2004) *Trouble Shooting Guide* (CD:ROMs). Berkshire: Edwards Lifesciences Ltd.

Faber P and Klein A (2009) Acute kidney injury and renal replacement therapy in the intensive care unit. *Nursing in Critical Care* 14(4): 207–212.

General Medical Council (2013) *Good Medical Practice*. London: GMC. http://www.gmc-uk.org/gmp2013 [accessed 25 March 2013].

Gladwin MT, Slonim A, Landucci DL et al. (1999) Cannulation of the internal jugular vein: is post procedural chest radiography always necessary? *Critical Care Medicine* 27: 1819–1823.

Griffiths L and Kanagasundaram NS (2011) Assessment and initial management of acute kidney injury. *Medicine* doi:10.1016/j.mpmed.2011.04.010.

Hall NA and Fox AJ (2006) Renal replacement therapies in critical care. *Continuing Education in Anaesthesia Critical Care and Pain* 6(5): 196–202.

Health and Care Professions Council (2012) *Standard of Conduct, Performance and Ethics*. London: HCPC. http://www.hcpc.uk.org/assets/documents/10003B6EStandardsofconduct,performanceandethics.pdf [accessed 16 November 2012].

Hilton PJ, Taylor J, Forni LG and Treacher DF (1998) Bicarbonate-based haemofiltration in the management of acute renal failure with lactic acidosis. *Quarterly Journal of Medicine* 91(4): 279–283.

Hilton R (2006) Acute renal failure. *British Medical Journal* 333: 786–790.

Kanagasundaram NS (2007) Renal replacement therapy in acute kidney injury: an overview. *British Journal of Hospital Medicine* 68(6): 292–297.

Kidney Disease: Improving Global Outcomes (KDIGO) (2012) Clinical Practice Guidelines for Acute Kidney Injury. *Kidney International Supplements* 2(1). http://www.kdigo.org/clinical_practice_guidelines/pdf/KDIGO%20AKI%20Guideline.pdf [accessed January 2013].

Langford S, Slivar S, Tucker SM and Bourbonnais FF (2008) Exploring CRRT practices in ICU: a survey of Canadian hospitals. *Canadian Association of Critical Care Nurses* Spring: 18–23.

Lee SJ, Park HS, Im EY and Sim YM (2008) A warming method to prevent hypothermia in patients treated using continuous venovenous hemodiafiltration. *Nephrology Nursing Journal* 35(2): 177.

Levy J, Brown E, Daley C and Lawrence A (2009) *Oxford Handbook of Dialysis* (3e). Oxford: Oxford University Press.

Levy J, Morgan J and Brown E (2004) *Oxford Handbook of Dialysis* (2e). Oxford: Oxford University Press.

Lewington A and Kanagasundaram S (2011) *Clinical Practice Guidelines Acute Kidney Injury*. Final version 8 March 2011. http://www.renal.org/Clinical/GuidelinesSection/AcuteKidneyInjury.aspx [accessed 5 December 2011].

Mehta RL (2001) Fluid management in CRRT. In: Ronco C Bellomo R and La Greca G (eds) *Blood Purification in Intensive Care*, pp. 335–348. Basel: Karger.

Mehta RL, Mcdonald B, Gabbal FB et al. (2001) A Randomised clinical trial of continuous versus intermittent dialysis for ARF. *Kidney International* 60: 1154–1163.

Mental Capacity Act (2005) http://www.legislation.gov.uk/ukpga/2005/9/pdfs/ukpga_20050009_en.pdf [accessed 9 February 2012].

Nursing and Midwifery Council (2008) *The Code: standards of conduct, performance and ethics for nurses and midwives*. London: NMC. http://www.nmc-uk.org/Documents/Standards/The-code-A4-20100406.pdf [accessed 15 February 2012].

Pannu N and Gibney N (2005) Renal replacement therapy in the intensive care. *Therapeutics and Clinical Risk Management* 1(2): 141–150.

Pannu N and Mehta R (2006) Continuous renal replacement therapies. In: Murray P, Brady H and Hall J (eds) *Intensive Care in Nephrology*, pp. 199–212. Oxon: Taylor & Francis.

Pratt RJ, Pellowea CM and Wilsona JA et al. (2007) epic2: National evidence-based guidelines for preventing healthcare-associated infections in NHS hospitals in England. *Journal of Hospital Infection* 655: s1–s64.

Raggio J and Umans JG (2006) Diagnosis of acute renal failure. In: Murray P, Brady H and Hall J (eds) *Intensive Care in Nephrology*, pp. 99–112. Oxon: Taylor & Francis.

Ronco C, Bellomo R, Homel P et al. (2000) Effects of different doses in continuous veno-venous haemofiltration on outcomes of acute renal failure: a prospective randomised trial. *Lancet* 356 (9223): 26–30.

Sarkar S (2009) Continuous renal replacement. *The Internet Journal of Anaesthesiology* **21**(1). http://www.ispub.com/journal/the_internet_journal_of_anesthesiology/volume_21_number_1/article/continuous-renal-replacement-therapy-crrt.html [accessed 22 October 2010].

Schetz M (2007) Drug dosing in continuous renal replacement therapy: general rules. *Current Opinion in Critical Care* **13**: 645–651.

Teo BW, Kanagasundaram NS and Paganini EP (2007) Continuous renal replacement therapy. In: Parrillo J and Dellinger ARP (eds) *Critical Care Medicine Principles of Diagnosis and Management of the Adult*. St Louis, MO: Mosby.

Tortora GJ and Derrickson B (2011) *Principles of Anatomy and Physiology (13e)*. New Jersey: John Wiley & Sons.

Wooley JA, Btaiche IF and Good KL (2005) Metabolic and nutritional aspects of acute renal failure in critically ill patients requiring continuous renal replacement therapy. *Nutrition in Clinical Practice* **20**: 176–191.

Chapter 10

Assessment and monitoring of analgesia, sedation, delirium and neuromuscular blockade levels and care

Phil Laws and Nicola Rudall

Newcastle upon Tyne Hospitals NHS Foundation Trust, Newcastle upon Tyne, UK

Critical Care Manual of Clinical Procedures and Competencies, First Edition.
Edited by Jane Mallett, John W. Albarran, and Annette Richardson.
© 2013 John Wiley & Sons, Ltd. Published 2013 by John Wiley & Sons, Ltd.

Pain

Definitions

Pain is:

'an unpleasant sensory and emotional experience associated with actual or potential tissue damage, or described in terms of such damage'
(Merskey and Bogduk 1994)

'whatever the person experiencing pain says it is, existing whenever the person communicates or demonstrates (voluntarily or involuntarily) it does'
(DH 2010, adapted from McCaffery and Beebe 1989)

Analgesia is derived from Greek; it literally means 'to be without the feeling of pain'. An analgesic is a drug or intervention used to relieve pain.

Aims and indications

The aims of pain prevention and management are:

- pain should be anticipated in all patients
- pre-emptive analgesia should be given for potentially painful procedures or painless alternatives sought
- the 'right drug' should be given at the 'right dose at the right time'
- pain should be regularly assessed, and if present, prompt the use of analgesics.

Background

Pain may be acute (less than 12 weeks' duration or pain that occurs during the expected period of healing) or chronic (pain of more than 12 weeks' duration or pain that continues after the expected period of healing) (DH 2010). For the purpose of this chapter the focus will be on acute pain. Acute pain may be: somatic (skin, muscle, joints, or tendons), visceral (internal organs, viscera, or skeleton), or referred (experience of pain distant to the site of origin). The latter is important for the diagnosis of pain, for example a patient experiencing pain in the shoulder may have the source of the pain around the diaphragm. For more information on referred pain see Guyton and Hall (2010). In the Study to Understand Prognoses and Preferences for Outcomes and Risks of Treatment (SUPPORT), pain was reported to occur in nearly 50% of seriously ill patients interviewed and was described as severe in 15% of patients (Desbiens et al. 1996).

Anatomy and physiology

Pain is sensed when the depolarization threshold of a nociceptor, a sensory nerve that responds to potentially damaging stimuli, is reached. This results in an action potential which is conducted along the nerve to the spinal cord where it synapses with a secondary pain neurone. If the depolarization threshold for the secondary neurone is met, the signal is then conducted up the spinal cord in the spinothalamic tract to the thalamus. From here, further nerves pass the signal on to the cortex where the conscious sensation of pain is produced. The depolarization threshold of the nociceptor may be reached by the chemicals released during tissue damage, chemical, radiation, mechanical pressure and/or thermal change. Neuropathic pain results from disease processes that physiologically alter the nociceptors, resulting in abnormal physiological responses to painful stimuli, or trigger the pain pathway even in the absence of painful stimuli (and is beyond the scope of this Manual).

Painful stimuli are transmitted to the spinal cord by fast-conducting myelinated Aδ fibres or unmyelinated slow-conducting C fibre nociceptors (Figure 10.1). Pain fibres enter the spinal cord via the dorsal root and synapses in the lamina of the grey matter in the dorsal horns. Secondary neurones cross the spinal cord and relay the signal up the spinothalamic tract, branching off to the reticular activating system (area of the brain responsible for regulating wakefulness) before terminating in the thalamus. From the thalamus, the signal is sent to the cortex, where conscious perception of pain occurs, and to the limbic system, instigating the emotional response.

Descending pain fibres originating in the periaqueductal grey (with some contribution from the cortex and thalamus) pass on to the reticular formation of the medulla and then down the spinal cord eventually on to the interneurones in the lamina in the spinal cord (substantia gelatinosa). Connections with the interneurons can modulate the threshold at which a painful stimulus is sent on to the secondary neurone. *Gray's Anatomy* can be referenced for more detailed descriptions of the anatomical structures referred to in the pain pathway (Standring 2008).

Analgesics can act at any point of the pain pathway: initiation of the signal (non-steroidal anti-inflammatory drugs), propagation of the signal (local anaesthetics), central relay of the signal (opioids) and the descending pathway (opioids).

Assessment of pain

Pain should be anticipated in all patients and every action should be questioned for its potential to cause pain. However, nurses underestimate patients' pain in 35–55% of patients (Hamill-Ruth and Marohn 1999; Watt-Watson et al. 2001). Anticipation of pain allows alternative strategies to be considered or pre-emptive analgesics given. Potential sources of pain should be looked for and may include: incisions, trauma, cannulation, intubation, catheterization, turning, endotracheal suctioning, drain removal, dressing changes, bowel obstruction, hard beds, immobility, joint pain, myopathy and neuropathy (Gunning 2010). All patients requiring critical care should be assessed for pain on a regular basis.

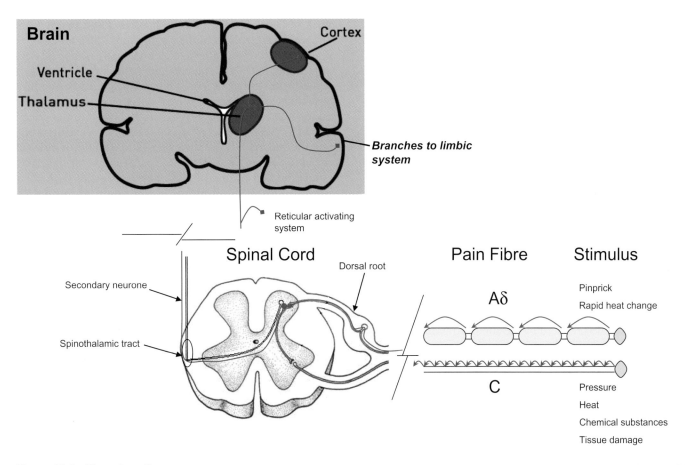

Figure 10.1 The pain pathway.

The frequency of pain assessment should be patient specific; this should be adjusted according to the risk of pain and be at least hourly in high-risk groups or patients managed with a patient controlled analgesic (PCA) device, epidural or nerve catheter. Pain should be reassessed after any change in therapy to assess the effectiveness of the intervention. Patient pain and discomfort can also be caused by monitoring and therapeutic devices (such as catheters, drains, non-invasive ventilating devices and endotracheal tubes), routine nursing care (such as airway suctioning, physical therapy, dressing changes and patient mobilization) and prolonged immobility (Jacobi et al. 2002).

The 'DOLOREA' prospective multicentred observational pain study compared critical care units where patients' pain was routinely scored compared with those units where it was not. This demonstrated both a reduction in duration of mechanical ventilation and length of critical care unit stay where scoring took place (Payen et al. 2009).

In view of the varied expression of pain, both behavioural and physiological indicators of pain should be sought. This involves looking for behavioural changes such as facial grimacing, ventilator dyssynchrony and limb flexion, along with physiological changes associated with pain, such as hypertension, tachycardia, tachypnoea and lacrimation. The

Society of Critical Care Medicine guidelines recommend that when a patient is able to cooperate, a numeric rating scale (NRS) should be used (Jacobi et al. 2002). The patient is asked to 'indicate on a scale from 0 to 10 where their pain is, with 0 being pain free and 10 being the worst pain you can imagine'. A score of 3 or less is the usual target, indicating mild pain at worst. A significant proportion of intensive care patients are unable to cooperate with this and require an alternative method of assessment. Hypertension, tachycardia, tachypnoea and lacrimation may all be associated with pain but are not sensitive or specific (that is, these signs are often present in the absence of pain and visa versa in the critical care patient population). Assessment of pain should include observation of pain-related behaviours (movement, facial expression and posturing) and physiological indicators (heart rate, blood pressure and respiratory rate), and the change in these parameters following analgesic therapy (Jacobi et al. 2002). The Behavioural Pain Scale (BPS) (Payen et al. 2001) was developed to allow a more quantifiable assessment of pain in patients unable to be assessed with a numeric rating scale. It is made up of three components: facial expression, degree of ventilator dyssynchrony and upper limb movement (see Table 10.1). A score of 5 or more was suggestive of pain in Payen's original study

Table 10.1 The Behavioural Pain Scale (adapted from Payen et al. 2001)

Facial expression	Relaxed	1
	Partially tightened (e.g. brow lowering)	2
	Fully tightened (e.g. eyelid closing)	3
	Grimacing	4
Upper limbs	No movement	1
	Partially bent	2
	Fully bent with finger flexion	3
	Permanently retracted	4
Compliance with ventilation	Tolerating movement	1
	Coughing but tolerating ventilation for most of the time	2
	Fighting ventilator	3
	Unable to control ventilation	4

Reproduced with permission from Elsevier.

as this score was reduced by the administration of analgesia. The scale is not perfect, as it may at times be unclear what category to place a patient into, in which case the best fit should be chosen. However, the BPS has been validated (Aissaoui et al. 2005), demonstrating construct validity, good inter-rater and internal reliability. Other assessment tools have been developed for non-communicative patients (Sessler et al. 2008). Some have been developed from paediatric tools such as the COMFORT scale and FLACC scale. The CCPOT scale has been developed for adult critically ill patients and has been validated in cardiac surgery patients.

So, as pain is by definition 'what the patient says it is', a numeric rating scale of the patient's perception of their level of pain should be used wherever possible in the first instance (Jacobi et al. 2002). When this is not feasible the limitations of physiological parameters in the assessment of pain have to be acknowledged and behavioural pain markers sought. Introduction of a formal system for assessing pain is associated with improved patient outcomes.

Management of pain

When pain is detected analgesics should be given following the World Health Organization analgesic ladder (WHO 1990), which states that it is important to give: 'the right drug at the right dose at the right time'. This guidance suggests starting with non-opioid analgesics, then, if the patient's pain is not appropriately managed, simultaneously administering weak opioids before escalating to strong opioids as necessary. In practice, certain groups of patients will have predictable pain requirements needing a combination of non-opioids and strong opioids to start with; elective laparotomies for example. It is important to consider reducing analgesia, especially continuous infusions of strong opiates, to prevent accumulation and side effects. Opioid infusions can be replaced by 'as required' boluses of opioids in the first instance, when the patient appears comfortable. If the patient requires regular boluses (hourly) or it is dif-

ficult to decrease pain levels with bolus doses, that is there are peaks and troughs in their pain scores, then an infusion is appropriate. For example, if a patient falls asleep and does not receive any 'as required' analgesic boluses and then wakes with significant pain, an infusion should be administered. It is important to ensure the patient is prescribed and taking regular enteral analgesics in keeping with the principles of the WHO analgesic ladder before commencing strong opiates, especially infusions. This is to ensure the risks of strong opiates are justified by the persistence of pain despite regular administration of non-opiate analgesics in the first instance. All analgesic infusions should be stopped on a daily basis to prevent drug accumulation such as may occur with sedatives unless there are specific contraindications to do so. (Refer to the section on sedation, below; *see also* Chapter 11.) Boluses should then be given to achieve analgesia prior to restarting the infusion at half its original rate and then titrating according to the patients needs. For further information on drugs used to treat pain, refer to the Treatment section later in the chapter.

Sedation

Definition

Sedation is an induced state of reduced consciousness in which verbal contact with the patient may be maintained. It is used to reduce anxiety and distress, and to facilitate compliance with invasive procedures such as mechanical ventilation.

Aims of sedation

The aims of sedation are to:

- allow essential procedures to be carried out, including intubation
- minimize distress to the patient (including to patients receiving neuromuscular blocking drugs)
- aid ventilation (for example to reduce oxygen consumption; if there is dyssynchrony with the ventilator)
- control delirium.

(Peck and Down 2009)

Sedation should be titrated appropriately to achieve these aims. This should include regular assessment of sedation level and incorporate sedation breaks where possible.

Background

A significant proportion of critical care patients will require a degree of sedation at some point during their stay. Although sedation relies on the use of appropriate drugs, there is no consensus on which drug or combination of drugs is best, and as such, usage varies widely between units. Increasingly, sedation is focused on an analgesia-based approach.

A level of light sedation, where the patient is either awake and settled, or lightly sleeping, is usually sufficient. Due to the potential risks of deep sedation, including hypotension, increased risk of ventilator-associated pneumonia and poor gastrointestinal absorption, it should only be used where the benefits are likely to outweigh the risks. For example:

- patients receiving neuromuscular blocking drugs
- head injury (for control of intracranial pressure)
- certain ventilator modes (see Chapter 5)
- refractory status epilepticus.

It is no longer considered good practice to continually sedate patients throughout their whole critical care stay. While there is clearly a need for patients to be sedated at times, depth of sedation varies in critical care according to its purpose. However, it should be noted that patients receiving deeper and lengthy periods of sedation are at higher risk of developing depression or post-traumatic stress disorder (PTSD) (Jones 2010). In addition, those with periods of amnesia or receiving long spells of sedation may be predisposed to developing delusional, sometimes very distressing, memories, which can also lead to PTSD. Patients allowed clear memories of their ICU stay are less likely to develop delusional memories, thereby reducing psychological problems in the longer term (Jones et al. 2001). This may be facilitated by withholding sedation for periods of time (see Sedation hold).

Sedation regimens should ideally be analgesic rather than hypnotic-based, that is opioid rather than benzodiazepine-based (Waldman 2010a). This can minimize the risk of over-sedation, and address pain, which may originate from a variety of sources (including mechanical ventilation, surgical procedures, or prolonged bed rest). Patients with inadequate analgesia may be agitated, and hypnotics alone, such as propofol or benzodiazepines, will not address this problem adequately. For further information on the drugs used in sedation, please refer to the Treatment section later in the chapter.

Sedation hold

Patients should have all continuous sedation drugs stopped daily (commonly known as a 'sedation hold') unless there are clinical contraindications such as muscle relaxation, unstable ventilation, or significantly raised intracranial pressure). Staff should be available during a 'sedation hold' in case the patient wakes up agitated and is difficult to manage. Patients requiring re-sedation should initially receive boluses to achieve control and the infusion should then be restarted at half the original rate (Kress et al. 2002). This is because restarting at a higher rate can lead to over-sedation. Many patients will tolerate an endotracheal tube while awake and it may not be necessary to restart the sedation if they are sufficiently comfortable.

Withholding sedation allows assessment of the patient's neurological status by ensuring they are not over-sedated, as well as minimizing the risks of ventilator-associated pneu-

monia and drug accumulation. Quantifiable benefits include reduced duration of mechanical ventilation, shorter length of stay and reduced alterations in mental status (Kress et al. 2002). Additionally, the use of sedation holds can be paired with spontaneous breathing trials, further reducing length of stay in critical care (Girard et al. 2008) (see also Chapter 5). In this study the spontaneous breathing trial (SBT) protocol was as follows: ventilatory support was removed and the patient was allowed to breathe through either a T-tube circuit or a ventilatory circuit with continuous positive airway pressure of 5 cm H_2O or pressure support ventilation of less than 7 cm H_2O. No change was made in FiO_2 or PEEP during the SBT. Patients failed the SBT if they developed:

- a respiratory rate of more than 35 or less than eight breaths/min for 5 minutes or longer
- hypoxaemia (SpO_2 less than 88% for equal to or greater than 5 minutes)
- abrupt changes in mental status
- an acute cardiac arrhythmia
- two or more signs of respiratory distress, including tachycardia (greater than 130 bpm), bradycardia (less than 60 bpm), use of accessory muscles, abdominal paradox, diaphoresis, or marked dyspnoea.

Patients who failed the SBT were ventilated immediately with the ventilator settings used before the trial. Patients passed the SBT if they did not develop any failure criteria during a 120-minute trial.

A Cochrane Collaboration review found that in units where protocols are used to manage sedation, there is a 25% reduction in length of mechanical ventilation, as well as reduction in time to wean and a shorter length of ICU stay (Blackwood et al. 2010). Addition of daily sedation holds with protocolized sedation in adult mechanically ventilated patients has not been shown to reduce the duration of mechanical ventilation or ICU stay (Mehta et al. 2012).

Regular sedation holds help patients to lay down clear memory from their time in critical care, which is important to their long term psychological recovery (Jones et al. 2001).

Withdrawal of sedation

It is estimated that up to 33% of patients receiving sedatives for seven or more days experience some degree of withdrawal effects (Borthwick et al. 2006). These are particularly associated with opioids and/or benzodiazepines, although there have been reports of propofol withdrawal. Patients at high risk of withdrawal effects include those sedated for longer than five days, and those receiving high doses (Devlin et al. 2010). Signs of withdrawal, which may include sweating, fatigue, tremor, agitation, cardiovascular instability and delirium, should be managed by gradual discontinuation of the offending drugs (Jacobi et al. 2002). The use of adjuncts such as clonidine to manage withdrawal may also be considered (Devlin et al. 2010). Acute withdrawal reactions generally last around 1–2 weeks, although somatic and psychiatric symptoms may persist for months (Borthwick et al. 2006).

Rescue sedation

In agitated, aggressive, or delirious patients, there may be a need to give intermittent sedation to calm the patient (usually referred to as 'rescue sedation'). This may be administered on an 'as needed' basis. The aim is to calm the patient without resorting to continual sedation. In aggressive or very agitated patients, rescue sedation may need to be given before the underlying cause can be treated.

The type of rescue sedation used depends on the underlying cause of the agitation. Where the cause is delirium, an antipsychotic is likely to be the most effective treatment, but different causes may require a different approach. For patients with delirium, haloperidol or olanzapine are the preferred choices (Borthwick et al. 2006; NICE 2010). Patients withdrawing from alcohol may require intermittent benzodiazepines such as chlordiazepoxide or lorazepam, whereas patients withdrawing from recreational drugs (usually psychoactive drugs) or nicotine may benefit from clonidine.

Staff in some units use physical restraint to manage agitated patients, such as bandaging of the hands to prevent essential tubes being pulled out. Some consider that physical restraint is ethically equivalent to chemical restraint with sedatives or other drugs (Nirmalan et al. 2004). It is sometimes considered reasonable to use physical restraints where the risks of drug-induced sedation (aspiration, increased infections, prolonged length of stay) outweigh the risks of physical restraint (patient anxiety and potential post-traumatic stress). This is a controversial area and it is advocated that physical restraint should only be used when all other methods have failed, and should also be used with caution (Bray et al. 2004). There is some concern that patients who have been physically restrained without sedation have shown an increased likelihood of post-traumatic stress disorder (PTSD) (Jones et al. 2007). However, this must be balanced against the recognized side effects and increased morbidity associated with sedative drugs.

The Mental Capacity Act 2005 (Department for Constitutional Affairs 2007) provides a legal framework whereby treatment may be given to a patient who lacks capacity to consent to it themselves. Attempts to restore capacity should be made where practical. The treatment must be in their overall benefit and the least incapacitating equally effective option should be chosen. Sedation is often required to facilitate interventions or treatments on critically ill patients who would otherwise resist such treatments. This is entirely acceptable practice if their resistance is due to a lack of capacity and the sedation is necessary to facilitate compliance with treatments that are in their overall benefit, such as invasive ventilation. In these situations any valid and applicable advance directives will need to be taken into account.

Assessment of sedation

Patients on critical care units should have their level of sedation recorded at least twice a day, to ensure that the patient is comfortable, cooperative and not over-sedated. Various scoring systems have been produced, some more complex than others. However, one that incorporates both sedation and agitation is helpful not only for assessing sedation, but as a first step in identifying possible delirium (Waldman 2010b).

Assessment tools should be quick and easy to use, with well-defined criteria and good inter-rater reliability and validity (Sessler 2004). Sedation scoring scales include:

- Ramsay (Ramsay et al. 1974)
- Sedation-Agitation Scale (SAS) (Riker et al. 1994)
- Motor Activity Assessment Scale (Devlin et al. 1999)
- Richmond Agitation and Sedation Scale (RASS) (Sessler et al. 2002)
- Adaption To Intensive Care Environment (De Jonghe et al. 2003).

The RASS is a frequently used scale that is currently endorsed by NICE clinical guideline 103 concerning delirium (NICE 2010) (see Box 10.1). RASS and SAS have excellent inter-rater correlation compared with Ramsay, which suffers from its limited descriptors. Whatever the choice of scale, the intention should be a calm and cooperative patient. Adoption of a systematic approach to the assessment of sedation has demonstrated reduced lengths of stay (Robinson et al. 2008).

Monitoring of sedated patients

An ideal sedative would, without any side effects, produce a calm and cooperative patient. However, no such drug exists. Consequently it is necessary to monitor patients not only for their level of sedation, but also for the other effects of the sedative drugs used.

As well as regular assessment of sedation levels, patients receiving sedative drugs should be monitored for side effects, including hypotension and dysrhythmias (Devlin et al. 2010). Lipid profiles for patients on prolonged periods of propofol (greater than 48 hours) and gastric motility (both absorption of feed and bowel movements) for those on opioids (Devlin et al. 2010) should be observed. Additionally, renal and hepatic function should be checked regularly to ensure doses are titrated to response and do not accumulate as a result of impaired clearance. While patients should be screened for delirium at least daily, this may need to be more frequent in patients receiving deliriogenic drugs.

The Bispectral Index (BIS) is a measure of the patient's level of consciousness by analysis of a patient's electroencephalogram (EEG), typically limited to unilateral frontal lobe analysis (see also Chapter 13). It is a statistically based, empirically derived (initially from around 1000 healthy adult volunteers) complex parameter, ranging from 0 (EEG silence) to 100 (fully awake), a level of 40–60 is recommended for general anaesthesia. Despite the Food and Drug Administration (FDA) in the USA clearing the BIS in 1996 for its use in monitoring the hypnotic effects of general

Box 10.1 Richmond Agitation and Sedation Scale (RASS) (adapted from Sessler et al. 2002)

Score term description

+4 Combative: Overtly combative, violent, immediate danger to staff

+3 Very agitated: Pulls or removes tube(s) or catheter(s); aggressive

+2 Agitated: Frequent non-purposeful movement, fights ventilator

+1 Restless: Anxious but movements not aggressive or vigorous

0 Alert and calm

−1 Drowsy: Not fully alert, but has sustained awakening (eye-opening/eye contact) to *voice* (greater than 10 seconds)

−2 Light sedation: Briefly awakens with eye contact to *voice* (less than 10 seconds)

−3 Moderate sedation: Movement or eye opening to *voice* (but no eye contact)

−4 Deep sedation: No response to voice, but movement or eye-opening to *physical* stimulation

−5 Unrousable: No response to *voice or physical* stimulation

Procedure for RASS assessment

1 Observe patient
  (a) Patient is alert, restless, or agitated. **(score 0 to +4)**
2 If not alert, state patient's name and *say* to open eyes and look at speaker.
  (b) Patient awakens with sustained eye opening and eye contact. **(score −1)**
  (c) Patient awakens with eye opening and eye contact, but not sustained. **(score −2)**
  (d) Patient has any movement in response to voice but no eye contact. **(score −3)**
3 When no response to verbal stimulation, physically stimulate patient by shaking shoulder and/or rubbing sternum.
  (e) Patient has any movement to physical stimulation. **(score −4)**
  (f) Patient has no response to any stimulation. **(score −5)**

Reproduced with permission from American Thoracic Society.

anaesthesia, its use remains globally controversial. A review of the BIS monitor in critical care (LeBlanc et al. 2006) found no randomized controlled trials demonstrating improved outcomes with BIS monitoring. In LeBlanc's review there was a low correlation between BIS and subjective sedation scales, and poor correlation between drug dosage and BIS, suggesting it is unhelpful in guiding sedation. At present BIS cannot be recommended for routine use in assessing conscious levels of patients receiving critical care, and further studies are required to determine its role in the assessment of sedation.

Delirium

Definition

Delirium is the acute onset of a fluctuating level of consciousness associated with confusion and inattention. It is formally defined by the Diagnostic and Statistical Manual of Mental Disorders IV –TR (American Psychiatric Association 2000), noting two equally prevalent distinct types.

- Hypoactive subtype with inhibition of behavioural and/ or locomotor activity, where the patient is unusually unresponsive to changes in their environment.
- Hyperactive subtype where the patient is abnormally and easily excitable or exuberant.

Occasionally a mixed type exists, where the patient may fluctuate from one subtype to the other. Due to its prevalence and significant impact in the critically ill it has been referred to as one of the vital signs (Flaherty et al. 2007).

Aims in treating patients with, or at risk of developing, delirium

The aims of treating patients with, or at risk of developing, delirium are to:

- regularly assess delirium status
- ensure possible causes of delirium are addressed, including drug causes
- orientate patients to time and place
- provide appropriate management (which may include drug therapy) of delirium, including removing causes where possible.

Background

Delirium may be found in 15–80% of critically ill patients and is associated with higher mortality, longer length of stay and greater likelihood of neuropsychological disturbance following hospital discharge (Borthwick et al. 2006). It often goes undetected, and therefore untreated, in patients receiving critical care. Delirium is characterized by an acute onset or fluctuating course of inattention, an altered level of consciousness and disordered thinking (NICE 2010). On waking, patients should be orientated in time and place and be within sight of a clock. They should also be given support, such as glasses and hearing aids, to ensure they can interact with people in their surroundings (NICE 2010).

There are several factors that can cause 'ICU delirium', some of which may be easily treated by, for example, adequate pain relief, explanation of circumstances and treatment plans, and regular review of drugs (Borthwick et al. 2006). Other causes include acidosis, sepsis, cerebral illness, constipation, unregulated diurnal rhythm, ventilator dysynchrony, previous drug abuse and advancing age.

Patients at risk of delirium include those with:

- age 65 years and over*
- pre-existing cognitive impairment*
- current hip fractures*
- severe illness* (a clinical condition that is deteriorating or is at risk of deterioration)
- coexisting medical conditions
- malnutrition or dehydration
- a history of, or active, alcohol abuse
- multiple drugs prescribed (polypharmacy)
- visual or hearing impairment
- immobility
- previous delirium episode(s)
- multiple psychoactive drugs
- poor sleep
- male gender.

*Risk factors listed in NICE clinical guidance 103 Delirium (NICE 2010).

Drugs and delirium

Many of the drugs used in critical care may contribute to delirium, and indeed several of the drugs traditionally used to treat agitation may exacerbate it. Deliriogenic drugs should be minimized, and when used, should be regularly reviewed to check they are still required (Borthwick et al. 2006). Drugs contributing to delirium include, among others:

- gastrointestinal drugs: ranitidine and metoclopramide
- cardiovascular drugs: atenolol, digoxin and furosemide
- central nervous system drugs: amitriptyline, diazepam, chlordiazepoxide, thiopental, codeine, fentanyl, morphine, pethidine, chlorpromazine and phenytoin
- endocrine drugs: steroids
- anticholinergic and antimuscarinic drugs: atropine and hyoscine.

For information on drugs used to treat delirium, refer to the Treatment section later in the chapter.

Assessment and monitoring of delirium

Delirium can be difficult to assess, due to the presence of a hypoactive, as well as a hyperactive, subtype. However, a delirium screen (a short clinical assessment for the presence of delirium) should be part of routine monitoring in critical care and should be performed at least once daily, preferably each shift. This is because patient's mental status may fluctuate, seeming lucid one moment and confused the next. Patients should also be formally screened if they are demonstrating behaviour that may be consistent with the definitions of hypoactive or hyperactive delirium.

Some sedation scoring systems may highlight a potentially delirious patient (see above), although further assessment will be required. An appropriate screening tool must be used, as without one, about two-thirds of delirium cases are missed. The recommended system by the NICE guidance on delirium (NICE 2010) is the Confusion Assessment Method for the Intensive Care Unit (CAM-ICU). The CAM-ICU tool has 98% accuracy and assessment can be completed, on average, in 2 minutes (Jacobi et al. 2002). The patient cannot be assessed if they are very unresponsive, that is a RASS (Sessler et al. 2002) of −4 or −5.

If a patient is assessed as being delirious, an underlying cause (opioid toxicity, polypharmacy, underlying condition, hyponatraemia, hypocalcaemia, hypoxaemia, infection, constipation, urinary retention, dehydration, sleep deprivation, pain, or stress) should be considered and treated where possible. In addition, deliriogenic drugs should be reviewed and stopped where appropriate. Rescue sedation may also be required if the patient is a danger to themselves or other people. As well as frequent monitoring of the delirium status, patients receiving antipsychotics as rescue sedation should have their cardiac rhythm checked frequently for arrhythmias, and those on older antipsychotics should be monitored for extrapyramidal symptoms.

Neuromuscular blockade

Definition

Neuromuscular blockade is the reversible impairment of neuromuscular transmission resulting in skeletal muscle relaxation. The word 'paralysis' should not be used as this suggests the irreversible loss of the ability to move a body part.

Aims and indications

The aim of neuromuscular blockade is to relax skeletal muscle, which may be of benefit:

- in facilitating mechanical ventilation where there is ventilator dyssynchrony or poor compliance
- in severe acute respiratory distress syndrome (Papazian et al. 2010) by increasing lung compliance
- during intubation and laryngoscopy to relax the mouth opening and optimize view of laryngeal inlet
- in head injury to minimize surges in refractory raised intracranial pressure
- in tetany to treat severe muscle spasms, including opithotonos (extreme rigid spasm of the body with the back completely arched with the heels and head bent back, seen occasionally in meningitis)
- in prolonged status epilepticus to prevent hyperthermia and rhabdomyolysis
- in reducing oxygen requirements by reducing muscle activity
- in sedation-resistant shivering during active cooling (that is, for clinical reasons) where the shivering is counterproductive, as it is thermogenic.

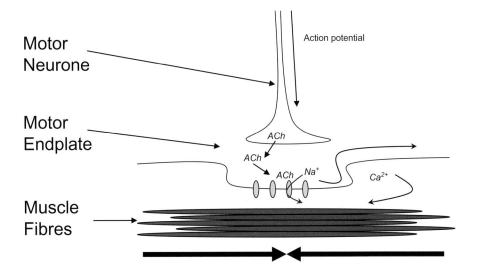

Figure 10.2 The neuromuscular junction.

It should be noted, however, that:

- neuromuscular blockade should only be used where absolutely necessary
- the effectiveness and degree of the blockade should be monitored via observation and a 'Train-of-Four Stimulator' (which measures depth of neuromuscular blockade; *see* Figure 10.3 and section below)
- some conditions interfere with the assessment of neuromuscular blockade, including critical illness polyneuropathy, Guillain-Barré syndrome and myasthenia gravis
- there should be prophylactic management to prevent other unwanted effects of neuromuscular blockade, including venous thromboses, skin and eye trauma.

Anatomy and physiology

Movement is produced by the contraction of muscle; the nerves supplying the muscles (motor neurones) release chemicals (neurotransmitters) to 'switch on' contraction. These chemicals attach to receptors in the muscle cells, which then open, starting a chain of events that results in muscle contraction.

Muscle contraction is instigated by a motor neurone. Subsequent depolarization at the nerve terminus releases acetylcholine (ACh) vesicles, each containing about 10 000 Ach molecules. The ACh transmitter diffuses across the 20 nm synaptic cleft and binds to the ligand-gated nicotinic ACh receptor on the motor endplate, resulting in depolarization of the muscle fibre, calcium release and subsequent muscle contraction. Neuromuscular blocking drugs (NMBDs) act at the nicotinic ACh receptors. Depolarizing NMBDs (DNMBDs) bind and activate the receptor leaving it in an 'on' position, hence inactivating it. Non-depolarizing NMBDs (NDNMBDs) also bind to the receptors but do not activate them, they act by competitive antagonism with the

ACh released from the motor neurone (Figure 10.2). The effects of DNMBDs are not reversible while the effects of NDNMBDs are reversible. More detail on the neuromuscular junction can be found in Guyton (Guyton and Hall 2010). For further information on drugs used for neuromuscular blockade, refer to the Treatment section later in the chapter.

Neuromuscular blockade

Neuromuscular blockade renders a patient unable to move. If the patient is conscious they will be able to see, hear and feel but not respond. This 'awareness' is potentially extremely distressing and is associated with a high incidence of post-traumatic stress disorder. The NMBDs potentially interact with other drugs and may produce adverse reactions. Therefore, neuromuscular blockade should be used only when alternative means of facilitating treatment have been tried without success. The goal is to obtain muscle relaxation without complete blockade. Patients must receive adequate analgesia and sedation before initiation of neuromuscular blockade, to ensure they are not distressed by the sensation of 'paralysis'. There should be prophylactic management to prevent other unwanted effects of neuromuscular blockade. These include: the development of venous thromboembolism and trauma to the skin from pressure ulceration (due to lack of movement), and damage to the eyes from direct trauma (due to an absent blink or corneal reflex) and dryness (due to lack of intermittent eyelid closure moving lacrimal fluid over the surface of the eye).

Neuromuscular blockade is no longer routinely used in conjunction with sedation in critically ill patients, although it does still have a place in selected cases. Prolonged neuromuscular blockade may increase the likelihood of neuropathy and myopathy developing (Pati et al. 2008). While continuous infusions of neuromuscular blocking agents may be used, boluses are a preferable alternative, reducing the chance of accumulation.

Prolonged infusions greater than 48 hours have been associated with acute quadriplegic myopathy syndrome. The incidence may rise with the concurrent administration of corticosteroids and it is reported in more than 30% of patients receiving prolonged infusions. There is inconsistent correlation between the incidence and the dose of steroid, but total doses during their intensive care admission greater than 1 g methylprednisolone or equivalent probably increase the risk (Murray et al. 2002). However, in the multicentre, blinded, placebo-controlled study of acute respiratory distress syndrome with cisatracurium or placebo infusion (Papazian et al. 2010), the rate of critical care unit-acquired 'paresis' was no higher with the infusion of muscle relaxant.

Assessment of neuromuscular blockade

Assessment of neuromuscular blockade is required if there is any doubt over the existence of residual blockade (NMBDs not fully metabolized and eliminated, hence having a residual effect or their action potentiated by hypermagnesaemia) prior to extubation of a patient or before undertaking tests to diagnose brainstem death. Observation of skeletal muscle movement and respiratory effort forms the foundation of clinical assessment of neuromuscular blockade. The Society of Critical Care Guidelines (Murray et al. 2002) recommend that patients receiving NMBDs should be assessed both via practitioners' observation of skeletal movement and respiratory effort, as well as by using more accurate, quantifiable methods, such as 'Train-of-Four' (TOF) monitoring to assess muscle tone (see Figure 10.3 and Table 10.2 for details).

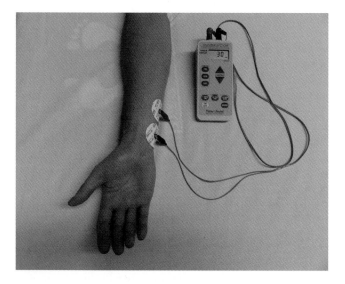

Figure 10.3 Train-of-Four Stimulator attached to electrodes placed over the ulnar nerve.

It is also important to observe for signs of distress from being aware of the inability to move due to the use of muscle-relaxing drugs with inadequate sedation. This may present as tachycardia, hypertension, sweating, or lacrimation. However, the presence of these signs when NMBDs are being used does not always indicate under-sedation as the signs are not sensitive or specific for awareness.

Extubation in the presence of residual blockade results in a 'partially reversed' patient (from the effects of the NMBD), and the patient will feel as if they cannot breath after extubation. This normally manifests as agitation and 'twitchy' movement of the patient and is an indication for the use of reversal agents despite the presence of four twitches on the TOF.

Treatment

Drugs for sedation, analgesia and neuromuscular blockade

A wide variety of drugs are used in critical care for the prevention and treatment of pain, sedation and delirium, and also to induce neuromuscular blockade. The following drugs may be used in other contexts in different ways; the indications discussed here relate to critically ill patients. *See* Table 10.3 for a summary table of commonly used drugs.

Sedation

Patients receiving continuous sedation on critical care will routinely get a combination of drugs; usually a strong opioid for analgesia and either an anaesthetic or sedative drug as an infusion.

The ideal sedation drug would be both analgesic and anxiolytic, with minimal side effects; short-acting with a rapid onset, easily administered and titrated. It would be cost-effective and unaffected by poor renal or liver function and have no active metabolites. It would also be readily reversible and would not interact with other drugs or therapies. In practice, no such drug exists, and hence a wide selection is used.

Anaesthetics

Propofol is a frequently used anaesthetic in critical care and is a lipid emulsion with a rapid onset and short duration of action. Its mechanism of action is unclear, but it appears to act on gamma-aminobutyric acid (GABA) receptors (Kress & Hall 2006). Propofol is widely distributed within the body and is metabolized by the liver, so care should be taken in severe hepatic impairment. As well as sedation, hypnosis and a degree of amnesia, it can cause significant hypotension – resulting in the need for vasopressors – and hyperlipidaemia due to the fatty nature of the drug (Devlin et al. 2010). When given concurrently with midazolam, blood levels of

Table 10.2 'Train-of-Four' (TOF) monitoring when using neuromuscular blockade drugs (NMBDs) for patients requiring level three care

Aim	To monitor degree of neuromuscular blockade and allow titration of drug dosing to a clinically appropriate level
Indications	To assess relaxation of muscle[*1] in order to: ■ adjust dosage of NMBDs to therapeutic levels ■ prevent build-up of residual NMBDs ■ minimize side effects of NMBDs ■ assess if brain stem death testing is valid *[*1] Particularly in the case of continuous infusion or repeated boluses*

Frequency of assessment	■ Hourly when using a continuous infusion
	■ When any doubt over residual blockade prior to:
	  ■ brain stem death testing
	  ■ extubation
	  ■ sedation hold

Method	■ Electrodes placed to stimulate peripheral nerve (ulnar [electrodes along the ulnar boarder of the forearm], facial [electrodes placed anterior to the tragus of the ear], or tibial [electrodes behind the medial maleolus]) ■ Delivery of four electrical impulses (each one every 0.5 s) to the peripheral nerve by the 'Train-of-Four' (TOF) nerve stimulator ■ Number of palpable twitches (T) of relevant muscle counted (TOF count) ■ Amplitude of the fourth twitch divided by the amplitude of the first (T4/T1) measured by acceleromyographic technique (TOF ratio). (This is not currently widely performed)
Results	Stimulation of the: ■ ulnar nerve will cause thumb abduction ■ facial nerve will cause contraction of the facial muscles[*2] ■ tibial nerve will cause flexion of the big toe The TOF ratio indicates the degree of neuromuscular block. A ratio of greater than, or equal to, 0.9 suggests little residual block exists and the patient is unlikely to have a sensation of muscle weakness or difficulty in breathing. The acceleration of the muscle contraction can be measured using an acceleromyograph[*3] The number of palpable muscular twitches (between 0 and 4) indicates the level of occupancy of the receptors by the NMBDs (Hughes and Griffiths 2002).[*4] Zero indicates complete clinical blockade. A count of three or fewer twitches indicates significant residual neuromuscular blockade, one or two twitches indicates a state of surgical relaxation (loss of abdominal muscle tone) and is the suggested target for the use of continuous infusions of NMBDs in patients receiving intensive care *[*2] It is possible to underestimate the degree of blockade using this method as direct stimulation of facial muscle is common (rather than stimulation of the facial nerve causing muscle twitching). This gives rise to a greater number of palpable facial twitches than may occur when stimulating the facial nerve alone* *[*3] Force = mass × acceleration. As the 'muscle' mass is constant, the acceleration is proportional to the force, therefore by measuring the acceleration of the first and fourth twitch the ratio can be calculated. The force of the contraction will produce a varying amplitude. However, the force of contraction is more closely linked to the degree of receptor blockade than to the amplitude of the resulting muscle contraction* *[*4] It should be noted that the absence of muscle twitching with electrical stimulation is possible with neuromuscular problems including: myasthenia gravis, Lambert-Eaton syndrome, Guillain-Barré Syndrome and critical illness polyneuropathy*
Clinical management	■ If the number of twitches is fewer than two, the dose can be reduced or the NMBDs interval increased or withdrawn ■ If the number of twitches is greater than two, the dose can be increased or interval shortened ■ If required, reversal of NDNMBDs with neostigmine is possible when two twitches are present. However, reversal it is much more likely to be successful when three or four twitches are present ■ Even when four twitches are counted, significant neuromuscular blockade may persist, so TOF is not helpful in deciding when not to reverse NDNMBDs. The timing of the last dose of NDNMBD is more helpful in this situation

343

propofol have been shown to be increased, and midazolam distribution and clearance reduced (Lichtenbelt et al. 2010). Propofol is licensed for critical care sedation for a maximum of 3 days, due to the risk of propofol infusion syndrome (PRIS); however, in practice it is frequently used for longer than this (Ostermann et al. 2000). PRIS is a rare syndrome causing lipaemia, acidosis, arrhythmias and rhabdomyolysis (Vasile et al. 2003). Risk factors for PRIS include high doses of propofol (greater than 5 mg/kg/h), age (it should not be used for critical care sedation in patients under 18 years old)

Table 10.3 Summary of commonly used drugs

Drug	Type	Use (in critical care)	Other Information
Alfentanil	Opioid	■ Continuous sedation	■ Short acting (half-life 1–2 h)*
Clonidine	Alpha-2-agonist	■ Rescue sedation (unlicensed use)	■ May be of particular use in certain withdrawal syndromes ■ Monitor BP carefully and taper dose slowly
Dexmedetomidine	Alpha-2-agonist	■ Continuous (light) sedation	■ Can be analgesic-sparing
Fentanyl	Opioid	■ Analgesia ■ Continuous sedation	■ Context-sensitive half-life ■ May accumulate in renal impairment
Haloperidol	Butyrophenone antipsychotic	■ Rescue sedation	■ May prolong QTc interval ■ May cause extrapyramidal side effects
Ibuprofen Diclofenac Naproxen	Non-steroidal anti-inflammatory drugs	■ Analgesia, particularly associated with inflammation	■ Nephrotoxic ■ Can cause cardiovascular problems ■ Increases bleeding risk
Lorazepam (infusion)	Benzodiazepine	■ Continuous sedation (unlicensed for this use)	■ Toxic solvents may accumulate
Midazolam	Benzodiazepine	■ Continuous sedation	■ Causes amnesia ■ May accumulate in renal impairment
Morphine	Opioid	■ Analgesia ■ Continuous sedation	■ May accumulate in renal impairment
Olanzapine Quetiapine Risperidone	'Atypical' antipsychotics	■ Rescue sedation	■ Better tolerated than older antipsychotics ■ Can cause hyperglycaemia
Paracetamol	Non-opioid analgesia	■ Analgesia	■ First-line analgesic ■ Well tolerated, although caution in liver impairment
Propofol	Anaesthetic	■ Continuous sedation	■ Rapid onset and short-acting (half-life 3–12 h) ■ High fat content
Remifentanil	Opioid	■ Continuous sedation ■ Very short term analgesia	■ Very short-acting (half-life 10–20 min) ■ Can cause respiratory depression
Thiopental	Barbiturate	■ Continuous sedation	■ Very long-acting (half-life 10–12 h) ■ May accumulate in hepatic impairment

*The elimination half-life of drugs stated throughout this chapter are to provide an *indication* of the normal length of action (www.medicinescomplete.com). However, the half-life has been estimated usually from healthy volunteers and is dependent on many factors, including, for example, genetic variation, length of infusion, and the impact of critical illness on pharmacokinetics and dynamics. Therefore, the half-life of any drug may vary considerably between patients in this group, and may well be considerably longer than stated.

and the concurrent use of corticosteroids and catecholamines (e.g. noradrenaline, adrenaline).

Benzodiazepines

Due to its licensing status, midazolam is the most frequently used benzodiazepine given as a continuous infusion in the UK, although lorazepam may also be given continuously (this is an unlicensed use). Benzodiazepines act on GABA receptors making them more likely to bind with GABA, the action of which is to inhibit transmission pathways (by raising the threshold for excitability) (Kress & Hall 2006). This produces the effects of sedation and anterograde amnesia. They also have an opioid-sparing effect (Jacobi et al. 2002). Benzodiazepines have fallen out of favour for various reasons, including accumulation of active metabo-

lites in renal and liver failure, drug interactions with midazolam, and their addictive potential, which can cause withdrawal in patients receiving them for longer than 48 h. Side effects include respiratory depression and over-sedation if not titrated properly. Benzodiazepines may worsen or precipitate delirium (Borthwick et al. 2006). Prolonged lorazepam infusions may lead to an accumulation of the solvents polyethylene glycol and propylene glycol, which can cause acute tubular necrosis, lactic acidosis and hyper-osmolar states (Jacobi et al. 2002).

Barbiturates

Thiopental is the only barbiturate anaesthetic given as a continuous infusion in critical care. It increases the effect of GABA, thereby causing sedation, by promoting opening of the chloride ion channel. Due to its half-life and its saturation of liver enzymes, thiopental takes a long time to clear from the body, making neurological assessment difficult. As such, it is rarely used as an infusion, although it may be of use in refractory status epilepticus or refractory raised intracranial pressure. It is metabolized by the liver via the cytochrome P450 system, giving rise to several drug interactions, and making it a poor choice in hepatically impaired patients. Side effects include increased infective complications, hypokalaemia, hypotension and histamine release, which can cause bronchospasm and oedema. Extravasation may cause tissue necrosis as the solution is highly alkaline (Pandit 2007).

Dexmedetomidine

Dexmedetomidine is gaining increasing focus as a critical care sedative in the UK. It is an alpha-2 agonist, causing sedation and anxiolysis, as well as decreased blood pressure and heart rate. It can also be analgesic-sparing. Dexmedetomidine causes a light sedation, from which patients are easily rousable (Coursin et al. 2001). It is more selective and shorter acting than its related drug, clonidine, and as such is given by continuous infusion. Dexmedetomidine appears to be less deliriogenic than benzodiazepines and also possibly opioids and propofol (Devlin et al. 2010). It has recently gained a licence in the UK.

Analgesia

Opioids

Strong opioids such as morphine, fentanyl, alfentanil and remifentanil may be used for continuous analgesia in ventilated patients. Some may also be given intermittently or as a patient-controlled infusion for analgesia. Weak opioids, such as codeine, though not routinely used in ventilated patients, may be of use in postoperative or mild to moderate pain. Opioids bind to the opioid receptors in the central nervous system, which are categorized as mu, delta or kappa, each having different properties. Mu receptors are found in the brain and delta in the peripheral nerves. Opioids bind to the receptors, resulting in analgesia by reduced transmission of pain signals along the pain pathway. Kappa receptors are found in the spinal column and cause regional analgesia as well as dysphoric effects. Opioids mimic naturally occurring endorphins (which modulate pain transmission), predominantly at the mu receptors (Pleuvry 2005). Older opioids such as morphine and fentanyl are renally excreted, and as such, may accumulate in renal failure. Fentanyl has a significant context-sensitive half-life, which means the longer it is infused, the longer its half-life and therefore duration of action (Liu and Gropper 2003). This makes it particularly prone to accumulation in longer-stay patients. Rarely it may also cause muscle rigidity. The newer opioid remifentanil is metabolized by non-specific esterases and therefore does not accumulate in renal or hepatic impairment.

Side effects of opioids include immune dysfunction (Roy and Loh 1996), respiratory depression, hypotension and decreased gastrointestinal motility leading to constipation and reduced absorption. In conscious patients, opioids may also cause hallucinations, dysphoria, delirium, nausea and vomiting (which are usually transient). Opioids can also cause histamine release.

Remifentanil in critical care

Due to its short half-life and lack of accumulation, remifentanil is increasingly being used in critical care for sedation, with the focus on adequate analgesia rather than just anxiolysis. While a meta-analysis showed no significant difference to standard sedatives in terms of ventilator days and length of critical care stay, the time from cessation of sedation to extubation is reduced (Tan and Ho 2009). Certain groups of patients are likely to benefit from remifentanil, especially those with multiple organ failure, due to its pharmacokinetic profile. However, to date, these patients have been excluded from most clinical trials so further trials are required to clarify its use.

Paracetamol

Paracetamol is the first-line analgesic for both acute and chronic pain (WHO 1990); it also works synergistically with opioids to give an opioid-sparing effect. The mechanism of action is relatively unknown. Paracetamol is generally very well tolerated, with few side effects, although due to its potential hepatotoxicity, care should be taken in severe liver impairment.

Non-steroidal anti-inflammatory drugs (NSAIDs)

NSAIDs are useful for treating mild to moderate pain, particularly when associated with inflammation. They inhibit the cyclo-oxygenase (COX) system, which is responsible for (among other things) the release of inflammatory mediators, as well as both vasodilatation and vasoconstriction of the blood vessels. NSAIDs also affect platelet aggregation, increasing the risk of bleeding. They are metabolized in the liver and excreted in the kidneys, making them a poor choice in renal and hepatic impairment. NSAIDs need to be used cautiously in critical care due to potential side effects, such as nephrotoxicity, bleeding, bronchospasm and cardiovascular problems, including heart failure.

Neuromuscular blockade

Depolarizing neuromuscular blockers (DNMBs)

DNMBs mimic acetylcholine, causing depolarization at the neuromuscular junction which leads to the loss of electrical excitability; suxamethonium is the only drug of this type in clinical use. Once it has diffused from the neuromuscular junction, it is metabolized by plasma cholinesterase. The effects of DNMBs cannot be reversed.

Suxamethonium is commonly used for intubation due to its rapid onset and short duration of action (usually less than 5 minutes). It causes a transient rise in serum potassium levels of around 0.5 mmol/L. This rise can be more significant and limit its use in renal failure, major burns, trauma with associated significant muscle injury, and spinal cord injury after the first 48 hours.

Non-depolarizing neuromuscular blockers (NDNMBs)

NDNMBs include atracurium, cisatracurium, vecuronium and rocuronium. They may be given as either boluses or continuous infusions in ventilated, sedated patients. They cause a flaccid neuromuscular blockade by competing at acetylcholine receptors, thereby preventing neuromuscular transmission. All NDNMBs, except vecuronium and to a lesser extent cisatracurium, cause histamine release, suggesting caution should be exercised if muscle relaxing an asthmatic or atopic patient. NDNMBs can be reversed by anticholinesterases such as neostigmine only after the majority of the drug has been metabolized or diffused away from the neuromuscular junction (i.e. when TOF monitoring elicits at least two twitches. However, the chance of successful reversal of the neuromuscular blockade is significantly higher if three or four twitches are present; *see* Table 10.2). Sugammadex, a complex-forming reversal agent, can reverse rocuronium and vecuronium at any time, although a significantly higher dose is required if immediate reversal is required.

Rescue sedation

Typical antipsychotics

The older, so-called 'typical' antipsychotics include butyrophenones (for example haloperidol) and phenothiazines (for example chlorpromazine). They block dopamine receptors, causing both sedation and extrapyramidal side effects (including rigidity and oculogyric crisis). While haloperidol is still widely used for the treatment of delirium in critical care, typical antipsychotics are not always well tolerated due to their extensive side effect profile. These include movement disorders, as well as arrhythmias (such as a prolonged QT interval) and hypotension. Intravenous haloperidol may be associated with fewer extrapyramidal effects than oral (Devlin et al. 2010). The older antipsychotics also have multiple drug interactions. They should not be used to treat patients with Parkinson's disease.

Atypical antipsychotics

Newer, 'atypical' antipsychotics include olanzapine, quetiapine and risperidone. All of these have been used for rescue sedation in critically ill patients, including the treatment of delirium. They block both serotonin and dopamine receptors, and are less associated with movement disorders; however, they can cause hyperglycaemia (Devlin et al. 2010). As such, they are generally better tolerated than the older antipsychotics, making them a potentially better choice for longer-term use (e.g. neurological patients).

Procedure guideline 10.1: **Assessment of pain (Gunning 2010)**

Procedure

Action	Rationale
1 Where possible, explain and discuss the procedure with the patient. If the patient lacks the capacity to make decisions the practitioner must act in the patient's best interests.	To ensure that the patient understands the procedure and gives their valid consent. To ensure the patient's best interests are maintained (Mental Capacity Act 2005).
2 Assess the risk of the patient developing pain.	To enable treatment and care to be provided to ameliorate pain (where possible) prior to pain developing or occurring.
3 Identify the source or potential source of pain. For example, ■ endotracheal suctioning, turning, presence of drains or dressings, ileus, constipation ■ incisions, trauma, cannulation, intubation, catheterization ■ hard beds, immobility, joint pain, myopathy, neuropathic.	To remove the cause or potential cause where possible. If removal not possible, to minimize pain with analgesics preferably pre-emptively where possible.

4 Observe for signs of pain
  ■ tachycardia
  ■ hypertension
  ■ tachypnoea
  ■ lacrimation
  ■ facial grimacing
  ■ limb flexion
  ■ ventilator dyssynchrony.
	To identify potential signs of pain and allow the degree of pain to be assessed in order to plan treatment.

5 Use a Numeric Rating Scale (NRS) to assess the degree of pain if the patient is able to cooperate. Ask the patient 'can you score your pain from 0 to 10, where 0 is no pain and 10 is the worst pain you could imagine.' A dynamic assessment (when the patient is active, for example when receiving physiotherapy) may also be necessary.	To assess the patient's perception of their level of pain using an NRS, the patient must be able to understand the question and to respond appropriately. To allow the need for analgesics to be assessed and to respond appropriately. NB An NRS for rest pain and dynamic pain may well be different. An NRS of less than 4 indicates mild pain. A suitable analgesic may be needed pre-emptively in patients with a greater than 4 dynamic pain score.
6 Use the Behavioural Pain Scale (BPS) (Payen et al. 2001) or alternative behavioural pain scale if the patient is not able to cooperate or communicate a NRS. Observe facial expression, arm position and ventilator dyssynchrony. Be aware of the limitations of this technique.	To provide an alternative means of assessing the level of pain when unable to obtain the patient's perspective of NRS. To provide pain management and reassessment if the assessment indicates pain. NB Physiological parameters alone are poorly predictive of pain in the critically ill so a patient's perspective or BPS should be used.

7 Titrate the analgesics to the patient following the WHO analgesic ladder (WHO 1990) and taking into account the patient's co-morbidities and the institution's usual selection of analgesics.	To enable an analgesic regimen tailored specifically to the patient. To take into account the:
	  ■ patient's pain levels
	  ■ suitability of analgesics (depending on the patient's allergies and altered pharmacokinetics during critical illness)
	  ■ the need to use drugs that the staff are familiar with to maximize safety.

8 Check for drug interactions.	To manage any interactions. For example, increasing analgesia may reduce sedative requirements and specific drugs may be contraindicated, such as paracetamol, which may cause or exacerbate hepatocellular dysfunction.

9 Document assessment and care provided.	To:
	  ■ provide an accurate record
	  ■ monitor effectiveness of procedure
	  ■ reduce the risk of duplication of treatment
	  ■ provide a point of reference or comparison in the event of later questions
	  ■ acknowledge accountability for actions
	  ■ facilitate communication and continuity of care.
	
	(NMC 2008; HCPC 2012; GMC 2013)

347

Procedure guideline 10.2: Sedation management: sedation holds and titration (Girard et al. 2008)

Procedure

Action	Rationale
1 Where possible, explain and discuss the procedure with the patient. If the patient lacks the capacity to make decisions the practitioner must act in the patient's best interests.	To ensure that the patient understands the procedure and gives their valid consent. To ensure the patient's best interests are maintained (Mental Capacity Act 2005).
2 Assess the patient for suitability for sedation hold. Contraindications include: ■ active seizures ■ alcohol withdrawal ■ agitation ■ use of paralytic agents ■ myocardial ischaemia ■ raised intracranial pressure.	To ensure that patient receives a daily sedation hold where possible and appropriate. To minimize the risk of oversedation and the complications that may result.
3 Ensure help is around should it be required.	To assist with managing patients who may wake up agitated and try to self-extubate or pose a danger to themselves or staff.
4 Stop the sedation and assess the need for providing, or providing a higher dose of, analgesia during the time of temporary withdrawal. It may be appropriate to leave some background analgesia running.	To enable full assessment of any build-up and residual effects of sedation during temporary withdrawal. To enable assessment of conscious level, pain and neurological function. To provide analgesia. For example, for surgical patients or those with chronic pain conditions.
5 As the patient wakes up, explain to them: ■ where they are and why ■ who you are ■ what is happening.	To minimize confusion to the patient and help to orientate them.
6 Monitor for signs that sedation needs to be restarted, including presence of: ■ anxiety, agitation. or pain (see below) ■ respiratory rate above 35 per minute ■ oxygen saturations below 88% ■ signs of respiratory distress ■ acute cardiac arrhythmias.	To ensure the safety of the patient and to appropriately manage their care.
7 Once the sedation is stopped, assess the patient's level of sedation/agitation against a suitable scoring chart (e.g. Richmond Agitation and Sedation Scale (RASS) [Sessler et al. 2002]): ■ observe patient ■ if not alert, speak patient's name and tell them to open their eyes and look at you ■ if still not responding, physically stimulate them by shaking their shoulder, then if still not responding, by rubbing their sternum.	To ascertain the alertness, agitation and comfort of the patient. If the patient is not alert, this suggests residual sedation effects. If the patient is agitated they may need further sedation. If the patient is comfortable then sedation can be withheld.
8 If the patient requires further sedation following the sedation hold, give a bolus dose to regain control of the patient's symptoms, then restart the infusion at half the previous rate (Kress et al. 2002).	To regain control of the patient's symptoms and reduce agitation or pain. To prevent over-sedation of the patient, which can lead to increased side effects, a greater risk of ventilator-associated pneumonia, an increased incidence of withdrawal effects and an increased risk of post-traumatic stress disorder (PTSD).

348

9 Reassess sedation and agitation levels at regular intervals (as specified by a senior practitioner).	To ensure that assessment of sedation and agitation levels are current as they may fluctuate. Reassessment allows for appropriate treatment.
10 Increase sedation in increments (one drug at a time) if assessment indicates that it needs to be increased.	To prevent over-sedation of the patient, which can lead to increased side effects, a greater risk of ventilator-associated pneumonia, an increased incidence of withdrawal and an increased risk of PTSD.
11 Patients receiving sedation should have regular monitoring. This should include: ■ sedation/agitation score ■ blood pressure.	To ensure appropriate levels of sedation and to monitor potential adverse effects of sedative drugs.
12 Document care provided.	To: ■ provide an accurate record ■ monitor effectiveness of procedure ■ reduce the risk of duplication of treatment ■ provide a point of reference or comparison in the event of later questions ■ acknowledge accountability for actions ■ facilitate communication and continuity of care. (NMC 2008; HCPC 2012; GMC 2013)

Procedure guideline 10.3: Assessing delirium (NICE 2010)

Procedure

Action	Rationale
1 Where possible, explain and discuss the procedure with the patient. If the patient lacks the capacity to make decisions the practitioner must act in the patient's best interests.	To ensure that the patient understands the procedure and gives their valid consent. To ensure the patient's best interests are maintained (Mental Capacity Act 2005).
2 Check the patient is awake and that they have their usual communication aids, e.g. glasses, hearing aids.	To ensure that the patient can communicate in order to be accurately screened for delirium.
3 Determine whether the patient has shown any signs of 'not being themselves,' plus demonstrated inattention, using the following test (Jacobi et al. 2002): ■ read out the following letters slowly, asking the patient to squeeze your hand every time the letter 'A' is said: SAVEAHAART.	To assess whether the patient is inattentive (which is a feature of delirium). If two or more mistakes are made in the exercise, this suggests inattention, and the patient should then be assessed further for delirium by assessing disorganized thinking (step 4) or altered level of consciousness (step 5). The patient is delirious if they have the following: ■ altered mental status ■ inattention ■ either disorganized thinking and/or altered level of consciousness.
4 Assess disorganized thinking. Ask the patient one of the following sets of questions and also ask them to follow your command. Set 1 ■ Will a stone float on water? ■ Are there fish in the sea? ■ Does 1 pound weigh more than 2? ■ Do you use a hammer to hit a nail? Set 2 ■ Will a leaf float on water? ■ Are there elephants in the sea? ■ Do 2 pounds weigh more than 1? ■ Do you use a saw to hit a nail?	To assess whether the patient answers the questions 'correctly' or has disorganized thinking (a feature of delirium).

(Continued)

Command
- Ask the patient to raise two fingers with one hand and then to do the same with the other hand.
  NB Do not instruct the patient to raise two fingers a second time, but instead instruct them to do the same with the other hand.

5 Assess whether the patient has an altered level of consciousness. Ascertain if the patient is anything other than awake and alert.	To assess whether the patient has an altered level of consciousness – a feature of delirium.
6 If the patient is delirious, assess for underlying cause and treat where possible. Consider starting antipsychotics.	To eliminate, where possible, causes of delirium. Some causes of delirium may be easily addressed (such as urinary retention). Untreated delirium can increase length of stay and is associated with increased mortality and morbidity.
7 Document assessment and care.	To: ■ provide an accurate record ■ monitor effectiveness of procedure ■ reduce the risk of duplication of treatment ■ provide a point of reference or comparison in the event of later questions ■ acknowledge accountability for actions ■ facilitate communication and continuity of care. (NMC 2008; HCPC 2012; GMC 2013)

Procedure guideline 10.4: Neuromuscular blockade assessment

Procedure

Action	Rationale
1 Assess the need for neuromuscular blockade.	To ensure that neuromuscular blockade is only used on patient if other strategies have failed or are clinically inappropriate.
2 Ensure patients receiving neuromuscular blockade drugs (NMBDs) have adequate analgesia and are sedated. Assess for signs of awareness such as tachycardia, tachypnoea, hypertension and lacrimation.	To prevent awareness and any related distress and associated psychological morbidity. Therefore, if signs of awareness are present then the dose of sedation and analgesia should be reviewed immediately and amended as appropriate.
3 Determine if the monitoring should be once only or continuous.	To provide appropriate monitoring. Once only assessment may be required to exclude significant residual blockade prior to brainstem death testing or extubation. Continuous monitoring should be in place with any patients on regular boluses or infusions of NMBDs.
4 Identify any possible co-existing neuromuscular problems that may interfere with Train-of-Four (TOF) monitoring.	To exclude any specific conditions that may interfere with TOF results, such as myasthenia gravis, Lambert-Eaton syndrome, Guillain-Barré syndrome and critical illness neuropathy.
5 Assess for clinical signs of muscle function, limb movement, breathing.	To ensure a full assessment. Practitioner's observations should be used in conjunction with TOF monitoring. This is because the presence of twitching does not necessarily indicate the patient does not have residual blockade.
6 Determine nerve to be stimulated and related movement to be counted.	To ensure the most appropriate nerve is utilized and the most accurate result obtained. Although the ulnar nerve is commonly used, this may not be appropriate for all patients. An awareness of the risk of false positive with the use of the facial nerve is necessary.

7	Place negative electrode (black) over the nerve and the positive electrode (red) 2–3 cm proximal to the negative electrode along the path of the nerve. For the ulnar nerve, black electrode in line with the smallest digit at the proximal skin crease of the wrist. Select 'TOF mode'.	Placing the black electrode over the nerve minimizes the electrical current required. TOF stimulation is the recommended monitoring modality.
8	Palpate and count the number of resultant twitches and adjust therapy accordingly.	To ensure the appropriate level of muscle blockade. The number of twitches indicates the level of neuromuscular blockade. For the ulnar nerve thumb twitching is observed. However, there may still be significant residual blockage with four twitches (normally manifested as agitation and twitch movement). Patients should have two to four twitches prior to reversal before considering extubation. The patient should have four twitches before brainstem death testing. A target of one to two twitches is recommended where infusions or repeated boluses are being used to maintain appropriate muscle relaxation for patient receiving intensive care.
9	Reassess hourly if the patient is on an infusion or multiple boluses of NMBDs.	To prevent overdosing or under-dosing of NMBDs.
10	Document care provided.	To: ■ provide an accurate record ■ monitor effectiveness of procedure ■ reduce the risk of duplication of treatment ■ provide a point of reference or comparison in the event of later questions ■ acknowledge accountability for actions ■ facilitate communication and continuity of care. (NMC 2008; HCPC 2012; GMC 2013)

Competency statement 10.1: Specific procedure competency statements for assessment of pain

Complete assessment against relevant fundamental competency statements (*see* Chapter 2, pp. 20, 21)	Evidence
Specific procedure competency statements for assessment of pain	**Evidence of competency for assessment of pain**
Demonstrate ability to: ■ teach and assess or ■ learn from assessment.	Examples of evidence of teaching, assessing and learning.
Identify reason(s) for assessing and treating (potential) pain, including knowledge of: ■ reasons for assessing pain ■ need for pre-emptive analgesia.	Discussion with supervisor/mentor. *May also include:* ■ teaching session for peers ■ completion of a workbook or training package.
Identify risks, potential problems and complications of pain and analgesics, including how to prevent or manage them, to include: ■ side effects of different analgesics ■ interactions of analgesics with other drugs commonly used in critical care. For example, sedatives and drugs that produce neuromuscular blockade ■ use of titration of drug against patient need.	Discussion with supervisor/mentor. *May also include:* ■ teaching session for peers ■ completion of a workbook or training package.

(Continued)

Demonstrate knowledge and understanding of local and national policies, guidance, and procedures in relation to pain assessment. including: ■ NICE guidance ■ local policy and procedure on assessment of pain in patients receiving critical care.	Discussion with supervisor/mentor. *May also include:* ■ teaching session for peers ■ completion of a workbook or training package.
Demonstrate knowledge and understanding of evidence base in relation to pain assessment, including: ■ anatomy and physiology of pain ■ how patient outcomes are effected by pain assessment ■ behavioural signs of pain ■ physiological signs of pain.	Case based discussion with supervisor/mentor. *May also include:* ■ teaching session for peers ■ completion of a workbook or training package.
Demonstrate skills that are required in relation to assessment and monitoring of pain, including: ■ ability to complete appropriately NRS with patient ■ ability to undertake a behavioural pain scale assessment appropriately ■ ability to identify side effects, drug interactions and contraindications to use ■ escalates or de-escalates analgesia in keeping with the WHO ladder in accordance to the results of the pain assessment.	Direct observation of procedure. *May also include:* ■ patient testimonial ■ reflection on practice.
Selects most appropriate tool in relation to pain assessment, treatment and monitoring, including: ■ medication required for patient ■ appropriate scoring system (NRS where appropriate or pain BPS [or alternative]).	Discussion with supervisor/mentor. Direct observation of procedure.
Demonstrate the correct technique for the procedure in relation to level of sedation and pain assessment tool used, including: ■ titration of medication ■ identification of side effects ■ assessment of sedation and pain ■ taking action to ameliorate side effects where possible.	Direct observation of procedure. *May also include:* ■ patient testimonial ■ reflection on practice.

Competency statement 10.2: Specific procedure competency statements for sedation management: sedation holds and titration

Complete assessment against relevant fundamental competency statements (*see* Chapter 2, pp. 20, 21)	Evidence
Specific procedure competency statement for sedation management: sedation holds and titration	**Evidence of competency for sedation management: sedation holds and titration**
Demonstrate ability to: ■ teach and assess or ■ learn from assessment.	Examples of evidence of teaching, assessing and learning.
Identify reason(s) for providing and titrating sedation and sedation holds, including to: ■ allow essential procedures to be carried out ■ minimize distress ■ provide analgesia ■ aid ventilation ■ control delirium ■ enable assessment of pain and delirium when withheld ■ prevent oversedation.	Discussion with supervisor/mentor. *May also include:* ■ teaching session for peers ■ completion of a workbook or training package.

Identify risks, potential problems and complications for titrating sedation and giving sedation holds and how to prevent or manage them, including: ▪ deep sedation ▪ hypotension ▪ ventilator-associated pneumonia ▪ poor gastrointestinal absorption ▪ assess agitation as appropriate ▪ monitor blood pressure and heart rate.	Discussion with supervisor/mentor. *May also include:* ▪ teaching session for peers ▪ completion of a workbook or training package.
Demonstrate knowledge and understanding of local and national policies, guidance, and procedures in relation to sedation titration and sedation holds.	Discussion with supervisor/mentor. *May also include:* ▪ teaching session for peers ▪ completion of a workbook or training package.
Demonstrate knowledge and understanding of evidence base in relation to sedation titration and 'sedation holds', including: ▪ side effects, such as delirium, delusional memories and post-traumatic stress syndrome ▪ need to maintain safety and control of patient's symptoms.	Discussion with supervisor/mentor. *May also include:* ▪ teaching session for peers ▪ completion of a workbook or training package.
Demonstrate skills that are required in relation to sedation titration and 'sedation holds', including: ▪ ability to assess sedation score ▪ ability to recognize and assess over-sedation, agitation, delirium and pain ▪ ability to manage over-sedation, agitation, delirium and pain.	Direct observation of procedure. *May also include:* ▪ patient testimonial ▪ reflection on practice.
Prepare equipment and staff required in relation to sedation titration and 'sedation holds': ▪ appropriate scoring system (e.g. RASS).	Discussion with supervisor/mentor. Direct observation of procedure.
Demonstrate the correct technique for the procedure in relation to sedation titration and sedation holds, including: ▪ accurate assessment of the patient in terms of contraindications for sedation holds ▪ ability to assess and manage consequences of sedation holds.	Direct observation of procedure. *May also include:* ▪ patient testimonial ▪ reflection on practice.

Competency statement 10.3: Specific procedure competency statements for assessing delirium

Complete assessment against relevant fundamental competency statements (*see* Chapter 2, pp. 20, 21)	Evidence
Specific procedure competency statement for assessing delirium	**Evidence of competency for assessing delirium**
Demonstrate ability to: ▪ teach and assess or ▪ learn from assessment.	Examples of evidence of teaching, assessing and learning.
Identify reason(s) for assessing and treating delirium, including: ▪ increased morbidity and mortality ▪ long-term psychological problems.	Discussion with supervisor/mentor. *May also include:* ▪ teaching session for peers ▪ completion of a workbook or training package.
Identify risks, potential problems and complications for assessing delirium and how to prevent or manage them: ▪ ensure patient's usual communication aids are available.	Discussion with supervisor/mentor. *May also include:* ▪ teaching session for peers ▪ completion of a workbook or training package.

(Continued)

Competency statement 10.3: *(Continued)*

Demonstrate knowledge and understanding of local and national policies, guidance, and procedures in relation to assessing delirium, including: ■ Diagnostic and Statistical Manual of Mental Disorders IV-TR (American Psychiatric Association 2000) ■ NICE guidance (2010).	Discussion with supervisor/mentor. *May also include:* ■ teaching session for peers ■ completion of a workbook or training package.
Demonstrate knowledge and understanding of evidence base in relation to delirium and assessing delirium: ■ definition of 'ICU delirium' ■ causes of delirium ■ predisposition to delirium ■ treatment options for delirium.	Discussion with supervisor/mentor. *May also include:* ■ teaching session for peers ■ completion of a workbook or training package.
Demonstrate skills that are required in relation to assessing delirium: ■ ability to screen for delirium.	Direct observation of procedure. *May also include:* ■ patient testimonial ■ reflection on practice.
Prepare equipment required in relation to assessing delirium: ■ CAM-ICU protocol ■ picture cards if being used.	Discussion with supervisor/mentor Direct observation of procedure.
Demonstrate the correct technique for the procedure in relation to assessing delirium including: ■ use of the CAM-ICU screening tool ■ appropriate frequency of assessment.	Direct observation of procedure. *May also include:* ■ patient testimonial ■ reflection on practice.

Competency statement 10.4: Specific procedure competency statements for neuromuscular blockade assessment

Complete assessment against relevant fundamental competency statements (*see* Chapter 2, pp. 20, 21)	Evidence
Specific procedure competency statements for neuromuscular blockade assessment	**Evidence of competency for neuromuscular blockade assessment**
Demonstrate ability to: ■ teach and assess or ■ learn from assessment.	Examples of evidence of teaching, assessing and learning.
Identify and discuss reason(s) neuromuscular blockade, including: ■ to facilitate mechanical ventilation ■ in severe acute respiratory distress syndrome ■ during intubation and laryngoscopy ■ in head injury ■ in tetany ■ in prolonged status epilepticus ■ to reduce oxygen requirements ■ in sedation-resistant shivering during active cooling.	Case based discussion with supervisor/mentor. *May also include:* ■ teaching session for peers ■ completion of a workbook or training package.
Identify risks, potential problems and complications for titrating neuromuscular blockade and how to prevent or manage them, including: ■ residual blockade ■ underestimation or overestimation of neuromuscular blockade ■ false positive by accidental direct stimulation off facial muscles ■ monitoring for signs of awareness.	Case based discussion with supervisor/mentor. *May also include:* ■ teaching session for peers ■ completion of a workbook or training package.

Demonstrate knowledge and understanding of local and national policies, guidance, and procedures in relation to neuromuscular blockade, including: ■ local policy in relation to diagnosing brainstem death.	Discussion with supervisor/mentor. *May also include:* ■ teaching session for peers ■ completion of a workbook or training package.
Demonstrate knowledge and understanding of evidence base in relation to neuromuscular blockade: ■ anatomy and physiology of neuromuscular blockade ■ action of depolarizing and non-depolarizing neuromuscular blockade drugs (NDNMDs) ■ reversal of NDNMDs.	Discussion with supervisor/mentor. *May also include:* ■ teaching session for peers ■ completion of a workbook or training package.
Demonstrate skills that are required in relation to assessment of neuromuscular blockade: ■ TOF measurement ■ observation of skeletal movement and respiratory distress.	Direct observation of procedure. *May also include:* ■ patient testimonial ■ reflection on practice.
Prepare equipment required in relation to neuromuscular blockade monitoring: ■ TOF monitor ■ correct placement of electrodes.	Discussion with supervisor/mentor. Direct observation of procedure.
Demonstrate the correct technique for the procedure in relation to TOF monitoring, including: ■ ability to identify false positive ■ ability to palpate and observe, or use equipment to assess, muscle contraction ■ ability to interpret results of TOF.	Direct observation of procedure. *May also include:* ■ patient testimonial ■ reflection on practice.

355

References and further reading

American Psychiatric Association (2000) *Diagnostic and Statistical Manual of Mental Disorders* (4e, text revision). Washington, DC: APA.

Aissaoui Y, Zeggwagh AA, Zekroui A et al. (2005) Validation of a behavioral pain scale in critically ill, sedated and mechanically ventilated patients. *Anesthesia and Analgesia* 101: 1470–1476.

Blackwood B, Alderdice F, Burns KE et al. (2010) The Cochrane Collaboration: protocolized versus non-protocolized weaning for reducing the duration of mechanical ventilation in critically ill adult patients (Review). *The Cochrane Library* Issue 7.

Barr J, Gilles FL, Puntillo K, et al. (2013) Clinical practice guidelines for the management of pain, agitation, and delirium in adult patients in the intensive care unit. *Critical Care Medicine* 41: 263–306.

Borthwick M, Bourne R, Craig M et al. (2006) *Detection, Prevention and Treatment of Delirium in Critically Ill Patients*. Leicester: United Kingdom Clinical Pharmacy Association.

Bray K, Hill K, Robson W et al. (2004) British Association of Critical Care Nurses position statement on the use of restraint in adult critical care units. *Nursing in Critical Care* 9(5): 199–212.

Bourne RS and Mills GH (2004) Sleep disruption in critically ill patients – pharmacological considerations. *Anaesthesia* 59: 374–384.

Coursin,DB, Coursin DB and Maccioli GA (2001) Dexmedetomidine. *Current Opinion in Critical Care* 7: 221–226.

Cullis B and Macnaughton P (2007) Sedation and paralysis in the ICU *Anaesthesia & Intensive Care Medicine* 8(1): 32–35.

De Jonghe B, Cook D, Griffith L et al. (2003) Adaptation to the Intensive Care Environment (ATICE): development and validation of a new sedation assessment instrument. *Critical Care Medicine* 31: 2344–2354.

Department for Constitutional Affairs (2007) Mental Capacity Act 2005 Code of Practice. London: The Stationery Office.

Department of Health (2010) *Essence of Care 2010*. London: The Stationary Office. http://www.dh.gov.uk/en/Publications andstatistics/Publications/PublicationsPolicyAndGuidance/DH_ 119969 [accessed 15 February 2012].

Desbiens NA, Wu AW, Broste SK et al. (1996) Pain and satisfaction with pain control in seriously ill hospitalized adults: Findings from the SUPPORT research investigations. *Critical Care Medicine* 24: 1953–1961.

Devlin JW, Boleski G, Mlynarek M et al. (1999) Motor Activity Assessment Scale: a valid and reliable sedation scale for use with mechanically ventilated patients in an adult surgical intensive care unit. *Critical Care Medicine* 27: 1271–1275.

Devlin JW, Mallow-Corbett S and Riker RR (2010) Adverse drug events associated with the use of analgesics, sedatives, and antipsychotics in the intensive care unit. *Critical Care Medicine* 38(6): S231–S243.

Flaherty JH, Rudolph J, Shay K et al. (2007) Delirium is a serious and under-recognized problem: why assessment of mental status should be the sixth vital sign. *Journal of the American Medical Directors Association* 8(5): 273–275.

General Medical Council (2013) *Good Medical Practice*. London: GMC. http://www.gmc-uk.org/gmp2013 [accessed 25 March 2013].

Girard TD, Kress JP, Fuchs BD et al. (2008) Efficacy and safety of a paired sedation and ventilator weaning protocol for mechanically ventilated patients in intensive care (Awakening and Breathing Controlled trial): a randomised controlled trial. *Lancet* **371**: 126–134.

Gunning K (2010) Management of pain in the intensive care patient. *Journal of the Intensive Care Society* **11**(supp 1): 4–7.

Guyton JE and Hall AC (2010) *Guyton and Hall Textbook of Medical Physiology* (12e). Philadelphia: Saunders Elsevier.

Hamill-Ruth RJ and Marohn ML (1999) Evaluation of pain in the critically ill patient. *Critical Care Clinics* **15**: 35–54.

Health and Care Professions Council (2012) *Standard of Conduct, Performance and Ethics*. London: HCPC. http://www.hcpc-uk.org/assets/documents/10003B6EStandardsofconduct,performance andethics.pdf [accessed January 2013].

Hughes S and Griffiths R (2002) Anaesthesia monitoring techniques. *Anaesthesia and Intensive Care Medicine* **3**: 477–480.

Jacobi J, Fraser GL, Coursin DB et al. (2002) Clinical practice guidelines for the sustained use of sedatives and analgesics in the critically ill adult. *Critical Care Medicine* **30** (1): 119–141.

Jones C (2010) Post-traumatic stress disorder in ICU survivors. *Journal of the Intensive Care Society* **11**(Supp 1): 12–14.

Jones C, Griffiths RD, Humphris G and Skirrow PM (2001) Memory, delusions, and the development of acute posttraumatic stress disorder-related symptoms after intensive care. *Critical Care Medicine* **29**(3): 573–580.

Jones C, Backman C, Capuzzo M et al. (2007) Precipitants of post-traumatic stress disorder following intensive care: a hypothesis generating study of diversity in care. *Intensive Care Medicine* **33**: 978–985.

Kress JP and Hall JB (2006) Sedation in the mechanically ventilated patient. *Critical Care Medicine* **34**(10): 2541–2546.

Kress JP, Pohlman AS and Hall JB (2002) Sedation and analgesia in the intensive care unit. *American Journal of Respiratory and Critical Care Medicine* **166**: 1024–1028.

LeBlanc JM, Dasta JF, Kane-Gill SL et al. (2006) Role of the Bispectral Index in sedation monitoring in the ICU. *Annals of Pharmacotherapy* **40**(3): 490–500.

Lichtenbelt BJ, Olofsen E, Dahan A et al. (2010) Propofol reduces the distribution and clearance of midazolam. *Anesthesia and Analgesia* **110**(6): 1597–1606.

Liu LL and Gropper MA (2003) Postoperative analgesia and sedation in the adult intensive care unit. *Drugs* **63**(8): 755–766.

McCaffery M and Beebe A (1989) *Pain: clinical manual for nursing practice*. St Louis, MO: CV Mosby.

Mehta S, Burry L, Cook D, et al. (2012) Daily sedation interruption in mechanically ventilated critically ill patients cared for with a sedation protocol: A randomized controlled trial. *Journal of the American Medical Association* **308**: 1985–1992.

Merskey H and Bogduk N (1994) *Classification of Chronic Pain* (2e). Seattle: IASP Task Force on Taxonomy, IASP Press.

Murray MJ, Corven J, DeBlock H et al. (2002) Clinical practice guidelines for sustained neuromuscular blockade in the adult critically ill patient. *Critical Care Medicine* **30**(1): 142–156.

National Institute for Clinical Excellence (2009) *Clinical Guidance 83: Rehabilitation after critical illness*. London: NICE.

National Institute for Health and Clinical Excellence (2010) *Clinical Guidance 103: Delirium*. London: NICE.

Nirmalan M, Dark PM, Nightingale P et al. (2004) Physical and pharmacological restraint of critically ill patients: clinical facts and ethical considerations. *British Journal of Anaesthesia* **92**: 789–792.

Ostermann ME, Keenan SP, Seiferling RA et al. (2000) Sedation in the intensive care unit: a systematic review. *Journal of the American Medical Association* **283**: 1451–1459.

Page V (2010) Optimum sedation and delirium assessment in ICU. *Journal of the Intensive Care Society* **11** (Supp 1): 8–11.

Pandit JJ (2007) Intravenous anaesthetic agents. *Anaesthesia and Intensive Care Medicine* **9**(4): 154–159.

Papazian L, Foren J-M, Gaucouin A et al. (2010) Neuromuscular blockers in early acute respiratory distress syndrome. *New England Journal of Medicine* **363**: 1107–1116.

Pati S, Goodfellow JA, Iyadurai S et al. (2008) Approach to critical illness polyneuropathy and myopathy. *Postgraduate Medical Journal* **84**: 354–360.

Payen J-F, Bru O, Bosson J-L et al. (2001) Assessing pain in critically ill sedated patients by using a behavioural pain scale. *Critical Care Medicine* **29**: 2258–2263.

Payen J-F, Changues G, Mantz J et al. (2007) Current practices in sedation and analgesia for mechanically ventilated critically ill patients. *Anesthesiology* **106**: 687–695.

Payen J-F, Bosson JL, Changues G et al. (2009) Pain assessment is associated with decreased duration of mechanical ventilation in the intensive care unit. *Anaesthesiology* **111**: 1308–1316.

Peck M and Down J (2009) Use of sedatives in the critically ill. *Anaesthesia & Intensive Care* **11**(1): 12–15.

Pleuvry BJ (2005) Opioid mechanisms and opioid drugs. *Anaesthesia & Intensive Care* **6**(1): 30–34.

Ramsay MA, Savege TM, Simpson BR et al. (1974) Controlled sedation with alphaxalone-alphadolone. *British Medical Journal* **2**: 656–659.

Riker RR, Fraser GL, Cox PM et al. (1994) Continuous infusion of haloperidol controls agitation in critically ill patients. *Critical Care Medicine* **22**: 433–440.

Robinson BR, Mueller EW, Henson K et al. (2008) An analgesia-delirium-sedation protocol for critically ill trauma patients reduces ventilator days and hospital length of stay. *Journal of Trauma* **65**: 517–526.

Roy S and Loh HH (1996) Effects of opioids on the immune system. *Neurochemical Res* **21**(11): 1375–1386,

Sessler CN (2004) Sedation scales in the ICU. *Chest* **126**(6): 1727–1730.

Sessler CN, Gosnell MS, Grap MJ et al. (2002) The Richmond Agitation-Sedation Scale: validity and reliability in adult intensive care patients. *American Journal of Respiratory and Critical Care Medicine* **166**: 1338–1344.

Sessler CN, Grap MJ and Ramsay MAE (2008) Evaluating and monitoring analgesia and sedation in the intensive care unit. *Critical Care* **12**(Suppl 3): S2.

Standring S (2008) *Gray's Anatomy, The Anatomical Basis of Clinical Practice* (40e). Philadelphia: Churchill Livingstone Elsevier.

Tan JA and Ho KM (2009) Use of remifentanil as a sedative agent in critically ill adult patients: a meta-analysis. *Anaesthesia* **64**: 1342–1352.

Vasile B, Rasulo F, Candiani A and Latronico N (2003) The Pathophysiology of propofol infusion syndrome: a simple name for a complex syndrome. *Intensive Care Medicine* **29**: 1417–1425.

Waldman C (2010a) Sedation management in the ICU: are we at a crossroads? *Journal of the Intensive Care Society* **11**(Suppl 1): 2–3.

Waldman C (2010b) Using and understanding sedation scoring systems *Journal of the Intensive Care Society* **11**(Supp 1): 15–17.

Watt-Watson JB, Stevens B, Garfinkel P et al. (2001) Relationship between nurses' knowledge and pain management outcomes for their postoperative cardiac patients. *Journal of Advanced Nursing* **36**(4): 535–545.

World Health Orgnization (1990) *Cancer Pain Relief and Palliative Care; report of a WHO expert committee*. World Health Organization Technical Report Series, 804. Geneva, Switzerland: WHO, pp. 1–75.

www.icudelirium.org

www.medicinescomplete.com/MC/martindale; Martindale, the Complete Drug Reference [accessed 20 February 2012].

Chapter 11

Assessment and monitoring of neurological status

Margaret A. Douglas[1] and Sarah E.C. Platt[2]

[1]*Northumbria University, Newcastle upon Tyne, UK*
[2]*Royal Victoria Infirmary, Newcastle upon Tyne, UK*

Critical Care Manual of Clinical Procedures and Competencies, First Edition.
Edited by Jane Mallett, John W. Albarran, and Annette Richardson.
© 2013 John Wiley & Sons, Ltd. Published 2013 by John Wiley & Sons, Ltd.

Definition

Neurological assessment is the evaluation of the integrity and function of an individual's nervous system (Rowley and Fielding 1991). Regular reassessment or monitoring of neurological status enables prompt detection of changes and allows early appropriate management to be instituted (Woodward and Mestecky 2011).

Aims and indications

The main aims of neurological assessment and monitoring are to:

- assess the patient's condition
- detect signs of neurological deterioration
- evaluate the impact of therapeutic interventions.

(Jennett and Teasdale 1981)

Neurological assessment is central to the care of all critically ill patients. Alteration in neurological status may be associated with head injury or other intracerebral pathology, but can also be caused by metabolic problems and systemic disease such as liver failure. Accurate assessment of neurological function enables the early recognition and treatment of deterioration and may ultimately improve outcomes.

Understanding and interpreting the significance of neurological assessment requires a sound understanding of the anatomy and physiology of the central nervous system.

Background anatomy and physiology of the central nervous system

The neurological or nervous system is the body's communication network. It coordinates and organizes the functions of all other body systems.

The two main divisions are:

- the central nervous system (CNS), made up of the brain and spinal cord – this is the body's control centre
- the peripheral nervous system (PNS), made up of the cranial and spinal nerves – these provide communication pathways between the CNS and peripheries.

The brain is divided into three main components (*see* Figure 11.1):

- the cerebrum
- the cerebellum
- the brainstem.

(Cutler and Cutler 2010)

Cerebrum

The cerebrum forms the bulk of the brain. The surface of the cerebrum is composed of billions of nerve cell bodies collectively described as grey matter. This is the cerebral cortex. Beneath the cerebral cortex lies the cerebral white matter, which consists of myelinated nerve axons. The cerebrum is divided into two hemispheres joined by the corpus callosum, a thick area of nerve fibres which facilitates inter-hemispheric communication. Each hemisphere has four lobes the frontal, parietal, occipital and temporal (Tortora and Derrickson 2011).

The frontal lobes' key functions relate to an individual's personality, judgement, abstract reasoning, social behaviour, language and expression. The motor cortex also lies within the frontal lobe. This area generates nerve impulses via motor neurones to muscle cells to initiate voluntary movement.

The parietal lobes' key functions involve spatial awareness. The sensory cortex also lies within the parietal lobe. This area receives and interprets stimuli via sensory neurones.

The temporal lobes are responsible for language and comprehension, and for memory.

The occipital lobes are responsible for the interpretation of visual stimuli (Cutler and Cutler 2010).

Cerebellum

The cerebellum receives input from peripheral nerves concerning body position and movement, and plays an important role in the integration of sensory perception and motor control. It facilitates coordination and fine tuning of muscle activity and is key to maintaining balance and posture (Tortora and Derrickson 2011).

Brainstem

The brainstem is a continuation of the upper part of the spinal cord, and conducts motor and sensory information between the cerebrum, cerebellum and cord. It is divided into the medulla oblongata, the midbrain and the pons. The brainstem contains vital centres that are responsible for automatic, elementary functions of the body, including control of the cardiovascular and respiratory systems. The cranial nerves arise from in and around the brainstem (Table 11.1).

Medulla oblongata

The medulla oblongata forms the inferior part of the brainstem and contains all ascending (sensory) and descending (motor) white matter 'tracts' that communicate between the brain and spinal cord. In the lower medulla, the majority of motor tracts cross over or 'decussate' to the opposite side of the body from which they originated. This results in motor areas of one side of the cerebral cortex controlling movement on the opposite side of the body. Ascending tracts responsible for the sensations of pressure, fine touch and vibration also decussate in the medulla.

Within the medulla there are vital centres responsible for special control functions, including some that are essential for preserving life.

358

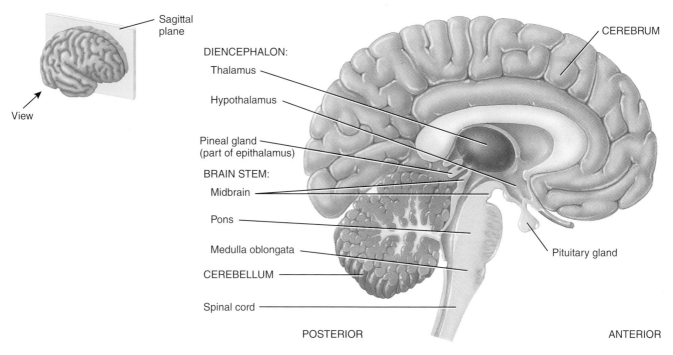

Sagittal plane

View

DIENCEPHALON:
Thalamus

Hypothalamus

Pineal gland
(part of epithalamus)

BRAIN STEM:
Midbrain

Pons

Medulla oblongata

CEREBELLUM

Spinal cord

CEREBRUM

Pituitary gland

POSTERIOR

ANTERIOR

(a) Medial view of sagittal section

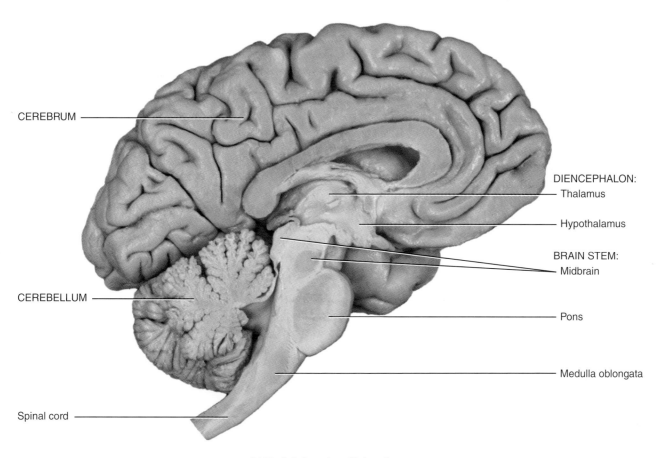

359

CEREBRUM

DIENCEPHALON:
Thalamus

Hypothalamus

BRAIN STEM:
Midbrain

CEREBELLUM

Pons

Medulla oblongata

Spinal cord

(b) Medial view of sagittal section

Figure 11.1 The brain (from Tortora and Derrickson 2011, reproduced with permission from Wiley).

Table 11.1 List of the twelve cranial nerves with motor and sensory functions

Cranial nerve	Motor or sensory	Key motor and sensory function
I Olfactory	Sensory function	Provides the sense of smell
II Optic	Sensory function	Conveys visual sensation
III Oculomotor	Motor function	Eye and upper eyelid movement, pupillary constriction
IV Trochlear	Motor function	Downward and inward eye movement
V Trigeminal	Sensory and motor function	Chewing, facial and scalp sensation, lacrimation
VI Abducens	Motor function	Lateral eye movement
VII Facial	Sensory and motor function	Facial expression, taste, lacrimation, salivation
VIII Vestibulocochlear	Sensory function	Hearing and balance
IX Glossopharyngeal	Sensory and motor function	Tongue and pharyngeal sensation, salivation and taste
X Vagus	Sensory and motor function	Sensation from larynx, pharynx and gastrointestinal tract, taste
XI Accessory	Motor function	Shoulder movement and head rotation
XII Hypoglossal	Motor function	Tongue movement

These centres include:

- the respiratory centre, which controls the rate and rhythm of breathing
- the cardiac centre, which regulates the rate and force of heart beat
- the vasomotor centre, which contributes to blood pressure regulation.

The swallow, cough, gag and sneeze reflexes also originate within the medulla oblongata in association with cranial nerves nine to twelve (Tortora and Derrickson 2011).

Pons

The pons forms a bridge connecting the medulla, midbrain and cerebellum. The transverse fibres in the pons connect with the cerebellum, while the longitudinal fibres belong to sensory and motor tracts connecting the spinal cord with the midbrain. Cranial nerves five to eight arise in the pons. Additional respiratory centres lie within the pons, which modulate breathing pattern in concert with those in the medulla oblongata (Tortora and Derrickson 2011).

Midbrain

The midbrain is involved in the control of eye movement, head and neck responses to visual and other stimuli (for example the blink reflex), and movements of the head and trunk in response to auditory stimuli (for example the startle reflex). The cerebral aqueduct passes through the midbrain connecting the third and fourth ventricles (*see* Ventricular pathways and cerebrospinal fluid (CSF) section). Cranial nerves three and four arise from the midbrain.

Reticular activating system (RAS)

The reticular activating system (RAS) is a diffuse system that extends from the lower brainstem to the cerebral cortex.

The RAS controls the sleep-wakefulness cycle, consciousness, focused attention and sensory perception, which may alter behaviour (*see also* Chapter 13). Consciousness is multifaceted and can be divided into two components:

- alertness or wakefulness, which reflects the activity of the RAS
- awareness or cognition, which reflects cerebral cortical activity (Hickey 2009).

Awareness or cognition is largely a cerebral cortical function, whereas alertness or wakefulness requires both brainstem and higher cortical function.

Meninges

The brain and spinal cord have three protective coverings which are collectively called the meninges (*see* Figure 11.2). The layers from the outermost layer inwards are called the dura mater, arachnoid mater and pia mater.

Dura mater

The dura mater is a tough double membrane. Its outer layer forms the periosteum of the inside of the skull; its inner layer separates to form folds, which protrude into the cranial cavity. There are four folds of dura mater within the skull, which support and protect the brain:

- the falx cerebri, which divides the two cerebral hemispheres
- the tentorium cerebelli, which separates the supratentorial space containing the cerebrum, from the infratentorial space containing the cerebellum and brainstem. The opening in the tentorium through which the brainstem emerges is called the tentorial notch

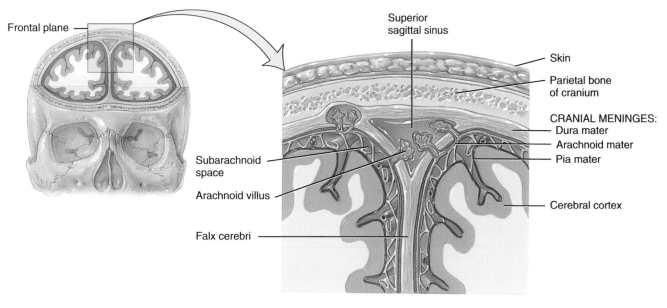

Frontal plane

Superior sagittal sinus

Skin

Parietal bone of cranium

CRANIAL MENINGES:
Dura mater
Arachnoid mater
Pia mater

Subarachnoid space

Arachnoid villus

Cerebral cortex

Falx cerebri

(a) Anterior view of frontal section through skull showing the cranial meninges

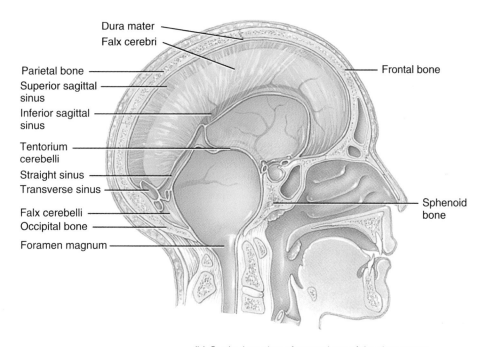

Dura mater
Falx cerebri

Parietal bone

Superior sagittal sinus

Inferior sagittal sinus

Tentorium cerebelli

Straight sinus

Transverse sinus

Falx cerebelli

Occipital bone

Foramen magnum

Frontal bone

Sphenoid bone

(b) Sagittal section of extensions of the dura mater

Figure 11.2 The meninges (from Tortora and Derrickson 2011, reproduced with permission from Wiley).

- the falx cerebelli, situated between the two lobes of the cerebellum
- the diaphragma sella, a small circular fold which creates a roof for the sella turcica.

The spinal dura mater is a continuation of the inner layer of the cerebral dura (Tortora and Derrickson 2011; Huether and McCance 2012).

Arachnoid mater

The arachnoid mater is a delicate layer containing blood vessels, which loosely encloses the brain. Beneath the arachnoid mater is the subarachnoid space, which consists of delicate spongy connective tissue between the arachnoid and pia mater. Cerebrospinal fluid flows in the subarachnoid space (Huether and McCance 2012).

Pia mater

The innermost layer of the meninges is the pia mater, which is a mesh-like vascular membrane covering the entire brain. It is closely adherent to the convolutions of the surface of the brain (Huether and McCance 2012).

The spinal meninges are a continuation of the layers of the cerebral meninges.

Ventricular pathways and cerebrospinal fluid

Within the skull, the brain is suspended in cerebrospinal fluid (CSF). This specialized fluid acts to confer mechanical protection to the brain by acting as a buffer after a blow to the head (Huether and McCance 2012). It also allows for delivery of nutrients to the brain and provides an excretory pathway for metabolic waste. CSF is produced from plasma and secreted primarily by the choroid plexi in the paired lateral ventricles, before circulating within the ventricular system (*see* Figure 11.3). The fluid passes first into the third ventricle via the two interventricular foramina (foramina of Munro), and on through the cerebral aqueduct (aqueduct of Sylvius) into the fourth ventricle. The majority of the CSF then flows through the two lateral foramina (of Luschka) and the central foramen (of Magendie) into the cerebellomedullary cistern (cisterna magna), situated below the cerebellar hemispheres. CSF then enters the subarachnoid space and flows around the spinal cord and brain. A small amount of CSF flows from the fourth ventricle down into the central spinal canal. Reabsorption of CSF occurs via the arachnoid villi (*see* Figure 11.2) into the venous sinuses, and via cerebral lymphatics (Zakharov et al. 2003). Approximately 500 mL of CSF is produced daily in the adult. With a capacity of only 125–150 mL, if the ventricular pathways become blocked with debris from infection or haemorrhage, or by swelling or tumour, accumulation of CSF can cause intracerebral pressure to rise (Hickey 2009).

Cerebral circulation

The brain receives about 15 to 20% of the cardiac output. Blood is supplied by two pairs of arteries: the internal carotid arteries and the vertebral arteries, which converge to form the cerebral arterial circle (Circle of Willis) (Figure 11.4). This is located at the base of the skull and is divided into anterior and posterior circulations as follows.

- Anterior – internal carotid arteries, anterior and middle cerebral arteries, and the anterior communicating artery, which connects the two anterior cerebral arteries.
- Posterior – vertebral arteries, basilar artery, posterior cerebral arteries and two posterior communicating arteries, which connect the middle cerebral arteries with the posterior cerebral arteries (Huether and McCance 2012).

Venous drainage occurs via the dural sinuses, which in turn empty into the jugular veins to return blood to the heart (Woodward and Mestecky 2011).

Autoregulation

In the normal brain, cerebral blood flow is maintained relatively constant through the process of autoregulation. The autoregulatory mechanism of the brain adjusts the diameter of the cerebral vessels to preserve constant cerebral blood flow despite changes in arterial pressure. In health, cerebral blood flow is unchanged over a mean arterial pressure (MAP) range of 60–160 mmHg (Sheppard and Wright 2006; Whitley et al. 2010). In areas of diseased or damaged brain autoregulation may be impaired (Mendelow and Crawford 1997), rendering cerebral blood flow dependent on mean arterial pressure (Figure 11.5).

The blood–brain barrier

In addition to protecting the brain from large alterations in cerebral blood flow, the brain must also be shielded from infection and toxins.

The blood–brain barrier describes the function of the thin, flat endothelial cells that form the walls of capillaries. Elsewhere in the body adjacent capillary endothelial cells have pores at their junctions, allowing free passage of water and electrolytes, and limited passage of proteins and larger molecules into the surrounding tissues. In the brain, the endothelial cells have tight, impermeable junctions, which block the passage of most substances except for essential metabolites, such as oxygen and water, from the blood to the brain. The blood–brain barrier plays an important part in maintaining homeostasis and cerebral protection, and may be damaged after brain injury (Fukuda et al. 1995).

Intracranial pressure

The skull is a rigid bony compartment that contains three components:

- brain (80%)
- cerebrospinal fluid (10%)
- arterial and venous blood (10%).

Intracranial pressure (ICP) reflects the volume of the intracranial contents. In health, the volume of brain tissue, CSF and blood remains nearly constant, and normal ICP varies between 0 and 15 mmHg. Should the volume of one component increase, the volume of one or both of the other components must decrease or an elevation in ICP will result – this is the 'Monro–Kellie hypothesis' (Monro 1783; Kelly 1824). In the early stages of brain swelling, compensation occurs as venous blood and CSF are displaced outside the skull, CSF reabsorption increases and venous sinuses are

POSTERIOR

ANTERIOR

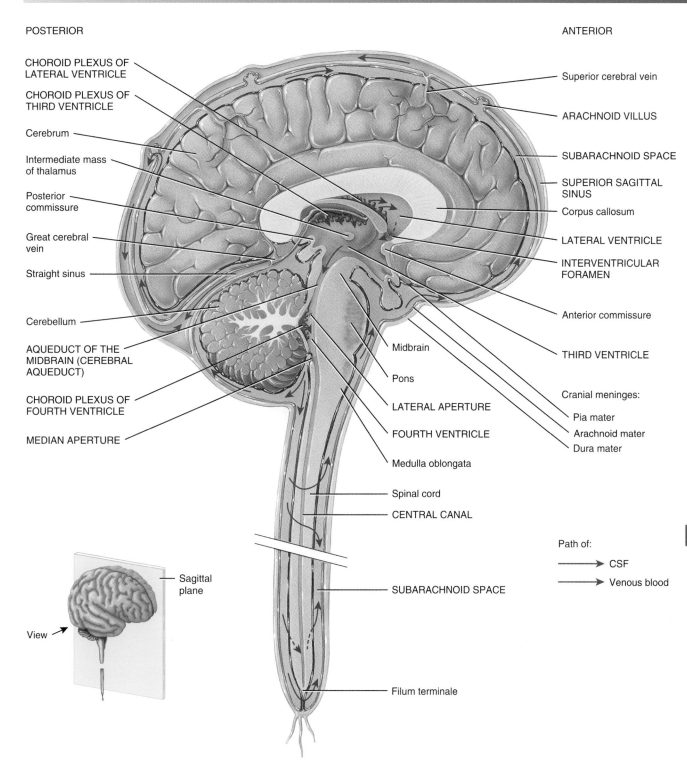

CHOROID PLEXUS OF LATERAL VENTRICLE

CHOROID PLEXUS OF THIRD VENTRICLE

Cerebrum

Intermediate mass of thalamus

Posterior commissure

Great cerebral vein

Straight sinus

Cerebellum

AQUEDUCT OF THE MIDBRAIN (CEREBRAL AQUEDUCT)

CHOROID PLEXUS OF FOURTH VENTRICLE

MEDIAN APERTURE

Superior cerebral vein

ARACHNOID VILLUS

SUBARACHNOID SPACE

SUPERIOR SAGITTAL SINUS

Corpus callosum

LATERAL VENTRICLE

INTERVENTRICULAR FORAMEN

Anterior commissure

THIRD VENTRICLE

Cranial meninges:
Pia mater
Arachnoid mater
Dura mater

Midbrain

Pons

LATERAL APERTURE

FOURTH VENTRICLE

Medulla oblongata

Spinal cord

CENTRAL CANAL

Sagittal plane

View

SUBARACHNOID SPACE

Path of:
→ CSF
→ Venous blood

Filum terminale

Figure 11.3 The ventricular pathways (from Tortora and Derrickson 2011, reproduced with permission from Wiley).

compressed (Sheppard and Wright 2006). This prevents a rise in intracranial pressure. As this compensation is exhausted, decompensation occurs and ICP will rise (Figure 11.6). Intracranial pressure that is persistently above 15 mmHg is termed intracranial hypertension. Intracranial hypertension causes reduction in cerebral blood flow and distortion or displacement of cerebral tissue. Current data support 20–25 mmHg as a threshold above which treatment to lower ICP should be initiated (Brain Trauma Foundation [BTF] 2007).

363

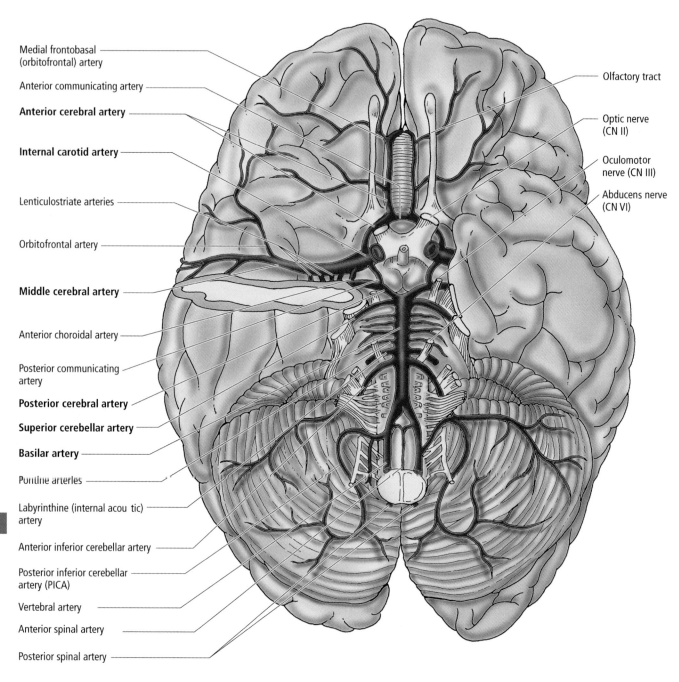

Medial frontobasal
(orbitofrontal) artery

Anterior communicating artery

Anterior cerebral artery

Internal carotid artery

Lenticulostriate arteries

Orbitofrontal artery

Middle cerebral artery

Anterior choroidal artery

Posterior communicating
artery

Posterior cerebral artery

Superior cerebellar artery

Basilar artery

Pontine arteries

Labyrinthine (internal acou tic)
artery

Anterior inferior cerebellar artery

Posterior inferior cerebellar
artery (PICA)

Vertebral artery

Anterior spinal artery

Posterior spinal artery

Olfactory tract

Optic nerve
(CN II)

Oculomotor
nerve (CN III)

Abducens nerve
(CN VI)

364

Figure 11.4 Cerebral circulation (from Patestas and Gartner 2006, reproduced with permission from Wiley).

Cerebral perfusion pressure

Cerebral perfusion pressure (CPP) is the pressure gradient between the systemic circulation and the pressure within the skull. It describes the pressure that is available to provide flow to the brain once the intracranial pressure has been accounted for. The equation to calculate cerebral perfusion pressure is:

$$CCP = MAP - ICP$$

Normal CPP is approximately 80 mmHg (Dinsmore and Hall 2006). Elevation in intracranial pressure results in a reduction in cerebral blood flow and consequently cerebral ischaemia. Cerebral blood flow is significantly impaired when CPP falls to around 50 mmHg. Impairment in delivery of glucose and oxygen further damages the already injured brain, and a cycle of raised ICP, impaired perfusion and further injury can result. In general, a target CPP of approximately 60 mmHg is recommended to minimize further brain injury (BTF 2007).

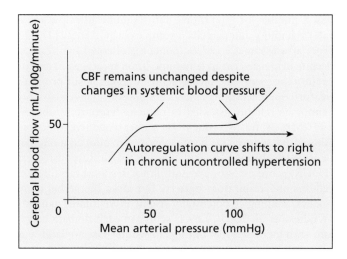

Figure 11.5 Changes in cerebral blood flow in response to changes in cerebral perfussion pressure (from Woodward and Mestecky 2011, reproduced with permission from Wiley).

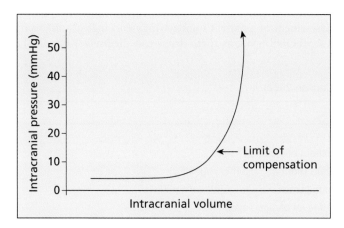

Figure 11.6 Pressure volume curve (from Woodward and Mestecky 2011, reproduced with permission from Wiley).

Assessment of neurological status

The assessment of neurological status aims to detect signs of injury to the brain and evidence of raised intracranial pressure, or impaired cerebral perfusion.

Assessment can be divided into clinical methods and use of invasive techniques.

Clinical methods

Vital signs

Control centres for respiration, blood pressure, pulse and temperature are located in the brainstem. Elevation in ICP may result in brainstem dysfunction with observable effects on a patient's vital signs. In addition, to optimize neurological function it is essential to ensure that mean arterial pressure and cerebral perfusion pressure are adequate and that the perfusing blood is well oxygenated.

Respiration

Control of respiration is mediated by several groups of neurons in different anatomical locations. In spontaneously breathing patients, damage at various points along the pathway gives rise to distinctive respiratory patterns. The rate, character and pattern of respiration should be noted (see Chapter 5). In practice, many patients in critical care will be sedated and mechanically ventilated, rendering clinical assessment of their respiratory patterns impossible.

Mechanical ventilation is a core component of management in this patient group. To limit continuing brain injury and reduce poor outcomes, close monitoring of arterial blood gases is essential. Hypoxia is an independent predictor of morbidity and mortality in head-injured patients (Jones et al. 1994). Cerebral blood flow is directly related to the partial pressure of carbon dioxide ($PaCO_2$) in the blood (see Chapter 5). Elevation in $PaCO_2$ causes cerebral vasodilatation, increase in cerebral blood flow and consequently increases intracranial pressure. $PaCO_2$ below the normal range causes cerebral vasoconstriction and inadequate cerebral perfusion. Current recommendations for practice advise keeping $PaCO_2$ at 4.0–4.5 kPa (McLeod 2004). Ventilatory parameters should be adjusted to ensure normal oxygenation and carbon dioxide levels.

Blood pressure

The vasomotor centre in the brainstem is responsible for regulating blood pressure. This area adjusts vascular tone in response to sensory inputs from peripheral receptors regarding current blood pressure (baroreceptors) and perfusion (chemoreceptors) (Hickey 2009). As ICP increases and global cerebral perfusion falls, there is a reflex increase in blood pressure in order to restore the cerebral perfusion pressure.

Ensuring blood pressure, and therefore cerebral perfusion pressure and cerebral blood flow are maintained adequately is essential to the management of this patient group. Episodes of hypotension have been associated with increased mortality (Chestnut et al. 1993; Manley et al. 2001).

Pulse

As the ICP increases and systemic blood pressure rises to preserve cerebral perfusion, the increase in arterial pressure is detected by the baroreceptors in the carotid arteries. These receptors interpret the systemic pressures as excessively high and this classically gives rise to a compensatory bradycardia. Hypertension with compensatory bradycardia and irregular respiration is termed the Cushing response, after the neurosurgeon who first described it in 1901 (Cushing 1901). This response is observed in critically elevated ICP.

Temperature

Hypothalamic dysfunction may be associated with disordered temperature regulation. Hyperthermia gives rise to increased cerebral metabolism and will increase oxygen requirements and carbon dioxide production. This causes cerebral vasodilatation, increased cerebral blood volume and consequently increased intracranial pressure. Temperature should be normalized in order to avoid compounding elevation in intracranial pressure (Waterhouse 2005).

Level of consciousness

Assessment of conscious level is a fundamental part of the assessment of neurological function. The Glasgow Coma Score (GCS) (Jennett and Teasdale 1974) assesses eye opening, motor and verbal responses, and is the most widely adopted tool (Table 11.2) (Fischer and Mathieson 2001). This score was developed for use in assessing patients with traumatic brain injury, but is in widespread use in populations in whom its validity is unproven. GCS has been shown to be associated with outcome in a number of clinical scenarios, including subarachnoid haemorrhage, anoxic coma and bacterial meningitis, with lower scores correlating with higher risk of death or severe disability (Qureshi et al. 2000; Booth et al. 2004; van de Beek et al. 2004). However, GCS

has a number of limitations, most significantly low inter-rater reliability and perceived complexity (Green 2011). The score also assumes each component is of equal significance, despite evidence that in traumatic brain injury, as in anoxic brain injury, only the motor score is a significant prognosticator (Zuercher et al. 2009). In addition, the verbal score cannot be reliably assessed in patients who are intubated, and there is no assessment of higher cognitive function. Alternative scores have been developed to address a number of these problems. The Full Outline of UnResponsiveness (FOUR) score assesses eye and motor responses, brainstem reflexes and respiratory pattern, but lacks the verbal component, making it potentially useful in ventilated patients (Wijdicks et al. 2005). Lower scores in each domain correlate with increased risk of mortality. Inter-rater reliability is reported as excellent (Iyer et al. 2009). The three-point Simplified Motor Score (SMS) describes only if a patient obeys commands, localizes pain, or worse. It has been shown to have greater inter-rater reliability, and equal validity in predicting outcome in traumatic brain injury in comparison to GCS (Gill et al. 2005; Thompson et al. 2011). Both scores are yet to be widely adopted.

Sedative and/or muscle relaxant agents may impact on the assessment of a patient's underlying neurological state using GCS/FOUR/SMS, as these drugs can themselves impair the

Table 11.2 The Glasgow Coma Score (Aucken and Crawford 1998; Carlson 2002)

Category	Score	Response
Eye opening		
Spontaneous	4	Eyes open spontaneously without stimulation
To speech	3	Eyes open to verbal stimulation (normal, raised or repeated)
To pain	2	Eyes open with painful/noxious stimuli
None	1	No eye-opening regardless of level of stimulation
Verbal response		
Orientated	5	Able to give accurate information regarding time, person and place
Confused	4	Able to answer in sentences using correct language but cannot answer orientation questions appropriately
Inappropriate words	3	Uses incomprehensible words in a random or disorganized fashion
Incomprehensible sounds	2	Makes unintelligible sounds, for example moans and groans
None	1	No verbal response despite verbal or other stimuli
Best motor response		
Obeys commands	6	Obeys and can repeat simple commands, for example arm raise or asking the patient to stick out their tongue
Localizes to pain	5	Purposeful movement to remove painful stimuli
Normal flexion	4	Withdraws extremity from source of pain, for example flexes arm at elbow without wrist rotation in response to painful stimuli
Abnormal flexion	3	Decorticate posturing (flexion of arms, hyperextension of legs) spontaneously or in response to noxious stimuli
Extension	2	Decerebrate posturing (limbs extended and internally rotated) spontaneously or in response to noxious stimuli
None	1	No response to noxious stimuli. Flaccid limbs

ability of a patient to respond by eye-opening or limb activity. However, deep sedation (Richmond Agitation and Sedation Scale [RASS] score less than −1) should only been targeted where a specific indication is present (for example raised ICP) (*see also* Chapter 10). Assessment of GCS/FOUR/SMS should remain possible with light sedation and during a break in sedation. Where deep sedation or muscle relaxants render level of consciousness assessment impossible, the additional clinical measures and invasive monitoring described in this chapter must be assessed.

Assessing GCS

Assessment should be made in steps, ensuring that a painful stimulus is not applied until spontaneous or verbally elicited responses are confirmed as absent (Waterhouse 2008). If it is necessary to apply a painful stimulus, care should be taken not to damage local tissues by using excess force. A central stimulus, either to the face or torso, may most reliably demonstrate the ability of the patient to localize pain. Common central stimuli are pressure on the supra-orbital notch or the trapezius muscle. If the patient does not reach purposefully towards the central stimulus, a peripheral stimulus, most commonly exerting pressure adjacent to the nail bed, can be used to establish the presence or absence of a withdrawal response. Assessment of the motor component of GCS includes a number of potential difficulties.

- A unilateral brain injury may give rise to an asymmetrical motor response. In this instance, the best response should be recorded as this is the most accurate indicator of overall brain function and conscious level (Edwards 2001). The poorer response may represent a localized injury to the motor area.
- The grasp reflex, a primitive response to stroking the palm, may be present in some patients in coma and may be mistaken for a voluntary movement. Two commands should be given – asking the patient to squeeze your fingers and then asking them to release (Shah 1999).
- Peripheral stimuli may provoke a spinal reflex. This response may resemble a purposeful withdrawal response but represents a reflex action mediated through the spinal cord. It does not require any cerebral function (Waterhouse 2008).

Assessment of the verbal response is not possible in patients who are intubated. In this case the overall score and the denominator may be adjusted to reflect this – for example 'GCS 8/10 (tube)'.

Pupillary responses

Normal pupils are spherical, usually at mid-position and have a diameter ranging from 2 to 5 mm (Shah 1999). As intracranial pressure increases, pressure is exerted on the oculomotor nerves (cranial nerve III). This may be detected clinically as asymmetrical, irregular, or dilated pupils, which are sluggish or unreactive to light (Table 11.3).

Table 11.3 Examination of pupils

Observation	Pupil size	Pupil reactivity	Possible indication
Pupils equal	Pinpoint	–	Opiates or pontine lesion
	Small	Reactive	Metabolic encephalopathy
	Mid-sized	Fixed	Midbrain lesion
		Reactive	Metabolic lesion
Pupils unequal	Dilated	Unreactive	3rd nerve palsy
	Small	Reactive	Horner's syndrome

Fuller (2004). Reproduced with permission from Elsevier.

Assessment of the pupil responses includes a number of potential difficulties.

- Facial swelling or eye injuries may prevent the assessor from opening the eyes.
- Assessment of reactivity may be difficult if the pupils are extremely constricted ('pinpoint') – for example as a result of opiate or barbiturate sedation.
- Alternative causes of pupillary abnormalities, including pre-existing medical problems and direct eye or orbital injuries, may confuse the clinical picture.

Herniation syndromes

Herniation occurs when raised intracranial pressure forces brain structures from one dural compartment into an adjacent compartment where pressure is lower (Suadoni 2009). Herniation syndromes are clusters of signs that occur during herniation. They can be broadly classified into supratentorial and infratentorial. Table 11.4 outlines the features and underlying mechanisms of these syndromes.

Progression of signs and symptoms

The signs and symptoms associated with raised intracranial pressure depend on the size, site and speed of onset of the causative lesion. In general, early signs and symptoms include:

- alteration in the level of consciousness
- headache
- vomiting.

Later findings comprise:

- continuing deterioration in the level of consciousness
- motor weakness
- abnormal posturing
- respiratory changes.

The development of pupillary dysfunction and Cushing's response are ominous signs seen in critically elevated intracranial pressure.

Table 11.4 Herniation syndromes

No herniation		Onset of raised intracranial pressure	Supratentorial herniation		Infratentorial herniation	
			Possible signs	Site of compression	Possible signs	Site of compression
Conscious level	Normal conscious level		Decreasing conscious level	Brainstem	Decreasing conscious level	Brainstem
Pupil reactions	Equal and reacting		Unilateral dilated pupil	Temporal lobe uncus compressing an oculomotor cranial nerve (III)	Bilateral dilation and fixation	Upward pressure on to an oculomotor cranial nerve (III)
Limb movements	Within normal limits for the patient		Abnormal posturing	Brainstem	Abnormal posturing	Direct pressure on to the brainstem
Blood pressure			Hypertension		Hypertension	
Pulse			Bradycardia		Bradycardia	
Respiration			Respiratory depression		Respiratory depression – apnoea	

Invasive monitoring

Both elevated ICP and inadequate CPP have been shown to correlate with poorer outcome in traumatic brain injury (Marmarou et al. 1991). Continuous ICP monitoring has become common in neurological critical care, despite the lack of robust evidence for its utility in improving outcome (Mauritz et al. 2008). It is most frequently used for patients with traumatic brain injury but may also be used for other pathologies where raised ICP may occur, for example meningitis, intracranial haemorrhage and encephalopathies (Mestecky et al. 2007). ICP monitoring allows the clinician to maintain adequate cerebral perfusion pressure, to evaluate a patient's responses to treatment and to identify interventions that precipitate increases in ICP (Mestecky 2007).

The Brain Trauma Foundation (BTF) and American Foundation of Neurosurgeons recommend ICP monitoring in patients with closed head injury and GCS 8 or below if:

- computerized tomography (CT) shows the brain is abnormal

OR

- CT shows the brain is normal but two or more of the following features are present:
  (i) age greater than 40
  (ii) unilateral or bilateral abnormal posturing
  (iii) systolic blood pressure below 90 mmHg

(BTF 2007)

ICP monitoring devices

The ideal ICP monitoring device is one that is accurate, reliable, cost-effective and causes minimal patient morbidity. The intraventricular catheter is conventionally regarded as the 'gold-standard' device in terms of cost-effectiveness and accuracy (BTF 2007), and has the advantage that CSF can be sampled or drained to help relieve ICP (Ross and Eynon 2005). However, significant risks and disadvantages remain, including catheter misplacement, infection, haemorrhage and obstruction. ICP may also be measured using a device placed within the brain tissue (intraparenchymal), or the subarachnoid, extradural, or subdural space. These monitoring devices can be fluid filled or non-fluid filled and each device has specific advantages and disadvantages (*see* Figure 11.7 and Table 11.5).

The most commonly used techniques for measuring ICP are intraventricular catheters and intraparenchymal devices.

ICP monitoring devices incorporating an external ventricular drainage system have the added advantage of being able to drain CSF, therefore treating, as well as measuring, raised ICP. If the patient's position is altered the drainage system should always be switched off prior to moving, then recalibrated (zeroed) afterwards before recommencing drainage (Woodward et al. 2002). Before opening the drainage system caution must be exercised to ensure that the height of the collecting/drip chamber is adjusted to the height prescribed whenever the patient is repositioned, otherwise inadvertent over- or under-drainage may occur (Jantzen 2007).

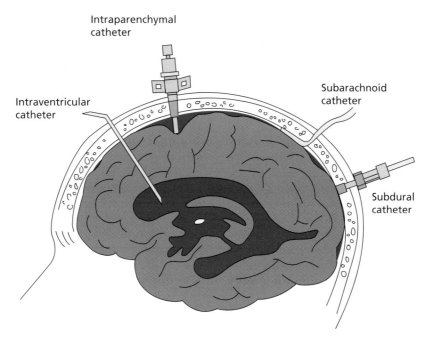

Figure 11.7 ICP devices situated in the lateral ventricle, intraparenchymal, subarachnoid and subdural spaces (adapted from Woodward and Mestecky 2011, reproduced with permission from Wiley).

Table 11.5 ICP monitoring devices, advantages and disadvantages

Device	Type	Advantages	Disadvantages
Intraventricular catheter	A small catheter inserted into the lateral ventricles through a burr hole. The catheter is 'tunnelled' under the scalp before being attached via fluid-filled tubing to a pressure transducer and drainage equipment	■ Accurate ■ Simple ■ Low cost ■ Can be recalibrated ■ Access to drain CSF ■ Access to instil drugs/contrast	■ Most invasive ■ Highest risk of infection ■ Risk of CSF leak ■ Catheter can block with blood clot or debris ■ Requires regular recalibration ■ Hemispheric reading may not reflect global ICP ■ Technically difficult in small ventricles
Subarachnoid catheter	A hollow metal shaft or screw inserted through a burr hole into the subarachnoid space. This is attached to fluid-filled pressure tubing and transducer equipment	■ Easy insertion ■ Does not penetrate brain tissue ■ Low risk of infection and haemorrhage	■ Less accurate ■ Easily blocked with blood clot or debris ■ Requires regular recalibration
Extradural or subdural catheters	A fibreoptic transducer-tipped catheter inserted into the extradural space through a burr hole	■ Easy insertion ■ Least invasive ■ Does not penetrate brain tissue ■ Low risk of infection and haemorrhage	■ Less accurate – dura may dampen the ICP reading ■ No access to CSF ■ Fragile catheter prone to damage
Intraparenchymal catheter	An electronic or fibreoptic-tipped catheter inserted through a subarachnoid bolt and advanced a few millimetres into the brain tissue	■ Easy insertion ■ Accurate ■ Low risk of infection and haemorrhage	■ Liable to become inaccurate over time ■ Local tissue reading may not reflect global ICP ■ No access to CSF ■ Complex system, risk of failure ■ Cannot be recalibrated once in situ

Arbour 2004; BTF 2007; Garner and Amin 2007; Mestecky et al. 2007; Hickey 2009; May 2009.

Strict aseptic technique must be adhered to at all times during any care associated with the external ventricular drainage system. Risk factors for infection include CSF leak around the insertion site, increased duration of catheter placement and device replacement (Hickey 2009; Mestecky et al. 2007). A sterile occlusive dressing should cover the monitoring device entry site to allow for inspection and early identification of signs of infection or CSF leak (Mestecky et al. 2007).

The subarachnoid, intraparenchymal, extradural and subdural monitors may be placed in the critical care unit due to the low infection risk. ICP monitoring devices can be connected to a dedicated ICP monitor or to most critical care monitors (Woodrow 2006; Mestecky et al. 2007).

ICP devices are generally inserted and calibrated by neurosurgeons. Following the insertion of the ICP monitoring device it is the responsibility of the practitioners caring for the patient to alert the neurosurgical team should there be any changes in neurological status or the monitoring parameters set by the neurosurgeons. Once the ICP monitoring device is in place the manufacturer's guidelines should be used for further guidance (Mestecky et al. 2007).

ICP waveforms

The shape of the ICP waveform is determined by interaction of the arterial pressure, intracranial contents and venous outflow (Kirkness et al. 2000). Individual waveforms have three characteristic peaks as described in Table 11.6.

A normal ICP wave appears as a descending sawtooth pattern, with each successive peak reducing in height. In contrast, a rising ICP appears as a progressive increase in P_2, giving the waveform a more rounded shape (Hickey 2009). In addition to the peaks within an individual waveform, the baseline of the normal ICP trace varies with the respiratory cycle (Figure 11.8) (see Problem solving table 11.1).

Problem solving table 11.1: ICP monitoring

Non-fluid-filled devices

Problem	Possible causes	Suggested action
No waveform or trace apparent on the monitor	■ Connections are not secure ■ Scale of the waveform on the monitor may not be set correctly ■ ICP device may not be positioned correctly inside the skull	■ Check the connections and ensure that they are connected properly ■ Check the scale set on the monitor ■ Attach to different monitor ■ Document and inform the neurosurgeons
Numerical reading present but no waveform apparent on the monitor	■ Scale of the waveform on the monitor may not be suitable for the pressure reading required ■ Faulty monitor	■ Check the scale set on the monitor ■ Attach to different monitor ■ Document and inform the neurosurgeons
Numerical reading present but waveform appears 'dampened on the monitor	■ Scale of the waveform on the monitor may not be set correctly	■ Check the scale set on the monitor ■ Document and inform the neurosurgeons
Fluid leakage around the insertion site of the ICP monitoring device	■ CSF leakage	■ Document and inform the neurosurgeons ■ Monitor the amount of leakage ■ Change the dressing as necessary using an aseptic technique ■ Monitor the patient for signs of infection

Fluid-filled devices – which may incorporate an external ventricular drainage system

Problem	Possible causes	Suggested action
Waveform appears 'dampened' and the pressure reading is lowered	■ The system may be open to the drip chamber, which will allow pressure to be dissipated and limit the peaks of pressure being registered by the transducer ■ Possible air bubble in drainage line or transducer. Care with the initial setting up of the system is essential to avoid this problem ■ The system may be blocked with debris or blood clot	■ Check the connections and if CSF drainage is not required then ensure that the system is closed to the drip chamber and open to the patient and transducer ■ Check the drainage line – if an air bubble is found or the system is blocked then the neurosurgeons should be informed

Table 11.6 ICP waveform

Order	Name	Origin and appearance
P_1	Percussion wave	Originates from the arterial pulsation transmitted from the choroid plexus to the ventricle. It has a sharp peak and a consistent amplitude
P_2	Tidal wave	Indicates the compliance of the surrounding brain tissue. Amplitude increases as compliance falls
P_3	Dicrotic wave	Arises due to closure of the aortic valve at the end of ventricular systole

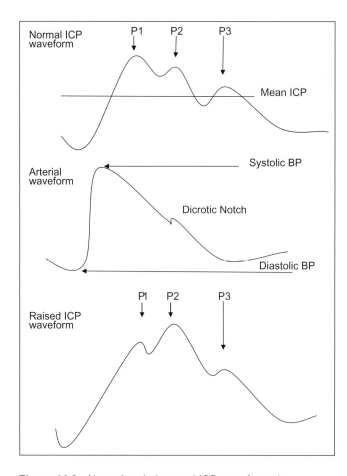

Figure 11.8 Normal and abnormal ICP waveforms in comparison to the arterial waveform.

Aspects of care impacting on intracranial pressure

In patients who are neurologically compromised, every effort should be made to maintain normal ICP and CPP, and reduce the risk of further brain injury and poorer neurological outcome (Kirkness et al. 2000). The critical care practitioner should be aware of the common causes of transient and reversible elevation in ICP in order to minimize their occurrence and duration, including:

- increased cerebral blood flow
- obstruction to venous outflow.

Increased cerebral blood flow

Hypoxia, hypercapnia and fever increase cerebral blood flow and may increase intracranial pressure in the injured brain. The importance of normal oxygenation and carbon dioxide levels, and of controlling fever, has been discussed above.

Increased arousal caused by pain and discomfort, noise and other external stimuli can also lead to increases in cerebral blood flow and consequently ICP. Appropriate use of analgesics and sedation, and control of environmental noise can help to minimize this problem (Cook 2008; Suadoni 2009).

Obstruction to venous outflow

Venous outflow may be obstructed by raised intrathoracic pressure or by mechanical obstruction of the jugular veins.

Raised intrathoracic pressure occurs during:

- coughing
- positive pressure ventilation
- straining
- positioning.

To reduce the risk of elevations in ICP, optimal sedation should be administered to minimize coughing and facilitate ventilator synchrony. A bolus of short-acting sedation may be required prior to endotracheal suctioning. On occasions, muscle relaxants may be employed to prevent surges in ICP occurring as a result of coughing. In addition, constipation should be prevented or treated (Hickey 2009; Suadoni 2009).

When positioning the patient, extreme hip flexion should be avoided as it can elevate intra-abdominal pressure, displacing the diaphragm upwards and increasing intrathoracic pressure and central venous pressure. This will in consequence reduce venous return and increase ICP (Woodward and Mestecky 2011).

Mechanical obstruction of the jugular veins may be caused by neck rotation and flexion (Cree 2003). Elevation of the head of the bed to 30° facilitates venous drainage with concurrent reduction in ICP (Hickey 2009). If the patient is hypovolaemic, elevating the head of the bed should be approached cautiously to limit hypotension. Ligatures around the neck, such as endotracheal or tracheostomy tube tapes, can impede venous return and should be avoided (Garner and Amin 2007). Care should be taken during activities such as positional change, personal hygiene and suctioning as they can result in an increase in ICP. Where the patient is ICP monitored then the effect of the activity can be established and the patient's care routine altered accordingly. Clustering of activities should be avoided as this can have a cumulative effect on ICP;

however, patient response to activities is variable (Mestecky 2007). Where patients are more physiologically stable it may be appropriate to cluster activities during the night to improve sleep (*see* Chapter 13).

Advanced neuromonitoring

In addition to ICP monitoring, further advanced techniques can be employed that allow measurement of physiological and metabolic parameters relating to brain perfusion.

Brain tissue oxygen tension can be directly measured using an electrode placed into brain tissue in the same manner as an intraparenchymal ICP measuring device. Low values of brain oxygen tension are similarly associated with worsened outcomes (BTF 2007).

More advanced intraparenchymal microdialysis probes can also be used to measure parameters such as glucose, lactate and pyruvate. These values are related to cerebral perfusion and may be correlated with secondary brain injury (Goodman et al. 2009).

Jugular venous oxygen saturation (SjV0₂)

To measure the oxygen saturation of the blood exiting the brain, a central venous catheter is inserted in a retrograde manner into the internal jugular vein to allow the tip to lie in the jugular bulb. Normal $SjVO_2$ is approximately 60%. Reduction in $SjVO_2$ to less than 50% for 10 minutes or more is associated with impaired CPP and poorer outcome (BTF 2007).

Procedure guideline 11.1: Neurological observations and assessment (adapted from Dougherty and Lister 2011)

Essential equipment

- Pen torch
- Thermometer
- Sphygmomanometer
- Alcohol handrub

Procedure

Action	Rationale
1 Where possible, explain and discuss the procedure to the patient. If the patient lacks the capacity to make decisions the practitioner must act in the patient's best interests.	To ensure that the patient understands the procedure and gives their valid consent. To ensure the patient's best interests are maintained (Mental Capacity Act 2005).
2 Wash and dry hands.	To minimize the risk of cross-contamination (Fraise and Bradley 2009).
3 Observe the patient. Note if they are alert, restless or drowsy.	To determine if the patient is behaving appropriately without stimulation.
4 Ask the patient their name, the day and date, and where they are.	To establish whether the patient's level of consciousness is deteriorating. If the patient is becoming disorientated, changes will occur in this order: (a) disorientation in time (b) disorientation in place (c) disorientation in person (Aucken and Crawford 1998). Call for immediate assistance from a senior practitioner if there is a deterioration in the patient's level of consciousness.
5 Ask the patient to squeeze and release your fingers with both hands, and then to stick out their tongue.	To evaluate motor responses and ensure that the responses are equal and are not reflexive (Carlson 2002).
6 If the patient does not respond, apply painful stimuli as previously described.	As the patient's level of consciousness deteriorates they may no longer localize and respond to pain in a purposeful way (Aucken and Crawford 1998).
7 Record the findings, including exactly what stimulus was used, where it was applied, how much pressure was required and the patient's best response.	Vague terms can be easily misinterpreted. Accurate recording will enable continuity of assessment and comply with professional guidelines (NMC 2008; HCPC 2012; GMC 2013).

8	Extend both hands and ask the patient to squeeze your fingers as hard as possible. Compare grip and strength.	To test grip and ascertain strength (Carlson 2002a).
9	Darken the room, if necessary, or shield the patient's eyes with your hands.	To enable a better view of the eye.
10	Ask the patient to open their eyes. If the patient cannot do so, hold the eyelids open and note the size, shape and equality of the pupils.	To assess the size, shape and equality of the pupils as an indication of brain function.
11	Hold each eyelid open in turn. Move pen torch from the side of the patient to shine directly into the eye.	To assess the reaction of the pupils to light (the pupil should constrict promptly) and the integrity of the neural pathway from eye to brainstem (Aucken and Crawford 1998).
12	Hold both eyelids open but shine the light into one eye only. Observe for bilateral pupillary constriction.	To assess consensual light reflex (Scherer 1986).
13	Record unusual eye movements.	To assess brain function (Aucken and Crawford 1998).
14	In spontaneously breathing patients, note the rate, character and pattern of the patient's respirations.	To assess for signs of injury to the respiratory centres of the brain (Carlson 2002).
15	Record the patient's temperature.	To monitor for change in temperature and ensure fever is avoided in order to maintain normal cerebral blood flow (CBF) and therefore intra cranial pressure (ICP). Damage to the hypothalamus or brainstem, the temperature-regulating centres in the brain, may be reflected in grossly abnormal temperatures (Fairley and McLernon 2005).
16	Record the patient's blood pressure and pulse.	To ensure central perfusion pressure (CPP) and hence CBF are monitored and maintained. To monitor signs of increased intracranial pressure (Scherer 1986; Tortora and Derrickson 2009).
17	Where patients are able to cooperate, ask them to hold the arms straight out in front, with palms upwards, for 20–30 s with their eyes closed. The weaker limb will 'fall away'.	To test arm strength. If one arm drifts downwards or turns inwards, it may indicate hemiparesis.
18	Where patients are able to cooperate, ask them to grasp your hands and to push and pull against resistance. Ask the patient to lie on their back in bed. Place your hand on the patient's extended legs. Instruct the patient to lift their legs in turn while you offer resistance.	To show any weakness and difference in limbs (Carlson 2002).
19	Document the observation recordings on the patient's chart.	To: ■ provide an accurate record ■ monitor effectiveness of procedure ■ reduce the risk of duplication ■ provide a point of reference or comparison in the event of later questions ■ acknowledge accountability for actions ■ facilitate communication and continuity of care. (NMC 2008; HCPC 2012; GMC 2013)
20	Report any abnormal findings to relevant senior practitioners.	To ensure deterioration is acted on appropriately.
21	Clean the equipment after use.	To prevent cross-infection (Fraise and Bradley 2009).

Procedure guideline 11.2: Recording intracranial pressure from an intracranial pressure monitor that incorporates an external ventricular drain (EVD)

Continuous CSF drainage and ICP measurements cannot be achieved simultaneously (follow the transducer manufacturer instructions for guidance on the proper use of their product) (Figure 11.9).

Equipment required
- Sterile gloves
- Apron
- Sterile caps × 1

Procedure

Action	Rationale
1 Where possible, explain and discuss the procedure with the patient. If the patient lacks the capacity to make decisions the practitioner must act in the patient's best interests.	To ensure that the patient understands the procedure and gives their valid consent. To ensure the patient's best interests are maintained (Mental Capacity Act 2005).
2 Put on an apron, then wash hands and apply sterile gloves.	To reduce the risk of microbial contamination (Pratt et al. 2007).
3 Rotate the tap to open the system between the patient and the transducer and switch off to the external ventricular (EVD) drainage bag.	To enable ICP recording.
4 Wait until the ICP waveform on the monitor is recognizable and the numerical display is constant.	To ensure the accuracy of the ICP recording.
5 The ICP pressure should be recorded and any deviation from the parameters set by the neurosurgeons reported.	To facilitate/initiate any further action that may be decided by the neurosurgeons. To: - provide an accurate record - monitor the effectiveness of procedure - reduce the risk of duplication - provide a point of reference or comparison in the event of later questions - acknowledge accountability for actions - facilitate communication and continuity of care. (NMC 2008; HCPC 2012; GMC 2013;)
6 If the patient is to continue to have CSF drained then the system should be turned off to the transducer and opened between the patient and CSF collection chamber.	To allow CSF drainage to recommence.

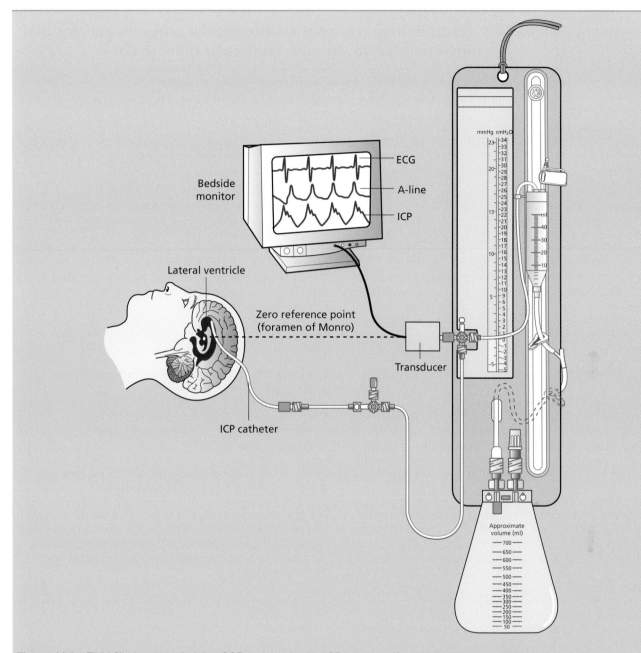

Figure 11.9 Fluid-filled system draining CSF and monitoring ICP pressure (from Mestecky et al. 2007, reproduced with permission from HFS Imaging).

Procedure guideline 11.3: Recalibrating (zeroing) an intracranial pressure monitor that incorporates an external ventricular drain (EVD)

(Follow the transducer manufacturer's instructions for guidance on the proper use of their product)

Equipment required

- Sterile gloves
- Apron

- Sterile caps × 1

Procedure

Action	Rationale
1 Where possible, explain and discuss the procedure with the patient. If the patient lacks the capacity to make decisions the practitioner must act in the patient's best interests.	To ensure that the patient understands the procedure and gives their valid consent. To ensure the patient's best interests are maintained (Mental Capacity Act 2005).
2 Refer to the manufacturer's guidance for information as to how frequently re-calibration (re-zeroing) should be performed.	Fluid-filled systems can become inaccurate over time and so must be recalibrated (zeroed) to the monitor at regular intervals (Mestecky et al. 2007).
3 Put on an apron, then wash hands.	To reduce the risk of microbial contamination (Pratt et al. 2007).
4 Check that all the connections and tubing are secure.	To ensure that accidental removal is avoided and that CSF does not leak out of drainage system.
5 Ensure that the section of tubing located between the drip chamber and the transducer is filled with fluid from end to end (see manufacturer's guidelines).	If the tubing is not completely filled with fluid the transducer cannot be accurately recalibrated to atmospheric pressure.
6 Ensure that the system is switched 'off' to the patient.	To prevent drainage of CSF while moving the system to recalibrate (re-zero) to atmospheric pressure.
7 Establish the correct 'zero' reference using the external auditory meatus as a landmark if the patient is lying on their back. If lying on their side, use the bridge of nose. Ensure that that the '0' pressure level on the pressure scale is in line with the landmark being used.	The external auditory meatus should be taken as the zero reference point, as this is at the level of the interventricular foramina (of Monro). The same reference point should be used each time to ensure consistency (Woodward et al. 2002; Hickey 2009).
8 Lower the drip chamber until the dropper in the drip chamber is in line with the '0' position on the pressure scale.	To ensure accurate recalibration to zero.
9 Wash hands and apply sterile gloves.	To reduce the risk of infection.
10 Using an aseptic no-touch technique remove the cap from the second three-way tap hub which is to be opened to facilitate zeroing.	To open up access to the transducer to facilitate zeroing to atmospheric pressure while reducing the risk of microbial contamination (Pratt et al. 2007).
11 Press the zero button on the monitor. Depending on the monitor in use, beeps may be heard and/or a visual display '0' will be seen on the monitor (see manufacturer's guidelines).	To recalibrate the transducer to zero.
12 Place a sterile cap on the hub which has been opened to atmospheric pressure using an aseptic no-touch technique.	To reduce the risk of microbial contamination (Pratt et al. 2007).

(Continued)

13 If the patient is to continue to have CSF drained via the external ventricular drain (EVD) following recalibration (zeroing), then the drip chamber should be returned to the original setting.	To recommence CSF draining at the height prescribed by the neurosurgeons to prevent over or under CSF drainage.
14 Once the chamber is at the correct position, if the patient is to continue to have CSF drained then the system should be turned off to the transducer and opened between the patient and CSF collection chamber.	This will allow for CSF drainage to recommence.
15 Document care provided.	To: ■ provide an accurate record ■ monitor the effectiveness of procedure ■ reduce the risk of duplication ■ provide a point of reference or comparison in the event of later questions ■ acknowledge accountability for actions ■ facilitate communication and continuity of care. (NMC 2008; HCPC 2012; GMC 2013)

Competency statement 11.1: Specific procedure competency statements for recording intracranial pressure from an intracranial pressure monitor that incorporates an external ventricular drain (EVD)

Complete assessment against relevant fundamental competency statements (*see* Chapter 2, pp. 20, 21)	Evidence
Specific procedure competency statements for recording intracranial pressure from an intracranial pressure monitor that incorporates an external ventricular drain (EVD)	**Evidence of competency for recording intracranial pressure from an intracranial pressure monitor that incorporates an external ventricular drain (EVD)**
Demonstrate the ability to: ■ teach and assess ■ learn from assessment.	Examples of evidence of teaching, assessing and learning.
Demonstrate an understanding of the anatomy and physiology of the brain and related structures and their relevance to the ICP system in use.	*May be demonstrated by:* ■ discussion with supervisor/mentor ■ teaching session for peers.

Discuss the rationale for the use of the ICP monitoring device.
■ Monitoring of raised intracranial pressure secondary to:
  ○ head injury
  ○ intracerebral haemorrhage
  ○ intracerebral infection.
	May be demonstrated by:
	■ discussion with supervisor/mentor
	■ teaching session for peers.

Identify the risks, potential problems and complications of the ICP monitoring device: ■ infection ■ haemorrhage ■ CSF leakage.	*May be demonstrated by:* ■ discussion with supervisor/mentor ■ teaching session for peers.

377

(Continued)

Competency statement 11.1: (*Continued*)

Correctly prepare to record the ICP pressure.
■ Ensures that the following are available:
  ○ sterile gloves
  ○ apron
  ○ sterile caps × 1.
	May be demonstrated by:
	■ observation of correct preparation, procedure in practice by supervisor/mentor
	■ teaching session for peers.

Demonstrate knowledge and skills of the correct procedure: ■ aseptic non-touch technique ■ follows manufacturer's instructions ■ correctly closes the ICP system off to the external ventricular drain (EVD) prior to procedure ■ waits until the patient's ICP waveform is recognizable and the numerical display is constant ■ correctly measures the patient's ICP ■ correctly re-establishes EV drainage if appropriate.	*May be demonstrated by:* ■ observation of correct preparation, procedure in practice by supervisor/mentor ■ teaching session for peers.
Demonstrate understanding and skill to correctly document: ■ ICP readings ■ time of recording.	*May be demonstrated by:* ■ discussion with supervisor/mentor ■ observation of documentation by supervisor/mentor ■ teaching session for peers.

Competency statement 11.2: Specific procedure competency statements for recalibrating (zeroing) an intracranial pressure monitor that incorporates an external ventricular drain (EVD)

Complete assessment against relevant fundamental competency statements (*see* Chapter 2, pp. 20, 21)	Evidence
Specific procedure competency statements for recalibrating (zeroing) an intracranial pressure monitor that incorporates an external ventricular drain (EVD)	**Evidence of competency for recalibrating (zeroing) an intracranial pressure monitor that incorporates an external ventricular drain (EVD)**
Demonstrate the ability to: ■ teach and assess ■ learn from assessment.	Examples of evidence of teaching, assessing and learning.
Demonstrate an understanding of the anatomy and physiology of the brain and related structures and their relevance to the ICP system in use.	*May be demonstrated by:* ■ discussion with supervisor/mentor ■ teaching session for peers.

Discuss the rationale for the use of the ICP monitoring device.
■ Monitoring of raised intracranial pressure secondary to:
  ○ head injury
  ○ intracerebral haemorrhage
  ○ intracerebral infection.
	May be demonstrated by:
	■ discussion with supervisor/mentor
	■ teaching session for peers.

Identify the risks, potential problems and complications of the ICP monitoring device: ■ infection ■ haemorrhage ■ CSF leakage.	*May be demonstrated by:* ■ discussion with supervisor/mentor ■ teaching session for peers.

Correctly prepares to recalibrate/re-zero the ICP device.
■ Ensures that the following are available:
  ○ sterile gloves
  ○ apron
  ○ sterile caps × 1.
	May be demonstrated by:
	■ observation of correct preparation, procedure in practice by supervisor/mentor
	■ teaching session for peers.

Demonstrate knowledge and skills of the correct procedure: ■ aseptic non-touch technique ■ follows manufacturer's instructions ■ correctly closes the ICP system off to the patient prior to procedure ■ locates the correct measuring position ■ recalibrates (re-zero) the transducer ■ correctly measures the patient's ICP ■ adjusts the drainage system correctly to the required parameters ■ reopens the system to recommence CSF drainage if required.	*May be demonstrated by:* ■ observation of correct preparation, procedure in practice by supervisor/mentor ■ teaching session for peers.
Demonstrate knowledge and skills to safely problem solve: ■ any changes in the ICP parameters/waveform ■ CSF leakage ■ communicates the problem effectively to colleagues when necessary.	*May be demonstrated by:* ■ Discussion of problems and causes with supervisor/mentor ■ Observation of actions to prevent and solve problems associated with ICP monitoring in practice by supervisor/mentor ■ Teaching session for peers.
Demonstrate understanding and skill to correctly document: ■ ICP readings ■ time of recalibration (zeroing).	*May be demonstrated by:* ■ discussion with supervisor/mentor ■ observation of documentation by supervisor/mentor ■ teaching session for peers.

References

Arbour R (2004) Intracranial hypertension: monitoring and nursing assessment. *Critical Care Nurse* **24**: 19–32.

Aucken S and Crawford B (1998) Neurological observations. In: Guerrero D (ed.) *Neuro-Oncology for Nurses*, pp. 29–65. London: Whurr.

Booth CM, Boone RH, Tomlinson G and Detsky AS (2004) Is this patient dead, vegetative, or severely neurologically impaired? Assessing outcome for comatose survivors of cardiac arrest. *Journal of the American Medical Association* **291**: 870.

Brain Trauma Foundation (2007) Guidelines for the management of severe traumatic brain injury, 3rd edition. *Journal of Neurotrauma* **24**(Suppl) 1.

Carlson BA (2002) Neurologic clinical assessment. In: Urden L, Stacy K and Lough M (eds) *Critical Care Nursing: diagnosis and management* (4e), pp. 645–657. St Louis, MO: Mosby.

Chestnut RM, Marshall LF, Klauber MR et al. (1993) The role of secondary brain injury in determining outcome from severe head injury. *Journal of Trauma* **34**(2): 216–222.

Cook NF (2008) Emergency care of the patient with subarachnoid haemorrhage. *British Journal of Nursing* **17**(10): 624–629.

Cree C (2003) Acquired brain injury: acute management. *Nursing Standard* **18**(11): 45–54.

Cushing H (1901) Concerning a definite regulatory mechanism of the vasomotor centre which controls blood pressure during cerebral compression. *Bulletin of the Johns Hopkins Hospital* **126**: 289–292.

Cutler LR and Cutler JM (eds) (2010) *Critical Care Nursing Made Incredibly Easy!* Philadelphia: Wolters Kluwer/Lippincott Williams & Wilkins.

Dinsmore J and Hall G (2006) *Neuroanaesthesia: anaesthesia in a nutshell*. Oxford: Butterworth-Heinemann.

Edwards S (2001) Using the Glasgow Coma Scale: analysis and limitations. *British Journal of Nursing* **10**(2): 92–101.

Fairley S and McLernon S (2005) Neurological problems. In: Adam S and Osborne S (eds) *Critical Care Nursing: science and practice* (2e), pp. 285–327. Oxford: Oxford University Press.

Fischer J and Mathieson C (2001) The history of the Glasgow Coma Scale: implications for practice. *Critical Care Nursing Quarterly* **23**(4): 52–58.

Fraise AP and Bradley T (eds) (2009) *Ayliffe's Control of Healthcare-associated Infection: a practical handbook* (5e). London: Hodder Arnold.

Fukuda K, Tanna H, Okimura Y et al. (1995) The blood–brain barrier disruption to circulating proteins in the early period after fluid percussion brain injury in rats. *Journal of Neurotrauma* **12**(3): 315-324. doi:10.1089/neu.1995.12.315.

Fuller G (2004) *Neurological Examinations Made Easy* (3e). Edinburgh: Churchill Livingstone.

Garner A and Amin Y (2007) The management of raised intracranial pressure: a multidisciplinary approach. *British Journal of Neuroscience Nursing* **3**(11): 516–521.

General Medical Council (2013) *Good Medical Practice*. London: GMC. http://www.gmc-uk.org/gmp2013 [accessed 25 March 2013].

Gill M, Windemuth R, Steele R and Green SM (2005) A comparison of the Glasgow Coma Scale score to simplified alternative scores for the prediction of traumatic brain injury outcomes. *Annals of Emergency Medicine* 45(1): 37–42.

Goodman JC and Robertson CS (2009) Microdialysis: is it ready for prime time? *Current Opinion in Critical Care* 15(2): 110.

Green SM (2011) Cheerio, laddie! Bidding farewell to the Glasgow Coma Scale. *Annals of Emergency Medicine* 58(5): 427–430. Epub 2011 Jul 30.

Health and Care Professions Council (2012) *Standard of Conduct, Performance and Ethics*. London: HCPC. http://www.hcpc-uk.org/assets/documents/10003B6EStandardsofconduct,performance andethics.pdf [accessed January 2013].

Hickey JV (2009) *The Clinical Practice of Neurological & Neurosurgical Nursing* (6e). Philadelphia: Lippincott Williams & Wilkins.

Huether SE and McCance KL (2012) *Understanding Pathophysiology* (5e). Missouri: Elsevier Mosby.

Iyer VN, Mandrekar JN, Danielson RD et al. (2009) Validity of the FOUR score coma scale in the medical intensive care unit. *Mayo Clinic Proceedings* 84: 694–701.

Jantzen J-P (2007) Prevention and treatment of intracranial hypertension. *Best Practice & Research Clinical Anaesthesiology* 21(4): 517–538.

Jennett B and Teasdale G (1974) Assessment of coma and impaired consciousness: a practical scale. *Lancet* 2: 81–84.

Jennett B and Teasdale G (1981) *Management of Head Injuries*. Philadelphia: FA Davis Company.

Jones, PA, Andrew PJ, Midgely S et al. (1994) Measuring the burden of secondary insults in head-injured patients during intensive care. *Journal of Neurosurgical Anesthesiology* 6(1): 4–14.

Kelly G (1824) Appearances observed in the dissection of two individuals; death from cold and congestion of the brain. *Transactions of the Medico-chirurgical Society of Edinburgh* 1: 84–169.

Kirkness CJ, Mitchell PH, Burr RL et al. (2000) Intracranial pressure waveform analysis: clinical and research implications. *Journal of Neuroscience Nursing* 32(5): 271–277.

Manley G, Knudson MM, Morabito D et al. (2001) Hypotension, hypoxia, and head injury: frequency, duration, and consequences. *Archives of Surgery* 136: 1118–1123.

Marmarou A, Anderson RL, Ward JD et al. (1991) Impact of ICP instability and hypotension on outcome in patients with severe head trauma. *Journal of Neurosurgery* 75: S59–S66.

Mauritz W, Steltzer H, Bauer P et al. (2008) Monitoring of intracranial pressure in patients with severe traumatic brain injury: an Austrian prospective multicenter study. *Intensive Care Medicine* 34(7): 1208.

May K (2009) The pathophysiology and causes of raised intracranial pressure. *British Journal of Nursing* 18(15): 911–914.

McLeod A (2004) Traumatic injuries to the head and spine 2: nursing considerations. *British Journal of Nursing* 13(17): 1041–1049.

Mendelow AD and Crawford PJ (1997) Primary and secondary brain injury. In: Reilly P and Bullock R (eds) *Head Injury*. London: Chapman & Hall, Chapter 4.

Mental Capacity Act (2005) http://www.legislation.gov.uk/ukpga/2005/9/pdfs/ukpga_20050009_en.pdf [accessed 9 February 2012].

Mestecky A (2007) Management of severe traumatic brain injury: the need for a knowledgeable nurse. *British Journal of Neuroscience Nursing* 3(1): 7–13.

Mestecky A-M, Brunker C, Connor J and Hanley C (2007) Understanding the monitoring of intracranial pressure: a benchmark for better practice. *British Journal of Neuroscience Nursing* 3(6): 276–281.

Monro A (1783) *Observations on the Structure and Function of the Nervous System*. Edinburgh: Creech & Johnson.

Nursing and Midwifery Council (2008) *The Code: standards of conduct, performance and ethics for nurses and midwives*. London: NMC. http://www.nmc-uk.org/Documents/Standards/The-code-A4-20100406.pdf [accessed 15 February 2012].

Nursing and Midwifery Council (2009) *Record Keeping: guidance for nurses and midwives*. London: NMC.

Patestas MA and Gartner LP (2006) *A Textbook of Neuroanatomy*. Oxford: Wiley.

Pratt RJ, Pellowea CM, Wilsona JA et al. (2007) epic2: National evidence-based guidelines for preventing healthcare-associated infections in NHS hospitals in England. *Journal of Hospital Infection* 655: s1–s64.

Qureshi AI, Sung GY, Razumovsky AY et al. (2000) Early identification of patients at risk for symptomatic vasospasm after aneurysmal subarachnoid hemorrhage. *Critical Care Medicine* 28: 984.

Ross N and Eynon MD (2005) Intracranial pressure monitoring. *Current Anaesthesia and Critical Care* 16: 255–261.

Rowley G and Fielding K (1991) Reliability and accuracy of the Glasgow Coma scale with experienced and inexperienced users. *Lancet* 331(8740): 535–538.

Scherer P (1986) The logic of coma. *American Journal of Nursing* 86: 542–549.

Shah S (1999) Neurological assessment. *Nursing Times* 13: 49–56.

Sheppard M and Wright M (2006) *Principles and Practice of High Dependency Nursing* (2e). London: Baillière Tindall.

Suadoni MT (2009) Raised intracranial pressure: nursing observations and interventions. *Nursing Standard* 23(43): 35–40.

Thompson DO, Hurtado TR, Liao MM et al. (2011) Validation of the simplified motor score in the out-of-hospital setting for the prediction of outcomes after traumatic brain injury. *Annals of Emergency Medicine* 58(5): 417–425.

Tortora GJ and Derrickson BH (2011) *Principles of Anatomy & Physiology Volume 1* (13e). New Jersey: Wiley International.

van de Beek D, de Gans J, Spanjaard L et al. (2004) Clinical features and prognostic factors in adults with bacterial meningitis. *New England Journal of Medicine* 351: 1849.

Waterhouse C (2005) The Glasgow Coma Scale and other neurological observations. *Nursing Standard* 19(33): 56–64.

Waterhouse C (2008) An audit of nurses' conduct and recording of observations using the Glasgow Coma Scale. *British Journal of Neuroscience Nursing* 4(10): 492–499.

Whitley SM, Bodenham A and Bellamy MC (2010) *Churchill's Pocket Book of Intensive Care* (3e). Edinburgh: Churchill Livingstone.

Wijdicks EF, Bamlet WR, Maramattom BV et al. (2005) Validation of a new coma scale: the FOUR score. *Annals of Neurology* 58: 585–593. DOI:10.1002/ana.20611. PMID 16178024.

Woodrow P (2006) *Intensive Care Nursing* (2e). London: Routledge.

Woodward S, Addison C, Shah S et al. (2002) Benchmarking best practice for external ventricular drainage. *British Journal of Nursing* 11(1): 47–53.

Woodward S and Mestecky A (2011) *Neuroscience Nursing Evidence-based Practice*. Oxford: Wiley-Blackwell.

Zakharov A, Papaiconomou C, Djenic J et al. (2003) Lymphatic CSF absorption pathways in neonatal sheep revealed by subarachnoid injection of Microfil. *Neuropathology and Applied Neurobiology* 29(6): 563–573.

Zuercher M, Ummenhofer W, Baltussen A and Walder B (2009) The use of Glasgow Coma Scale in injury assessment: a critical review. *Brain Injury* 23(5): 371–373.

Chapter 12

Assessment and care of tissue viability, and mouth and eye hygiene needs

Philip Woodrow,[1] Judy Elliott[1] and Pauline Beldon[2]

[1]*East Kent Hospitals University NHS Foundation Trust, Kent, UK*
[2]*Epsom and St Helier University Hospitals NHS Trust, Surrey, UK*

Critical Care Manual of Clinical Procedures and Competencies, First Edition.
Edited by Jane Mallett, John W. Albarran, and Annette Richardson.
© 2013 John Wiley & Sons, Ltd. Published 2013 by John Wiley & Sons, Ltd.

Tissue viability

Definition

Living tissue is an organization of cells. Animal tissues can be grouped into four basic types:

- connective
- muscle
- nervous
- epithelial (Tortora and Derrickson 2011).

Viable tissue is that which is healthy, capable of living, and undergoes normal growth and development.

Tissue viability needs are the requirements necessary to keep tissue viable, including to:

- keep tissue healthy, alive, growing and developing
- prevent tissue damage
- facilitate repair of damaged tissue
- promote hygiene.

Indications

Tissue viability support is required whenever there is potential or actual challenge to tissue health. Tissue health is affected by both intrinsic and extrinsic risk factors, therefore reducing these threats promotes tissue health. Some intrinsic factors, such as the ageing process, are irreversible. Others, such as poor perfusion, oxygenation and nutrition, are reversible and are likely to be found in critically ill patients (please refer to Chapters 5–8). However, the focus in this text is on reducing extrinsic factors, such as pressure and shear stresses, that can cause pressure ulceration and delay wound healing[1].

Anatomy and physiology

The skin consists of two layers:

- epidermis
- dermis.

(*See* Figure 12.1)

Epidermis

The epidermis forms the tough outer layer of the skin (Marieb and Hoehn 2013) and creates a barrier to water loss and invasion by microorganisms and toxic chemicals (Weller et al. 2008). It consists of four or five layers:

- stratum corneum (outermost layer)
- stratum lucidum (only in thicker skin areas such as finger tips, palms of hands and soles of feet)
- stratum granulosum (also known as the granular layer)
- stratum spinosum (or the 'prickle' layer)
- stratum basale (innermost layer) (Tortora and Derrickson 2011).

These layers consist of closely packed cells known as stratified squamous epithelium (Tortora and Derrickson 2011). The epithelium varies in thickness in different parts of the body. It is mostly 0.075–0.150 mm thick, but areas experiencing greater 'wear and tear' (such as palms and soles) are 0.4–0.6 mm thick (Penzer and Ersser 2010). Cells from the basal layer constantly divide by mitosis, moving towards the outer (dead) surface (Weller et al. 2008). This journey takes 30–60 days (Weller et al. 2008). As the cells (keratinocytes) travel to the surface they differentiate through the stratum spinosum where they synthesize keratins. The keratinocytes then enter the stratum granulosum, where they flatten out and die to form the top horny layer of corneocytes, which are coated with keratin. (The corneocytes may be likened to 'bricks' in a wall, and are separated by intracellular lipids, which are similar to 'mortar'.) This creates a barrier to water loss and invasion by infectious agents and toxic chemicals (Weller et al. 2008). The process ends with desquamation of dead cells at the skin surface (Tortora and Derrickson 2011).

More than 90% of the epidermis is keratinocyte cells (Thibodeau and Patton 2007; Penzer and Ersser 2010), with the remaining epidermal cells including:

- melanocytes (which produce the pigment melanin) (Butcher and White 2005; Clancy and McVicar 2009; Tortora and Derrickson 2011)
- Langerhans cells (which produce antigens to activate the immune system) (Butcher and White 2005; Marieb and Hoehn 2013)
- Merkel cells (involved in tactile perception) (Butcher and White 2005; Marieb and Hoehn 2013).

The epidermis lacks a direct blood supply (Marieb and Hoehn 2013), so receives nutrients and oxygen via diffusion from blood vessels in the papillary dermis, which is immediately below the epidermis.

In health, the dermis and epidermis are inextricably linked by interlocking ridges (rete pegs – which form fingerprint lines). Separation of dermis and epidermis causes a blister.

Dermis

The thickness of the dermis ranges from approximately 1 mm at the eyelids to 5 mm on the back and thighs. It weighs approximately 2.5–3.5 kg (15 to 20% of total body weight), and has a surface area of approximately 20 square feet.

The dermis consists of two layers:

---

[1] Patients with complex tissue damage requiring specialized care, such as those with severe chemical or burns damage, are beyond the remit of this Manual.

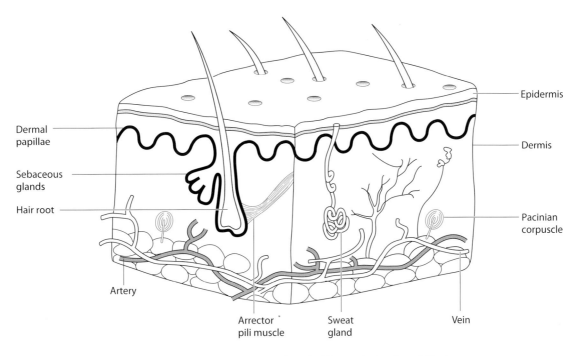

Figure 12.1 Cross-section of the skin (from Ousey 2005, reproduced with permission from Wiley).

- papillary dermis (a thin superficial layer underneath the epidermis)
- reticular dermis (a thicker deeper layer attached to the subcutaneous layer) (Tortora and Derrickson 2011).

The papillary dermis consists predominately of connective tissue, consisting of thin collagen and fine elastin fibres. The reticular dermis consists of thick collagen and coarse elastin fibres (Tortora and Derrickson 2011). This gives the skin its tensile strength and stretch, and allows it to recoil back into shape (Tortora and Derrickson 2011).

The dermis is also rich in hyaluronic acid, a carbohydrate polymer that is the main component of a viscous gel. This provides cushioning against pressure (Balasz 2004; Weller et al. 2008), can absorb and expel water like a sponge (Timmons 2006) and enables the transfer of nutrients, blood cells and waste products (Weller et al. 2008).

The dermis also contains:

- fibroblasts – cells that enable growth of new tissue, and so are fundamental to wound healing
- blood vessels (Weller et al. 2008);
- nerves (which stimulate to touch, pain, warmth and coolness)
- hair follicles, sebaceous and sweat glands (Marieb and Hoehn 2013)
- macrophages (Tortora and Derrickson 2011).

Subcutaneous layer

Underneath the dermis is the subcutis or subcutaneous layer. This is loose connective tissue and abundant fat, which acts as a shock absorber, calorie reserve and provides insulation (Weller et al. 2008).

Functions of the skin

Skin has many functions, including the following.

- Thermoregulation:
  - thermoreceptors in the dermis can sense changes in temperature (Timmons 2006). Thermoregulation is controlled by the hypothalamus in response to core body temperature via the autonomic nervous system. Signals relayed from peripheral thermoreceptors in the skin and centrally in the body core, assist in this process
  - heat can be lost by evaporation of sweat and vasodilatation (the latter promotes loss by convection and conduction)
  - heat can be conserved by vasoconstriction and trapping insulating air over the skin. This is achieved by activation by autonomic nerves of arrector pili muscles at hair follicles, which cause the hairs to rise (Marieb and Hoehn 2013).
- Immunity:
  - Langerhans cells, mast cells and other mechanisms trigger inflammatory responses to protect against infection and promote tissue repair (Timmons 2006). The inflammatory response causes release of vasoactive mediators, which (i) attract white cells into blood; (ii) vasodilate in the area of inflammation; (iii) increase capillary leak. This results in more white

383

cells being carried to the area of damage and leaking into the surrounding tissues, which enables destruction of (most) invading microorganisms.

- Absorption:
  - drugs, such as glyceryl trinitrate (GTN), fentanyl and nicotine can be absorbed by the skin.
- Vitamin D synthesis:
  - ultraviolet rays in sunlight modify 7-dehydrocholesterol (a precursor of vitamin D) in the skin to cholecalciferol (D_3). This is converted via the liver and kidneys to calcitrol (the active form of vitamin D) (Tortora and Derrickson 2011).
- Protection:
  - sensory nerves warn of temperature changes or other painful stimuli, which may cause injury. Melanocytes produce melanin, which provides a barrier against sunburn (Marieb and Hoehn 2013).
- Communication:
  - facial expression and touch enable humans to communicate. Skin damage may affect communication, impair relationships and harm self-image (Penzer and Ersser 2010).

The outermost layer of skin is visible and is taken very much for granted, until trauma or injury occurs.

Challenges to health of skin

Healthy cells normally repair themselves and recover from transient damage. Cells use energy in the form of adenosine triphosphate (ATP), which the mitochondria of cells produce from energy sources (normally glucose, metabolized using oxygen). ATP synthesis produces metabolic waste (mainly carbon dioxide, water and acids) (Marieb and Hoehn 2013). Cell health therefore necessitates:

- adequate supply of nutrients, water and oxygen
- adequate removal of potentially toxic waste
- prevention of damage from any external factors.

Viability of any tissue may threaten health, but skin damage breaches the body's protective barrier between its internal and external environments.

Cell, and therefore skin, health is threatened by:

- poor oxygenation of cells (hypoxia, hypoperfusion)
- poor nutrition
- poor hydration
- poor removal of carbon dioxide and waste products.

In addition, ageing leads to generalized atrophy of skin, making it increasingly thin, fragile and prone to injury, pressure damage and delayed healing.

Patients who are critically ill will have many challenges to skin tissue viability and may very quickly develop pressure ulcers (Tortora and Derrickson 2011).

Pressure ulcers

Definition

A pressure ulcer (previously also called 'pressure sore' or 'decubitus ulcer') is localized injury to skin and/or underlying tissue, usually over a bony prominence, caused by pressure, or pressure in combination with shear (European Pressure Ulcer Advisory Panel and National Pressure Ulcer Advisory Panel EPUAP/NPUAP 2009a, b).

Pressure area care is a range of interventions aimed at preventing or healing pressure ulcers.

Indications

Tissue viability management is important in patients who are critically ill as they have many of the risk factors for developing tissue damage.

Many, although not all, pressure ulcers are preventable (Orsted et al. 2010), and those that develop can usually be healed (Shahina et al. 2009). Patients who develop pressure ulceration while in critical care units are more likely to remain longer in the unit, and their chances of survival are reduced (Compton et al. 2008). Factors correlating with skin breakdown include:

- severity of illness (Bell 2008)
- poor tissue perfusion due to haemodynamic instability (Elliott et al. 2008; Terekeci et al. 2009)
- co-morbidities (Bell 2008), especially vascular disease (Nijs et al. 2009)
- use of inotropes (Theaker et al. 2000; Elliott et al. 2008; Nijs et al. 2009)
- renal replacement therapy (Nijs et al. 2009)
- malnutrition (Elliott et al. 2008; Terekeci et al. 2009)
- pyrexia above 38.5°C (Compton et al. 2008; Nijs et al. 2009)
- faecal incontinence (Lowery 1995; Theaker et al. 2000)
- immobility (Bours et al. 2001; Bell 2008; Elliott et al. 2008)
- use of sedatives (Elliott et al. 2008; Nijs et al. 2009).

Background

Pressure ulcers pose challenges to practitioners, are time consuming and can cause suffering (Fleurence 2005; NHS Institute for Innovation and Improvement 2009; Alderden et al. 2011). They also incur high financial and potential litigation costs (Bennett et al. 2004).

Incidence

Incidence of pressure ulcers varies considerably between different studies, hospitals, countries and clinical areas

(Elliott et al. 2008): Reddy et al. (2006) cite ranges between 0.4% and 38%, the highest figure being in acute care. Critically ill patients are at especially high risk of pressure ulcer formation (Hassanin and Tantawey 2011). Most pressure ulcers occur in older people (Terekeci et al. 2009; Kelly and Isted 2011), and most critically ill patients are aged over 65 (Pisani 2009). Therefore older critically ill patients are at especially high risk. About one-fifth of critically ill patients develop pressure ulcers (Pender and Frazier 2005; Nijs et al. 2009), and the incidence is increasing (Eachempati et al. 2001; Alderden et al. 2011). Therefore all critically ill patients need pressure area care.

Pressure ulcer grading

The European Pressure Ulcer Advisory Panel (EPUAP), and in the USA the National Pressure Ulcer Advisory Panel (NPUAP), classify pressure ulcers into four categories (*see* Table 12.1), depending on factors such as their depth. Category one ulcers are the most superficial.

Table 12.1 Pressure ulcer classification (adapted from EPUAP/NPUAP 2009a,b)

Category of pressure ulcer*	Description
Category 1	*Intact skin with non-blanchable redness of a localized area usually over a bony prominence* A category 1 ulcer does not demonstrate blanching of the reddened area (erythema). Blanching erythema is an area of erythema that turns white on light finger pressure. This is a natural response to tissue damage (reactive hyperaemia) but not capillary damage. It is a warning that pressure and shear forces are causing damage, and therefore, more frequent repositioning may be needed to prevent ulcer development (Clark and Stephen-Haynes 2005)
Category 2	*Partial thickness loss of dermis* A category 2 ulcer has partial thickness skin loss resulting in a shallow open ulcer with a red/pink wound bed without slough. This may also present as an intact or ruptured blister filled with serous or serosanguinous fluid
Category 3	*Full thickness tissue loss* A category 3 ulcer has full thickness tissue loss involving damage necrosis of subcutaneous tissue that may extend down to, but not through, underlying fascia. Bone, muscle or tendon are not visible. Slough may be present but does not obscure depth of tissue loss
Category 4	*Full thickness tissue loss with exposed bone, tendon or muscle* A category 4 ulcer involves full thickness tissue loss with bone, tendon or muscle being exposed. These ulcers can extend into muscle and/or supporting structures. However, the depth varies by anatomical location. The bridge of the nose, ear, occiput and malleolus do not have (adipose) subcutaneous tissue and these ulcers can be shallow

*If the wound bed is obscured with slough or eschar, it cannot be fully categorized until debrided.

Extrinsic factors

Two main extrinsic factors directly contribute to pressure ulceration:

- pressure
- shear

(EPUAP/NPUAP 2009a,b)

with arguably a third factor:

- friction.

These factors must be eliminated or minimized to reduce the risk to the patient (NICE 2005).

Pressure

Pressure is a perpendicular force directly on tissue that causes compression (Takahashi et al. 2010). Average mean capillary pressure within dermal tissue is 17 mmHg, although like all blood pressures this varies considerably between individuals and different parts of the body (Barrett et al. 2010; Tortora and Derrickson 2011). (For example, the pressure gradient can be greater in deeper than in superficial [visible], tissue.) Any intense or prolonged pressure, usually from body weight, deprives skin and soft tissue cells of oxygen and nutrients (Hampton and Collins 2004). This can, therefore, cause necrosis.

Shear force

Shear results from two parts of body tissue moving in opposing (parallel) directions (Gunnewicht and Dunford 2004; Reger et al. 2010). This is typically created by gravity when patients are in a sitting position: the dermis and epidermis are held by the external surface (such as a chair or linen), while gravity causes deeper tissue (such as subcutaneous fat and muscle) to be pulled downwards (Hampton and Collins 2004). This can result in the soft tissue becoming deformed and compressed between the support surface and bone. Older people are at greater risk from shear, as reduced skin elasticity and turgor increase skin displacement. Shear doubles the effect of pressure on tissue damage (Reger et al. 2010). Irregularly shaped pressure ulcers and wound dressings that repeatedly peel off at one edge indicate shear damage (Reger et al. 2010). Shear can be reduced by ensuring patients are sufficiently supported.

Friction

'Friction' is caused by two objects rubbing against the other (Reger et al. 2010), although its role in causing pressure damage is debated. Friction is influenced by:

- nature of textile (rougher textiles cause more friction)
- moisture

- ambient humidity (high humidity increases skin moisture).

(Reger et al. 2010)

Friction can result from poor moving and handling technique; friction injuries cause abrasions, superficial ulceration and blistering.

Moisture

Shear and friction damage are exacerbated if skin is moist (Elliott et al. 2008; Berlowitz et al. 2011). Moisture, such as perspiration, urine, faeces, or wound exudates, can weaken crosslinks between collagen fibres in the dermis and soften the stratum corneum (Mayrovitz and Sims 2001). Maceration exposes blood vessels to the effects of pressure and shear (Clark et al. 2004), making wounds larger (Elliott et al. 2008). Patients with diarrhoea (for example due to *Clostridium difficile*) are at especially high risk of skin breakdown (European Wound Management Association, EWMA 2005), as excoriation initiates inflammatory responses, which, together with factors such as existing irritation, moisture lesions, or infection, makes superficial damage more likely (Reger et al. 2010).

Moisture lesions or incontinence-associated dermatitis may occur independently or in conjunction with pressure damage. Incontinence or moisture lesions are frequently confused with category 2 or 3 pressure damage (Defloor and Schoonhoven 2004), so identifying causes enables accurate diagnosis and treatment (*see* Table 12.2).

Assessment

Assessing risk and implementing appropriate prevention strategies can reduce pressure ulcer incidence (Terekeci et al. 2009). Although many assessment tools have been developed, none is designed specifically for critically ill patients (Cox 2011). EPUAP/NPUAP (2009a,b) recommend assessing risk of pressure ulceration by using clinical judgement in combination with an assessment tool and skin assessment. Risk assessment should be initially undertaken within 6 hours of admission to the hospital and/or critical care unit and repeated on any change in the patient's condition (NICE 2005).

Any assessment tools used should identify risks for patients receiving critical care (de Laat et al. 2006). In the UK, most critical care areas (and most wards) use the Waterlow risk assessment, which Sayar et al. (2009) suggest is effective for critically ill patients. However, others argue it is too insensitive as it identifies most critically ill patients as 'high risk' (Sollars 1998).

Skin inspection

Skin should be inspected at least once every shift and documented in the patient's notes. Bony prominences should be

Table 12.2 Identifying pressure ulcers and moisture lesions (after Bale et al. 2005)

	Pressure ulcer	Moisture lesion	Combined pressure/moisture
Causes	Pressure and or shear	Moisture, for example, shiny wet skin caused by urinary incontinence or diarrhoea	Moisture, pressure and shear present simultaneously
Location	Often over bony prominence	Anal cleft, perianal region, skin folds	Pressure may occur in skin folds, wounds and fleshy areas
Shape	Tend to be regular and localized	Diffuse superficial spots or 'kissing ulcer' (ulcers anatomically opposite each other) ('copy' or 'mirror' lesion)	Irregular
Depth	May be superficial or deep	Superficial – infection may lead to depth	Friction may be exerted on a moisture lesion causing skin loss with torn, jagged skin fragments

inspected on repositioning the patient, to evaluate effectiveness of repositioning regimens. Skin should be inspected for:

- persistent erythema
- non-blanching hyperaemia
- localized induration
- purplish/bluish localized areas
- localized coolness
- blisters
- localized heat
- localized oedema.

(NICE 2005)

Additional risk areas for critically ill patients may include:

- pre-existing trauma or surgical wounds
- mechanical damage to eyes, from linen (a particular risk when the patient is lying in a prone position [Guerin et al. 2004]), periorbital oedema, impairment of blink reflexes and any tapes or tubes lying across the eye surface (Farrell and Wray 1993)
- prolonged occipital pressure (head resting back on pillows)
- areas in contact with endotracheal tube or tracheostomy tapes (sides of the lips being especially vulnerable) (Kite and Pearson 1995). Ulcers of the tongue or other oral mucosa should not be classified as pressure ulcers (EPUAP/NPUAP 2009a,b)
- any parts of the body near or on cables, tubing, or other equipment
- equipment (such as administration set tubing) lying on bedding but underneath the patient.

Alderden et al. (2011) found that two-fifths of pressure ulcers developing in critical care units occurred in areas not generally associated as high-risk parts of the body, such as the back, head and neck.

While some risk-reducing measures may generally be in place for all patients (such as alternating pressure relief mattresses), individual patient risk assessment enables individualized interventions. If early signs of pressure damage are found, avoid positioning on the ulcer and review skincare plan. Options include:

- increasing frequency of repositioning
- enhancing support surfaces
- adjusting positioning techniques.

Any tissue damage should be documented.

Prevention

Preventing harm by maintaining skin integrity is a fundamental role for all practitioners, so pressure ulcer prevention is a multidisciplinary responsibility (Beldon 2007; General Medical Council 2009; Health and Care Professions Council 2012; Nursing and Midwifery Council 2008). The multidisciplinary EPUAP and the NPUAP, representing the USA, have collaborated to produce guidelines for prevention and treatment of pressure ulceration (EPUAP/NPUAP 2009a,b).

Pressure ulcer prevention aims to reduce an individual's risk of pressure ulcer development by identification and modification of all risk factors involved by all of the multidisciplinary team (Gould 2002). All modifiable risk factors should be reduced as much as possible. Skin integrity and health are promoted by:

- maintaining good hygiene
- avoiding prolonged contact with moisture
- optimizing hydration
- optimizing nutrition
- optimizing oxygenation
- reducing pressure, shear and friction forces
- early mobilization.

(Bell 2008; Penzer and Ersser 2010; Reddy et al. 2006)

Maintaining good hygiene and avoiding maceration of skin

Maintaining good hygiene and avoiding maceration reduces external risk factors. Washing skin with pH-balanced emollients helps promote a lipid moisture barrier (Bliss et al. 2006; Reger et al. 2010). Protective barrier film dressings are sometimes also needed to provide a barrier against moisture (Falanga 2004; Reger et al. 2010), especially in the perianal area.

Optimizing hydration

Dehydration impairs perfusion (Wakefield et al. 2009), so optimizing hydration reduces this intrinsic risk factor.

Optimizing nutrition

Although the outer layer of skin is 'dead', basal layers are living cells and therefore need nutrients for normal (healthy) replacement of cells. Wound repair increases metabolic demand. Glucose is normally the main energy source for cells (Marieb and Hoehn 2013), but micronutrients, especially phosphate, are also important for cell health (Adams 2005). Malnutrition increases incidence, and cost, of pressure ulcers (Terekeci et al. 2009; Banks et al. 2010). Enteral nutrition can reduce incidence of pressure ulcers by 25% (Stratton et al. 2005).

Optimizing oxygenation

Without oxygen, cells resort to anaerobic metabolism, which, like metabolism of alternative energy sources, produces relatively little ATP but increases waste (Clay et al. 2001). This creates a toxic environment for cells.

While levels of oxygen in blood can be easily measured, assessing tissue oxygenation is problematic, and can be affected by:

- oedema (which creates a fluid barrier between capillaries and cells – oxygen is not very soluble, and so diffusion is impaired by oedema)
- poor perfusion from systemic hypotension
- microcirculatory (capillary blood flow) imbalance (for example as in distributive shock, such as from sepsis [Hinds and Watson 2008]).

Tissue oedema commonly occurs with critical illness due to capillary leak. Tissue oedema is often visibly obvious, but difficult to reverse. Diuretics usually only have transient effects, and may exacerbate hypotension.

Pressure redistributing equipment

In health, most people reposition themselves every 15–20 minutes, even during sleep (Myers 2008). Prolonged pressure on skin can be reduced by frequent changes of position and the use of pressure redistribution and relieving equipment (such as alternating pressure mattresses). Shear and friction forces can be reduced by supportive positioning and protective dressings.

High specification foam mattresses are suitable for many at-risk patients, but those at higher risk will need a powered support surface (Takahashi et al. 2010). Most critical care units can access specialized mechanical pressure-redistributing equipment; selection should be based on individual risk assessment, the care setting and the clinical condition (Bell 2008). A wide variety of dynamic or active mattresses are available, each with individual features (*see* Table 12.3).

Electric profiling beds, standard on most critical care units, can augment repositioning programmes, as body weight may be redistributed by adjusting the back and leg supports. Electric profiling beds reduce pressure ulcer incidence and facilitate patient independence (Birtles and Williams 2004; Rush 2005).

Heels are particularly at risk of pressure damage, due to:

- higher pressures are exerted over a smaller area
- peripheral shutdown and/or poor perfusion due to critical illness, and use of vasopressors (e.g. noradrenaline)
- oedema
- co-morbidities, such as peripheral arterial disease, diabetes mellitus.

EPUAP/NPUAP (2009a,b) recommend support surfaces to ensure the heels are free from the surface of the bed. This may be achieved by heel-protector devices or placing a pillow under the calves.

Pressure damage is related to the intensity and duration of the applied pressure (Takahashi et al. 2010). Pressure reducing/relieving equipment can reduce, but not eliminate, pressure, so patients still need regular repositioning (Beldon 2007; Winkelman and Chiang 2010). However, as evidence supporting a single time interval for all patients (for example the traditionally cited 2 hours) is lacking (Winkelman and Chiang 2010), frequency should be individually assessed for each patient, not by ritualistic practice (NICE 2005; EPUAP/ NPUAP 2009a,b).

Positioning

To reduce shear and friction:

- decrease tangential forces – for example minimize elevation of head of bed, avoid patient sliding downwards and or forwards when in sitting positions
- avoid actions that induce tissue distortion – for example sliding or dragging the patient
- maximize contact area with support surface.

(Reger et al. 2010)

Useful equipment for repositioning may include:

- slide sheet (full length)
- hoist
- hoist sling
- electric profiling bed
- pillows.

See the Procedure guidelines in Chapter 14 for repositioning critically ill patients for more detail.

If critically ill patients are too unstable to reposition, a careful risk assessment should be made by the multidisciplinary team to formulate an individual plan of care (Takahashi et al. 2010).

Table 12.3 Pressure-redistributing equipment

Equipment and mode of action	Patient indication	Rationale
Alternating cell mattress Air-filled cushions that alternate between inflation and deflation. Inflated cells support the patient, while deflated ones facilitate perfusion. Available in mattress overlay or replacement Examples include: Solo™, Autologic™, Quattro™, Nimbus 3™	Suitable for most critically ill patients Check operating weight limit is compatible with patient's body weight Contraindicated in spinal injury and unstable fractures	Reduces incidence of pressure ulcer formation in critically ill patients (Shahina et al. 2009) Mattress movement stimulates vascular supply (Rithalia and Kenney 2000)
Low air loss mattress Cells into which air is constantly pumped. The patient's body weight causes slow air loss through the vapour permeable surround. The effect is slight deflation of cells, so the mattress conforms to and supports the body. Examples include: Duo™, Breeze™	For severely injured patients, those at high risk of pressure damage or patients who have category 3 or 4 pressure ulcers Patients with low body weight Check operating weight limit is compatible with patient's body weight Contraindicated in spinal injury and unstable fractures	The patient may not be able to tolerate regular repositioning and so requires additional support (EPUAP/NPUAP 2009a,b) Patients unable to tolerating alternating mattresses Low air loss mattresses assists in micro-climate control by decreasing skin temperatures (air escapes through minute pores in the mattress surface)
Pillow under calves Acts to 'float heel' over the edge of the pillow while leg supported under the calf *Heel protection devices* Examples include: Leeder Boot™, Prevalon boot™, Repose boot™	Patients at risk of, or who have developed, pressure ulceration at the heel and who are, for example: ■ immobile, heavily sedated or unconscious ■ diabetic, have vascular or renal disease ■ oedematous legs Patients on bedrest Not always suitable for patients with contractures Ensure knee is slightly flexed to avoid pressure on the popliteal vein (EPUAP/ NPUAP 2009a,b)	Provides total pressure off-loading to the heels Additional protection of heels
Bariatric mechanical support surfaces These may be alternating pressure or low air loss Examples include: Bariair™, Bari-Breeze™ Some equipment has features that assist repositioning. For example, Bari-Breeze is a low air loss mattress with in-built mechanical lateral-tilt facility	Patients whose weight cannot be accommodated on usual equipment (check manufacturer's instructions) Patients who require wider mattress to assist lateral tilt and or repositioning	Able to provide sufficient inflation and pressure redistribution at higher weights, for example 540 kg Allows patient to be repositioned due to wide dimensions
Continuous lateral rotation ('kinetic therapy) Examples include: Linnet Multicare™, RotoRest™	Usually used to treat and or prevent pulmonary complications (Swadener-Culpepper et al. 2008) Also used to help promote skin integrity (Goldhill et al. 2007)	Prolonged immobility causes difficulty moving bronchial secretions (Welch 2002) Limited evidence supports prevention and healing of skin breakdown (Wanless and Aldridge 2012) But rotation can cause: ■ tachycardia (McLean,2001) ■ hypotension (McLean 2001) ■ desaturation (McLean 2001) ■ discomfort, necessitating sedation (Kennedy 2004)

Postures should be comfortable for the patient, minimize pressure on bony prominences and avoid positioning directly on a pressure ulcer (NICE 2005). Postures found to create the highest localized pressures are sitting and 90° degree side-lying (Sewchuk et al. 2006). Flatter postures are preferable as body weight is distributed more evenly over the surface, reducing localized pressure. While semi-recumbency reduces the risk of ventilator-associated pneumonia (VAP) (Drakulovic et al. 1999), pressure ulcer prevention necessitates changes of position. For side-lying, EPUAP/NPUAP (2009a,b) recommend a tilt of 30°, which places less stress on the bony hip prominence.

The angle of the back strongly influences shear stresses in tissues. All angles except horizontal cause shear stresses as the body slides downwards. Sitting with bed backrests at more than a 30° angle should be avoided, as it causes excessive shear stress and pressure to buttocks and sacrum (Reger et al. 2010). If sitting patients at more than 30° upright, consider more frequent repositioning. Shear forces can be reduced by positioning patients to prevent slouching or sliding down the bed, supporting knees by either profiling the electric bed or using a pillow under the calves.

When sitting in chairs, shear and pressure forces should be minimized by ensuring the chair is sufficiently supportive (correct height and width). Knees should be vertical, with feet on the floor, and shoulders and arms supported (Beldon 2007). Acutely ill patients, or those at risk of developing pressure damage, should be restricted to 2 hours maximum sitting in a chair (EPUAP/NPUAP 2009a,b), and they should be repositioned at least every hour.

Specific conditions may necessitate or preclude specific positions, but the more commonly used positions used in critical care units are listed in Table 12.4.

Healing pressure ulcers

If a pressure ulcer develops the aims of treatment and care are to:

- minimize or remove pain
- promote healing
- prevent infection from microorganisms in the atmosphere or surrounding skin surface.

The main aspects of wound assessment are outlined in Table 12.5.

Dressings

There are four stages to wound healing:

- inflammatory
- granulation
- epithelization
- remodelling/maturation.

(Russell 2002)

Dressings are not usually advised for reducing risk of pressure ulcers. However, open wounds need protective dressings. Choice of dressings is restricted in most hospitals, and many will produce guidelines for which types of dressing to apply to particular wounds. Types and frequency of dressings should assist progression to the next stage of healing. Wounds heal best in a moist environment (Russell 2002), although excessive exudates should be removed. Adherent dressings will remove some granulation tissue with each dressing change, especially if skin is friable. Table 12.6 outlines the main groups of dressings, although there are often differences between different products within each group. For complex dressings, advice should always be sought from tissue viability specialists (some units have 'link' staff for tissue viability).

Topical negative pressure therapy (TNPT) applies a pumped vacuum below a wound dressing to remove exudate (Dealey and Cameron 2008), and therefore accelerates wound healing (Xie et al. 2010).

Reporting pressure ulcers

Pressure ulcers category 2 and above should be reported as an adverse clinical incident (NICE 2005). Currently, all hospital reported hospital-acquired pressure ulcers are reported to the National Reporting and Learning Service (NRLS), part of the National Patient Safety Agency. All avoidable category 3 or 4 pressure ulcers are reportable via the Strategic Executive Information System (STEIS), and the STEIS reports are forwarded to the primary care trust. Root cause analysis should identify the origin, rather than the superficially apparent cause, of problems (NHS Institute for Improvement and Innovation 2008).

Conclusion

Skin has many functions, including providing a barrier between the body's internal and external environments. Promoting skin integrity is therefore fundamental to health. Any signs of actual or potential problems should be assessed and recorded, and appropriate action taken to encourage healing and prevent further damage.

Useful websites

European Pressure Ulcer Advisory Panel: http://www.epuap.org/

National pressure Ulcer Advisory Panel (USA): http://www.npuap.org/

Mouth care

Definition

Mouth care refers to measures that maintain oral health (mouth hygiene) and or comfort. Mouth hygiene is 'effective

Table 12.4 Common positions for critically ill patients (for further details see Chapter 14)

Position		Manoeuvres	Rationale	Main risks
Sitting in bed, semi-recumbent, at a 30–45° angle		■ Ensure patient's buttocks are in line with the fold of the bed ■ Use bed mechanism to sit the patient up ■ If patient is likely to slide down (creating a shear force), raise the foot section of the bed ■ Position pillows to support patient's head and arms, as appropriate ■ Ensure tracheostomy and administration set tubing are clear from possible obstruction	Semi-recumbency significantly reduces ventilator-associated pneumonia (Drakulovic et al. 1999)	Increases risks breakdown of skin over the coccyx (Bell 2008)
Lateral 30° tilt	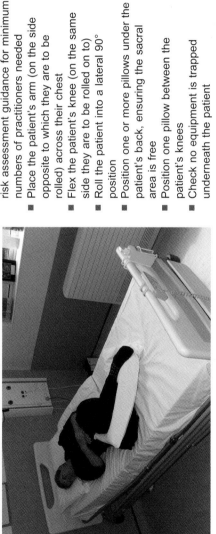	■ Follow individual moving and handling risk assessment guidance for minimum numbers of practitioners needed ■ Place the patient's arm (on the side opposite to which they are to be rolled) across their chest ■ Flex the patient's knee (on the same side they are to be rolled on to) ■ Roll the patient into a lateral 90° position ■ Position one or more pillows under the patient's back, ensuring the sacral area is free ■ Position one pillow between the patient's knees ■ Check no equipment is trapped underneath the patient	■ Minimizes risk of pressure ulceration (Defloor 2000) ■ Removes pressure from body prominences (Hampton and Collins 2004) ■ Angles significantly greater than 30° may place pressure on the greater trochanter (Myers 2008) ■ This position can be tolerated for more hours than any other without causing skin damage (Hampton and Collins 2004)	May place pressure on the lower elbow

(Continued)

Table 12.4 (*Continued*)

Position	Manoeuvres	Rationale	Main risks
Sitting in chair	■ Follow individual moving and handling risk assessment guidance for minimum numbers of practitioners needed, or whether to use a hoist ■ Place chair near bed, and cover it with a sheet ■ Encourage patients to do as much for themselves as they safely can ■ Place slippers on the patient's feet (if they do not have slippers, remove TEDS from the soles of feet, as these could cause the patient to slip) ■ Unless hoisted, the patient should sit up and move to the end of the bed. With appropriate numbers of staff, they should then stand up and transfer to the chair ■ Support the patient's head and arms with pillows; offer them a blanket for warmth and dignity	■ To encourage mobilization and normality ■ Assists breathing, as diaphragm moves down with gravity	■ Increases risks breakdown of skin over the coccyx (Bell 2008) ■ Most chairs place significant pressures on skin, so limit to 2 hours maximum sitting in a chair (EPUAP/NPUAP 2009a,b)

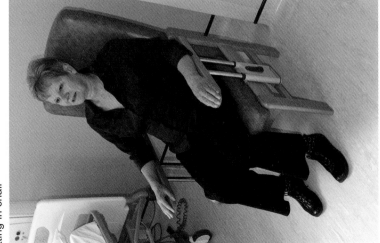

Table 12.5 Wound assessment

Wound observation and assessment	Actions	Rationale
Wound size Assess approximate wound size in square centimetres	▪ Complete initial documentation of wound assessment, using hospital proformas ▪ If possible, draw or photograph wound ▪ Categorize the ulcer using EPUAP/NPUAP (2009a,b) guidance (see Table 12.1)	▪ To provide baseline information to assess future progress ▪ To assist in the choice of dressings and pressure relieving equipment ▪ To provide regular measurements to indicate rate of wound healing or deterioration
Exudate The colour and consistency of exudate indicates wound health. Serous exudate (straw colour) is most healthy, and thicker, viscous purulent exudate is indicative of wound infection The amount of exudate guides the absorbency required of wound dressing	▪ Record quantity* and quality (colour, odour) ▪ If the amount of exudate is large, cover with absorbent dressings ▪ If wound appears infected, swab for microscopy, culture and sensitivity to identify microorganisms. Antimicrobial agents will probably be needed (microbiologists will advise practitioners about this)	▪ Moderate exudate stimulates cell proliferation and healing (Dealey and Cameron 2008) ▪ A large amount of exudate is a medium for bacterial growth (Jones et al. 2005), and can excoriate or macerate surrounding skin ▪ Purulent or malodorous exudate indicates infection
Necrotic tissue Assess for presence and size of necrotic tissue	▪ Debride necrotic tissue (Dealey and Cameron 2008). This is usually achieved by autolytic debridement (body shedding tissue naturally), which is helped by dressings which create a moist wound environment ▪ Extensive necrotic tissue may necessitate surgical debridement	▪ Necrotic tissue is dead and healing will not occur until it is removed. Dead tissue may also provide a medium for bacterial growth ▪ Dry, necrotic tissue at the heels should not be debrided without a full vascular assessment and can often be left dry to debride by desiccation
Surrounding skin Observe whether surrounding skin is: ▪ healthy ▪ macerated (saturated, white looking) ▪ inflamed (red) ▪ has localized erythema (if more than 2 cm around wound this may indicate spreading systemic infection)	Prevent damage by selecting appropriate: ▪ dressings ▪ skin barrier products (e.g. Cavilon™) Observe for signs of infection as indicated by periwound erythema	▪ If skin is friable, adhesive dressings may cause extension of the wound with each dressing change

(Continued)

Table 12.5 (*Continued*)

Wound observation and assessment	Actions	Rationale
Infection Assess for signs of infection. This includes: ■ cellulitis ■ change in nature of the pain ■ crepitus ■ increase in exudate volume ■ pus ■ serous exudate with inflammation ■ spreading erythema ■ viable tissues become sloughy ■ warmth in surrounding tissues ■ wound stops healing despite relevant measures ■ wound enlarging despite pressure relief ■ erythema ■ friable granulation tissue that bleeds easily ■ malodour ■ oedema (EWMA 2005)	■ If wound appears infected, swab for microscopy, culture and sensitivity to identify microorganisms	■ Antimicrobial agents will probably be needed (microbiologists will advise practitioners about this) ■ Systemic antimicrobials may be augmented by local antimicrobials. For example some dressings have silver impregnated into the dressing

*It is difficult to accurately ascertain and describe the amount of exudate relative to the expected amount, as this is dependent on various factors such as the type and size of the wound. In addition, different assessors may have varying perceptions of what constitutes, for example, a small, moderate or large amount of exudate. However, the following may be useful.

■ Small amount of exudate – there is just a detectable discharge when the dressing is removed, less than 33% of the dressing surface
■ Moderate amount of exudate – there is discharge covering more than 33% and less than 67% of the dressing surface
■ Large amount of exudates – there is discharge covering more than 67% of the dressing surface (adapted from Baranoski and Ayello [2008])

Table 12.6 Wound management dressings and their modes of action

Dressing	Mode of action	Rationale for use	Type of wound	Application and frequency of dressing change
Film dressings Examples include: Mepore Film™, Tegaderm™, Opsite™	■ High moisture vapour transmission rates that protect the skin without causing maceration (Russell 2002; Takahashi et al. 2006)	Reduces friction and shear forces against skin (Ohura et al. 2007)	■ Category 1 pressure ulcers ■ Useful if patients are restless or agitated and constantly moving in bed	■ Apply over clean, dry skin ■ Overlap skin 4–5cm beyond the wound surface (Dealey and Cameron 2008)
Hydrogel dressings Examples include: Granugel™, Intrasite™, Curagel™ OR *Hydrogel sheets* Examples include: Actiform Cool™, Geliperm™	■ As water is the main constituent of these dressings, they rehydrate dry, necrotic tissue (Russell 2002) ■ Debride and clean (Russell 2002) ■ Soothing (Russell 2002)	Provides moist wound environment to facilitate autolytic debridement by the body. Reduces numbers of microorganisms (Reger et al. 2010; Bruggisser 2005)	Pressure ulcers with dry necrotic tissue (do not use with a large amount of exudate)	■ A thin application of hydrogel is advised, too much and the dressing will need to be changed more frequently ■ If a hydrogel sheet is used, apply over the edges of the wound and change every 2–3 days ■ Cover hydrogel with a secondary dressing, such as an absorbent pad (Dealey and Cameron 2008)
Hydrocolloid dressings Examples include: Duoderm Signal™, Tegaderm™, Activheal™, carboxymethylcellulose (CMC) dressings	■ Provides warm, moist environment (Russell 2002) ■ Impermeable to moisture, liquids and bacteria (Russell 2002) ■ Promotes granulation (Russell 2002)	Provides moist environment to facilitate autolytic debridement by the body (Shahina et al. 2009)	■ Pressure ulcers with dry necrotic tissue ■ Hydrocolloids are the secondary dressing of choice to a hydrogel	■ If dressing is used directly on the wound may be left in place for up to 7 days ■ If hydrocolloid is used over a hydrogel then change every 3–4 days ■ May need to be cut to assure good conformability

(Continued)

Table 12.6 (Continued)

Dressing	Mode of action	Rationale for use	Type of wound	Application and frequency of dressing change
Foam dressings Examples include: Allevyn™, Biatain™, Mepilex™	■ Maintains a moist environment (Russell 2002) ■ Absorbs exudate (Russell 2002) ■ Non-adherent (Russell 2002)	Removing exudate reduces risks of maceration or excoriation of the surrounding skin Exudate provides a medium for bacterial growth (Jones et al. 2005), and can also macerate or excoriate surrounding skin (Elliott et al. 2008)	Exudating wounds (a large amount of exudate is often produced by pressure ulcers which are healing and exhibiting granulation tissue)	■ Change when exudate staining begins to show on the outside
Hydrofibre dressing Examples include: Aquacel™	■ Provides a moist environment (Russell 2002) ■ Highly absorbent, removes exudate and 'locks' away by binding water molecules within the dressing (Jones et al. 2005) ■ Non-adherent	As foam dressings (above)	Exudating wounds	■ Change once dressing is fully saturated with exudate ■ Available in flat sheet dressings and cavity ribbon
Other absorbent dressings include: Sorbion Sachet S™	Highly absorbent, removes exudate, permanently locks away exudate into the dressing (Sharp 2010). Facilitates rapid epithelialization (Kaya et al. 2005)	Removing exudate reduces risks of maceration or excoriation of the surrounding skin	Exudating wounds	■ Once the dressing is fully saturated with exudate it should be changed ■ Can be inserted into cavity wounds ■ Available in different sizes

removal of plaque and debris to ensure the structures and tissues of the mouth are kept in a healthy condition' (Department of Health 2010: 182). Dental plaque is a film on teeth, usually including bacteria and breakdown products from food, including acid.

Aims and indications

Critical illness, and treatments, may compromise oral health. Mouth hygiene should:

- maintain comfort
- remove plaque and debris
- prevent damage and complications.

If patients are unable to maintain their own mouth hygiene, practitioners should plan and implement appropriate care.

Background

Critically ill patients are vulnerable and often unable to maintain their own hygiene. While patients rarely require critical care because of oral pathologies, some have problems on admission, and all are at potential risk of developing complications.

Mouth hygiene is specifically identified as a benchmark of personal hygiene in the Department of Health's *Essence of Care* (2010). For many people, oral comfort is an important component of psychological wellbeing (O'Reilly 2003; Abidia 2007). Unfortunately, oral care is poorly researched (O'Reilly 2003; Berry and Davidson 2006; Berry et al. 2007), and sometimes poorly practised (Cutler and Davis 2005; Ross and Crumpler 2007; Kearns et al. 2010). The weak research base results in conflicting evidence, with some recommendations being based on little more than custom and practice and most aspects continuing to generate debate. Berry et al.'s (2007) literature review identifies many controversies and unresolved debates, such as whether sterile or tap water should be used for oral hygiene.

The oral cavity includes mucous membranes, teeth and lips. In health, most people maintain oral health and comfort by:

- drinking
- salivation
- brushing teeth/cleaning dentures

and often by additional methods, such as:

- mouthwashes (many of which are antibacterial)
- flossing
- lip balm.

Poor oral hygiene can cause or contribute to complications ranging from short-term (e.g. ventilator-associated pneumonia) to long-term (tooth loss). Oral discomfort from dryness, fungal infection, or other problems can also cause distress.

Anatomy and physiology

The mouth is lined with mucosa (Marieb and Hoehn 2013). In health, the oral cavity is lubricated with drinks and by saliva (Barrett et al. 2010). Saliva, which assists digestion and swallowing, is secreted from salivary glands by a parasympathetic-mediated reflex response caused by presence of food (or other substances) in the mouth (Marieb and Hoehn 2013). However, production of saliva is strongly dependent on blood flow to the salivary glands – a reduction in systemic blood volume of 8% causes near-total cessation of saliva production (de Almedia et al. 2008). Secretion of saliva is also affected by many other factors, including posture – most saliva is secreted when upright and least when lying down (Davies 2005).

Saliva is mostly (more than 97%) water (Marieb and Hoehn 2013), but also includes important antibacterial chemicals such as lysozyme (Barrett et al. 2010) and lactoferrin (Berry et al. 2007). It also buffers the acids which demineralize teeth (de Almedia et al. 2008).

The mouth is not sterile. It is normally colonized by hundreds of species of microbes, which can contribute to plaque formation and caries (cavities), both causes of tooth decay. In health, oral microbes are seldom pathogenic. In ill health, the normally aerobic oral biofilm is usually replaced mainly with gram-negative organisms (Kearns et al. 2010). These are more likely to become respiratory pathogens (Cutler and Davis 2005), and if aspirated may cause pneumonia (Paju and Scannapieco 2007).

In health, saliva or other fluids collecting in the oropharynx would stimulate a reflex swallowing action (Marieb and Hoehn 2013). However, endotracheal/tracheostomy tube cuffs often cause dysphagia (Romero et al. 2010), so critically ill patients are less likely to swallow pooled secretions. The warm, moist and static environment of pooled secretions creates an ideal medium of bacterial (or other microbes) growth. Endotracheal and tracheostomy cuffs are seldom water-tight (Young and Ridley 1999), so secretions and microbes can usually bypass cuffs into the lungs, contributing to development of ventilator-associated pneumonia (Mori et al. 2006; Cason et al. 2007; Gastmeier and Geffers 2007; Ross and Crumpler 2007; Chao et al. 2009). Subglottic drainage (*see also* Chapter 5) can remove these secretions, and so reduce ventilator-associated pneumonia (Lorente et al. 2007).

Lips form the entrance to the oral cavity. They lack both the protective keratin and sebaceous glands of the adjacent skin, so rely on frequent lubrication with saliva to prevent them becoming dry and cracked (Marieb and Hoehn 2013). They are also highly innervated, making dry or cracked lips very uncomfortable. Lips are normally kept moist by periodic lubrication from the tongue; many people also use commercial lip balm. Critically ill patients are often unable to lubricate their own lips, so lip care should form part of mouth care.

397

Oral pathophysiology

Plaque is a calcified film formed from bacteria, sugar and other debris; the bacteria and acids in plaque can cause caries (Marieb and Hoehn 2013), but can also be a source for further colonization and infection (O'Reilly 2003; Munro and Grap 2004), especially pneumonia (El-Solh et al. 2004). Poor oral hygiene and plaque are the main causes of periodontitis (de Oliveira et al. 2010) – inflammation extending from the gum (gingival) to connective tissue and bone supporting teeth. Periodontitis is an irreversible bacterial infection (Tolle 2010), the main cause of adult tooth loss (Marieb and Hoehn 2013), and a major source for ventilator-associated pneumonia (Paju and Scannapieco 2007).

Plaque is not water-soluble, so cannot be removed by mouthwash solutions or foam swabs (Berry and Davidson 2006). Toothbrushes (with or without toothpaste) remain the best way to clean patients' teeth (Abidia 2007; Rello et al. 2007; Kelly et al. 2010), loosening debris trapped between teeth and removing plaque. Teeth should be brushed at least twice daily.

An early sign of poor oral health may be *gingivitis* – sore, red and bleeding gums. This occurs within ten days of plaque formation (Kite and Pearson 1995), and is often detected when brushing teeth causes bleeding. Tooth decay and loss usually begins as gingivitis, so although progression is not inevitable, gingivitis should prompt reassessment of oral health and care.

Problems in critical illness

In addition to general health problems, critical illness may cause or exacerbate:

- xerostomia (dry mouth)
- trauma from oral intubation

while sedation, weakness, or limited mobility prevents patients from being able to maintain their own hygiene and comfort.

Xerostomia

The sensation of a dry mouth is usually caused by lack of saliva (Davies 2005). Dryness of the normally moist mucous membranes can lead to ulceration, and colonization by microbes. Other factor that contribute to xerostomia in critically ill patients often include:

- dysphagia (see above)
- absence of oral intake
- convection
- side effects of drugs.

Hydration and nutrition rightly receive attention in critical care, but these are usually supplied through nasogastric or intravenous routes. Drinks directly lubricate the mouth, while food in the mouth stimulates salivary secretion. Swallowing food and drink also helps remove transient microbes that may be colonizing the oral cavity. Absence of oral intake therefore predisposes patients to developing discomfort from a dry mouth and oral infection. Even if patients are not mouth-breathing, fear that they have halitosis may also cause them distress (Abidia 2007).

Critically ill patients usually produce insufficient saliva (Dennesen et al. 2003), although oral intubation can stimulate hypersecretion (Helm et al. 2006). Reduced salivary volume increases its viscosity (Marieb and Hoehn 2013) and acidity (de Almedia et al. 2008). (Saliva is normally slightly acidic [pH 6 to 7], but its pH can range from 7.9 with peak secretion flow to 5.3 with low flow [de Almedia *et al*, 2008]. Treloar [1995] found mean salivary pH was 5.3 in critically ill patients.) Quantity and quality of saliva is therefore often poor in the critically ill, causing xerostomia, which increases the risk of oral infections (Abidia 2007), and accelerating tooth decay.

If critically ill patients are orally intubated, much of the front of the oral cavity is exposed to the atmosphere, resulting in convection of moisture. Problems may be exacerbated if:

- the atmosphere is hot and/or dry (often the case in critical care units)
- tapes for securing oral endotracheal tubes also wedge the mouth open
- patients are nursed in supine positions or at only a slight angle.

It has been suggested that more than half of drugs cause salivary gland dysfunction (Davies 2005). Drugs commonly used in critical care that reduce salivary secretion include opioids (Wiener et al. 2010) and diuretics (Abidia 2007). Sympathetic stimulation, for example from noradrenaline, reduces volume of saliva secreted.

Foam sticks are useful for moistening the mouth but do not remove plaque (Pearson 1996; Grap et al. 2003), and so are a supplement to tooth-brushing, not a replacement for it.

Trauma from oral intubation

Intubation is necessarily a quick procedure, and so may cause unintentional trauma. Emergency intubation may be especially traumatic. While trauma may be caused to almost any part of the mouth, the cavity can be easily seen and the durability of the hard pallet (roof of the mouth) usually prevents many potential problems. However, loose teeth or crowns may be dislodged. Any damage from intubation should be recorded as a clinical incident.

Oral endotracheal tubes inevitably place pressure on parts of the oral cavity, including the tongue. While oral damage from prolonged pressure is relatively rare, the oral cavity should be inspected for signs of any problems.

Tapes used to secure oral endotracheal tubes can cause trauma, sores and lacerations, especially to the corners of mouth. If possible, tapes should avoid corners of the lips. Tapes should be changed at least daily, with a slightly different position in relation to oral tissue with each change. There are various tube holders and sponge covers marketed that may reduce trauma from endotracheal tube tape (Figure 12.2).

Moist tapes, and tissue adjacent to tubes, can encourage microbial growth (Hayes and Jones 1995). Frequent mouth care and daily change of tapes reduce these risks.

Assessment and care of oral cavity

The oral cavity should normally be assessed each time the mouth is cleaned (usually twice daily) (see Problem-solving table 12.1).

Problem-solving table 12.1: Oral assessment

Problem	Possible causes	Prevention	Suggested action
Oral cavity (all parts, especially tongue) ■ Colonization by microorganisms, especially *Candida albicans* (commonly known as thrush) (Muzyka 2005; Schelenz 2008). *Candida* typically presents as a white coating of the tongue	■ Immunocompromise ■ Lack of oral intake	■ Regular moisturizing of mouth	■ Document ■ Prescribe/administer appropriate antimicrobial agents (*Candida* is usually treated with nystatin: 1 mL 4 times each day; this should be instilled after mouth care)
Lips ■ Ulceration ('cracking')	■ Dryness, unhumidified oxygen via facemask ■ Damage from endotracheal tape/holder	■ Provided there are no signs of infection, apply a lubricant such as yellow soft paraffin ■ Humidify face-mask oxygen ■ If possible, prevent equipment (such as endotracheal tubes) being in contact with ulcers	■ Document ■ Increase frequency of lip care
Teeth ■ Damaged (e.g. broken) ■ Caries	■ Trauma ■ Poor oral hygiene	■ Clean teeth with toothbrush and toothpaste (usually twice daily)	■ Document – including in discharge summary
Gums ■ Gingivitis ■ Bleeding	■ Trauma ■ Poor oral hygiene	■ When cleaning teeth, include brushing margin of tooth and gum at 45° angle (see Figure 12.3)	■ Document – including in discharge summary
Saliva ■ Excess ■ Lack of ■ High viscosity	■ Objects in mouth (e.g. ETT) ■ Dehydration	■ Moisten mouth if dry	■ Increase frequency of moistening mouth
Tongue ■ Dark colour ■ Dry	■ Poor perfusion ■ Dehydration	■ Poor perfusion and dehydration are systemic problems	■ Document and report
Hard palate ■ Bleeding ■ Ulceration	■ Trauma		■ Document and report
Soft tissue ■ Necrosis	■ Poor perfusion		■ Document and report

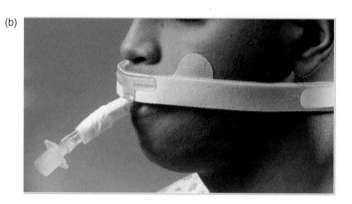

Figure 12.2 (a) Anchor Fast oral endotracheal tube fastener (courtesy of Hollister Inc., Libertyville, Illinois, USA). (b) Dale endotracheal tube holder (courtesy of Dale Medical Products Inc.).

If patients are able to clean their own teeth, they should be encouraged to do so. Procedure guidelines 12.1–12.3 are for intubated patients, but may sometimes apply in whole or part for non-intubated patients.

Dentures

About half of older people are endentitious (Watson 2001). Although the number of endentitious older people continues to decline, substantial numbers still have dentures (Heath et al. 2011).

Eye care

Definition

Eye care refers to measures that maintain ocular health and/or comfort. In critical care this usually means care given to protect eye surfaces from potential harm. It can also include treatments for specific problems (acute or chronic) and care of visual aids, such as glasses and contact lenses.

Aims and indications

While many critically ill patients may not need active interventions, the aim of eye care is to:

- prevent potential harm/trauma
- treat any identified problems
- replace any physiological functions that are compromised/absent
- care for and clean any visual aids.

Background

Vision is one of the main senses and means of communication for most people. Impaired vision, therefore, can contribute to delirium. Ocular disease or treatment rarely necessitates critical care admission, and pre-existing conditions are unlikely to be significantly affected by critical illness, although may need continuing treatment (such as eye drops) (Dawson 2005). Treatments for critical illness, especially sedation and paralysis, may impair a patient's ability to maintain their own ocular health. Identified ocular problems should be treated (if possible), but more often eye care will be prophylactic, and ensuring availability of patients' own visual aids.

Eye care is listed in the DH (2010) indicators of good practice, although no specific aspects are identified. Like mouth hygiene, eye care for critically ill patients is poorly researched and often poorly practised (Dawson 2005). Not all critically ill patients will need active interventions, but ocular health needs and risks should be assessed to identify whether or not interventions are needed.

Anatomy and physiology

The eye is normally protected by external structures such as eyelids and eyelashes. Eyelashes have a particularly rich nerve supply, and if touched will normally elicit a protective blink reflex (Marieb and Hoehn 2013). Adjacent to the eyelids are tarsal glands, which secrete an oily substance to prevent eyelids from sticking together (Marieb and Hoehn 2013). Blinking spreads this lubricant, and the moisture from tears, across the eye surface.

The eye surface, and inner aspect of eyelids, is covered with the conjunctiva, a transparent mucous membrane

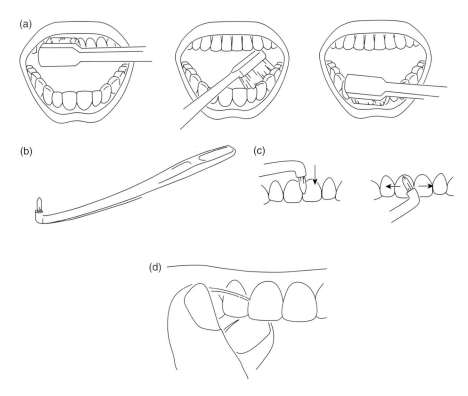

Figure 12.3 (a) The 'Bass' method of toothbrushing using a small-headed toothbrush. (b) Interspace brush. (c) The tip of the brush is placed in to the gingival margin and follows the contour of the teeth. (d) Interdental cleaning. (From Pritchard and Mallett 1992, reproduced with permission from Wiley).

(Marieb and Hoehn 2013). Below this is the cornea, a transparent fibrous layer that forms the outer part of the eyeball over the anterior chamber of the eye (Marieb and Hoehn 2013). Both the conjunctiva and cornea lack blood vessels (Marieb and Hoehn 2013), as blood vessels would obstruct vision. Supply of oxygen and other nutrients is therefore relatively poor, predisposing damaged eye surfaces to slow (or no) healing. The cornea has the highest concentration of nerves of any body tissue, making it very sensitive to irritation and pain (Agarwal 2006) (*see* Figure 12.4). Impaired consciousness may impair blink reflexes, exposing eye surfaces to potential trauma from equipment, such as ventilator tubing, endotracheal tube tapes, or bedding.

Like saliva, tears contain antimicrobial chemicals such as lysozymes and antibodies (Marieb and Hoehn 2013). The cornea will therefore not normally harbour microbes (Parkin and Cook 2000), but insufficient tear production or spread across the eye exposes patient's eyes to potential infection. Clean gloves should be worn by the practitioner giving eye care to prevent transferring skin-surface microorganisms into the patient's eye.

Intraocular pressure is normally about 15 mmHg (Guyton and Hall 2005), but if drainage from the anterior chamber of the eye is impaired, intra-ocular pressure can increase significantly (Marieb and Hoehn 2013). Pressures exceeding 25–30 mmHg can cause blindness (Guyton and Hall 2005). In critical illness and its care, acutely raised intraocular pressure may be caused by:

- positive pressure ventilation
- anything impeding venous return from the cranium
- hypercapnia (Patil and Dowd 2000).

'Ventilator eye' (conjunctival oedema) impairs eye closure (Rosenberg and Eisen 2008), so exposing the eye surface to drying. It occurred in more than half of patients receiving ventilation studied by Suresh et al. (2000). Sitting upright improves ocular drainage, so reduces 'ventilator eye'.

Problems

Frequent problems occurring in patients' eyes in critical care include:

- *keratitis* (corneal inflammation)
- *blepharitis* (inflammation of eyelash follicles and sebaceous glands).

What may appear as minor irritations can progress to serious complications such as:

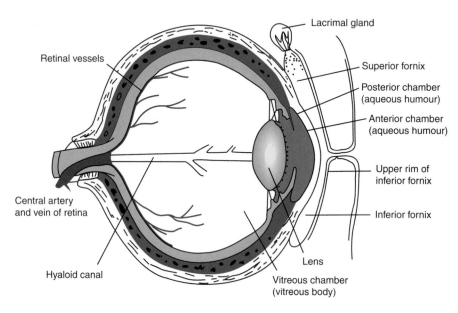

Figure 12.4 Diagram of the eye (from Dougherty and Lister 2011, reproduced with permission from Wiley).

- microbial keratitis (Parkin and Cook 2000)
- corneal abrasions and or erosions (Imanaka et al. 1997).

Keratitis and corneal erosions can lead to blindness, unless corneal transplantation is available (Garg et al. 2005).

Factors that expose eyes to potential damage in critical care may include:

- inability to protect own eyes
- impaired tear production
- intraocular hypertension
- drying with oxygen from face masks (unhumidified oxygen or non-invasive ventilation)
- deep sedation (Parkin and Cook 2000), which impairs blink reflexes and possibly tear production
- trauma from equipment (e.g. ventilator tubing, tapes to secure endotracheal tube, linen).

'Dry eye' is the most common problem in critically ill patients (Oh et al. 2009). Patients may have pre-existing problems with 'dry eye', but tear production may be impaired by drugs, such as atropine, antihistamines, muscle relaxants and paralysing agents.

Drying may be caused by:

- incomplete eyelid closure
- loss of blink reflexes.

(Suresh et al. 2000)

Dry corneal surfaces lack the antibacterial protection of tears. Exposure to opportunist organisms is therefore more likely to cause infection (Parkin et al. 1997). Acute bacterial conjunctivitis ('pink eye') is the most common eye disease in the general population (Høvding 2008) and is highly contagious (Marieb and Hoehn 2013). Most mechanically ventilated patients (77%) develop bacterial colonization of eye surfaces after one week (Mela et al. 2010). Infection may appear as:

- 'red eye'
- stickiness
- discharge
- crusts (dried mucus).

Dry eye surfaces, and especially eye surfaces exposed to hardened substances (e.g. crusts), can cause corneal abrasions. Abrasions occur in up to one-fifth of critically ill patients, and can develop within 48 hours to one week (Joanna Briggs Institute 2002). Intact corneas, like skin, provide a barrier against microbes, but damaged corneas can harbour microbes, progressing to microbial ketatitis (Parkin and Cook 2000). Keratitis can lead to corneal ulceration (Dawson 2005) – an acutely painful condition. It may also cause loss of vision, unless urgent keratoplasty is performed (Parkin and Cook 2000).

Anything touching the eye surface, such as ointment or drops, should therefore be sterile. Excess moisture should be removed with a clean swab. Gauze fibres can damage the corneal surface, so swabs should be soft, such as non-woven or low-linting gauze; available swabs are popularly called 'gauze swabs', although seldom are now made from gauze. Separate eye drops and pads should be used for each eye, to prevent microorganisms being transferred between eyes.

Keratitis (inflammation of the cornea) may be caused by any irritant, and is more likely to occur if eye surfaces are dry. Deeply unconscious and or sedated patients often develop dry, red eyes (Oh et al. 2009). Keratitis can also be caused by microbes (see below). Keratitis can progress to *keratopathy* (corneal damage). Exposure keratophy, from drying of corneal surfaces, occurs relatively frequently (20–42% (Rosenberg and Eisen 2008) in critically ill patients and can cause permanent damage (Joanna Briggs Institute 2002).

Blurred vision may be caused by critical illness or other factors. Problems should be recorded, but vision usually normalizes with recovery, so patients and families should be reassured that this is probably a temporary problem.

Ocular health should therefore be assessed and interventions may be needed if:

- blink reflexes are absent or poor
- tear secretion is poor ('dry eyes')
- ocular pathophysiologies are noted.

Suspected ocular infection should be recorded and communicated to relevant practitioners. Swabs may need to be taken and topical antibiotics prescribed.

Prone positioning places eyes at high risk of damage, so prophylactic interventions are needed to keep eye surfaces clear from bedding or other objects.

Assessment and care

Although seldom life threatening, eye problems frequently occur in critically ill patients, so preventative eye care should be commenced on admission (Oh et al. 2009). Both eyes should be clearly visualized for assessment. A good light is therefore needed (Cooke et al. 2011); ambient light may be sufficient, but if using a torch this should not be shone directly into the patient's eyes, as this could cause distress (Cooke et al. 2011).

If the patient normally uses visual aids (glasses, contact lenses), this should be documented, together with whether aids are present or absent. If present, but not being used, they should be stored safely. Aids should only be used if the patient wishes, if they are conscious and in a suitable position (e.g. upright), as glasses can be broken and contact lenses lost. Contact lenses can also provide a medium for corneal surface infection, and if patients are unconscious, they are unable to communicate pain, which would indicate a potential problem.

Aids should be cleaned using one of the options below:

- patient's own cleaning solution and cloth
- glasses may be cleaned under running water, then dried with a lint-free cloth or soft tissue
- hard contact lenses may be cleaned by soaking in 0.9% sodium chloride, then dried with a tissue
- soft contact lenses are normally only cleaned weekly (Cooke et al. 2011). Advice is inconsistent (Wu et al. 2010), but manufacturer's instructions should be followed and lenses stored in a sterile solution (Cooke et al. 2011) to prevent them drying out. Contact lenses should be rubbed to remove bacteria to reduce the risk of keratitis (Sweeney et al. 2009).

Gloves should be worn when handling contact lenses, to prevent cross-infection (*see also* Problem-solving table 12.2).

Problem-solving table 12.2: **Care of the eye**

Problem	Cause	Preventation	Suggested action
Eyelid			
■ Unable to fully close, which can cause drying, ulceration and trauma (Oh et al. 2009) ■ Absent blink reflex	■ Periorbital oedema or high intraocular pressure may prevent full closure ■ Blink reflex will be absent if paralysing agents are given, and may be absent with deep coma	■ Regular cleaning of eye ■ Cover eye surface with (non-adhesive) hydrocolloid dressings or polyethylene (cling wrap) (Koroloff et al. 2004). If using hydrocolloid, change 4 to 6 hourly, and whenever eye looks dry ■ Cover eyes with swabs soaked in sterile water (Sivasankar et al. 2006) ■ Ensure ventilator tubing, ETT tapes and other equipment is kept away from eyes	■ Document and report any problems ■ Treat 'dry eye' with lubricants (see below, Tears)

(Continued)

Problem-solving table 12.2: *(Continued)*

Conjunctiva

▪ Ulceration ▪ Infection ('red eye') ▪ Pain	▪ Trauma ▪ Infection	▪ If patient is unable to blink, perform regular eye care ▪ If infection is suspected, swab infected area for microbiology, culture and sensitivity	▪ Document and report any problems ▪ Ulceration should be reported to specialist practitioners in ophthalmology ▪ Infection should be treated with topical antimicrobials (usually choramphenicol [Høvding 2008]) ▪ Assess nature of pain, and any activities it is related to. This could indicate an ocular emergency, such as a corneal laceration (ulcer), so record and urgently communicate to relevant practitioners

Tears

▪ Inadequate to prevent drying of corneal surfaces	▪ Dehydration ▪ Positioning ▪ Muscle paralysing agents		▪ Instil sterile lubricant (e.g. 'artificial tears') – see below for technique. Frequency will vary with need and lubricant; Dawson (2005) suggests 1 to 4 hourly

'Crusts' at corner of eye or on eyelid

▪ May traumatize corneal surface ▪ May provide a medium for bacterial growth	▪ Inadequate tear production ▪ Possible infection	▪ Remove with sterile swabs and water, to prevent crusts causing trauma to cornea ▪ Consider need for regular eye drops ▪ Use a new swab for each eye and discard after single use, to prevent introducing infection on to the corneal surface	▪ Document and communicate to relevant practitioner – this may be a sign of infection

Surrounding muscles

▪ Weakness	▪ Probably a short-term complication of critical illness and drugs used, but could indicate an unidentified problem		▪ Document and communicate to relevant practitioners

Retina

▪ Patient reports seeing flashing lights, sudden showers of red/dark spots, unilateral visual defect (Field and Tillotson 2008)	▪ Possible retinal detachment		▪ Urgent ophthalmic review is needed within 24 hours, as ophthalmic surgery may be needed to save sight (Field and Tillotson 2008)

Procedure guideline 12.1: Assessment of oral cavity

Equipment

- Pen torch

Procedure

Action	Rationale
1 Where possible, explain and discuss the procedure with the patient. If the patient lacks the capacity to make decisions the practitioner must act in the patient's best interests.	To ensure that the patient understands the procedure and gives their valid consent. To ensure the patient's best interests are maintained (Mental Capacity Act 2005).
2 Follow any oral assessment tool available within your critical care unit (*see* Problem-solving table 12.1).	To ensure consistency between staff and facilitate a thorough examination.
3 Ensure sufficient light (a pen torch is usually useful).	To visualize as much of the oral cavity as possible
4 Ensure head is appropriately supported (e.g. with pillows) to prevent trauma or discomfort.	To protect the oral cavity from damage.
5 Ensure linen is not touching mucous membranes (e.g. lips).	Linen can cause drying and discomfort.
6 Document care and report any abnormalities.	To: ■ provide an accurate record ■ monitor effectiveness of procedure ■ reduce the risk of duplication of treatment ■ provide a point of reference or comparison in the event of later questions ■ acknowledge accountability for actions ■ facilitate communication and continuity of care. (NMC 2008; HCPC 2012; GMC 2013)

Procedure guideline 12.2: Care of the oral cavity

Equipment

- Small headed paediatric toothbrush
- Fluoride toothpaste
- Sterile water
- 5 mL syringe
- Rigid oropharyngeal suction catheter (for example a Yankauer catheter)

- Chlorhexidine 0.1%
- Soft suction catheter
- Foam sticks or ice chips
- Lubricant (such as yellow soft paraffin)
- Tapes to hold endotracheal tube/Endotracheal holder

Procedure

Action	Rationale
To clean teeth:	
1 Where possible, explain and discuss the procedure with the patient. If the patient lacks the capacity to make decisions the practitioner must act in the patient's best interests.	To ensure that the patient understands the procedure and gives their valid consent. To ensure the patient's best interests are maintained (Mental Capacity Act 2005).

(Continued)

Procedure guideline 12.2: (Continued)

2 Sit patient upright (unless contraindicated).	To assist removal, and minimize oropharyngeal accumulation, of fluid.
3 Brush teeth with a small-headed paediatric toothbrush (Fitch et al. 1999; Jones 2004).	To facilitate more effective intra-dental cleaning. To more easily manipulate toothbrush around oral endotracheal tubes (Berry and Davidson 2006).
4 Clean teeth at least twice each day (Barnason et al. 1998) with fluoride toothpaste, using sterile water (Berry and Davidson 2006).	Brushing removes plaque (Abidia 2007; Rello et al. 2007; Kelly et al. 2010). Fluoride toothpaste helps prevent plaque formation (Rattenbury et al. 1999; Abidia 2007; Walsh et al. 2010).
5 Unless contraindicated (for example in the case of disseminated intravascular coagulation) teeth should be brushed vigorously (Grap et al. 2003).	To assist plaque removal and reduce risk of ventilator-associated pneumonia.
6 Brush teeth away from gums.	To remove plaque from gingival crevices.
7 Rinse mouth with water during and after cleaning (a 5 mL syringe may be useful).	To remove toothpaste – if left in mouth toothpaste can cause drying (Jones 2004; Berry and Davidson 2006). 5 mL syringes provide a moderate volume of water, while usually being small enough to manipulate into corners of the mouth.
8 After each rinse, suction oral cavity with a rigid oropharyngeal suction catheter, for example a Yankauer catheter.	To remove waste water and debris. To enable visualization of teeth.
9 If brushing causes bleeding, continue brushing vigorously, unless the patient has a coagulopathy/ low platelets or bleeding gums.	Bleeding is often caused by gingivitis, so vigorous brushing is needed to remove the plaque causing gingivitis (Frenkel et al 2002). With coagulopathies, over-vigorous brushing could cause bleeding (Berry and Davidson 2006).
10 Rinse daily with oral antiseptics, such as chlorhexidine 0.12% (NICE 2008).	To reduce the risk of ventilator-associated pneumonia (Mori et al. 2006; Cason et al. 2007; Gastmeier and Geffers 2007, Ross and Crumpler 2007; Chao et al. 2009).
11 If tongue or gum is heavily coated, gently brush with toothbrush.	To remove biofilm (O'Reilly 2003; Berry and Davidson 2006).
12 Remove fluid and secretions in the trachea with a soft suction catheter if necessary.	To remove microbes that may cause pneumonia.
13 At the end of the procedure, clean toothbrush under running water.	To remove microbes (Cooke et al. 2011).
To moisten mouth between brushing:	
14 Use foam sticks (or other appropriate aid) soaked in sterile water (O'Reilly 2003). Alternatively, ice-chips may be used (Trieger 2004).	To maintain oral comfort.

Lip care:

15	Moisten lips frequently (as necessary) with lubricant (e.g. yellow soft paraffin [Winslow and Jacobson 1998; Bowsher et al. 1999]).	To prevent drying and cracking (Berry and Davidson 2006).
16	If possible, prevent tape securing oral endotracheal tube from touching lips (especially at the corners of the mouth). If not possible, change position of tapes on lips at least daily and use any available aids to reduce trauma.	To prevent sores, lacerations and/or trauma from tape.
17	Document care and any abnormalities.	To: ■ provide an accurate record ■ monitor effectiveness of procedure ■ reduce the risk of duplication of treatment ■ provide a point of reference or comparison in the event of later questions ■ acknowledge accountability for actions ■ facilitate communication and continuity of care. (NMC 2008; HCPC 2012; GMC 2013)

Procedure guideline 12.3: Denture hygiene

Equipment

- Clean gloves
- Denture cleaning fluid or sodium hypochlorite
- Toothbrush
- Labelled denture pot
- Mouth wash

Procedure

Action	Rationale
1 Where possible, explain and discuss the procedure with the patient. If the patient lacks the capacity to make decisions the practitioner must act in the patient's best interests.	To ensure that the patient understands the procedure and gives their valid consent. To ensure the patient's best interests are maintained (Mental Capacity Act 2005).
2 Remove dentures from unconscious patient (use clean gloves, remove lower set first).	To prevent obstruction of airway. Denture plates may be displaced towards the back of the mouth. To facilitate cleaning.
3 Remove dentures overnight from patients who are conscious.	To facilitate cleaning.
4 If possible, follow patient's preferred practice.	To maintain comfort of patient.

(Continued)

Procedure guideline 12.3: (Continued)

5 Use preparations preferred by the patient (Xavier 2000) (check time indicated by product). If this not available, soak overnight in cold water (Xavier 2000; Clay 2002; O'Reilly 2003) or sodium hypochlorite (Cooke et al. 2011).	To facilitate cleaning of teeth.
6 Brush dentures with a toothbrush.	To remove debris (Yoon and Steele 2007).
7 Rinse under running cold water and dry thoroughly (Cooke et al. 2011).	Dentures can be damaged if left dry or cleaned in hot water (Clarke 1993).
8 If not worn by patient during the day, store safely (e.g. in a labelled denture pot, within the patient's own property).	To protect dentures and avoid loss.
9 If tongue coated, clean gently with a toothbrush (O'Reilly 2003).	To remove coating.
10 Offer mouthwash, and if patient unable to rinse mouth, rinse with water and remove with suction (see Procedure guideline 12.2).	To provide comfort.
11 Document care and report any abnormalities.	To: ■ provide an accurate record ■ monitor effectiveness of procedure ■ reduce the risk of duplication of treatment ■ provide a point of reference or comparison in the event of later questions ■ acknowledge accountability for actions ■ facilitate communication and continuity of care. (NMC 2008; HCPC 2012; GMC 2013)

Procedure guideline 12.4: Assessing the eye

Equipment

■ Pen torch

Procedure

Action	Rationale
1 Where possible, explain and discuss the procedure with the patient. If the patient lacks the capacity to make decisions the practitioner must act in the patient's best interests.	To ensure that the patient understands the procedure and gives their valid consent. To ensure the patient's best interests are maintained (Mental Capacity Act 2005).
2 Follow any eye assessment tool already used within your critical care unit.	To ensure consistency between staff and facilitate a complete assessment.
3 Ensure sufficient light (a pen torch is usually useful).	To visualize all external surfaces of the eye.
4 Ensure the patient's head is supported at a sufficient angle to enable periorbital drainage.	To prevent periorbital oedema and intraocular hypertension.
5 Ensure any tapes or tubing around the face do not restrict venous drainage.	Prone positioning places eyes at risk of potential damage, so cover eyes with occlusive dressings and ensure the final position leaves the eye clear of risk of trauma.

6 Ensure linen (especially seams) and equipment are not in direct contact with either eye.	Anything touching the eye surface can cause trauma.
7 Document care and report any abnormalities.	To: ■ provide an accurate record ■ monitor effectiveness of procedure ■ reduce the risk of duplication of treatment ■ provide a point of reference or comparison in the event of later questions ■ acknowledge accountability for actions ■ facilitate communication and continuity of care. (NMC 2008; HCPC 2012; GMC 2013)

Procedure guideline 12.5: Cleansing the eyes

Equipment

- Water (open a new bottle of sterile water each day, document date and time of opening)
- 2 gallipots (one per eye; change daily)
- Sterile soft swab
- Clean gloves

Procedure

Action	Rationale
1 Where possible, explain and discuss the procedure with the patient. If the patient lacks the capacity to make decisions the practitioner must act in the patient's best interests.	To ensure that the patient understands the procedure and gives their valid consent. To ensure the patient's best interests are maintained (Mental Capacity Act 2005).
2 Tilt head backwards (Cooke et al. 2011) where possible and lower bottom eyelid.	To enable the eye to be seen and keep solution in the eye.
3 With gloved hands, clean along eyelashes, using a soft cloth or swab soaked in sterile water, removing any crusts. ■ Do not drag debris across surface of the eye. ■ Use each swab only once.	To remove crusts which will minimize risks of trauma. To avoid trauma. Sterile water and single-use swabs are to prevent spreading infection.
4 Gently brush the fornix with new swab moistened in water, removing any crusts.	To remove crusts which may cause trauma. To prevent the spread of infection.
5 Once the fornix is clear of any crusts, brush moistened sterile swab from the fornix very gently across the eyelids, avoiding contact with the cornea.	To moisten and clean the eye surface. To prevent trauma.
6 Repeat until eye appears clean.	To ensure thorough cleansing.
7 Remove excess moisture with dry swab.	To avoid irritation.
8 Clean other eye in the same way. If one eye looks or is known to be infected, clean that eye last.	To reduce the risk of cross-infection to the uninfected eye.

Procedure guideline 12.6: Instillation of eye drops

Equipment

- Water (open a new bottle of sterile water each day, document date and time of opening)
- 2 gallipots (one per eye; change daily)
- Sterile soft swab
- Clean gloves

Procedure

Action	Rationale
1 Where possible, explain and discuss the procedure with the patient. If the patient lacks the capacity to make decisions the practitioner must act in the patient's best interests.	To ensure that the patient understands the procedure and gives their valid consent. To ensure the patient's best interests are maintained (Mental Capacity Act 2005).
2 Ensure eye drops are clearly labelled for the individual patient and (if appropriate) which eye. If medicinal, ensure they are prescribed. Ensure they have been stored appropriately (e.g. some preparations state they should be stored in a fridge). Check expiry date and (if appropriate) date of opening.	To optimize safety for the patient by ensuring they obtain the correct type and dose of medication at the correct time in the correct eye. To ensure efficacy of preparations.
3 Clean eye surface (as above) with sterile water and swab.	To optimize efficacy of eye drops.
4 Instil eye drops into fornix of eye (*see* Figure 12.5).	To avoid fluid dropping directly on to the corneal surface, which is usually painful.
5 Remove excess moisture with sterile swab.	To avoid irritation.
6 Return eye drops to appropriate storage areas.	To ensure continuing efficacy of preparations.
7 Document care and any abnormalities.	To: - provide an accurate record - monitor effectiveness of procedure - reduce the risk of duplication of treatment - provide a point of reference or comparison in the event of later questions - acknowledge accountability for actions - facilitate communication and continuity of care. (NMC 2008; HCPC 2012; GMC 2013)

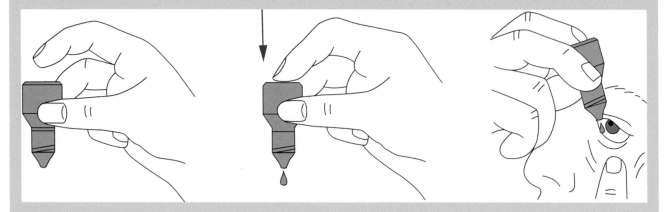

Figure 12.5   How to instil eye drops (from Dougherty and Lister 2011, reproduced with permission from Wiley).

Competency statement 12.1: Specific procedure competency statements for pressure ulcer prevention

Complete assessment against relevant fundamental competency statements (*see* Chapter 2, pp. 20, 21)	Evidence

Specific procedure competency statements for pressure ulcer prevention	**Evidence of competency for pressure ulcer prevention**
Demonstrate ability to: ■ teach and assess or ■ learn from assessment.	Examples of evidence of teaching, assessing and learning.
Identify patients at risk of pressure ulcer development: ■ knowledge of risk factors for pressure ulcer prevention and management ■ undertake a risk assessment using clinical judgement ■ undertake a risk assessment using a pressure ulcer risk assessment tool, e.g. Waterlow ■ undertake a skin assessment and identify potential and present signs of pressure ulcer development.	There are a number of ways in which competency can be judged. These include: ■ direct observation of procedure ■ testimonial from people, carer and or staff members ■ teaching session for peers ■ completion of a reflective text, workbook or educational package ■ examination ■ test ■ discussion with supervisor/mentor.
Develop and implement a pressure ulcer prevention care plan to address individual risk factor modification including: ■ facilitating patient involvement and concordance with care plan ■ strategies to address holistic risk factors ■ interventions for minimizing pressure, shear and friction ■ choice of support surfaces ■ moving and handling techniques ■ positioning techniques ■ use of appropriate medical devices, e.g. active mattress systems, heel boots ■ maintaining healthy skin, e.g. hygiene, emollients, moisture control ■ prevention of moisture lesions, e.g. pH balance cleanser, continence promotion, skin barriers ■ identification of signs of potential and actual pressure damage ■ evaluation of care plan and review in response to skin assessment ■ provision of nutritional support and hydration maintenance.	In relation to repositioning in a 30° tilt: ■ observation of moving and handling techniques ■ use of appropriate postures for positioning to reduce pressure and shear ■ use of pressure redistributing equipment, e.g. active mattress systems ■ taking appropriate action in response to tissue damage, e.g. avoiding positioning on the ulcer site, increasing frequency of repositioning ■ demonstrate rapport with patient, which facilitates communication and cooperation ■ provides explanations to patient and family ■ ensures patient comfort and dignity ■ encourages self-care where possible ■ documents accurately ■ keeps records of repositioning.
Demonstrate knowledge and understanding of evidence base in relation to pressure ulcer prevention, including: ■ NICE Guidelines (2005) ■ EPUAP/NPUAP Pressure Ulcer Prevention Guidelines (2009a) ■ EPUAP/NPUAP Pressure Ulcer Treatment Guidelines (2009b).	Demonstrates: ■ appropriate wound assessment and dressing selection ■ use of off-loading techniques ■ undertakes a wound dressing using aseptic non-touch techniques ■ assesses patient for painful stimuli pre-procedure, during and post procedure, and ensures adequate analgesia ■ documents on wound assessment form ■ maintains patient's dignity ■ provides explanations to patient as appropriate ■ ensures patient comfort.
Demonstrate knowledge and understanding of local and national policies, guidance and procedures, including those in relation to: ■ pressure ulcer prevention ■ moving and handling ■ infection control ■ repositioning regimes for those at risk of developing pressure ulcers ■ use of medical devices ■ wound dressings formulary.	

411

Competency statement 12.2: Specific procedure competency statements for assessing and managing pressure ulcers in patients who are critically ill

Complete assessment against relevant fundamental competency statements (*see* Chapter 2, pp. 20, 21)	Evidence
Specific procedure competency statements for assessing pressure ulcers in patients who are critically ill	**Evidence of competency for assessing pressure ulcers in patients who are critically ill**
Demonstrate ability to: ■ teach and assess or ■ learn from assessment.	Examples of evidence of teaching, assessing and learning.
Identify reason(s) for assessing pressure ulcers, including: ■ pressure, shear and friction forces ■ general risk factors ■ risk factors specific to critically ill patients ■ risk factors specific to critical treatment ■ appropriate treatment.	There are a number of ways in which competency can be judged. These include: ■ direct observation of procedure ■ testimonial from people, carer and or staff members ■ teaching session for peers ■ completion of a reflective text, workbook or educational package ■ examination ■ test ■ discussion with supervisor/mentor.
Identify risks, potential problems and complications for assessing pressure ulcers and how to prevent or manage them, including: ■ inappropriate identification of cause ■ underlying cause not adequately treated ■ inappropriate assessment of category of pressure ulcer ■ inappropriate treatment prescribed.	
Demonstrate knowledge and understanding of pressure ulcer wound management. ■ pressure ulcer classification ■ pressure off-loading techniques ■ holistic and local wound assessment and management ■ aseptic non-touch technique ■ observations of signs of infection and referral to other agencies as appropriate ■ pain assessment and monitoring.	In relation to assessing pressure ulcers: ■ observation of wound assessment ■ appropriate positioning and off-loading techniques at the pressure ulcer site ■ application of wound dressing using an aseptic non-touch technique
Demonstrate knowledge and understanding of evidence base in relation to developing, assessing and managing pressure ulcers, including: ■ pressure ulcer assessment tool ■ NICE Guidelines 2005 ■ EPUAP/NPUAP Pressure Ulcer Prevention Guidelines 2009a ■ EPUAP/NPUAP Pressure Ulcer Treatment Guidelines 2009b ■ local reporting of pressure ulcer incidence and prevalence.	■ assessing the wound for complications ■ completing the wound assessment form ■ referring to appropriate agencies ■ ensuring patient is comfortable and monitoring pain ■ ensuring rapport and cooperation ■ providing adequate explanations to patient ■ completes appropriate documentation.

412

Demonstrate skills that are required in relation to assessing pressure ulcers, including:
- TISSUE: viable or non viable (debridement techniques)
- EXUDATE: colour, amount and consistency (choice of wound dressing, symptom of infection)
- DIMENSIONS: length, width, depth, undermining, tunnelling (measurements to guide healing or deterioration)
- PERI-WOUND SKIN: maceration, inflammation, spreading erythema, cellulitis
- PAIN: symptom of infection, pain control
- INFECTION: clinical signs.

Demonstrate skills of wound care ensuring maintenance of aseptic non-touch technique (ANTT):
- wound assessment
- wound dressing selection
- undertake procedure
- pain control/monitoring.

Prepare equipment required in relation to assessing pressure ulcers:
- dressing trolley
- selection of wound dressings
- wound assessment chart
- non-touch aseptic technique packs
- apron and gloves.

Demonstrate the correct technique for the procedure in relation to assessing pressure ulcers, including:
- measuring wound surface area and depth
- pressure ulcer classification
- treatment and care of pressure ulcer
- ascertaining appropriate type of dressing
- care of surrounding skin
- infection control procedures
- identification of wound deterioration
- knowing when to refer to specialist.

Competency statement 12.3: Specific procedure competency statements for mouth care for critically ill patients

Complete assessment against relevant fundamental competency statements (*see* Chapter 2, pp. 20, 21)	Evidence
Specific procedure competency statements for mouth care for critically ill patients	**Evidence for competency for mouth care for critically ill patients**
Demonstrate ability to: - teach and assess or - learn from assessment.	Examples of evidence of teaching, assessing and learning.
Demonstrate reason(s) for mouth care, including: - replacing normal functions that patient is currently unable to perform - individualized assessment of needs, e.g. patient's own preferred oral care, existing problems, dentures.	*May be demonstrated by:* - providing appropriate mouth care that meets individual patients' needs - documentation identifies needs, appropriate assessment and actions - ability to discuss rationale for interventions.

(Continued)

Competency statement 12.3: (*Continued*)

Identify risks, potential problems and complications for oral health, and how to prevent or manage them, including: ■ potential complications (short-term and long-term) ■ potential effects of treatments/procedures on oral health ■ risk of developing ventilator-associated pneumonia ■ potential dislodgement of endotracheal tube.	*May be demonstrated by:* ■ documented assessment of risks, potential problems and complications ■ appropriate prophylactic interventions ■ discussion of risks, potential problems and complications, including ventilator-associated pneumonia.
Demonstrate knowledge and understanding of local and national policies, guidance, and procedures in relation to mouth care.	*May be demonstrated by:* ■ discussion of policies, guidance and procedures ■ evidence from documentation ■ observation of practice.
Demonstrate knowledge and understanding of evidence base in relation to mouth care, including: ■ potential effect of critical care interventions and patient-specific interventions on oral health.	*May be demonstrated by:* ■ discussing supporting evidence/rationale for planned interventions.
Demonstrate skills that are required in relation to mouth care.	*May be demonstrated by:* ■ providing care in a safe and appropriate manner.
Prepare equipment required in relation to mouth care, including: ■ to remove plaque and other film effectively and safely (e.g. toothbrush, paste, sterile water, a rigid oropharyngeal suction catheter, such as a Yankauer catheter) ■ to provide comfort between cleaning (e.g. rinses, sponges).	*May be demonstrated by:* ■ observing appropriate equipment is assembled to meet individual patient needs.
Demonstrate the correct technique for the procedure in relation to mouth care. With orally intubated patients, demonstrate how to clean parts of the oral cavity obstructed by the endotracheal tube.	*May be demonstrated by:* ■ adhering to appropriate procedures and guidelines ■ delivering mouth care in a safe and effective manner ■ patient's mouth appears clean following the procedure.

Competency statement 12.4: Specific procedure competency statements for eye care for critically ill patients

Complete assessment against relevant fundamental competency statements (*see* Chapter 2, pp. 20, 21)	Evidence
Specific procedure competency statements for eye care for critically ill patients	**Evidence of competency for eye care for critically ill patients**
Demonstrate ability to: ■ teach and assess or ■ learn from assessment.	Examples of evidence of teaching, assessing and learning.
Identify reason(s) for eye care, for example: ■ incomplete closure of eyelid ■ insufficient tear production ■ pre-existing problems and any aids (e.g. glasses, contact lenses).	*May be demonstrated by:* ■ providing appropriate eye care that meets individual patients' needs ■ documentation identifies needs, appropriate assessment and actions ■ ability to discuss rationale for interventions.

Identify risks, potential problems and complications for ocular health, and how to prevent or manage them, including: ■ risks of opportunist infection, especially if open suction is used (Parkin et al. 1997) ■ potential complications (short-term and long-term) ■ potential effects of treatments/procedures on ocular health.	*May be demonstrated by:* ■ documented assessment of risks, potential problems and complications ■ appropriate prophylactic interventions ■ ensuring suction catheter is kept away from eyes.
Demonstrate knowledge and understanding of local and national policies, guidance, and procedures in relation to eye care: ■ potential effect of critical care interventions and patient-specific interventions on ocular health.	*May be demonstrated by:* ■ discussion of policies, guidance and procedures ■ evidence from documentation ■ observation of practice.
Demonstrate knowledge and understanding of evidence base in relation to eye care.	*May be demonstrated by:* ■ discussing supporting evidence/rationale for planned interventions.
Demonstrate skills that are required in relation to eye care.	*May be demonstrated by:* ■ providing care in a safe and appropriate manner.
Prepare equipment required in relation to eye care, including: ■ clean and or sterile equipment ■ sufficient equipment to avoid re-use of swab or tissues.	*May be demonstrated by:* ■ observing appropriate equipment is assembled to meet individual patient needs.
Demonstrate the correct technique for the procedure in relation to eye care.	*May be demonstrated by:* ■ adhering to appropriate procedures and guidelines ■ delivering eye care in a safe and effective manner ■ patient's eyes appears clean.

References and further reading

Abidia RF (2007) Oral care in the intensive care unit: a review. *Journal of Contemporary Dental Practice* 8(1): 76–82.

Adams K (2005) Anatomy and physiology of the renal system. In: Morton PG, Fontaine DK, Hudak CM and Gallo BM (eds) *Critical Care Nursing: a holistic approach* (8e), pp. 629–639. Philadelphia: Lippincott Williams & Wilkins.

Agarwal A (2006) Anatomy and physiology of the ocular surface. In: Agarwal A (ed.) *Dry Eye*, pp. 3–12. Thorofare: SLACK Inc.

Alderden J, Whitney JD, Taylor SM and Zaratkiewicz S (2011) Risk profile characteristics associated with outcomes of hospital-acquired pressure ulcers: a retrospective review. *Critical Care Nurse.* 31(4): 30–42.

Balasz EA (2004) The visco-elastic properties of hyaluronan and its therapeutic use. In: Garg H and Hales C (eds) *Chemistry and Biology of Hyaluronan*, Chapter 20. London: Elsevier.

Bale S (2005) Incontinence care. Chapter 6: p 107–121. In: White R (ed.) *Skin Care in Wound Management: assessment, prevention and treatment*. Aberdeen: Wounds UK Publishing.

Bale S, Dealey C, Defloor T et al. (2007) The experience of living with a pressure ulcer. *Nursing Times* 103(15): 42–43.

Banks MD, Graves N, Bauer JD and Ash S (2010) The costs arising from pressure ulcers attributable to malnutrition. *Clinical Nutrition* 29(2): 180–186.

Barnason S, Graham J and Wild MC (1998) Comparison of two endotracheal tube securement techniques on unplanned extubation, oral mucosa, and facial skin integrity. *Heart Lung* 27(6): 409–417.

Baranoski S and Ayello E (2008) *Wound Care Essentials, practice principles* (2e). Philadelphia: Lippincott Williams & Wilkins USA.

Barrett KE, Barman SM, Boitano S and Brooks HL (2010) *Ganong's Review of Medical Physiology* (23e). New York: McGraw Hill Lange.

Beldon P (2007) Pressure ulcer prevention and management; using mattresses and cushions. *Wound Essentials* 2: 92–100.

Bell L (2008) Evaluation of and caring for patients with pressure ulcers. *American Journal of Critical Care* 17(4): 348.

Bennett G, Dealey C and Posnett J (2004) The cost of pressure ulcers in the UK. *Age & Ageing* 33(3): 230–235.

Berlowitz D, Berman RS, Schmader KE and Collins KA (2011) Pressure ulcers: epidemiology; pathogenesis; clinical manifestations; and staging. *Up-To-Date.* http://www.uptodate.com/contents/pressure-ulcers-epidemiology-pathogenesis-clinical-manifestations-and-staging?source=search_result&search=pressure+ulcers&selectedTitle=2%7E96 [last 17 October 2011].

Berry AM and Davidson PM (2006) Beyond comfort: oral hygiene as a critical nursing activity in the intensive care unit. *Intensive and Critical Care Nursing* 22(6): 318–328.

Berry AM, Davidson PM, Masters J and Rolls K (2007) Systematic literature review of oral hygiene practices for intensive care patients receiving mechanical ventilation. *American Journal of Critical Care* 16(5): 552–562.

Birtles M and Williams S (2004) An ergonomics evaluation of hospital backrests. *The Column* 16(2): 18–20.

Bliss DZ, Savik K, Harms S et al. (2006) Prevalence and correlates of perineal dermatitis in nursing home residents. *Nursing Research* 55(4): 243–251.

Bours GJJW, De Laat E, Halfens RJG and Lubbers M (2001) Prevalence, risk factors and prevention of pressure ulcers in Dutch intensive care units. *Intensive Care Medicine* 27(10): 1599–1605.

Bowsher J, Boyle S and Griffiths J (1999) Oral care. *Nursing Standard* 13(37): 31.

Bruggisser R (2005) Bacterial and fungal absorption properties of a hydrogel dressing with a superabsorbent polymer core. *Journal of Wound Care* 14(9): 438–444.

Butcher M and White R (2005) The structure and functions of the skin. In: White R (ed.) *Skin Care in Wound Management; assessment, prevention and treatment.* Aberdeen: Wounds UK Publishing.

Cason CL, Tyner T, Saunders S and Broome L (2007) Nurses' implementation of guidelines for ventilator-associated pneumonia from the centers for disease control and prevention. *American Journal of Critical Care* 16(1): 28–37.

Chao Y-FC, Chen Y-Y, Wang K-WK et al. (2009) Removal of oral secretions prior to position change can reduce the incidence of ventilator-associated pneumonia for adult ICU patients. *Journal of Clinical Nursing* 18(1): 22–28.

Clancy J and McVicar AJ (2009) *Physiology & Anatomy: a homeostatic approach* (3e). London: Hodder Arnold.

Clark M, Schols J M G A, Benati G et al. (2004) Pressure ulcers and nutrition: a new European guideline. *Journal of Wound Care* 13(7): 267–272.

Clarke G (1993) Mouthcare and the hospitalised patient. *British Journal of Nursing* 2(4): 225–227.

Clark M and Stephen-Haynes J (2005) Superficial pressure ulcers. Chapter 2, p. 17–46. In: White R (ed.) *Skin Care in Wound Management: assessment, prevention and treatment.* Aberdeen: Wounds UK Publishing.

Clay AS, Behina M and Brown KK (2001) Mitochondrial disease. *Chest* 120(2): 634–648.

Clay M (2002) Assessing oral health in older people. *Nursing Older People* 14(8): 31–32.

Compton F, Hoffman F, Hortig T et al. (2008) Pressure ulcer predictors in ICU patients: nursing skin assessment versus objective parameters. *Journal of Wound Care* 17(10): 417–424.

Cooke K, Doyle N and Farley A (2011) Patient comfort. In: Dougherty L and Lister S (eds) *The Royal Marsden Hospital Manual of Clinical Nursing Procedures* (8e), pp. 417–532. Oxford: Wiley-Blackwell.

Cox J (2011) Predictors of pressure ulcers in adult critical care patients. *American Journal of Critical Care* 20(5): 364–375.

Cutler CJ and Davis N (2005) Improving oral care in patients receiving mechanical ventilation. *American Journal of Critical Care* 14(5): 389–394.

Davies A (2005) Salivary gland dysfunction. In: Davies A and Finlay I (eds) *Oral Care in Advanced Disease.* Oxford: Oxford University Press.

Dawson D (2005) Development of a new eye care guideline for critically ill patients. *Intensive and Critical Care Nursing* 21(2): 118–122.

de Almedia PVD, Trindade AM, Machado MAN et al. (2008) Saliva composition and functions: a comprehensive review. *Journal of Contemporary Dental Practice* 9(3): 72–80.

De Laat EHEW, Schoonhoven L, Pickkers P and van Achterberg T (2006) Epidemiology, risk and prevention of pressure ulcers in critically ill patients, a literature review. *Journal Wound Care* 15(6): 269–275.

de Oliveira C, Watt R and Hamer M (2010) Toothbrushing, inflammation, and risk of cardiovascular disease: results from Scottish Health Survey. *British Medical Journal* 340(7761): 1400.

Dealey C and Cameron J (2008) *Wound Management.* Chichester: Wiley-Blackwell.

Defloor T and Schoonhoven L (2004) Inter-rater reliability of the EPUAP pressure ulcer classification system using photographs. *Journal of Clinical Nursing* 13(8): 952–959.

Defloor T (1999) The risk of pressure sores; a conceptual scheme. *Journal of Clinical Nursing* 8(2): 206–216.

Defloor T (2000) The effect of position and mattress on interface pressure. *Applied Nursing Research* 13(1): 2–11.

Dennesen P, van der Ven A, Vlasveld M et al. (2003) Inadequate salivary flow and poor oral mucosal status in intubated intensive care unit patients. *Critical Care Medicine* 31(3): 781–786.

Department of Health. 2010. *Improving Quality, Increasing Cost Efficiency.* http://www.dh.gov.uk/en/Publicationsandstatistics/Bulletins/Chiefnursingofficerbulletin/July2010/DH_118126 [accessed 6 December 2011].

Dougherty L and Lister S (eds) (2011) *The Royal Marsden Hospital Manual of Clinical Nursing Procedures* (8e). Oxford: Wiley-Blackwell.

Drakulovic MB, Torres A, Bauer TT et al. (1999) Supine body position as a risk factor for nosocomial pneumonia in mechanically ventilated patients: a randomised trial. *Lancet* 354(9193): 1851–1858.

Eachempati SR, Hydo LJ and Barie PS (2001) Factors influencing the development of decubitus ulcers in critically ill surgical patients. *Critical Care Medicine* 29(9): 1678–1682.

El-Solh AA, Pietrantoni C, Bhat A et al. (2004) Colonization of dental plaques: a reservoir of respiratory pathogens for hospital-acquired pneumonia in institutionalized elders. *Chest* 126(5): 1575–1582.

Elliott R, McKinley S and Fox V (2008) Quality improvement program to reduce the prevalence of pressure ulcers in an intensive care unit. *American Journal of Critical Care* 17(4): 328–334.

EPUAP/NPUAP (European Pressure Ulcer Advisory Panel and National Pressure Ulcer Advisory Panel) (2009a) *Prevention and treatment of pressure ulcers: quick reference guide.* Washington DC: National Pressure Ulcer Advisory Panel.

EPUAP/NPUAP (European Pressure Ulcer Advisory Panel and National Pressure Ulcer Advisory Panel) (2009b) *Treatment of Pressure Ulcers: Quick Reference Guide.* Washington DC: National Pressure Ulcer Advisory Panel.

EWMA (2005) *Position Document: Identifying Criteria for Wound Infection.* London: European Wound Management Association. Medical Education Partnership.

Falanga V (2004) Would bed preparation: science applied to practice. In: European Wound Management Association (EWMA) *Position Document: Wound Bed Preparation in Practice*, pp. 2–5. London: Medical Education Partnership Ltd.

Farrell M and Wray F (1993) Eye care for ventilated patients. *Intensive and Critical Care Nursing* 9(2): 137–141.

Field D and Tillotson J (2008) *Eye Emergencies: the practitioner's guide.* Keswick: M&K Update.

Fitch JA, Munro CL, Glass CA and Pellegrini JM (1999) Oral care in the adult intensive care unit. *American Journal of Critical Care* 8(5): 314–318.

Fleurence RL (2005) Measuring quality of life in patients with pressure ulcers to include in economic evaluations. *Journal Wound Care* 14(3): 129–131.

Frenkel H, Harvey I and Needs K (2002) Oral health care education and its effect on caregivers' knowledge and attitudes: a randomised controlled trial. *Community Dentistry and Oral Epidemiology* 30(2): 91–100.

Garg P, Krishna PV, Stratis AK and Gopinathan U (2005) The value of corneal transplantation in reducing blindness. *Eye* 19: 1106–1114.

416

Gastmeier P and Geffers C (2007) Prevention of ventilator-associated pneumonia: analysis of studies published since 2004. *Journal of Hospital Infection* **67**(1): 1.

General Medical Council (2013) *Good Medical Practice*. London: GMC. http://www.gmc-uk.org/gmp2013 [accessed 25 March 2013].

Goldhill DR, Imhoff M, McLean B and Waldmann C (2007) Rotational bed therapy to prevent and treat respiratory complications: a review and meta-analysis. *American Journal of Critical Care* **16**(1): 50–61.

Gould D (2002) Using replication studies to enhance nursing research. *Nursing Standard* **16**(49): 33–36.

Grap MJ, Munro CL, Ashtiani B and Bryant S (2003) Oral care interventions in critical care: frequency and documentation. *American Journal of Critical Care* **12**(2): 113–118.

Guerin C, Gaillard S, Lemasson S et al. (2004) Effects of systematic prone positioning in hypoemic acute respiratory failure. *Journal of the American Medical Association* **292**(19): 2379–2387.

Gunnewicht B and Dunford C (2004) *Fundamentals of Tissue Viability Nursing*. London: MA Healthcare.

Guyton AC and Hall JE (2005) *Textbook of Medical Physiology* (11e). Philadelphia: Elsevier Saunders.

Hampton S and Collins F (2004) *Tissue Viability*. London: Whurr Publishers.

Hassanin AA and Tantawey NM (2011) Pressure ulcer prevention and management guideline: comparison between intensive care unit and general word at Mansoura University Hospital. *Journal of American Science* **7**(9): 110–117.

Hayes J and Jones C (1995) A collaborative approach to oral care during critical illness. *Dental Health* **34**(3): 6–10.

Health and Care Professions Council (2012) *Standard of Conduct, Performance and Ethics*. London: HCPC. http://www.hcpc-uk.org/assets/documents/10003B6EStandardsofconduct,performance andethics.pdf [accessed January 2013].

Heath H, Sturdy D, Edwards T et al. (2011) *Promoting Older People's Oral Health*. London: Nursing Standard.

Helm M, Hossfeld B, Schäfer S et al. (2006) Factors influencing emergency intubation in the pre-hospital setting – a multicentre study in the German Helicopter Emergency Medical Service. *British Journal of Anaesthesia* **96**(1): 67–71.

Herbert RA (2006) The biology of human ageing. In: Redfern SJ and Ross FM (eds) *Nursing Older People* (4e), pp. 57–81. Edinburgh: Churchill Livingstone Elsevier.

Hinds CJ and Watson D (2008) *Intensive Care: a concise textbook* (2e). London: WB Saunders.

Høvding G (2008) Acute bacterial conjunctivitis. *Acta Ophthalmologica Scandinavia* **86**(1): 5–17.

Imanaka H, Taenaka N, Nakamura J et al. (1997) Ocular surface disorders in the critically ill. *Anesthesia & Analgesia* **85**(2): 343–346.

Jamieson EM and McCall JM (1992) *Guidelines for Clinical Nursing Practice* (2e). Edinburgh: Churchill Livingstone.

Joanna Briggs Institute (2002) Eye care for intensive care patients. *Best Practice* **6**(1): 1–6.

Jones CV (2004) The importance of oral hygiene in nutritional support. In: White R (ed.) *Trends in Oral Health Care*, pp. 72–83. Dinton: Quay Books.

Jones S, Bowler PG and Walker M (2005) Antimicrobial activity of silver-containing dressings is influenced by dressing conformability with a wound surface. *Wounds* **17**(9): 263–270.

Kaya AZ, Turani N and Alküz M (2005) The effectiveness of a hydrogel dressing compared with standard management of pressure ulcers. *Journal of Wound Care* **14**(1): 42–44.

Kearns R, Brewer A and Booth MG (2010) The introduction of an oral surgical service in an intensive care unit serving a deprived inner city population. *Journal of the Intensive Care Society* **11**(4): 237–239.

Kelly J and Isted M (2011) Assessing nurses' ability to classify pressure ulcers correctly. *Nursing Standard* **26**(7): 62–71.

Kelly T, Timmis S and Twelvetree T (2010) Review of the evidence to support oral hygiene in stroke patients. *Nursing Standard* **24**(37): 35–38.

Kennedy MS (2004) Kinetic therapy: in search of the evidence: it may prevent some pulmonary complications. *American Journal of Nursing* **104**(12): 22.

Kite K and Pearson L (1995) A rationale for mouth care: the integration of theory with practice. *Intensive and Critical Care Nursing* **11**(2): 71–76.

Koroloff N, Boots R, Lipman J et al. (2004) A randomised controlled study of the efficacy of hypromellose and Lacri-Lube combination versus polyethylene/cling wrap to prevent corneal epithelial breakdown in the semiconscious intensive care patient. *Intensive Care Medicine* **30**(6): 1122–1126.

Lorente L, Lecuona M, Jiménez A et al. (2007) Influence of an endotracheal tube with polyurethane cuff and subglottic secretion drainage on pneumonia. *AJRCCM* **176**(11): 1079–1083.

Lowery MT (1995) A pressure sore risk calculator for intensive care patients: the Sunderland experience. *Intensive and Critical Care Nursing* **11**(6): 344–353.

Marieb EN and Hoehn K (2013) *Human Anatomy and Physiology* (9e). Boston: Pearson.

Mayrovitz HN and Sims N (2001) Biophysical effects of water and synthetic urine on skin. *Advances in Skin and Wound Care* **14**(6): 302–308.

McLean B (2001) Rotational kinetic therapy for ventilation/perfusion mismatch. *Connect* **1**(4): 113–118.

Mela EK, Drimtzias EG, Christofidou MK et al. (2010) Ocular surface bacterial colonisation in sedated intensive care unit patients. *Anesthesia and Intensive Care* **38**(1): 190–193.

Mental Capacity Act (2005) http://www.legislation.gov.uk/ukpga/2005/9/pdfs/ukpga_20050009_en.pdf [accessed 9 February 2012].

Mori H, Hirasawa H, Oda S et al. (2006) Oral care reduces incidence of ventilator-associated pneumonia in ICU populations. *Intensive Care Medicine* **31**(2): 230–236.

Munro CL, Grap MJ, Jones DJ et al. (2009) Chlorhexidine, toothbrushing, and preventing ventilator-associated pneumonia in critically ill adults. *American Journal of Critical Care* **18**(5): 428–437.

Munro CL and Grap MJ (2004) Oral health and care in the intensive care unit: state of the science. *American Journal of Critical Care* **13**(1): 25–34.

Muzyka BC (2005) Oral fungal infections. *Dental Clinics of North America* **49**(1): 49–65.

Myers BA (2008) *Wound Management*. New Jersey: Pearson Prentice Hall.

NHS Institute for Innovation and Improvement (2008) http://www.institute.nhs.uk/creativity_tools/creativity_tools/identifying_problems_-_root_cause_analysis_using5_whys.html [accessed 14 December 2011].

NHS Institute for Innovation and Improvement (2009) *High Impact Actions for Nursing & Midwifery*. http://www.institute.nhs.uk/images/stories/Building_Capability/HIA/NHSI%20High%20Impact%20Actions.pdf [accessed 14 December 2011].

National Institute for Health and Clinical Excellence (2005) *The Management of Pressure Ulcers in Primary and Secondary Care; a clinical practice guideline*. London: NICE.

National Institute for Health and Clinical Excellence (2008) *Technical Patient Safety Solutions for Ventilator-associated Pneumonia in Adults*. London. NICE.

417

Nijs N, Toppets A, Defloor T et al. (2009) Incidence and risk factors for pressure ulcers in the intensive care unit. *Journal of Clinical Nursing* **18**(9): 1258–1266.

Nursing and Midwifery Council (2008) *The Code; standards of conduct, performance and ethics for nurses and midwives.* London: NMC. http://www.nmc-uk.org/Documents/Standards/The-code-A4-20100406.pdf [accessed 15 February 2012].

O'Reilly M (2003) Oral care of the critically ill: a review of the literature and guidelines for practice. *Australian Critical Care* **16**(3): 101–109.

Oh EG, Lee WH, Yoo JS et al. (2009) Factors related to incidence of eye disorders in Korean patients at intensive care units. *Journal of Clinical Nursing* **18**(1): 29–35.

Ohura T, Ohura N Jr and Oka H (2007) Incidence and clinical symptoms of hourglass and sandwich-shaped tissue necrosis in stage IV pressure ulcers. *Wounds* **19**(11): 310–319.

Orsted HL, Ohura T and Harding K (2010) Pressure, shear, friction and microclimate in context. In: Baharestani M, Black J, Clark M et al. (eds) *International Review. Pressure Ulcer Prevention: pressure, shear, friction and microclimate, a consensus document*, p.1. London: Wounds International.

Ousey K (ed.) (2005) *Pressure Area Care*. Oxford: Wiley-Blackwell.

Paju S and Scannapieco F (2007) Oral biofilms, periodontitis, and pulmonary infections. *Oral Diseases* **13**(6): 508–512.

Parkin B and Cook S (2000) A clear view: the way forward for eye care on ICU. *Intensive Care Medicine* **26**(2): 155–156.

Parkin B, Turner A and Moore E (1997) Bacterial keratitis in the critically ill. *British Journal of Ophthalmology* **81**: 1060–1063.

Patil BB and Dowd TC (2000) Physiological functions of the eye. *Current Anaesthesia & Critical Care* **11**(6): 291–298.

Pearson LS (1996) A comparison of the ability of foam swabs and toothbrushes to remove dental plaque: implications for nursing practice. *Journal of Advanced Nursing* **23**(1): 62–69.

Pender LR and Frazier SK (2005) The relationship between dermal pressure ulcers, oxygenation and perfusion in mechanically ventilated patients. *Intensive & Critical Care Nursing* **21**(1): 29–38.

Penzer R and Ersser SJ (2010) *Principles of Skin Care*. Chichester: Wiley-Blackwell.

Pisani MA (2009) Considerations in caring for the critically ill older patients. *Intensive Care Medicine* **24**(2): 83–95.

Pritchard AP and Mallett J (1992) *The Royal Marsden Hospital Manual of Clinical Nursing Procedures* (3e). Oxford: Blackwell Publishing.

Rattenbury N, Mooney G and Bowen J (1999) Oral assessment and care for inpatients. *Nursing Times* **95**(49): 52–53.

Reddy M, Gill SS and Rochon PA (2006) Preventing pressure ulcers: a systematic review. *Journal of the American Medical Association* **296**(8): 974–984.

Reger SI, Ranganathan VK, Orsted HL et al. (2010) Shear and friction in context. In: Baharestani M, Black J, Clark M et al. (eds) *International Review. Pressure Ulcer Prevention: pressure, shear, friction and microclimate, a consensus document*, pp. 11–18. London: Wounds International.

Rello J, Koulenti D, Blot S et al. (2007) Oral care practices in intensive care units: a survey of 59 European ICUs. *Intensive Care Medicine* **33**(6): 1066–1070.

Rithalia SVS and Kenney L (2000) Mattresses and beds: reducing and relieving pressure. *Nursing Times* **96**(36 suppl): 9–10.

Romero CM, Marambio A, Larrondo J et al. (2010) Swallowing dysfunction in nonneurologic critically ill patients who require percutaneous dilational tracheostomy. *Chest* **137**(6): 1278–1282.

Rosenberg JB and Eisen LA (2008) Eye care in the intensive care unit: narrative review and meta-analysis. *Critical Care Medicine* **36**(12): 3151–3155.

Ross A and Crumpler J (2007) The impact of an evidence-based practice education program on the role of oral care in the prevention of ventilator-associated pneumonia. *Intensive and Critical Care Nursing* **23**(3): 132–136.

Rush A (2005) Purchasing electric profiling beds: benefits and challenges. *International Journal of Therapy and Rehabilitation* **12**(12): 559–562.

Russell L (2002) Understanding physiology of wound healing and how dressings help. In: White R and Harding K (eds) *Trends in Wound Care*, pp. 3-15. Dinton: Quay Books.

Sayar S, Turget S, Do an H et al. (2009) Incidence of pressure ulcers in intensive care unit patients at risk according to the Waterlow scale and factors influencing the development of pressure sores. *Journal of Clinical Nursing* **18**(5): 765–774.

Schelenz S (2008) Management of *candidiasis* in the intensive care unit. *Journal of Antimicrobial Chemotherapy* **61**(Suppl 1): i31–i34.

Sewchuk D, Padula C and Osborne E (2006) Prevention and early detection of pressure ulcers in patients undergoing cardiac surgery. *AORN Journal* **84**(1): 75–96.

Shahina ESM, Dassena T and Halfens RJG (2009) Incidence, prevention and treatment of pressure ulcers in intensive care patients: a longitudinal study. *International Journal of Nursing Studies* **46**(4): 413–421.

Sharp C (2010) Managing the wound with Hydration Response technology. *Wounds UK* **6**(2): 112–115.

Sivasankar S, Jasper S, Simon S et al. (2006) Eye care in ICU. *Indian Journal of Critical Care Medicine* **10**(1): 11–14.

Sollars A (1998) Pressure area risk assessment in intensive care. *Nursing in Critical Care* **3**(6): 267–273.

Stratton RJ, Ek A-C, Engfer M et al. (2005) Enteral nutritional support in prevention and treatment of pressure ulcers: a systematic review and meta-analysis. *Ageing Research Reviews* **4**(3): 422–450

Suresh P, Mercieca F, Morton A and Tullo AB (2000) Eye care for the critically ill. *Intensive Care Medicine* **26**(2): 162–166.

Swadener-Culpepper L, Skaggs RL and VanGilder CA (2008) The impact of continuous lateral rotation therapy in overall clinical and financial outcomes of critically ill patients. *Critical Care Nursing Quarterly* **31**(3): 270–279.

Sweeney D, Holden B, Evans K et al. (2009) Best practice contact lens care: a review of the Asia Pacific Contact Lens Care Summit. *Clinical and Experimental Optometry* **92**(2): 78–89.

Takahashi J, Yokota O, Fujisawa Y et al. (2006) An evaluation of polyvinylidine film dressing for treatment of pressure ulcers in older people. *Journal of Wound Care* **15**(10): 449–454.

Takahashi M, Black J, Dealey C and Gefen A (2010) Pressure in context. In: Baharestani M, Black J, Clark M et al. (eds) *International Review. Pressure Ulcer Prevention: pressure, shear, friction and microclimate, a consensus document*, pp. 2–10. London: Wounds International.

Terekeci H, Kucukardali Y, Top C et al. (2009) Risk assessment study of the pressure ulcers in intensive care unit patients. *European Journal of Internal Medicine* **20**(4): 394–397.

Theaker C, Mannan M, Ives N and Soni N (2000) Risk factors for pressure sores in the critically ill. *Anaesthesia* **55**(1): 221–224.

Thibodeau GA and Patton KT (2007) *Anatomy & Physiology* (6e). St Louis, MO: Mosby Elsevier.

Timmons J (2006) Skin function and wound healing physiology. *Wound Essentials* **1**: 8–17.

Tolle SL (2010) Periodontal and risk assessment. In: Darby ML and Walsh MM (eds) *Dental Hygiene: theory and practice*, pp. 305–347. St Louis. MO: Saunders Elsevier.

Torra I Bou JE, Rueda López J, Camañes G et al. (2002) Heel pressure ulcers, comparative study between heel protective bandage and hydrocellular dressing with special form for heel. *Revista de Enfermeria* **25**(5): 50–56.

Tortora GJ and Derrickson B (2011) *Principles of Anatomy and Physiology* (13e). New Jersey: John Wiley & Sons.

Treloar DM (1995) Use of a clinical assessment tool for orally intubated patients. *American Journal of Critical Care* **4**(5): 355–360.

Trieger N (2004) Oral care in the intensive care unit. *American Journal of Critical Care* **13**(1): 24.

Wakefield BJ, Mentes J, Holman JE and Culp K (2009) Postadmission dehydration: risk factors, indicators and outcomes. *Rehabilitation Nursing* **34**(5): 209–216.

Walsh T, Worthington HV, Glenny AM et al. (2010) Fluoride toothpastes of different concentrations for preventing dental caries in children and adolescents. *Cochrane Database of Systematic Reviews* 2010, Issue 1. Art. No.: CD007868. DOI: 10.1002/14651858.CD007868.pub2.

Wanless S and Aldridge M (2012) Continuous lateral rotation therapy – a review. *Nursing in Critical Care* **17**(1): 28–35.

Watson R (2001) Assessing gastrointestinal (GI) tract functioning in older people. *Nursing Older People* **12**(10): 27–28.

Welch, J. 2002. Kinetic therapy. *Care of the Critically Ill.* **18** (6): centre insert.

Weller RPB, Hunton JAA, Savin JA and Dahl MV (2008) *Clinical Dermatology* (4e). Oxford: Blackwell Publishing.

Wiener RC, Wu B, Crout R et al. (2010) Hyposalivation and xerostomia in dentate older adults. *Journal of the American Dental Association* **141**(3): 279–284.

Winkelman C and Chiang C-L (2010) Manual turns in patients receiving mechanical ventilation. *Critical Care Nurse* **30**(4): 36–44.

Winslow EH and Jacobson AF (1998) Dispelling the petroleum jelly myth. *American Journal of Nursing* **98**(11): 16.

Wu Y, Carnt N, Willcox M and Stapleton F (2010) Contact lens and lens storage case cleaning instructions: whose advice should we follow? *Eye & Contact Lens: Science & Clinical Practice* **36**(2): 68–72.

Xavier G (2000) The importance of mouth care in preventing infection. *Nursing Standard* **14**(18): 47–51.

Xie X, McGregor M and Dendukuri N (2010) The clinical effectiveness of negative pressure wound therapy: a systematic review. *Journal of Wound Care* **19**(11): 490–495.

Yoon M and Steele C (2007) The oral care imperative: the link between oral hygiene and aspiration pneumonia. *Topics in Geriatric Rehabilitation* **23**(3): 280–288.

Young PJ and Ridley SA (1999) Ventilator-associated pneumonia. *Anaesthesia* **54**(12): 1183–1197.

Chapter 13

Assessment of sleep and sleep promotion

Annette Richardson, Micheala Allsop and Elaine Coghill

Newcastle upon Tyne Hospitals NHS Foundation Trust, Newcastle upon Tyne, UK

Critical Care Manual of Clinical Procedures and Competencies, First Edition.
Edited by Jane Mallett, John W. Albarran, and Annette Richardson.
© 2013 John Wiley & Sons, Ltd. Published 2013 by John Wiley & Sons, Ltd.

Definition

Sleep is 'unconsciousness from which the person can be aroused by sensory or other stimuli' (Guyton and Hall 1997). During sleep, the body rests and does not respond to the environment, but a person can be aroused by external stimuli, such as being called, physical touch, bright lights and noise (Kryger et al. 2000).

Indications

Sleep is an essential function of the human body and is a basic physiological need for all humans' survival (Honkus 2003). Although all the functions are not clearly understood, sleep is necessary for the maintenance of good health and wellbeing (Dogan et al. 2005).

Background

The stages of sleep

Sleep is a complex process involving two distinct states known as rapid eye movement (REM) and non-REM sleep (Shapiro and Flanigan 1993). Non-REM sleep comprises of four stages, progressing from stage 1 to stage 4, followed by a fifth stage of REM sleep. Stages 1 to 5 are known as the 'sleep cycle', which starts over and repeats throughout the period of sleep (*see* Figure 13.1). Stage 1 is light sleep, eyes move very slowly and also muscle activity reduces; if woken people recall fragmented visual images (American Sleep Association 2007). In stage 2, eye movements stop and brain activity becomes slower; this activity is only detectable with an electroencephalograph (EEG) monitor. There are

also occasional bursts of activity called sleep spindles (American Sleep Association 2007). By stage 3 the brain exhibits very slow brain waves called delta waves, with occasional smaller faster waves. During stage 4 the brain almost exclusively produces delta waves.

It is very difficult to wake someone from stages 3 and 4, and together they are called deep sleep (American Sleep Association 2007). The fifth, or last, stage is REM sleep where heart rate increases, arousal remains difficult and if woken, dreaming is often reported (Reid 2001). REM sleep is shortened or suppressed by medications and alcohol (American Sleep Association 2007). A complete sleep cycle takes on average 90–110 minutes and the time spent in each stage changes throughout the night. At night, the first sleep cycle contains short REM periods and long periods of deep sleep, and as the night progresses, REM sleep periods increase in length while deep sleep decreases. By morning, nearly all sleep time is in stages 1, 2 and REM (American Sleep Association 2007).

Why is sleep important?

Sleep is thought to contribute to physiological and psychological conservation and restoration (Hodgson 1991). During slow delta wave sleep energy is conserved as basal metabolic rate is lowered, resulting in reduced oxygen consumption, heart rate and body temperature (Shapiro and Flanigan 1993). The lowering of basal metabolic rate is also thought to help restore the body as it provides a period of increasing protein synthesis and cellular division for repairing and renewing epithelial cells (Shapiro and Flanigan 1993).

The amount of sleep needed depends on many factors, but on average infants require about 16 hours/day, teenagers about 9 hours/day and most adults 7–8 hours/night, although as little as 5 hours or as many as 10 hours of sleep per day can occur (American Sleep Association 2007).

In addition to sleep quantity, quality is important. Complaints related to sleep quality are common (Dogan et al. 2005) and low sleep quality is an indicator of many illnesses (Buysse et al. 1989). Sleep quality defects can cause problems with a person's feelings, thoughts and motivation (Dogan et al. 2005), which can cause a multitude of problems, such as tiredness, loss of concentration, weariness, low pain threshold, anxiety, nervousness, irrational thoughts, hallucinations, loss of appetite, constipation and an increased tendency for the occurrence of accidents (Closs 1988).

Lack of sleep and interrupted sleep are main sources of patient complaints while in hospital (Dogan et al. 2005). Disturbances at night time have been reported in patient satisfaction surveys as one of the causes of inpatient dissatisfaction while in hospital (Commission for Patient and Public Involvement in Health 2007). The dissatisfaction is not always about quantity of sleep, it can be from broken sleep and feeling exhausted in the morning (Reid 2001).

The effects of sleep deprivation on critical care patients are wide ranging and include:

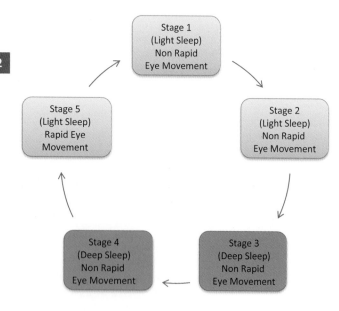

Figure 13.1 Five stages of sleep.

- behavioural changes occurring within a 48-hour period, such as irritability, restlessness, tiredness and disorientation (Dines-Kalinowski 2002)
- psychotic behaviour (Hobson 1995)
- confusion (Dogan et al. 2005)
- decreased pain tolerance (Weitzman et al. 1974)
- long-term health problems and an increase in patient morbidity (Tamburri et al. 2004)
- stress (Aurell and Elmqvist 1985; Wilson 1987; Soehren 1995; Perez de Ciriza et al. 1996; Novaes et al. 1997)
- development of delirium (Xie et al. 2009)
- delayed recovery from illness (Redeker et al. 2004).

Assessment of sleep

Traditionally, sleep assessment in critical care has been performed unsystematically and largely based on inaccurate staff perceptions of the patient's sleep (Richardson et al. 2007a). Sleep assessment needs to be conducted systematically, as it provides an understanding of the patient's own routines and habits in this area of daily living. It can:

- reveal usual sleep patterns
- reveal routines and habits prior to going to sleep
- identify variations with normal sleep and factors influencing sleep
- measure and monitor the success of interventions to promote sleep.

A number of different approaches to assessing patients' sleep exist and they can be categorized into physiological and non-physiological methods. Physiological sleep methods are often referred to as objective measurements of sleep and non-physiological methods as subjective measurements. The latter method usually involves gaining the patient's perception of their sleep or an observer's perception of the patient's sleep (Closs 1988). Examples of both types include:

- physiological
  - polysomnography
  - actigraphy
- non- physiological
  - observation (for example, sleep charts)
  - self-reporting (for example spontaneous reporting, diaries, or questionnaires).

Physiological sleep assessment methods

Polysomnography

Polysomnography is the study of sleep involving a range of methods to measure different physiological parameters during sleep stages. Polysomnographic recordings include:

- an electroencephalogram (EEG), the recording of electrical brain activity
- an electromyogram (EMG), the recording of muscle activity
- an electroculogram (EOG), the recording of eye movements.

(Bourne et al 2007; Beecroft et al 2008)

This has been found to be the most effective and accurate way to assess the physiological attributes of sleep (Chuman 1983; Tamburri et al. 2004; Bourne et al. 2007). However, polysomnography methods are normally used in detailed medical research studies and are difficult to use outside the laboratory setting (Snyder-Hapern and Verran 1987; Beecroft et al 2008) as they are expensive and difficult to access (Richardson 1997; Beecroft et al. 2008), limiting their use in critical care areas (Tamburri et al. 2004) on a daily basis. In addition, polysomnography is cumbersome, and requires electrode placement by experienced technicians (Redeker 2000; Bourne et al. 2007) so is an impractical method for everyday practice (Beecroft et al. 2008).

Actigraphy

Actigraphy involves using a small measuring device attached to the wrist or leg that is capable of sensing and storing information regarding patient movement. Computer software translates the movement data into sleep–wake periods but it does not provide any information related to sleep stages or quality of sleep (Bourne et al. 2007). This has similar interpretation and access problems to other polysomnography methods (Tamburri et al. 2004), limiting its application for regular use in critical care.

In addition, it should be noted that while polysomnography measures physiological parameters associated with sleep, it cannot provide an indication of how the patient receiving critical care perceives the quality and quantity of their sleep.

Non-physiological sleep assessment methods

Observation

Staff observation of patients' sleep requires no participation on the part of the patient and no equipment and technician expertise. Therefore this approach can be seen as an easy way to assess patients who are unable to communicate their own experiences of sleep. However, this method is often unreliable as staff may over- or underestimate patients' sleep (Aurell and Elmqvist 1985; Richardson et al. 2007a). Overestimation is most likely in patients in critical care who are not moving or have their eyes closed due to their critical illness. Conversely, an observer can underestimate sleep, for example when there is a high level of activity in a critical care unit throughout the night. Staff can presume this activity has impacted on their patients' sleep. Consequently the

423

data obtained using this method is open to observer bias (Redeker 2000).

Self-reporting

Self-reporting requires the patient to report their perception of their sleep. This can be in the form of a questionnaire or diary and can be recorded by the patient or a member of staff. The reporting includes responses that address features of sleep during a specific night, and are designed to gain general information over a period of time. A number of questionnaires and tools have been developed and tested in a range of clinical settings (Ellis et al. 1981; Snyder-Hapern and Verran 1987; Richardson et al. 2007a) to assess sleep.

Non-physiological sleep assessment tools

An early sleep tool, called the St Mary's Hospital Sleep Questionnaire, was designed specifically to assess patients' sleep while in hospital. This tool was very detailed and included 11 items as a multiple-choice instrument. It was found to be comprehensive when tested on patients from surgical, medical and psychiatric wards (Ellis et al. 1981). However, the tool was not tested on critically ill patients and due to its long and detailed nature (along with a number of questions inappropriate for critically ill patients who are in bed for 24 hours such as 'how clear headed did you feel after getting up this morning?') would not be relevant for patients in critical care.

Another detailed sleep assessment tool developed by Snyder-Hapern and Verran (1987) is a 15-item visual analogue scale to measure patients' perception of sleep for the preceding night. Each item is scored from 0 to 100, and the tool contains three main sleep scales:

- disturbance (interruptions and delays in sleep)
- effectiveness (how well sleep-refreshed is the individual)
- supplementation (napping).

When this tool was tested in the hospital environment patients reported many difficulties using the visual analogue scale. These included problems seeing and reading the tool because of medication side effects, difficulties in using reading glasses due to the patient's body position, as well as their attached tubes and dressings, and difficulties in writing because the patient's hands and arms were often immobilized by monitoring equipment, treatment and illness (Richardson 1997). The tool was further tested with quadriplegic patients and was applied by a nurse who held the scale at right angles to the patient's face to make it easier to read, and each item was read to them. The nurse then indicated

the position on the scale with a pencil once confirmed by the patient. This method was found to be a useful approach in the critical care clinical environment, but it was very long and time-consuming (Richardson 1997).

Other rating scales have been developed for clinicians to assess patients' sleep with the critically ill. Olsen et al. (2001) used a tool where nurses were asked to indicate patients' sleep following a 5-second observation of patients at eight pre-determined periods throughout 24 hours. Difficulties with this tool were experienced because of staff requirements to be constantly close to the patient, often resulting in waking the patient during their sleep. These early sleep assessment tools were problematic for critically ill patients mainly due to difficulties experienced in communicating and recalling information. Additionally, patients often have difficulty writing due to limb weakness.

More recently, three simple and easy to understand sleep rating scales have been designed to measure both quality and quality of patients' sleep (Richardson et al. 2007a). A study was conducted to determine the usefulness of these simple tools with lucid critically ill patients by establishing the patient's preferences with regard to the scales and also how the patient's perception of their sleep compared with the nurse's judgement. Each scale was printed in enlarged font for easy patient viewing and patients were supplied with a bedside clock. The data were collected between 07.00 and 09.30 hrs from the patient and the nurse caring for the patient by a researcher not directly involved in patient care. Nurses and patients provided separate and independent assessments of the patient's sleep. The three tools were:

- Newcastle Sleep Assessment Tool 1 (NSAT1): quantity of sleep banded in hours
- Newcastle Sleep Assessment Tool 2 (NSAT2): quality of sleep compared to their normal sleep
- Newcastle Sleep Assessment Tool 3 (NSAT3): overall quality rating of sleep on a numerical 1–10 scale.

Statistical analysis demonstrated that there was a weak correlation between the nurses' judgements and the patients' experiences of their sleep, suggesting it would be inappropriate to rely solely on nurses' judgements. The greatest association between nurses and patients related to the quality of patients' sleep compared with their normal sleep (NSAT2). The analysis also indicated that patients preferred the tools that rated the sleep in hours (NSAT1) and assessed the comparative quality of sleep (NSAT2). The Newcastle Sleep Assessment Tool has been amended to take account of these findings (see Figure 13.2). It is also recommended that for the purposes of determining quality and quantity sleep in critically ill patients, wherever possible, the patients' perceptions should be ascertained and acted on as being the most likely to provide a valid assessment. The authors, however, emphasize that although experience has shown the new two-

Patient's Assessment of Number of Hours of Sleep

Please tick box to indicate the number of hours of sleep. This should be completed at the end of your normal sleep period. If required a clinician can assist with writing your answers on this sheet.

	0 to 2 hours	More than 2 hours to 4 hours	More than 4 hours to 6 hours	More than 6 hours to 8 hours	More than 8 hours
Patient's Assessment					

Patient's Assessment of Quality of Their Sleep Compared to Normal Quality of Sleep

Please tick box to indicate quality of sleep at the end of your normal sleep period. If required a clinician can assist with writing your answers on this sheet.

	Much less than normal quality of sleep	Less than normal quality of sleep	Normal quality of sleep	More than normal quality of sleep	Much more than normal quality of sleep
Patient's Assessment					

Figure 13.2 Newcastle Sleep Assessment Tool.

part tool to be useful, it requires further research to assess reliability and validity.

Factors that disrupt and promote sleep

Several factors have been found to disrupt sleep and some are more difficult to overcome in critical care, such as severity of illness. However, many strategies have been tested to promote sleep (Table 13.1) and should be considered as part of the care of the critically ill. A small number of assessments can be undertaken in order to establish patient's preferred sleeping regimens, which can then be incorporated as part of their care to promote sleep. The following patient preferences should be assessed.

1   Where they sleep – this can vary between in a bed or in a chair (in a chair may not be possible due to their critical illness and safety requirements).
2   How many pillows, sheets, blankets and/or duvets are used.
3   The time they go to sleep and wake up.
4   Medications, herbal remedies, or other means (such as milky drinks) used to help improve their sleep.

Table 13.1 Factors that disrupt and promote sleep

Sleep disruption factors	Sleep promotion strategy
Severity of illness	
▪ Inflammatory mediators produced in sepsis (Friese 2008)	▪ Procedures such as taking blood samples should, where possible, be completed prior to the planned sleep time. It is recognized that with any critically ill patient the specific frequency and timings of blood sampling will need to be reviewed continually and will depend on the patient's condition
▪ Numerous arousals with regular assessment of haemodynamic status, for example blood sampling for assessment or use of automated sphygmomanometer	
Mechanical ventilation	▪ Procedures such as taking blood samples should, where possible, be completed prior to the planned sleep time
▪ Numerous arousals with the regular assessment of respiratory status (Cooper et al. 2000; Gabor et al. 2003), for example blood sampling for gas analysis	▪ Ensure the ventilation tubing is free from excess water. This will prevent noise from water in the tubes and associated alarms being set off in the ventilator alarms
▪ Numerous arousals in order to maintain a clear airway and good ventilation	▪ Set alarm limits appropriate to prevent unnecessary high alarm noise
▪ Greater sleep fragmentation in patients receiving pressure support than assisted controlled ventilation (Parathasarthy and Tobin 2004)	
Noise	▪ Use single rooms where possible as these may reduce noise intensity (Gabor et al. 2003)
▪ Prolonged, intermittent and loud noise (Freedman et al. 2001; Xie et al. 2009). This can be from a number of sources, including	▪ Provide a quiet environment by fitting drawers and bin lids with foam pads to minimise noise on closing
▪ staff conversation (Gabor et al. 2003)	▪ Fit and maintain doors correctly to ensure they close quietly
▪ technical equipment with safety alarms and alerts initiated when patients' observations and respiratory function move outside safe parameters, e.g. haemodynamic monitors and ventilators (Gabor et al. 2003)	▪ Adjust monitor alarms and parameters to reduce noise levels and to avoid unnecessary alarms (NB Alarms must always be heard to detect changes in the patient's condition)
	▪ Consider switching telephones to vibrate or turning down the volume. If telephones are located in patient bed spaces transferring calls to these bed spaces should be avoided overnight
	▪ Request staff to wear soft-soled shoes
	▪ Ensure staff discussions are kept to a minimum and away from the patients' bed areas
	▪ Reduce noise peaks, during the night or a rest period, by turning off televisions and radios (Mann et al. 1986) and asking visitors to leave
	▪ Offer earplugs to patients as a way of reducing the noise levels. Earplugs should be considered with lucid and oriented patients and assistance given to insert and remove them to ensure them comfortable (Richardson et al. 2007b)
	▪ Consider suitability of masking sounds, for example by using music or white noise such as ocean waves (Gragert 1990)
	▪ Soundproof incubators with acoustic foam (Johnson 2001) or replace ceiling tiles (Blomkvist et al. 2005)

Light and darkness	■ Constant light – which affects the body's ability to sleep. The body's circadian rhythm relies on periods of light and darkness for sleep and wakefulness to be maintained (Hood et al. 2004) ■ Bright lights are often required 24 hours/day to enable accurate assessment of patient observations. Raising of light levels occurs in order to carry out procedures and patient care activities, such as venous or arterial catheter replacements, chest drain insertions and essential pressure area care, when patients are admitted or transferred out, and emergency events ■ The degree to which night light is dimmed is dependent on the stability of the patient	■ Use light to strengthen the circadian timing system (Campbell et al. 1993; Shochat et al. 2000; Wakamura and Tokura 2001) ■ Open blinds and curtains to allow daylight in during awake periods to reinforce the circadian rhythms. During waking hours consider increasing the patient's physical activity within the level of ability (Alessi et al. 2005) ■ Dim lights at night, where possible, to an appropriate level (NB The clinician must be able to adequately assess the patients' condition, colour and skin at all times, including throughout the night) ■ Consider drawing curtains around the patient to shield from unnecessary light. (NB To ensure patients can be observed at all times curtains should not be fully closed) ■ Avoid switching on lights whenever possible ■ Offer eye masks to lucid, oriented patients who must be able to remove them on their own (Richardson et al. 2007b)
Ambient temperature	■ High temperatures – due to the large amount of heat generating equipment (Tembo and Parker 2009) ■ High summertime temperatures – resulting in high critical care unit temperatures (Richardson et al. 2007b)	■ Adjust room temperatures and/or air conditioning to ensure patient comfort ■ Consider using other cooling devices, such as a fan (Richardson et al. 2007b)
Clinical interventions and procedures	■ Positioning for nocturnal X-rays, monitoring or administering medications, and unblocking of intravenous catheters (Bartick et al. 2010) ■ Constant disruption through the night (Tamburri et al. 2004) to carry out essential care, such as eye care, mouth care and pressure area care	■ Consider offering a 90-minute block of uninterrupted sleep (quiet time/rest period) to increase the amount of sleep during the day (Lower et al. 2003). A period between 13.00 and 16.00 hrs is best as this is one of the natural lows in the body circadian rhythm (Lower et al. 2003) ■ Appropriately manage and coordinate procedures (Bartick et al. 2010). For example, activities such as mouth care, changing bed linen and positioning the patient to ensure comfort for sleeping (Bartick et al. 2010) ■ Where possible (patients whose conditions are more physiologically stable) cluster patient care activities and procedures throughout the night to allow for complete sleep cycles (Bartick et al. 2010). These activities can include: turning, taking a temperature, non-invasive blood pressure, removal of blood samples and administering drugs (Inouye et al. 2000) ■ At night try to allow at least 2 hours (based on a complete sleep cycles) between the sleep-disturbing interventions to provide opportunities to improve sleep (Lower et al. 2003)

(Continued)

427

Table 13.1 *(Continued)*

	Sleep disruption factors	Sleep promotion strategy
Medication	A wide variety of drugs to treat sleep disorders do not always improve patients' sleep (Bourne and Mills 2004) ■ Benzodiapines – shorten the time taken to fall asleep and increase the length of sleep (Drouot et al. 2008), but reduce the amount of the last stage of sleep (REM sleep). This decreases the physiological benefits of sleep (Tembo and Parker 2009) ■ Beta-blockers – such as metoprolol easily cross the blood brain barrier and can precipitate nightmares (Friese 2008) ■ Methyldopa – similar affects to metoprolol (Honkus 2003) ■ Catecholomines – disrupt sleep (Parathasarthy and Tobin 2004) ■ Inotropes – used in continuous infusions, stimulate the reticular activating system (Friese 2008), thus reducing REM sleep ■ Diuretics – can disturb sleep in uncatheterized patients as they awake to urinate (Pandharipande and Ely 2006)	■ Sedatives and analgesics can be used to assist patients to sleep in critical care units (Tembo and Parker 2009) ■ Pharmacological use in isolation will not prevent or resolve the majority of sleeping problems (Bourne and Mills 2004) ■ Medication considerations should be examined on a continuous basis – checking and discussing the prescribed drugs and whether any omissions or modifications could be made (Bourne and Mills 2004). For example, could nightmare-inducing beta-blockers be reduced. (NB Some drugs in use due to the critical illness are necessary and alterations are not always possible or appropriate [Bourne and Mills 2004])

Pain and stress	■ Pain – ranked as one of the most stressful problems in intensive care units and a major contributor to sleep deprivation (Drouot et al. 2008)
	■ Pain – interrupts sleep from the illness processes and the clinical procedures used to monitor and maintain patients (Tembo and Parker 2009)
	■ Inability to lie comfortably – clinicians should assume uncomfortable beds contribute to discomfort and sleep disruption (Tembo and Parker 2009)
	■ Stress – from the experience of being hospitalized. For example:
	  ○ patients' temporary loss of income
	  ○ social isolation
	  ○ inability to perform domestic tasks
	  ○ care of pets
	all impact on sleep (Humphries 2008)
		■ Often complete pain relief in patients is difficult to achieve (Coyer et al. 2007)
		■ Assess and treat with the most suitable pain relief
		■ Ensure the patient's anxieties or worries are minimized prior to sleep (Humphries 2008)
		■ Encourage patients to relax all muscles, using relaxing mental imagery, such as imaging peaceful images and surroundings and or the use of relaxing music (Chlan and Tracy 1999)

Procedure guideline 13.1: **Sleep assessment and promotion**

Staff caring for critically ill patients should have the knowledge, skills and expertise to assess and promote sleep.

Action	Rationale
1 If appropriate, and where possible, explain and discuss the planned care with the patient. If the patient lacks the capacity to make decisions the practitioner must act in the patient's best interests.	To ensure that the patient understands the planned care and gives their valid consent. To ensure the patient's best interests are maintained (Mental Capacity Act 2005).
2 Ascertain patients' sleeping preferences: ■ where they would like to sleep ■ number of pillows and blankets, etc. ■ sleeping position ■ what time they go to sleep ■ what time they wake.	To gather information on which to base care to promote sleep. For example, by mirroring home comforts, sleep maybe more easily achieved (Bartick et al. 2010).
3 Assess quality and quality of sleep activity, by asking the patient.	To ensure the patient's perception is obtained. Staff observation is unreliable as staff underestimate patients' sleep (Aurell and Elmqvist 1985; Richardson et al. 2007a).
4 Record the outcome of the assessment of sleep on a daily basis.	To ensure accurate record keeping and to assess outcome of sleep promotion activities.
5 Ensure environmental noise minimized. Consider using the following: ■ ensure bins, doors and drawers close quietly ■ change telephones to vibrate or minimize volume ■ adjust alarms noises to appropriate levels and parameters ■ request staff wear soft-soled shoes ■ reduce staff conversation to a minimum ■ offer earplugs to reduce noise perception ■ turn off televisions and music or provide head sets for patient wishing to listen.	To reduce the risk of sleep disruption. Patients have a greater tendency to sleep disruption when sound levels are increased (Xie et al. 2009). ■ Conversation is one of the most disruptive noises (Gabor et al. 2003). ■ Earplugs increase sleep quality and quantity (Richardson et al. 2007b).
6 Ensure light and darkness rhythms are applied to match the body's circadian rhythm. Consider using the following. ■ Dim lights to an appropriate level at night. ■ Draw curtains around patients' bed spaces to reduce light exposure. ■ Avoid switching on lights. ■ Offer eye masks to reduce light exposure.	To strengthen the circadian rhythm. Using light and darkness strengthens the circadian rhythm and increases the quality of subsequent night-time sleep (Campbell et al. 1993; Shochat et al. 2000; Wakamura and Tokura 2001). Eye masks increase sleep quality and quantity (Richardson et al. 2007b).
7 Deliver care in clusters ('clustered care') leaving a 90-minute to 2-hour gap between interventions. Consider clustering the following cares: turning, taking temperature, non-invasive blood pressure, blood gases and administering drugs.	To allow the patient time for a complete sleep cycle. A complete sleep cycle lasts 90 minutes therefore allowing 2 hours between the sleep disturbing interventions provides opportunities to improve chances for sleep (Lower et al. 2003).
8 Offer a 90-minute to 2-hour block of uninterrupted sleep (quiet time/rest period) at a period between 13.00 and 16.00 hrs.	To use the body's circadian rhythm to promote sleep. Between 13.00 and 16.00 hrs is one of the natural lows in the body's circadian rhythm (Lower et al. 2003).
9 Control environment temperature to that suitable for sleep by altering heating, air conditioning, using fans, offering extra blankets.	To assist patients to maintain their temperature. People are unable to regulate temperature during REM sleep (American Sleep Association 2007), therefore being too cold or hot will cause the patient to unnecessarily awaken.

429

(Continued)

Procedure guideline 13.1: (Continued)

10 Provide analgesics or use other means to ameliorate or remove pain.	To ensure the patient is not in any pain. Pain is ranked as one of the most stressful problems in 'intensive care' units and a major contributor to sleep deprivation (Drouot et al. 2008)
11 Encourage relaxation or relaxation techniques.	To reduce psychological stress. Psychological stress can affect sleep, therefore ensure the patient's anxieties or worries are minimized prior to sleep (Humphries 2008).
12 Document assessment and care provided.	To: ■ provide an accurate record ■ monitor effectiveness of procedure ■ reduce the risk of duplication of treatment ■ provide a point of reference or comparison in the event of later questions ■ acknowledge accountability for actions ■ facilitate communication and continuity of care. (NMC 2008; HCPC 2012; GMC 2013)

Competency statement 13.1: Specific procedure competency statements for sleep assessment

Complete assessment against relevant fundamental competency statements (see Chapter 2, pp. 20, 21)	Evidence
Specific procedure competency statements for sleep assessment	**Evidence of competency for sleep assessment**
Demonstrate ability to: ■ teach and assess or ■ learn from assessment.	Examples of evidence of teaching, assessing and learning.
Demonstrate knowledge and understanding of the importance of sleep and sleep assessment including: ■ physiological methods ■ non-physiological methods.	
Identify risks, potential problems and complications of sleep deprivation, including: ■ confusion ■ hallucinations ■ irritability ■ decreased pain tolerance ■ delirium ■ delayed recovery from illness.	
Demonstrate skills that are required in relation to assessing a patient's sleep, including: ■ patient preference ■ communication.	
Demonstrate the correct technique for the procedure to undertake sleep assessment, including: ■ use of tools ■ documentation.	

Competency statement 13.2: Specific procedure competency statements for sleep promotion

Complete assessment against relevant fundamental competency statements (*see* Chapter 2, pp. 20, 21)	Evidence
Specific procedure competency statements for sleep promotion	**Evidence of competency for promoting sleep**
Demonstrate ability to: ■ teach and assess or ■ learn from assessment.	Examples of evidence of teaching, assessing and learning.
Identify reason(s) for promoting sleep, including: ■ prompt recovery from illness ■ patient satisfaction with levels of sleep.	
Identify risks, potential problems and complications of sleep deprivation sleep, including: ■ confusion ■ hallucinations ■ irritability ■ decreased pain tolerance ■ delirium ■ delayed recovery from illness.	
Demonstrate knowledge and understanding of local and national policies, guidance, and procedures in relation to sleep assessment and promotion, including: ■ local policy in relation to 'quiet' and 'rest' times in critical care.	
Demonstrate knowledge and understanding of evidence base in relation to promoting sleep, including: ■ clustering procedures and minimizing disruptions ■ medication timings ■ noise-reduction strategies ■ appropriate application of earplugs and eye masks.	
Demonstrate knowledge and understanding of the evidence base in relation to environmental factors that promote sleep, e.g. mirroring patient's home routine, protecting quiet time, reducing noise levels from bins, drawers and telephones, using light and curtains appropriately.	
Demonstrate knowledge and understanding of staff actions that may promote sleep, e.g. impact of wearing soft-soled shoes, applying quiet staff discussion away from the patients bed area.	
Demonstrate ability to alter monitor alarms to a safe and appropriate level, during the wake/sleep cycle.	

References and further reading

Alessi CA, Martin JL, Webber AP et al. (2005) Randomised, controlled trial of a nonpharmacological intervention to improve abnormal sleep/wake patterns in nursing home residents. *Journal of the American Geriatrics Society* 53(5): 803–810.

American Sleep Association (2007) *What is Sleep?* http://www.sleepassociation.org/index.php?p=whatissleep [accessed 12 March 2011].

Aurell J and Elmqvist D (1985) Sleep in the surgical intensive care unit: continuous polygraphic recording in nine patients receiving postoperative care. *British Medical Journal* 190: 1029–1032.

Bartick MC, Thai X, Schmidt T et al. (2010) Decrease in as-needed sedative use by limiting night time sleep disruptions from hospital staff. *Journal of Hospital Medicine* 5(3): 20–24.

Beecroft JM, Ward M, Younes M et al. (2008) Sleep monitoring in the intensive care unit: comparison of nurse assessment, actigraphy and polysomnography. *Intensive Care Medicine* 34: 2076–2083.

Blomkvist V, Eriksen CA and Theorell T (2005) Acoustics and psychosocial environment in intensive coronary care. *Occupational Environment Medicine* 62: e1.

Bourne RS and Mills GH (2004) Sleep disruption in critically ill patients-pharmacological considerations. *Anaesthesia* 59: 374–384.

Bourne RS, Minelli C, Mills GH and Kandler R (2007) Clinical review: sleep measurement in critical care patients: research and clinical implications. *Critical Care* 11: 226.

Buysse DJ, Reynolds CF, Monk TH et al. (1989) The Pittsburgh Sleep Quality Index: a new instrument for psychiatric practice and research. *Psychiatry Research* 28: 193–213.

Campbell SS, Dawson D and Anderson MW (1993) Alleviation of sleep maintenance insomnia with timed exposure to bright light. *Journal of American Geriatric Society* 41: 829–836.

Chlan L and Tracy MF (1999) Music therapy in critical care. Guidelines for intervention. *Critical Care Nurse* 19(3): 35–42.

Chuman MA (1983) The neurological basis of sleep. *Heart and Lung* 12: 177–181.

Closs J (1988) Assessment of sleep in hospital patient: a review of methods. *Journal of Advanced Nursing* 12: 501–510.

Commission for Patient and Public Involvement in Health (2007) *Care Watch: National survey of patient's views on privacy and dignity in the NHS.* Birmingham: Commission for Patient and Public Involvement in Health.

Cooper AB, Thornley KS, Young GB et al. (2000) Sleep in critically ill patients requiring mechanical ventilation. *Chest* 117: 809–818.

Coyer MF, Wheeler KM, Wetzig MS and Couchman AB (2007) Nursing care of the mechanically ventilated patient: what does the evidence say? *Intensive and Critical Care Nursing* 23(2): 71–80.

Culpepper-Richards K (1988) Sleep in the ICU: a description of night sleep patterns in the critical care unit. *Heart and Lung* 17: 35–42.

Dines-Kalinowski CM (2002) Nature's nurse: promoting sleep in the ICU. *Dimensions of Critical Care Nursing* 21: 32–35.

Dogan O, Ertekin S and Dogan S (2005) Sleep quality in hospitalized patients. *Journal of Clinical Nursing* 14: 107–113.

Drouot X, Cabello B, d'Ortho MP and Brouchard L (2008) Sleep in the intensive care unit. *Sleep Medicine Review* 12(5): 391–403.

Edwards GB and Schuring LM (1993) Pilot study: validating staff nurses's observations of sleep and wake states among critically ill patients using polysomnography. *American Journal of Critical Care* 2: 125–131.

Ellis BW, Lancaster R, Raptopoulos P et al. (1981) The St Mary's Hospital sleep questionnaire: a study of reliability. *Sleep* 4: 93–97.

Freedman NS, Gazendam J, Levan L et al. (2001) Abnormal sleep/wake cycles and the effect of environmental noise on sleep disruption in the intensive care unit. *American Journal of Respiratory and Critical Care Medicine* 163: 451–457.

Friese RS (2008) Sleep and recovery from critical illness and injury: a review of theory, current practice, and future directions. *Critical Care Medicine* 36(3): 697–705.

Gabor JY, Cooper AB, Crombach SA and Lee B (2003) Contribution of the intensive care unit environment to sleep disruption in mechanically ventilated patients and healthy subjects. *American Journal of Respiratory and Critical Care Medicine* 167: 708–721.

Gragert MD (1990) The use of a masking signal to enhance sleep of men and women 65 years of age and older in the critical care environment. PhD thesis. The University of Texas at Austin. Cited in Xie H, Kang J and Mills GH (2009) Clinical review: the impact of noise on patients' sleep and the effectiveness of noise reduction strategies in intensive care units. *Critical Care* 13: 208.

General Medical Council (2013) *Good Medical Practice*. London: GMC. http://www.gmc-uk.org/gmp2013 [accessed 25 March 2013].

Guyton AC and Hall JE (1997) *Human Physiology and Mechanisms of Disease (6e)*. Philadelphia: Saunders.

Health and Care Professions Council (2012) *Standard of Conduct, Performance and Ethics*. London: HCPC. http://www.hcpc-uk.org/assets/documents/10003B6EStandardsofconduct,performanceandethics.pdf [accessed January 2013].

Hobson JA (1995) *Sleep*. Scientific American Library, USA.

Hodgson LA (1991) Why do we need sleep? Relating theory to nursing practice. *Journal of Advanced Nursing* 16: 1503–1510.

Honkus VL (2003) Sleep deprivation in critical care units, *Critical Care Nursing Quarterly* 26: 179–189.

Hood B, Bruck D and Kennedy G (2004) Determinants of sleep quality in the healthy aged: the role of physical, psychological, circadian and naturalistic light variables. *Age and Ageing* 33: 159–165.

Humphries JD (2008) Sleep disruption in hospitalised adults. *Medsurg Nursing* 17(6): 391–396.

Inouye SK, Bogardus ST Jr, Baker DI et al. (2000) The Hospital Elder Life Program: a model of care to prevent cognitive decline and functional decline in older hospitalized patients. *Journal of American Geriatric Society* 48: 1697–1706.

Jensen DP and Herr KA (1993) Sleeplessness. *Nursing Clinics of North America* 28: 385–405.

Johnson AN (2001) Neonatal response to control noise inside the incubator. *Paediatric Nursing* 27: 600–605.

Knabb B and Engel-Sittenfeld P (1983) The many facets of poor sleep. *Neuropsychobiology* 10: 141–147

Kryger M, Roth T and Dement W (2000) *Principles: sleep medicine (3e)*. Philadelphia: Saunders.

Lower J, Bonsack C and Guion J (2003) Peace and quiet. *Nursing Management* 34(4): 40.

Mann NP, Haddow R, Stokes L et al. (1986) Effect of night and day on preterm infants in a newborn nursery: randomised trial. *British Medical Journal* 293: 1265–1267.

McGonigal K (1986) The importance of sleep and the sensory environment to critically ill patients. *Intensive Care Nursing* 2: 73–83.

Mental Capacity Act (2005) http://www.legislation.gov.uk/ukpga/2005/9/pdfs/ukpga_20050009_en.pdf [accessed 9 February 2012].

Meza S, Mendez M, Ostrowski M and Younes M (1998) Susceptibility to periodic breathing with assisted ventilation during sleep in normal subjects. *Journal of Applied Physiology* **85**: 1929–1940.

Novaes MAFP, Aronovich A, Ferraz MB and Knobel E (1997). Stressors in ICU: patients' evaluation. *Intensive Care Medicine* **23**: 1282–1285.

Nursing and Midwifery Council (2008) *The Code: standards of conduct, performance and ethics for nurses and midwives.* London: NMC. http://www.nmc-uk.org/Documents/Standards/The-code-A4-20100406.pdf [accessed 15 February 2012].

Olsen D, Borel C, Laskowitz and McConnell E (2001) Quiet time: a nursing intervention to promote sleep in neurocritical care units. *The American Journal of Critical Care* **10**: 74–78.

Pandharipande P and Ely WE (2006) Sedative and analgesic medications: risk factors for delirium and sleep disturbances in the critically ill. *Critical Care Clinics* **22**: 313–327.

Parathasarthy S and Tobin MJ (2004) Sleep in the intensive care unit. *Intensive Care Medicine* **30**: 197–206.

Perez de Ciriza A, Otamendi S, Ezenarro A and Asiain MC (1996) Factors causing stress in patients in intensive care units. *Enfermeria Intensiva* **7**: 95–103.

Redeker NS, Tamburri L and Howland CL (1998) Prehospital correlates of sleep in patients hospitalised with cardiac disease. *Research in Nursing and Health* **21**: 27–37.

Redeker RS (2000) Sleep in acute care settings: an integrative review. *Journal of Nursing Scholarship* **32**: 31–49.

Redeker RS, Ruggiero JS and Hedges C (2004) Sleep is related to physical function and emotional well being after cardiac surgery. *Nursing Research* **53**(3): 154–162.

Reid E (2001) Factors affecting how patients sleep in the hospital environment. *British Journal of Nursing* **10**(14): 912–915.

Richardson A, Crow W, Coghill E and Turnock C (2007a) A comparison of sleep assessment tools by nurses and patients in critical care. *Journal of Clinical Nursing* **16**: 1660–1668.

Richardson A, Coghill E and Allsop M (2007b) Earplugs and eye masks: do they improve critical care patients' sleep? *Nursing in Critical Care* **12**(6): 278–286.

Richardson A, Thompson A, Coghill E et al. (2009) Development and implementation of a noise reduction intervention programme: a pre- and post audit of three hospital wards. *Journal of Clinical Nursing* **18**: 3316–3324.

Richardson SJ (1997) A comparison of tools for the assessment of sleep pattern disturbance in critically ill adults. *Dimensions of Critical Care Nursing* **16**: 223–239.

Shapiro CM and Flanigan MJ (1993) Function of sleep. *British Medical Journal* **306**: 383–385.

Shochat T, Martin J and Marler M (2000) Illumination levels in nursing home patients: effects on sleep and activity rhythms. *Journal of Sleep Research* **9**: 373–379.

Simpson T, Lee E and Cameron C (1996) Patients' perceptions of environmental factors that disturb sleep after cardiac surgery. *American Journal of Critical Care* **5**: 173–181.

Snyder-Hapern R and Verran JA (1987) Instrumentation to describe subjective sleep characteristics in healthy subjects. *Research in Nursing and Health* **10**: 155–163.

Soehren P (1995) Stressors perceived by cardiac surgical patients in the intensive care unit. *American Journal of Critical Care* **5**: 71–76.

Tamburri LM, DiBrienza R and Zozula R (2004) Nocturnal care interactions with patients in critical care units. *American Journal of Critical Care* **13**: 102–112.

Tembo AC and Parker V (2009) Factors that impact on sleep in intensive care patients. *Intensive and Critical Care Nursing* **25**: 314–322.

Wakamura T and Tokura H (2001) Influence of bright light during daytime on sleep parameters in hospitalised elderly patients. *Journal of Physiology, Anthropology, and Applied Human Science* **20**: 345–351.

Wallace CJ, Robins J, Alvord LS and Walker JM (1999) The effects of earplugs on sleep measures during exposure to simulated intensive care unit noise. *American Journal of Critical Care* **8**: 210–219.

Weitzman ED, Nogliere AB, Perlow CD et al. (1974) Effects of prolonged 3-hour sleep-wake cycle on sleep stages, plasma cortisol, growth hormone and body temperature in man. *Journal of Clinical Endocrinology and Metabolism* **38**: 1018–1030.

Wilson VS (1987) Identification of stressors related to patients' psychologic response to the surgical intensive care unit. *Heart and Lung* **16**: 267–273.

Xie H, Kang J and Mills GH (2009) Clinical review: the impact of noise on patients' sleep and the effectiveness of noise reduction strategies in intensive care units. *Critical Care* **13**: 208.

Chapter 14

Physical mobility and exercise interventions for critically ill patients

D.J. McWilliams[1] and Amanda Thomas[2]

[1]University Hospitals Birmingham NHS Foundation Trust, Birmingham, UK
[2]The Royal London Hospital, London, UK

Critical Care Manual of Clinical Procedures and Competencies, First Edition.
Edited by Jane Mallett, John W. Albarran, and Annette Richardson.
© 2013 John Wiley & Sons, Ltd. Published 2013 by John Wiley & Sons, Ltd.

Definitions

Physical morbidity is the deterioration in physical wellbeing, resulting from disease, illness, injury, or sickness. When associated with critical illness and restricted mobility, this morbidity relates to a multitude of physical complications commonly seen within a critical care population. These include muscle wasting and weakness, reduced cardiovascular and respiratory fitness, a reduced bone density and neurological changes.

Mobility and exercise interventions in critically ill patients incorporate a range of care activities, including passive movements and positioning for those still in the acute phase of illness, to walking and active exercise for those who are awake or in the recovery phase.

Aims and indications

Mobility and exercise interventions are essential components for all critically ill patients due to the short- and long-term complications of a period of critical illness and the associated period of potentially prolonged bed rest (McWilliams et al. 2011). These interventions should be instituted as early as possible to limit the degree of physical morbidity. This can include the implementation of preventative and/or maintenance strategies, or the early mobilization of critically ill patients to limit the level of physical morbidity and maximize physical recovery. When instituted they specifically aim to:

- assess for early changes and institute early and appropriate interventions
- prevent or limit the onset of joint contractures and muscle shortening
- regain muscle strength and function
- maximize functional ability
- aid airway clearance though optimization of posture and increased lung volumes
- improve cardiorespiratory fitness and facilitate independence/reliance from mechanical ventilation (commonly known as 'weaning')
- prevent formation of thrombi (e.g. deep vein thrombosis).

Background anatomy and physiology

The causes of the negative physical effects of critical illness are multifactorial, including, but not limited to:

- bed rest and prolonged immobility – due to muscular inactivity, reduced neurological stimulation and reduced weight bearing on joints and bones
- sepsis – which has been linked to a higher incidence of critical illness polyneuromyopathy (CIPNM)
- malnutrition – due to a reduced calorie intake or a higher metabolic demand
- use of certain medications – for example corticosteroids or neuromuscular blocking agents, which have been associated with the onset of CIPNM

- corresponding neuropathies – for example critical illness polyneuropathy, which are associated with greater degrees of physical morbidity and longer periods of recovery (Op De Coul et al. 1991; Garnacho-Montero et al. 2005).

Muscles

Muscle wasting and weakness is common. When present it can take many months to recover, especially with prolonged periods of mechanical ventilation. It has been identified that those patients staying more than 10 days on level 3 care facilities and over 50 years of age are particularly at risk (Jones and Griffiths 2000). Muscle mass has been shown to decrease at a rate of between 2 and 4% per day during the first 2–3 weeks of ICU admission (Helliwell et al. 1998; Brower 2009), although in some patients the loss is as much as 6% per day (Bloomfield 1997). As well as a reduction in muscle mass there can also be a deterioration in terms of muscle performance. Maximal knee extensor contraction (that is, maximal strength) has been shown to decrease by 22% after 14 days of bed rest (Hespel et al. 2001) and as much as 53% after 28 days of limb immobilization (Veldhuizen et al. 1993). Muscular decline is particularly evident in the anti-gravity muscles of the lower limbs and torso, leading to problems with balance. This muscle weakness is closely associated with a reduced capacity to perform functional activities such as rolling, self-care and walking. In follow-up studies, muscular dysfunction and impaired functional status have been found to be still present at one year post hospital discharge (Herridge et al. 2003).

Respiratory

From a respiratory perspective, in a patient who is mechanically ventilated, partial or complete atelectasis (collapse) of the left lower lobe can occur and be apparent on chest X-ray within 48 hours of recumbency (Talmore et al. 2006). In addition, in the presence of critical illness there is a reduction in diaphragmatic activity, where atrophy and contractile dysfunction have been identified as early as 18 hours following the onset of mechanical ventilation (Levine et al. 2008). This reduction in lung volume and diaphragmatic function results in decreased respiratory capacity and adversely impacts on secretion clearance and successful 'weaning' from mechanical ventilation.

Cardiovascular

The heart is also affected by a period of critical illness and immobility, demonstrating a 28% reduction in stroke volume after just 10 days of bed rest (Convertino et al. 1982). To meet resting oxygen demands this would require an increase in resting heart rate and an increased ejection fraction (percentage of blood expelled by the heart in each beat). The reduction in both cardiovascular and respiratory function has a subsequent effect on overall fitness, with a reduction in the maximal oxygen consumption (VO_2 max) at a rate of 0.9% per day (Kashihara et al. 1994). VO_2 max refers to the maximum capacity of an individual's body to transport and use oxygen during aerobic exercise, reflecting the physical fitness of the individual. This reduced exercise capacity could contribute to delayed physical recovery and prolonged weaning from mechanical ventilation.

Bone

During a period of critical illness there is a degree of bone demineralization as a result of reduced activity levels. Studies have shown a loss of 6 mg of calcium per day from bone tissue, which equates to approximately 2% of total bone density after just one month of immobility (Zerwekh et al. 1998). It can take up to two years to return to the prior level of bone density. Clinically, this may leave the skeletal system weaker and more brittle in survivors of critical illness.

Neurological

Alongside the deterioration in the muscles there have been observed changes specifically related to the neurological system. Patients often present with paraesthesia, which may be reported as numbness or pins and needles, tingling or burning. There is also an observed reduction in proprioception, which is the person's ability to know where their limbs are in space. This can cause problems with coordination and balance.

Long term

In an analysis of a group of acute respiratory distress syndrome (ARDS) survivors at one year post level 3 care facility discharge, functional status (assessed via the 6-minute walk test) was found to be only 66% of that compared with normal values achieved by a healthy population (Herridge et al. 2003). This supported an earlier study by Eddleston et al. (2000), which demonstrated that it frequently takes 9–12 months for patients to return to employment. Prolonged mechanical ventilation has also been associated with impaired health related quality of life (assessed via the SF36 quality of life questionnaire) up to 3 years after discharge, even when patients are living independently at home (Coombes et al. 2003). This results in an increased dependence on both carers and secondary care services.

Evidence and current debates

Both the degree and impact of physical morbidity associated with critical illness have been increasingly recognized in recent times (Griffiths and Jones 2007). In view of this, rehabilitation within critical care has been made a high priority by the government, evident in the publication of *Quality Critical Care* (DH 2005). This document states that hospitals must provide structured rehabilitation services for critically ill patients within level 3 care facilities, on the wards, and in the community and/or outpatient setting. More recently the NICE short clinical guideline 83, *Rehabilitation after Critical Illness* (NICE 2009), emphasizes the importance of starting rehabilitation as early as clinically possible for patients who are critically ill. This process involves the identification of high-risk patients (for example those with pre-existing physical or psychological problems) and providing early and structured rehabilitation to optimize recovery while encouraging ongoing assessment and screening of patients throughout their recovery period (*see also* Chapter 16).

Early mobilization has been shown to decrease the time taken for patients to breathe independently from their ventilator (weaning time) and reduce length of stay (LOS) in a critical care facility (McWilliams et al. 2008; Morris et al. 2008). This ultimately leads to a shorter stay in hospital (Schweickert et al. 2009). Early and structured rehabilitation has also been associated with reduced incidence of delirium and improvements to respiratory and peripheral muscle strength in comparison with control subjects receiving no physiotherapy (Chiang et al. 2006). However, these results need to be interpreted with a degree of caution, as the majority of data is taken from North America and Asia, where physiotherapy is not routinely provided on a daily basis, instead patients are only seen when referred by the medical team. In the Morris et al, (2008) study only 13% of control subjects received any form of physical therapy while on a critical care facility. It is therefore unclear as to whether the enhanced effects achieved via these mobility protocols are really superior or transferable to a UK population where daily physiotherapy and rehabilitation are a part of usual care. It does, however, provide evidence that structured and regular physiotherapy for critically ill patients is more effective than no input at all.

Review of components of physical mobility and exercise

Assessment of readiness to mobilize

Much has been made of 'early rehabilitation' within critical care, but it is perhaps important to understand what this term really means. Early rehabilitation does not refer to a specific time point (e.g. day 5). Instead, rehabilitation commences, or should commence, as soon as the patient is able to participate and should be individualized and specific to the patient's needs. Even with the move towards earlier waking and active rehabilitation programmes, some disease processes, such as severe sepsis and ARDS, will lead to unavoidable periods of prolonged mechanical ventilation and possibly periods of deep sedation (Navarrete-Navarro et al. 2000). To assess patient readiness a number of mobilization protocols have been produced (Stiller 2000), although these may in fact serve to delay mobilization inappropriately (Thomas et al. 2009).

Table 14.1 Early mobilization: parameters for decision making

Parameter	Examples of considerations (Note: these examples do not preclude early mobilization but should be considered as part of an assessment of readiness)

Cardiovascular stability	■ Unstable heart rhythm within last 24 h
	   ■ fast atrial fibrillation (AF)
	   ■ raised troponin T
	■ Pulmonary arterial catheter in situ
	■ Hypotension requiring the use of inotropic support and/or noradrenaline

Respiratory stability/reserve	■ Airway concerns
	   ■ poor tolerance of endotracheal tube
	   ■ unstable tracheostomy tube in situ
	■ High work of breathing (WOB)
	   ■ increased respiratory rate
	   ■ accessory muscle use

Paralytic agents and or sedation	■ Use of muscle paralysing medications ■ Degree of sedation NB No restriction if patient is minimally sedated and/or is able to follow simple commands
Fractures (unstable)	■ Position of fracture ■ Instability of fracture Seek specific orthopaedic advice
Haematological status and/or deranged clotting	■ Platelets less than 20×10^9/L ■ Hb less than 8.0 g/dL (or following sudden drop in Hb, e.g. 2 g/dL over 24 h)
Agitation and/or deliruim	■ Degree of agitation and or delirium There may need to be some restrictions with patients who are unable to follow command or with unpredictable behaviour
Abdominal wound dehiscence	■ Risk to further wound dehiscence Consider the use of a corset or vacuum therapy

Interventions

During the acute phases of illness

If a patient is physiologically not ready or it is not appropriate for them to mobilize, other rehabilitation measures should be initiated where possible. In view of the protracted recovery period associated with physical morbidities, prevention or limitation of exposure to the many associated risk factors is an essential starting point in improving outcomes for patients requiring critical care. Measures such as ensuring early and sufficient nutrition, glycaemic control and avoidance of the use of neuromuscular blocking agents where possible may reduce the degree of muscle weakness (McWilliams et al. 2011). To this end, a more proactive approach to the removal of sedation has been advocated to facilitate earlier waking (Kress et al. 2000). This would, therefore, allow earlier and more active rehabilitation with the aim of combating the negative impact outlined previously. For example, even short periods of decreased sedation

to allow spontaneous breathing on the ventilator, even for as few as 5 minutes regularly throughout the day, has been demonstrated to decrease the degree of diaphragmatic contractile dysfunction (Gayan-Ramirez et al. 2005). This would then go some way to preserving respiratory muscle strength and function and enable shorter ventilator weaning times.

Rehabilitation for patients unable to sit on the edge of the bed (i.e. 'bed bound')

Passive movements and active exercise

It is particularly important throughout this acute stage of illness that rehabilitation occurs to prevent/reduce the risk of physical morbidity (see Table 14.2). The most commonly used intervention to achieve this is through passive limb movements, which aim to maintain muscle length and joint range of motion (ROM), although there is still much debate with regard to their effectiveness within critical care. There is some evidence, however, that the use of continuous passive motion (CPM) devices prevent some degree of muscle loss. CPM involves placing a limb (upper or lower) in a device that will passively move through a pre-set range of move-

Table 14.2 Benefits and precautions of mobility and exercise interventions for critically ill patients

Benefits	Precautions
Passive movements (commenced after 24 hours on critical care unit once patient stable)	
■ Ability to assess joint range and any limitations ■ Maintains joint range of movement (ROM) and prevents contractures ■ Utilizes muscle pump (i.e. aids drainage of oedema)	■ Will not effect muscle strength ■ Can damage flaccid and unprotected joints ■ Need to know normal joint range ■ Be aware of attachments (e.g. avoid kinking arterial tubing, haemofiltration tubing, etc.)
Active assisted/Active exercise	
■ Ability to assess muscle power ■ Maintains/increases muscle strength and function ■ Increases exercise tolerance ■ Maintains joint ROM and prevents contractures ■ Utilizes muscle pump	■ Be aware of attachments (e.g. avoid kinking arterial tubing, haemofiltration tubing, etc.)
Chair position/Upright sitting in bed	
■ Upright posture encourages basal lung expansion ■ Improves trunk stability ■ Prevents/addresses postural hypotension ■ Better view for patient/psychological benefits	■ Weary or agitated patients (slumping) ■ Abdominal distension – may be difficult or uncomfortable ■ Should still be in conjunction with active exercises
Sitting on the edge of the bed	
■ Ability to assess sitting balance (static and dynamic) ■ Ability to assess bed mobility ■ Psychological benefits ■ May be able to assess/progress to sit to stand ■ Prerequisite to transfers (weight bearing through lower limbs) ■ Increases exercise tolerance	■ Attachments, ventilator tubing, etc. ■ Cardiovascular stability ■ Needs at least 2–3 people ■ Postural hypotension
Sitting out in a chair	
■ Further psychological benefits as patient's level of mobility progresses ■ Full weight bearing ■ Upright posture encourages basal lung expansion and increases functional residual capacity (FRC) ■ Improves bowel function ■ Increases muscle strength ■ Increases exercise tolerance	■ Inotropes ■ Use of aids if unable to transfer (hoist, standing hoist, banana board etc.) ■ Attachments ■ Needs at least 2–3 people
Mobilization/Ambulation	
■ Increases exercise tolerance ■ Promotes active deep breathing (increased lung volumes) ■ Enables secretion mobilization ■ Improves bowel function ■ Increases FRC facilitates weaning as a result of above	■ Intensity (BORG breathlessness scale [Borg 1982]) ■ Tubing, ventilator tubing, etc ■ Monitor patient closely (HR, BP, oxygen saturations)

439

ment for a directed time period. This technique has been widely used in orthopaedic rehabilitation. Griffiths et al. (1995) observed the use of CPM in a group of sedated and paralysed, ventilated trauma patients. Each patient's uninjured leg was placed in the CPM device for up to 9 h/day with the other leg acting as control. Due to the effect of the neuromuscular blocking agents, no muscle contraction was possible and, as such, the specific effect of mechanical stretch could be assessed independent of any muscular activity. It was observed that the control leg muscle wasted much faster and demonstrated some fibre necrosis compared with the leg that had been passively moved. The leg that had undergone CPM also retained more protein and a better, healthier

structure, the effects of which were more pronounced in the slow type 1 muscle fibres (used for aerobic activity). Whether passive movements (specific movement of joints through the patient's ROM) performed by physiotherapists have the same benefit is unknown as there are no clinical studies that set out to specifically determine the benefits within a critically ill population (Stiller 2000). However, Griffiths et al. (1995) demonstrated the physiological harm of immobility and the potential benefit of passive movements, while also demonstrating the importance of implementing active exercise programmes as early as possible to try to maintain or improve muscle strength. The use of splinting may also be of benefit in preserving both joint range and muscle length, particularly for ankles, wrists and hands. A variety of splints are available to meet this aim and can be obtained from orthotic services, although consideration needs to be given to underlying skin integrity. During this acute phase of illness and the associated immobility there would also be an increased risk of developing venous thromboembolism (VTE). To combat this, prophylactic treatment would be indicated and may be managed through the use of anti-embolism stockings, intermittent pneumatic compression devices (e.g. Flowtron) and or anticoagulation therapies.

Electrical muscle stimulation

In the acute stage of a patient's illness, while they may still be deeply sedated or even paralysed, active exercise is obviously not an option. There is some debate, however, over the benefit of electrical muscle stimulation (EMS) devices as a method of maintaining muscle strength. This process involves the elicitation of muscle contractions using electric impulses to prevent the muscle loss associated with a period of bed rest. The electrical impulses are delivered through electrodes attached to the skin in direct proximity to the muscle to be contracted. A number of clinical trials have demonstrated smaller reductions in muscle strength for the specific muscles stimulated when compared with non-stimulated muscles in the same subject (Zanotti et al. 2003; Gerovasili et al. 2009). As yet no effect has been demonstrated in a reduction of critically ill patients' length of stay, ventilator weaning times and mortality rates, or an increase in functional status. Therefore the role of EMS remains in question, with the benefits of maintaining only the specific muscles that can be accessed for EMS unknown. EMS may still have some utility in the early rehabilitation of those patients unable to participate in active therapy measures.

Positioning

If a patient cannot be mobilized from the bed to sit on the bed edge or out in a chair, the high sitting (that is, when the patient is sat upright) posture can be attempted. Electronically controlled beds that provide multiple bed shapes and which can tilt the whole bed are particularly suited to assisting this procedure. In healthy individuals, upright postures are associated with a larger functional residual capacity (FRC, the volume of air left in the lungs at the end of normal passive expiration) when compared with recumbent postures (Blair and Hickam 1955; Jenkins et al. 1988). As the FRC becomes larger, the point on the lung's pressure volume curve at which ventilation occurs moves upwards, leading to increased lung compliance and decreased lung resistance (Navajas et al. 1988). In other words, the higher volume of air inside the lungs acts to keep airways open, preventing collapse and decreasing the work of breathing. Importantly, this increase in FRC with the associated alterations in body posture to the upright (or vertical) position is mechanical, allowing both an increase in overall ventilation and tidal volume (Sasaki et al. 1977). In the intubated and ventilated patient, upright postures and the associated increase in FRC enhance the matching of ventilation with pulmonary blood flow (V/Q ratio; see also Chapter 5) in all dependent lung regions (Woodrow 2000). This leads to enhanced overall tissue oxygenation (Jones and Dean 2004). In addition, backrest elevation of 30–45° (compared with supine lying) reduces the incidence of pneumonia in ventilated patients by reducing the risk of aspiration of gastric or oropharangeal secretions, which may be colonized by bacteria (Drakulovic et al. 1999; Hubmayr 2002;). This position is, therefore, recommended as the position of choice for ventilated patients (Grap et al. 2003; Vollman 2004). The upright posture may also represent an orthostatic challenge to the cardiovascular system, eliciting an increase in both heart rate and blood pressure (Jones et al. 2004). Therefore, the high sitting posture may be used as a precursor to more advanced mobility techniques as the patient's tolerance to upright sitting is enhanced. However, the inability to maintain an effective upright position in the semi-conscious patient may limit its physiological effectiveness. Assessing the patient's tolerance and maintenance of the vertical sitting position should be ascertained by careful monitoring throughout and following the procedure.

Critically ill patients with specific clinical presentations can also benefit from positioning strategies. For example, correct positioning of the patient with known or suspected raised intracranial pressure (e.g. the patient with head injury or liver failure) can prevent or minimize secondary brain injury associated with cerebral oedema, hypoxia and hypotension (Sullivan 2000). Positioning these patients is aimed at reducing intracranial pressure (ICP) and maintaining this pressure for as long as possible within set parameters (Griffiths and Gallimore 2005). A reduction in ICP is achieved by promoting cerebral venous drainage (Feldman et al. 1992). Elevation of the head of the bed by 30° above the level of the heart is considered important for reducing ICP (Sullivan 2000; Winkelman 2000) (see also Chapter 11). However, the effect of this position on mean arterial pressure, cerebral perfusion pressure, cardiovascular and respiratory parameters should be constantly monitored since alterations from normal or required parameters can be a secondary cause of brain injury (Fan 2004; Christie 2008) (see also Table 14.3).

In addition to the supine bed posture, the side lying posture can be a useful position for patients with the following presentations:

1 Compromised venous return, e.g. pelvic/abdominal mass, pregnancy. Side lying allows the abdominal contents to fall forwards and towards the bed, resulting in a decreased mechanical impedance to blood flow in the descending thoracic and lumbar aorta.

2 Reduced conscious levels leading to decreased airway patency. The side lying position will allow the airway to remain unobstructed in the event that a patient with reduced conscious levels vomits their gastric contents.

Table 14.3 Type of physical position, use and location

Position	Use	Reference
High sitting in bed	■ Provides an orthostatic challenge ■ Reduces the incidence of pneumonia in ventilated patients ■ Increases functional residual capacity (FRC) compared with supine or slumped postures ■ Enhances the matching of ventilation with pulmonary blood flow	Chapter 14
Semi-recumbent sitting	■ Semi-recumbency significantly reduces ventilator-associated pneumonia	Chapter 12
Positioning for raised ICP	■ Prevents or minimizes secondary brain injury associated with cerebral oedema, hypoxia and hypotension ■ Promotes cerebral venous drainage	Chapter 14
Positioning for a chest X-ray	■ Improves visualization of all anatomical details	Chapter 14
High side lying	■ Decreases mechanical impedance to blood flow in descending thoracic and lumbar aorta ■ Elicits active and stabilization muscle contractions throughout the body ■ Alleviates pain and discomfort associated with immobility ■ For pressure area care ■ Reduces stretch or tension on muscles and tendons ■ Enables gravity assisted drainage of pulmonary secretions ■ Optimizes pulmonary ventilation and perfusion matching	Chapter 14
Lateral 30° tilt	■ Minimizes risk of pressure ulceration ■ Removes pressure from body prominences	Chapter 12
Side lying	■ Decreases mechanical impedance to blood flow in descending thoracic and lumbar aorta ■ Elicits active and stabilization muscle contractions throughout the body ■ Alleviates pain and discomfort associated with immobility ■ For pressure area care ■ Reduces stretch or tension on muscles and tendons ■ Enables gravity-assisted drainage of pulmonary secretions ■ Optimizes pulmonary ventilation and perfusion matching	Chapter 14
Prone positioning	■ Elicits alveolar recruitment ■ Enhances ventilation perfusion matching ■ Relieves hypoxia	Chapter 5
Sitting on the bed edge	■ Enables early assessment of acute response to exercise ■ Enables assessment of sitting balance ■ Enables assessment of readiness to sit out of bed	Chapter 14
Chair sitting	■ Encourages mobilization ■ Assists breathing, as diaphragm moves down with gravity	Chapters 12 and 14
Hoist transfer to chair	■ Facilitates a daily seating programme ■ Enhances lung volume ■ Promotes muscular strength and endurance	Chapter 14
Log rolling	■ Allows physical examination of the back, transfer on and off specialized spinal boards, and pressure area care in a patient with known or suspected spinal injury	Chapter 14
Tilt table	■ Facilitates weight bearing in the lower limb ■ Prevents joint contractures and muscle shortening in the lower limb ■ Improves lower limb strength and endurance ■ Increases arousal ■ Elicits a physiological strain and activates the oxygen transport pathway	Chapter 14
Ambulation	■ Improves muscle strength ■ Increases endurance ■ Benefits the patient's psychological status ■ Promotes independence	Chapter 14

3 Global muscle weakness. Side lying postures elicit active and stabilization muscle contractions throughout the body. In particular, moving body parts into a changed relationship with respect to gravity allows a variety of different muscle actions (Weissman and Kemper 1993) and joint positions to be elicited, and can help to alleviate pain and discomfort associated with immobility and muscle weakness.

4 Known, developing, or at risk of pressure ulcers. Side lying is one of the positions chosen to reduce contact pressure along the spine, sacrum and buttocks.

5 Unilateral pelvic or lower limb pain. Side lying may alleviate pain by allowing some musculoskeletal structures to be positioned comfortably without excessive muscle stretch or tension.

6 Altered muscular tone. Positioning the lumbar spine, hips and knees in flexion can reduce generalized extensor tone.

7 Chest infection, for gravity-assisted drainage of pulmonary secretions. Positioning the patient in side lying positions alters the relationship of the main branches of the bronchial tree with respect to gravity. This may allow the gravity-assisted drainage of pulmonary secretions into the bronchus and facilitate the movement of secretions towards the mouth.

8 Lung pathology, to optimize ventilation and perfusion matching. In a patient who is breathing independently, a gravity-dependent gradient of pulmonary perfusion exists such that pulmonary perfusion is greatest in the lower lung. If the lower lung is affected by a pathological process that decreases the ventilation to that lung (e.g. pneumonia), a ventilation/perfusion mismatch will occur, since the blood is flowing to areas that are not receiving ventilation. In this instance, placing the affected lung uppermost places the healthy lung lowermost, allowing a matching of pulmonary ventilation and perfusion.

9 Abdominal distension, e.g. ascites, bulky disease, to optimize lung volume. Side lying allows the abdominal contents to fall forwards and away from the thoracic diaphragm. The resulting reduction in mechanical impedance to diaphragm descent during inspiration allows a greater tidal volume to be generated and may enhance functional residual capacity.

10 Careful appreciation of the multiple clinical benefits of alternative positioning strategies can assist to reduce complications and improve the outcome of a critical care admission. (Staudinger et al. 2010).

Correct patient positioning can also improve the outcome of frequently used critical care diagnostic tests. For example, the completion of an anteroposterior chest radiograph or portable chest X-ray in the critical care unit requires the patient to be positioned as upright as possible, with particular attention to symmetrical alignment of the trunk and spine. An X-ray taken when the patient is supine, slumped,

rotated, or asymmetrical will not provide adequate visualization of the lung fields and diaphragm, making interpretation of results ambiguous (Stewart 1992). Erect and semi-erect postures will improve visualization of all anatomical details and assessment of pulmonary vasculature in the presence of pleural fluid.

While positioning or moving patients who are critically ill can elicit many beneficial physiological effects, not all patients are able to be moved safely. Some patients may have restrictions on the degree of trunk and limb movements because of fractures involving the pelvis or spine. In these instances, specific procedures need to be implemented to allow safe movement for basic nursing care. For example, the 'log roll' is a manual handling procedure whereby the patient is moved from their back to their side while keeping the spine in neutral alignment. The log roll is used to allow physical examination of the back, transfer on and off specialized spinal boards and for pressure area care in a patient with known or suspected spinal injury (Griffiths and Gallimore 2005). Expert positioning and moving of the patient with suspected spinal injury is essential to prevent secondary spinal cord damage (Harrison 2007). The principle of log rolling is to constantly maintain neutral spinal alignment by preventing flexion or extension of the spine regardless of the level of injury (Grundy and Swain 2002; Griffiths and Gallimore 2005). The number of times a patient is rolled should be kept to an absolute minimum. Only suitably qualified and experienced health professionals should attempt this procedure. The log roll procedure requires five to six members of staff who are competent in the procedure and who work under the control of a team leader. The team leader is responsible for maintaining alignment of the patient's head and neck, and directing the procedure. The reader is referred to an excellent publication produced by the Spinal Cord Injury Centres of the United Kingdom and Ireland for an illustrated description of the log rolling procedure (Harrison 2007).

For some patients requiring a critical care admission, positioning may be employed as a management technique for their underlying physiological or system failure. For example, the prone position may be employed as one element of the management for severe hypoxic respiratory failure secondary to acute lung injury, e.g. acute respiratory distress syndrome (ARDS). The technique of prone positioning is covered in Chapter 5 in relationship to prone ventilation and details the indications, mechanisms of improved ventilation, risks and practical considerations for using this extreme position.

Rehabilitation for patients deemed ready to sit on the edge of the bed

Once a patient is deemed ready, the process of sitting on the edge of the bed forms an important part of the early physical assessment and subsequent provision of a structured rehabilitation programme and seating plan. This process can be labour intensive, particularly for those patients who are obese, have low arousal, or profound weakness, where it may take four or five members of staff to transfer the patient on to the edge of the bed. However, this process provides vital information with regard to the patient's sitting balance and readiness for sitting out of bed. In addition, it demonstrates their physiological stability in response to activity and positional change, as well as providing many other specific physical and psychological benefits (*see* Table 14.2). The assessment of physiological stability should include observation of any changes in the patient's heart rate, blood pressure, respiratory rate, tidal volume and any issues with pain or discomfort (Figure 14.1).

Once physiological stability has been determined an individualized seating programme can be devised utilizing the bed in an upright position or a full body sliding board (such as a Patslide®) to place the patient on to a stretcher chair where there is insufficient trunk control. For those patients who have a basic level of trunk stability, transfers out of bed are deemed appropriate and sitting out in a chair is advised. Transfer from bed to chair may be through the use of specialist equipment such as hoists that transfer the patient in a seated position, hoists that transfer a patient in standing position, or physically assisted standing transfers to the chair regularly throughout the day. As indicated previously (Chapter 12) sitting out should generally be limited for those patients at risk of developing pressure ulcers to a maximum

of 2 hours. For those patients who could tolerate longer periods it would be beneficial to increase the frequency of sitting in a chair (as opposed to the duration) after this point. Appropriate seating and pressure relief is fundamental to ensure that patients of varying physical abilities can sit out safely, comfortably and in a well-supported position. A tilt table may also be used to enable early standing, with the aim of facilitating weight bearing, preventing joint contractures, improving lower limb strength and to increase arousal, although no quantitative evidence is currently available to support their use with critical care patients (Chang et al. 2004).

Ambulation

Once a seating plan has been formulated and the patient is sitting out on a daily basis, progression can be made to more active exercise, mobilization and ambulation. This may initially consist of mobilization around the bed space or transfer on to a portable ventilator to allow ambulation over greater distances. As the patient's muscle strength and stamina increase, so does the level of functional independence (Schweickert et al. 2009). This also will have beneficial effects on the patient's psychological status as they become more independent and the improvements become more tangible (Figure 14.2). The process of mobilization does, however, bring additional safety considerations, such as:

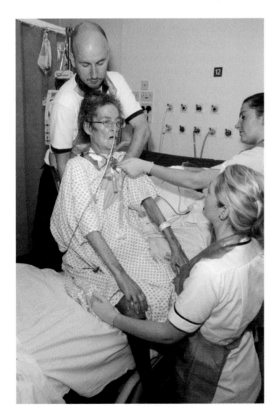

Figure 14.1 Early mobilization of critically ill patient: sitting on edge of bed.

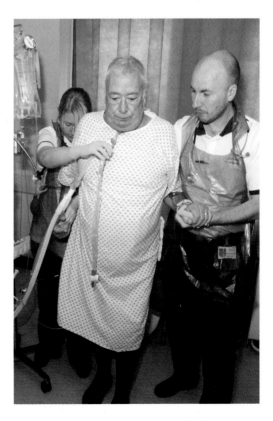

Figure 14.2 Early mobilization of a critically ill patient: ambulation.

- airway stability
- portability of equipment, such as the use of portable ventilators and suction devices
- management of multiple attachments
- reduced level of monitoring.

Monitoring of the intensity level of the activity and the patient's physiological response is vital to ensure the safety of these interventions. Portable oxygen saturation monitors and the BORG breathlessness scale (a visual analogue scale of the patient's perception of breathlessness [Borg 1982]) provide quick and simple methods of achieving ongoing monitoring during mobilization and ambulation.

The process of early rehabilitation can be enhanced through involvement of the multidisciplinary team (MDT), with the aim of restoring function, facilitating independence from mechanical ventilation and maximizing physical status at hospital discharge (Martin 2002). This is a key recommendation set out in the NICE critical illness rehabilitation guideline (NICE 2009), which highlights the importance of coordination of care as well as regular multiprofessional assessments and formalized goal setting (*see* Chapter 16). For example, weekly discussion and MDT goal setting for those patients with longer stays in critical care provide an ideal forum to achieve this aim. This was demonstrated in a study by Black et al, (2007), where, following the introduction of meetings to discuss longer-term patients, mortality was reduced by 22% for those with a stay in critical care facilities of more than 14 days and by 53% with a length of stay of greater than 50 days. Involvement of, for instance, occupational therapists may also be useful in improving patient outcomes. For example, sitting on the edge of the bed or in the chair provides an excellent opportunity to engage the patient in functional activities such as grooming, which may be associated with increased levels of functional independence at hospital discharge (Schweickert et al. 2009).

Post-critical care rehabilitation

Due to the significant degree of physical morbidity it is important that rehabilitation is an ongoing process and not one that finishes as patients leave a critical care unit or indeed hospital. For many survivors of critical illness recovery is a slow process and can often be incomplete, leading to reduced functional independence and thus quality of life. The use of structured, self-directed rehabilitation programmes (in the form of a self-help manual), which commence in hospital and extend into the community setting, have shown some benefit in improving physical function and quality of life (QoL) at 6 months post discharge. However, this was observed to be lower than the mean QoL for somebody with a severe illness (Jones et al. 2003). Structured exercise programmes such as exercise classes are successfully utilized in many other clinical areas with a variety of patients (Siebens et al. 2000); however, self-directed programmes may be limited by patient motivation and when utilized may not be sufficient to address the psychological sequelae of critical illness. More recently exercise class-based rehabilitation programmes have been advocated to optimize the recovery of patients following discharge from hospital. These programmes of cardiovascular exercise and education have shown significant improvements in patient's physical function, with improved walking distances of 48% and 76% on the 6-minute walk test and incremental shuttle walk test respectively over an 8-week period. These physical improvements were also associated with significant reductions in both anxiety and depression scores (McWilliams et al. 2009). At present more research is needed to assess the effectiveness of these interventions in promoting full and long-term recovery.

Measurement of manual handling risk

The moving and handling of patients and equipment in the critical care environment by manual force is a necessary and important aspect of critical care practice. However, manual handling can place the practitioner at significant risk of musculoskeletal injury. It is therefore a legislated requirement that risks associated with manual handling of patients and equipment are eliminated or reduced to the lowest practicable level (Health and Safety Executive 1992). Acute care settings invariably operate a manual handling policy that involves the least amount of manual moving and handling possible, with full recognition of the need to balance the risk of undertaking a manual handling task with the necessity for the task to be performed. Decisions regarding any manual handling activity should be based on the result of a comprehensive manual handling risk assessment. The risk assessment process is particularly important for those manual handling tasks that are classified as therapeutic or rehabilitative in nature, since these tasks often require significant manual effort to elicit active patient participation.

Best practice for the measurement of manual handling risk involves the completion of a standardized risk assessment designed specifically for the clinical setting and common tasks encountered by the critical care practitioner. The risk assessment may incorporate an evaluation of the components relating to the nature of the task and the load, the individual completing the task and the environment in which the task is taking place. An assessment that follows this model is known as the TILE assessment (Task, Individual, Load and Environment), an example of components that may be included in the TILE assessment is given in Table 14.4.

A list of commonly used manual handling equipment and specialist seating is provided in Table 14.5.

Table 14.4 Components that may be included in the TILE assessment

Component	Points to evaluate
The TASK	*Does the task involve:* ■ Holding the load away from the body? ■ Twisting or stooping? ■ Reaching upwards? ■ Large vertical movements? ■ Carrying the load over long distances? ■ Strenuous pushing or pulling? ■ Unpredictable movement of the load? ■ Repetitive movements? ■ Prolonged postures? ■ An imposed speed of movement? ■ Movements hindered by clothing or personal protective equipment? ■ The need for multiple staff?
The INDIVIDUAL capacity	*Does the individual require:* ■ Unusual capabilities? ■ Special information or training to complete the task safely? ■ Specific assistance due to a pre-existing (medical) condition that places them at risk, e.g. pregnancy?
The LOAD itself	*Is the load:* ■ Heavy? ■ Bulky/unwieldy? ■ Difficult to grasp? ■ Unstable/unpredictable? *Is or does the patient:* ■ Overweight? ■ Totally dependent? ■ Able to assist the movement? ■ Uncooperative? ■ Confused? ■ In pain? ■ Have poor skin integrity? ■ Prone to falls? ■ Have movement restrictions due to their injury, medical condition or treatment?
The ENVIRONMENT	*Is the environment:* ■ Hot/humid or cold? ■ Poorly lit? ■ Cramped? ■ At a safe working height? ■ On steps/stairs or uneven floor surfaces? ■ On a slippery floor? ■ Obstructed by furniture?

The reader should locate relevant risk assessment procedures within their own working environments.

Assessment of the characteristics of a manual handling task will enable the identification of control measures that may be employed to reduce risk. These measures may include the use of manual handling equipment (sliding sheets, boards, lifting aids and mechanical aids), the provision of specialist training, an identification of the minimum skill levels of staff and modifications of the task that may reduce the risk involved. Such risk reduction measures should be adequately documented for each patient and reviewed regularly. If unacceptable levels of risk are involved in the task the critical care practitioner should consult their organization's manual handling department for advice prior to attempting the task.

Table 14.5 Moving and handling equipment

Equipment and mode of action	Patient indication	Rationale
Overhead hoist May be a mobile hoist which can be moved to the bedside or a ceiling hoist	Suitable for most critically ill patients who are unable to stand and transfer either independently or with assistance A variety of hoists and slings are available to accommodate patients of varying weights and sizes	Allows transfer of patients to a chair earlier in their rehabilitation pathway
Standing hoist A hoist that assists the patient to transfer between two seating surfaces, e.g. from sitting on the edge of the bed to a chair or commode An example of one such device is the ARJO standing and raising aid (Encore)	For those patients with a basic level of trunk control and leg strength but who are unable to stand without assistance Once in standing position can also be used to facilitate transfers to the chair It is also possible to remove the foot plate and allow walking in a supported position	Allows weight bearing through the upper and lower limbs to maintain/improve muscle strength and prevent bone demineralization Assists patients into standing and can facilitate walking (with footplate removed)
Tilt table A flat plinth-like device that allows a patient to be gradually raised from supine to a standing position	Commonly used for neurological patients and those with prolonged stays in level 3 critical care facilities	Movement of patients into a standing position in order to: ■ facilitate weight bearing ■ prevent muscle contractures ■ improve lower limb strength ■ increase arousal
Stretcher chairs Chairs that can be made completely flat, allowing patients to be transferred out of bed using a Patslide	Critically ill patients who are not suitable for hoisting, including those with: ■ external pelvic fixation ■ cardiovascular instability/risk of postural drop as bed can be laid flat ■ significantly reduced muscle tone	Promotes earlier mobilization and the benefits of sitting for those patients who otherwise would be unable to sit out
Recliner chairs Chair that can be adjusted into a more reclined position and allow elevation of the legs	Patients who have absent or insufficient trunk control to maintain an upright posture Patients with postural hypotension as it allows the seating position to be tailored according to cardiovascular stability	Promotes earlier mobilization and the benefits of sitting for those patients who otherwise would be unable to sit out
Patslide Full body sliding board that is designed to be used when transferring patient in a semi reclined or lying position	Primarily used to transfer patients from one bed to another Also used to transfer on to other flat surfaces such as tilt tables and stretcher chairs	Reduces risk of injury to staff and patients for transfers
Sliding sheets	For all patients unable to move themselves independently in bed	Reduces friction between the patient and the mattress reducing the load to be moved

Procedure guideline 14.1: Positioning a patient in high sitting (adapted with permission from the Royal Marsden Hospital Manual of Clinical Nursing Procedures)

Equipment

- Electronically controlled bed
- 2 members of staff
- Pillows

- Manual handling equipment may be required, e.g. sliding sheets or a hoist, depending on local best practice standards

Procedure

Action	Rationale
1 Where possible, explain and discuss the procedure with the patient. If the patient lacks the capacity to make decisions the practitioner must act in the patient's best interests.	To ensure that the patient understands the procedure and gives their valid consent. To ensure the patient's best interests are maintained (Mental Capacity Act 2005).
2 Ensure the bed brakes are on and position the bed at a safe working height for all team members.	To promote health and safety of team members.
3 Starting in the supine position with the bed flat, position the patient with their hips over the hinge of the automatic bed elevator or backrest of the bed.	To ensure postural alignment and hip flexion when sitting up in the bed. To prevent lumbar spine flexion when sitting up in the bed.
4 (a) Place a pillow under the patient's knees or use the electrical control of the bed to bend the patient's hips and knees to 30° if possible. (b) The degree of hip and knee flexion will be determined by: range of movement; any pain experienced on flexion; any underlying trauma or disease (such as fractures involving the femur or pelvis, leg oedema, abdominal distension); whether the patient is confused or agitated; or by the existence of equipment (such as femoral catheters or other medical devices).	(a) To reduce lumbar spine strain when sitting erect. (a) Bending the knees reduces the stretch on the hamstrings in the long sitting position (i.e. the trunk is flexed but the knees remain in extension) making the position more comfortable. (a) To assist the maintenance of the erect sitting position. (b) To avoid causing tissue damage, pain, or discomfort due to excessive stretch or compression of lower limb structures. (b) To reduce the risk of dislodging any medical devices.
5 (a) Elevate the head of the bed to bend the patient at the hips such that the trunk is as erect as possible. (b) The angle of elevation may be limited by hip or abdominal pain, fracture involving the femur or pelvis, abdominal distension, or confusion/agitation.	(a) To increase basal lung expansion (Pryor and Webber 2002). (a) To optimize end expiratory lung volume by assuming a near vertical position of the trunk (Navajas et al. 1988; Jenkins et al. 1988). (a) To increase physiological and muscular tolerance to the head up posture. (b) To avoid causing tissue damage due to excessive stretch or compression of lower limb structures.
6 (a) Place a pillow to support both upper limbs. (b) Extra care should be taken for patients with chest drains, upper limb and trunk weakness, surgery involving the shoulder/upper limb/breast/thorax, lymphoedema, or fractures of the ribs or upper limbs.	(a) To provide upper limb alignment and support. (a) To maintain trunk alignment. (b) To provide additional support for the upper limbs. (b) To avoid causing tissue damage due to excessive stretch or compression of upper limb or trunk structures.

(Continued)

Procedure guideline 14.1: (Continued)

Action	Rationale
7 (a) Tilt the whole bed in a foot down direction to achieve a close to vertical position of the trunk.	(a) To encourage basal lung expansion (Pryor and Webber 2002).
(b) The degree of foot down tilt may be modified by pain, abdominal distension and head, trunk, or upper limb weakness. Physically weak patients may not be able to manage the very vertical posture and extra care should be taken to ensure the patient can maintain head alignment and control when placed in this position.	(a) To optimize end expiratory lung volume by assuming a near vertical position of the trunk (Navajas et al. 1988; Jenkins et al. 1988). (a) To encourage active head shoulder girdle and trunk muscular activity and control. (a) To provide an orthostatic stress (Jones and Dean 2004).
8 Document care.	To: ■ provide an accurate record ■ monitor effectiveness of procedure ■ reduce the risk of duplication of treatment ■ provide a point of reference or comparison in the event of later questions ■ acknowledge accountability for actions ■ facilitate communication and continuity of care. (NMC 2008; HCPC 2012; GMC 2013)

NB Care should be taken when high sitting the patient with poor skin integrity or reduced sensation as this position increases the risk of developing pressure damaged areas or ulcers. In addition, high sitting postures will elicit fatigue due to an increase in head, shoulder and trunk muscle activity, and should be utilized for short specified periods only. The semi-conscious patient may be unable to maintain this position effectively. Care should be taken to immediately reposition the patient once postural alignment is unable to be maintained.

Procedure guideline 14.2: Positioning a patient in high side lying (adapted with permission from the Royal Marsden Hospital Manual of Clinical Nursing Procedures)

Equipment
■ Pillows
■ Towels
■ Manual handling equipment may be required, e.g. sliding sheets or a hoist

Procedure

Action	Rationale
1 Where possible, explain and discuss the procedure with the patient. If the patient lacks the capacity to make decisions the practitioner must act in the patient's best interests.	To ensure that the patient understands the procedure and gives their valid consent. To ensure the patient's best interests are maintained (Mental Capacity Act 2005).
2 Ensure the bed brakes are on and position the bed at a safe working height for all team members.	To promote health and safety of team members.
3 Starting in the supine position roll the patient to their side. (a) Ensure patient is positioned in the centre of the bed with hips over the hinge of the automatic mattress elevator or backrest of the bed. (b) Place one or two pillows under the patient's head. Pillows should ensure alignment of the head with the spine, avoiding excessive neck rotation. (c) Place pillows against the length of the patient's spine. (d) Extra care should be taken for those patients with a tracheostomy, central venous catheters, or recent head and neck surgery.	(a) To prevent lateral flexion of the trunk. NB If the patient's hips are not correctly aligned, elevation of the bed head will cause trunk side flexion, which is both anatomically limited and uncomfortable. (b) To ensure the airway remains patent. (b) To support the head in the mid-position. (b) To support the shoulder contours. (c) To provide support and stability and prevent rolling. (d) To prevent any medical devices being dislodged.

4 (a) Semi-flex the underneath leg at the hip and the knee.	(a) To support the patient in a stable position and prevent rolling on to their back.
(b) Extra care should be taken with the degree of flexion for those patients who have hip or knee pain or loss of movement, fracture involving the femur or pelvis, leg oedema, femoral CVC, or other venous access devices.	(b) To reduce the risk of causing pain and further tissue damage. (b) To prevent any medical devices being dislodged.
5 (a) Semi-flex the uppermost leg at the hip and knee.	(a) To prevent lumbar spine rotation when the bed head is elevated.
(b) Place a pillow between the patient's knees.	(b) To reduce the risk of excessive pressure on the skin between the knees.
6 (a) Place the underneath arm in front of the patient's body with scapula protracted (this would not be appropriate for patients with shoulder pathology).	(a) To promote patient comfort.
(b) Flex elbow.	(b) To promote shoulder alignment.
(c) Extra care should be taken for patients with low tone in the affected arm, lymphoedema, or who have venous or arterial access cannula or catheters in that arm.	(c) To avoid causing soft tissue damage, pain and discomfort due to excessive stretch or compression of structures which lack active muscular control. (c) To reduce the risk of dislodging medical devices.
7 Place a pillow between the uppermost arm and the trunk.	To allow a natural position of the shoulder and arm. To promote patient comfort.
8 (a) Elevate the head of the bed.	(a) To elevate the patient's trunk. (a) To optimize ventilation and perfusion matching in the dependent lung (Dean 1985). (a) To optimize gravity-assisted drainage of pulmonary secretion (Ross et al. 1992; Cecins et al. 1999).
(b) The angle of elevation will be influenced by pain, abdominal distension, fracture involving the femur or pelvis, the positioning of femoral CVCs or other venous access devices.	(b) To reduce the risk of further tissue damage and of dislodging medical devices.
9 Inspect the patient's position from the foot of the bed to ensure correct alignment of the head, shoulders and trunk. Adjust posture as required using additional pillows.	To promote patient comfort. To minimize soft tissue damage, pain and discomfort.
10 Document care and any observations.	To: ■ provide an accurate record ■ monitor effectiveness of procedure ■ reduce the risk of duplication of treatment ■ provide a point of reference or comparison in the event of later questions ■ acknowledge accountability for actions ■ facilitate communication and continuity of care. (NMC 2008; HCPC 2012; GMC 2013)

NB Care should be taken in lying the patient directly over the greater trochanter and other bony prominences as this increases the risk of developing pressure ulcers (Hawkins et al. 1999).

Procedure guideline 14.3: Positioning a patient in side lying (adapted with permission from the Royal Marsden Hospital Manual of Clinical Nursing Procedures)

Equipment

- Pillows
- Manual handling equipment may be required, e.g. sliding sheets or a hoist

Procedure

Action	Rationale
1 Where possible, explain and discuss the procedure with the patient. If the patient lacks the capacity to make decisions the practitioner must act in the patient's best interests.	To ensure that the patient understands the procedure and gives their valid consent. To ensure the patient's best interests are maintained (Mental Capacity Act 2005).
2 Ensure the bed brakes are on and position the bed at a safe working height for all team members.	To promote health and safety of team members.
3 Starting in the supine position roll the patient to their side. (a) Place one or two pillows under the patient's head ensuring the airway remains patent. (b) Extra care should be taken for those patients with a tracheostomy, central venous cannulas, or recent head and neck surgery. (c) Place pillows against the length of the patient's spine. (d) Extra care should be taken for those patients with a tracheostomy, central venous catheters, or recent head and neck surgery.	(a) To support the head in the mid-position. (a) To support the shoulder contours. (b) To avoid dislodging any medical device. (c) To provide support and stability and prevent rolling. (d) To prevent any medical devices being dislodged.
4 (a) Semi-flex the underneath leg at the hip and the knee. (b) Extra care should be taken with the degree of flexion for those patients who have hip or knee pain or loss of movement, fracture involving the femur or pelvis, leg oedema. (c) Extra care should be taken for those patients who have femoral tubing or other venous access devices.	(a) To support the patient in a stable position and prevent rolling. (b) To avoid causing pain and or any further tissue damage. (c) To avoid dislodging any medical devices.
5 (a) Semi-flex the uppermost leg at the hip and knee. (b) Place a pillow between the patient's knees.	(a) To prevent lumbar spine rotation. (a) To support the pelvic girdle. (b) To reduce the risk of excessive pressure on the skin between the knees.
6 (a) Place the underneath arm in front with scapula protracted (this would not be appropriate for patients with shoulder pathology). (b) Flex elbow. (c) Extra care should be taken with patients with low tone in the affected arm, lymphoedema, or who have access tubing in that arm.	(a) To promote patient comfort. (b) To promote shoulder alignment. (c) To avoid causing soft tissue damage, pain and discomfort due to excessive stretch or compression of structures that lack active muscular control. (c) To avoid dislodging any medical devices.
7 Document care and any observations.	To: - provide an accurate record - monitor effectiveness of procedure - reduce the risk of duplication of treatment - provide a point of reference or comparison in the event of later questions - acknowledge accountability for actions - facilitate communication and continuity of care. (NMC 2008; HCPC 2012; GMC 2013)

Note: Care should be taken in lying the patient directly over the greater trochanter as this increases pressure at this interface and the risk of developing pressure ulcers (Hawkins *et al*, 1999)

Procedure guideline 14.4: Positioning a patient with raised intracranial pressure (30° tilt) (adapted with permission from the Royal Marsden Hospital Manual of Clinical Nursing Procedures)

Equipment	
■ Pillows ■ 2 to 4 members of staff	■ Manual handling equipment may be required e.g. sliding sheets or a hoist

Procedure

Action	Rationale
1 Where possible, explain and discuss the procedure with the patient. If the patient lacks the capacity to make decisions the practitioner must act in the patient's best interests.	To ensure that the patient understands the procedure and gives their valid consent. To ensure the patient's best interests are maintained (Mental Capacity Act 2005).
2 Ensure the bed brakes are on and position the bed at a safe working height for all team members.	To promote health and safety of team members.
3 Starting in the supine position with the bed flat, position the patient with their hips over the hinge of the automatic mattress elevator or backrest of the bed.	To ensure postural alignment when sitting up in the bed. To prevent lumbar spine flexion when sitting up in the bed.
4 (a) Elevate the head of the bed no greater than 30°. (b) If the patient has injuries that prevent elevation of the head of the bed (e.g. unstable spinal or pelvic fractures), tilt the whole bed 30° from the horizontal with the head end uppermost.	(a) Cerebral venous drainage is a passive process whereby the higher the head, the greater the effect of gravity on the flow of venous blood. (b) However, as the head is raised, gravity will also decrease arterial pressure, which will reduce the pressure of blood perfusing the brain. A 30° head elevation improves venous drainage with minimal affect on arterial pressure (Winkelman 2000).
5 (a) Place the patient's head in alignment with the trunk and ensure it is not rotated or excessively flexed. (b) Assess whether a flat pillow or a towel under the back of the head is required to ensure correct neck alignment.	(a) Neck rotation and flexion have been shown to narrow the internal jugular vein. Any obstruction to jugular venous drainage will reduce jugular venous flow and increase intracranial pressure (Williams and Coyne 1993). (b) To avoid too much neck flexion.
6 Ensure that any circumferential endotracheal or tracheostomy tapes do not impede blood flow to the head. It may be necessary to consider alternative methods of securing an airway that does not involve circumferential bindings.	To ensure venous drainage is not obstructed by circumferential airway tapes (Williams and Coyne 1993). To reduce intracranial pressure (Winkelman 2000).
7 Support the upper limbs on pillows. Extra care should be taken for patients with chest drains, weakness, surgery involving the shoulder/upper limb/breast/thorax, lymphoedema, or fractures of the ribs or upper limbs.	To reduce the risk of increased intramuscular pressures. Excessive muscle activity in the shoulders and neck may elicit increased intramuscular pressures associated with reduced arterial and venous blood flow. The increased muscular activity and associated tension causes a restriction to both cerebral perfusion and venous return. Supporting the upper limbs helps to maintain a neutral trunk alignment and reduces tension in the muscular structures around the neck and shoulders, reducing pain and promoting venous return from the head.

451

(Continued)

Procedure guideline 14.4: (*Continued*)

8 Document care and observations.	To: ■ provide an accurate record ■ monitor effectiveness of procedure ■ reduce the risk of duplication of treatment ■ provide a point of reference or comparison in the event of later questions ■ acknowledge accountability for actions ■ facilitate communication and continuity of care. (NMC 2008; HCPC 2012; GMC 2013)

NB Check with local policy and procedures regarding the use of circumferential tapes to secure airways in the patient with raised intracranial pressure. Alternative methods of securing the airway may be required to prevent impediment of cerebral venous drainage and the resultant increase in intracranial pressure. Since increases in intra-abdominal pressure can elicit increases in ICP and it is recommended that extreme hip flexion should be avoided.

Procedure guideline 14.5: Log rolling a patient with suspected spinal injury to lay on their right side

Equipment

■ Up to 6 members of staff including a team leader identified as the person controlling the patient's head
■ Manual handling equipment may be required, e.g. sliding sheets or spinal board or scoop

■ Thin pillow
■ Towel

Procedure

Action	Rationale
1 Where possible, explain and discuss the procedure with the patient. If the patient lacks the capacity to make decisions the practitioner must act in the patient's best interests.	To ensure that the patient understands the procedure and gives their valid consent. To ensure the patient's best interests are maintained (Mental Capacity Act 2005).
2 Ensure the bed brakes are on and position the bed at a safe working height for all team members.	To promote health and safety of team members.
3 Assess and record the patient's motor and sensory function.	To establish baseline neurological function prior to the procedure.
4 A semi-rigid collar should be left in place during the log roll procedure.	To assist in the maintenance of head and neck alignment and prevent secondary spinal cord compression, impingement or vascular disruption.
5 (a) Team leader: From the head of the bed apply a 'Manual Cervical Spine Immobilization Technique'. This is achieved by standing at the head end of the bed and sliding both hands downwards behind the patient's head so that the thumbs rest below the patient's jawline or above the patient's clavicle with the fingers spread behind the neck encompassing the C7 vertebra. (b) Team leader: Bring forearms together at either side of the back of the patient's head ensuring the ears are not covered. If sandbags or head blocks are used either side of the patient's head these should be removed one at a time and the team leader should bring each hand into position individually (Harrison 2007).	(a) To maintain continuous head and neck alignment to prevent secondary spinal cord compression, impingement or vascular disruption (Harrison 2007). (a) To comply with the head hold technique endorsed by the Multidisciplinary Association of Spinal Cord Injury Professionals (MASCIP). (b) To maintain effective communication with the patient at all times.

6 Second assistant: (a) Stand on the right side of the patient and position both of the patient's arms across the chest but (b) above the diaphragm.	(a) To prevent injury to the shoulder joint. (b) To allow movement of the diaphragm and prevent respiratory compromise.
7 Third assistant: Stand on the right side at the level of the patient's abdomen, and place your left hand under the patient's left shoulder and your right hand under the patient's left hip.	To enable control of trunk alignment during the log roll (Harrison 2007).
8 Fourth assistant: Stand on the right side at the level of the patient's thigh, and place your left hand at the patient's hip alongside the third assistant and your right hand underneath the patient's left thigh close to the knee joint.	To enable control of pelvic alignment during the log roll (Harrison 2007).
9 Fifth assistant: Stand on the right side at the level of the patient's knee, and place your left hand under the patient's left knee and your right hand under the patient's left ankle.	To enable control of the legs during the log roll (Harrison 2007).
10 Log roll the patient to lay on their right side Team leader: (a) Check that the team are in position and ready to roll the patient. Team leader: (b) Clarify the command for the log roll before the patient is moved, e.g. 'We will log roll the patient to his right on the word roll, ready . . . steady . . . roll.' Team leader: (c) When the team are ready and the command clarified give the instruction to roll the patient. Team leader and assistants: (d) Log roll the patient.	(a) To ensure that the team leader remains in control of the procedure at all times. (b),(c),(d) To ensure coordinated team movement and promote patient safety.
11 Team leader: Hold the nose, chin and sternum in alignment during the roll. Support the head using the right forearm and hand. A thin pillow or towel can be used to elevate the team leader's right forearm and maintain spinal alignment in patients with broad shoulders.	To maintain continuous head and neck alignment, forward flexion or rotation of the cervical spine to prevent secondary neurological damage (Turner 1989).
12 Return the patient to supine. Team leader: (a) Check that the team are in position and ready to roll the patient. Team leader: (b) Clarify the command for the log roll before the patient is moved, e.g. 'We will roll the patient to his back on the word roll, ready . . . steady . . . roll." Team leader: (c) When the team are ready and the command clarified give the instruction to roll the patient to supine. Team leader and assistants: (d) Return the patient to supine.	(a) To ensure that the team leader remains in control of the procedure at all times. (b),(c),(d) To ensure coordinated team movement thereby preventing uneven spinal rotation and ensuring correct spinal alignment.
13 Assistants: Remain in position on return to the supine position until the team leader has ensured that the head, torso, pelvis and legs are in alignment and gives the instruction to 'release all hand holds'.	To ensure that the team leader remains in control of the procedure at all times. To ensure correct spinal alignment. To ensure coordinated team movement and promote patient safety.
14 If sandbags or head blocks are used either side of the patient's head these should be replaced one at a time and the team leader should remove each hand individually.	To minimize the opportunity for spinal movement. To promote patient safety.

453

(Continued)

Procedure guideline 14.5: (Continued)

15 Inspect the patient's spinal alignment and adjust loading as required.	To ensure correct spinal alignment. To preserve skin integrity. For pressure area care.
16 Re-assess and record the patient's motor and sensory function.	To establish whether there has been a change in neurological function as a result of the procedure.
17 Document care and any observations.	To: ■ provide an accurate record ■ monitor effectiveness of procedure ■ reduce the risk of duplication of treatment ■ provide a point of reference or comparison in the event of later questions ■ acknowledge accountability for actions ■ facilitate communication and continuity of care. (NMC 2008; HCPC 2012; GMC 2013)

NB 'Manual Cervical Spine Immobilization can be achieved by several hand-hold techniques. The technique described above is endorsed by the Multidisciplinary Association of Spinal Cord Injury Professionals (MASCIP). If a patient has a plaster cast or external fixation of leg fractures a 6th assistant may be required to support the fractured limb.

Procedure guideline 14.6: Positioning a patient for a chest X-ray

Equipment

■ Pillows
■ 2 to 3 assistants

■ Manual handling equipment may be required, e.g. sliding sheets or a hoist

Procedure

Action	**Rationale**
1 Where possible, explain and discuss the procedure with the patient. If the patient lacks the capacity to make decisions the practitioner must act in the patient's best interests.	To ensure that the patient understands the procedure and gives their valid consent. To ensure the patient's best interests are maintained (Mental Capacity Act 2005).
2 Ensure the bed brakes are on and position the bed at a safe working height for all team members.	To promote health and safety of team members.
3 Starting in the supine position with the bed flat, position the patient with their hips over the hinge of the automatic mattress elevator or backrest of the bed.	To ensure postural alignment and hip flexion when sitting up in the bed. To prevent lumbar spine flexion when sitting up in the bed.
4 (a) Place a pillow under the patient's knees or use the electrical control of the bed to bend the patient's hips and knees to a comfortable angle. (b) The degree of hip and knee flexion will be determined by pain or loss of movement, fracture involving the femur or pelvis, leg oedema, the positioning/placement of femoral CVC, or of other venous access devices.	(a) Bending the knees reduces lumbar spine strain when sitting erect. (a) Bending the knees reduces the stretch on the hamstrings in the long sitting position making the position more comfortable. (a) To assist the maintenance of the erect sitting position. (b) To avoid causing tissue damage, pain, or discomfort due to excessive stretch or compression of lower limb structures. (b) To avoid dislodging any medical devices.

5 (a) Elevate the head of the bed bending the patient at the hips. The angle of elevation may be influenced by pain, fracture involving the femur or pelvis, abdominal distension, or confusion/agitation.

(b) Care must be taken when elevating the back rest to ensure the patient's head does not roll forward or to the side.

(a) To ensure the X-ray is taken in the erect position allowing enhanced visualization of anatomical details compared to the supine or slumped posture.

(b) To ensure that head position does not cause excessive trunk rotation leading to poor symmetry of the resulting X-ray.

(b) To prevent the skull shadow from obstructing visualization of the upper lung fields.

6 First and second assistant: (a) With the patient now sitting in an upright position, move to a position on either side of the patient and assist them to lean forward at the hips by using the sheet they are lying on to lift the shoulders and trunk away from the backrest of the bed. (b) Monitor patient's airway, venous access devices and head position.

(a) To ensure patient safety.

(b) To ensure all medical devices continue to work effectively throughout the procedure.

7 Third assistant: (a) Cover the surface of the image plate with two layers of sliding sheet. (b) Place the image plate between the patient's back and the bed. (c) The top edge of the plate should be at least 2.5 cm above the shoulders to ensure the plate is placed at the centre of the thorax.

(a) To allow the patient to be positioned on the plate as required.

(b) To ensure patient safety.

(b) To ensure the plate is positioned appropriately to capture the patient's full lung fields.

8 The first and second assistant: (a) Recline the patient against the image plate by lowering the sheets to the bed. (b) Monitor the patient's airway, venous access devices and head position. (c) Ensure the patient is positioned symmetrically on the image plate and adjust patient position as required.

(a) To ensure patient safety.

(b) To ensure all medical devices continue to work effectively throughout the procedure.

(c) To ensure the plate is positioned appropriately to capture the patient's full lung fields.

9 If the patient's condition allows place the patient's hands on their hips or support the arms forward and away from the body with a medial rotation using pillows placed along the side of the patient's trunk.

To protract the scapula around the rib cage to enable clear visualization of the lung fields.
To provide upper limb alignment and support.

10 Inspect the patient's position from the foot of the bed.

(a) To ensure correct alignment of the head, shoulders, arms and trunk.

(b) Adjust posture as required using additional pillows or folded towels.

(c) As far as possible move any tubing or drains from the view of the X-ray.

(a) To allow visualization of all anatomical details.

(b) To maintain trunk symmetry and alignment.

(b) To maintain head alignment.

(c) To reduce extraneous artefacts which may obscure the lung fields on the final image.

11 Document care and any observations.

To:

- provide an accurate record
- monitor effectiveness of procedure
- reduce the risk of duplication of treatment
- provide a point of reference or comparison in the event of later questions
- acknowledge accountability for actions
- facilitate communication and continuity of care.

(NMC 2008; HCPC 2012; GMC 2013)

Procedure guideline 14.7: Mechanical hoist transfer

Equipment

- Mechanical hoist
- Appropriate size and make of hoist sling
- Manual handling equipment as required, e.g. sliding sheets
- 3 assistants (more will be required if patient has a BMI greater than $25\,kg/m^2$)

Procedure

Action	Rationale
1 Where possible, explain and discuss the procedure with the patient. If the patient lacks the capacity to make decisions the practitioner must act in the patient's best interests.	To ensure that the patient understands the procedure and gives their valid consent. To ensure the patient's best interests are maintained (Mental Capacity Act 2005).
2 Prepare the working environment to allow the procedure to be conducted safely.	
(a) Remove furniture or equipment not required from the area.	(a) To prepare the patient and team members for a safe hoist procedure.
	(a) To allow space for the procedure to be conducted safely.
(b) check the hoist battery is charged clean and operational.	(b) To comply with health and safety regulations for use of mechanical equipment.
(c) Ensure the chair is suitable, operational.	(c) To comply with health and safety regulations regarding the use of safe seating systems.
(d) Cover chair with a bed sheet.	(d) To reduce the risk of cross-infection.
(e) Place any pressure relieving cushions on the chair if required.	(e) To increase patient comfort.
	(e) To prevent the development of pressure areas, pain, or tissue damage.
(f) Ensure the bed brakes are on and position the bed at a safe working height for all team members.	(f) To promote health and safety of team members.
3 Lower the head of the bed to position the patient in the supine position.	To allow the rolling to occur.
4 Disconnect any tubing, monitoring equipment and other attachments as safely possible.	To prevent any medical devices being dislodged or broken during the hoist procedure.
5 First assistant: Stand on the right side at the level of the patient's abdomen, and place your left hand under the patient's left shoulder and your right hand under the patient's left hip.	To enable control of trunk alignment during the roll.
6 Second assistant: Stand on the right side at the level of the patient's thigh, and place your left hand at the patient's hip alongside the third assistant and your right hand underneath the patient's left thigh close to the knee joint.	To enable control of pelvic alignment during the roll.
7 Team leader: (a) Stand on left side of patient and prepare the hoist sling by (b) orienting the sling, (c) checking the size, (d) checking the sling integrity including all hooks or material loops and (e) rolling one quarter of the sling longitudinally towards the centre of the front side.	To comply with health and safety regulations relating the safe use of mechanical slings.
	(a) To ensure the sling is on the side of the patient with most easy access, the assistants are standing on the right.
	(b) To ensure the sling is in the correct alignment with the patient.
	(c) To ensure the sling will fit the patient.
	(d) To ensure the sling is operational and that none of the parts will fail in use.
	(e) To prepare the sling ready for insertion under the patient.

8 Roll the patient to lay on their right side.
Team leader: (a) Check that the team are in position and ready to roll the patient.
Team leader: (b) Clarify the command for the roll before the patient is moved, e.g. 'We will roll the patient to his right on the word roll, ready . . . steady . . . roll.'
Team leader: (c) When the team are ready give the instruction to roll the patient.
(d) Extra care should be taken for those patients with a tracheostomy, central venous catheters, urinary catheters, bowel management systems or venous access devices.

a) To ensure that the team leader remains in control of the procedure at all times.
(b), (c) To ensure coordinated team movement and promote patient safety.

(d) To prevent any medical devices being dislodged or damaged during the hoist procedure.

9 Team leader: Place the folded hoist sling along the length of the patient's spine and neck such that (a) the folded area of the sling is touching the bed adjacent to the length of the patient's spine and neck and (b) the top end of the sling extends to the top of the patient's head so that it will support the patient's head and (c) the bottom end of the sling extends to the coccyx to ensure the sling will support the weight of the patient's trunk.

(a), (b) and (c) To comply with health and safety instructions regarding safe use of mechanical hoist equipment.
(a), (b) and (c) To ensure the sling is placed correctly and will support the patient's head and the trunk. Failure to place the sling correctly will result in the patient's buttocks protruding through the bottom of the sling when hoisted resulting in pain, discomfort and lack of dignity.

10 Return the patient to supine.
Team leader: (a) Check that the team are ready to roll the patient.
Team leader: (b) Clarify the command for the roll before the patient is moved, e.g. 'We will roll the patient to his back on the word roll, ready . . . steady . . . roll.'
Team leader: (c) Give the instruction to roll the patient to supine.
(d) Extra care should be taken for those patients with a tracheostomy, central venous catheters, urinary catheters, bowel management systems, or venous access devices.

(a) To ensure that the team leader remains in control of the procedure at all times.
(b), (c) To ensure coordinated team movement and promote patient safety.

(d) To prevent any medical devices being dislodged or damaged during the hoist procedure.

11 Assistant one and two retrieve the rolled quarter of the sling from under the left side of the patient and (a) ensure the patient has equal sling material at both sides to ensure body symmetry during the hoist process and (b) ensure the sling extends to the top of the patient's head to support the patient's head during the hoist process. (c) Draw the lower end of the sling on the right under the right thigh, (d) draw the lower end of the sling on the left under the left thigh, (e) reaching between the patient's upper thighs, retrieve both the lower ends of the sling from under the patient's thighs so that they rest between the patient's inner thighs in preparation for attaching the sling to the hoist.

(a), (b) To ensure the sling is placed correctly for safe hoist transfer. To ensure the safety and comfort of the patient during the hoist transfer.
(c), (d) and (e) To ensure the sling will support the weight of the legs and prevent the patient from falling through the sling when hoisted. The distal end of the sling is designed to support the legs while allowing the buttocks to be free of hoist material. This design facilitates toileting and hygiene needs if required.

457

(Continued)

12 Bring the mechanical hoist into position and secure the sling hooks/loops to the hoist arms as per manufacturers instructions. (a) Ensure each thigh is secured by the sling passing beneath it to prevent the patient from slipping through the bottom of the sling, (b) ensure all hooks/loops are securely fastened to the hoist, (c) ensure the patient's arms and hands are placed on the abdomen or holding the hoist itself (if possible), (d) ensure all tubing, catheters, drains and other attachments are free of obstructions or entanglement and or attached to the hoist itself (if possible).	To ensure the safety and comfort of the patient during the hoist transfer. (a) To prevent the patient from slipping through the bottom of the hoist sling. (b) To comply with safe operating instructions for a mechanical hoist. (c) To avoid tissue damage, pain and discomfort due to excessive stretch or compression of soft tissues. (d) To prevent any medical devices from being dislodged or damaged during the hoist procedure.
13 Raise the patient using the hoist until the patient is elevated above the bed. Team leader confirms that (a) assistants are ready, (b) all tubing are secured and (c) patient is informed that the hoist will commence. (d) Continually observe and communicate with the patient and assistants and monitor attachments throughout the hoist process. Assistants monitor tubing and attachments.	(a) To ensure that the team leader remains in control of the procedure at all times. (a) To ensure coordinated team movement and promote patient safety. (b) To prevent any medical devices being dislodged or damaged during the hoist procedure. (c) To promote patient comfort and confidence. (d) To ensure that the team leader remains in control of the procedure at all times.
14 Once the patient is clear of the bed the hoist should be wheeled to a position directly over the chair ensuring that (a) the buttocks will be placed as far back in the seat as possible and (b) the safety and integrity of all tubing, drains catheters and other attachments are constantly monitored.	(a) The patient will assume a symmetrical and erect posture when sitting. (b) To prevent any medical devices being dislodged or damaged during the hoist procedure.
15 Lower the patient into the chair. Team leader: ensure that (a) assistants are prepared and (b) patient is informed, and (c) the safety and integrity of all tubing, drains catheters and other attachments is maintained.	(a) To ensure that the team leader remains in control of the procedure at all times. (b) To promote patient comfort and confidence. (c) To prevent any medical devices being dislodged or damaged during the hoist procedure.
16 Once the patient is in the chair the hoist sling should be (a) disconnected from the hoist, (b) extracted from between the patient's legs and (c) removed by leaning the patient forward from the hips (using the sling edges) and sliding the sling upwards. (d) Support the patients head and arms with pillows and offer them a blanket.	(a), (b), (c) and (d) To promote patient safety comfort and confidence. (b), (c) To avoid tissue damage pain and discomfort due to excessive pressure caused by the sling. (b), (c) For pressure area care. (d) To ensure the patient's comfort, warmth and dignity.
17 Reconnect all tubing, monitoring and equipment.	To ensure patient safety and reinstigate continuous monitoring and treatment following the hoist procedure.
18 Clean the hoist and plug it back in so it is charged ready for its next use.	To adhere to best practice infection control guidelines.
19 Document care and any observations.	To: ■ provide an accurate record ■ monitor effectiveness of procedure ■ reduce the risk of duplication of treatment ■ provide a point of reference or comparison in the event of later questions ■ acknowledge accountability for actions ■ facilitate communication and continuity of care. (NMC 2008; HCPC 2012; GMC 2013)

NB Most chairs place significant pressures on skin, so limit to 2 hours maximum sitting in a chair (*see* Chapter 12)

Competency statement 14.1: Specific procedure competency statements for positioning a patient in high sitting

Complete assessment against relevant fundamental competency statements (see Chapter 2, pp. 20, 21)	Evidence
Specific procedure competency statements for positioning a patient in high sitting	**Evidence of competency for positioning a patient in high sitting**
Demonstrate ability to: ■ teach and assess or ■ learn from assessment.	Examples of evidence of teaching, assessing and learning.
Identify reason(s) for positioning a patient in high sitting.	*May be demonstrated by:* ■ discussion with supervisor/mentor.
Identify risks, potential problems and complications of positioning a patient in high sitting and how to prevent or manage them: ■ monitor pain levels ■ monitor cardiovascular stability ■ monitor respiration and blood oxygen levels ■ monitor skin integrity ■ monitor endurance and fatigue ■ monitor confusion and agitation ■ monitor any equipment that may be affected by the position chosen, e.g. femoral catheters ■ monitor level of consciousness.	*May be demonstrated by:* ■ direct observation of appropriate monitoring of physiological responses (e.g. heart rate, respiratory rate, blood oxygen levels and pain responses) during and following the procedure ■ demonstrate or describe corrective action in the event of deterioration ■ discussion with supervisor/mentor.
Demonstrate knowledge and understanding of local and national policies, guidance and procedures in relation to positioning a patient in high sitting.	*May be demonstrated by:* ■ teaching session for peers ■ completion of workbook or educational package ■ discussion with supervisor/mentor.
Demonstrate knowledge and understanding of evidence base in relation to positioning a patient in high sitting.	*May be demonstrated by:* ■ teaching session for peers regarding the physiological consequences of changes in body posture ■ completion of workbook or educational package ■ discussion with supervisor/mentor.
Demonstrate skills that are required in relation to positioning a patient in high sitting: ■ moving and handling ■ positioning correctly with respect to the bed hinge ■ correct use of the bed.	*May be demonstrated by:* ■ direct observation of procedure ■ practical examination ■ peer practice.
Prepare equipment required in relation to positioning a patient in high sitting: ■ operating a bed manually or by using the electronic controls ■ collecting appropriate manual handling equipment ■ demonstrate safe and effective use of this equipment.	*May be demonstrated by:* ■ direct observation of procedure ■ practical examination.
Demonstrate the correct procedure for positioning a patient in high sitting, including: ■ moving the patient without risk to skin integrity ■ positioning correctly with respect to the bed hinge ■ supporting the upper limbs ■ tilting the bed to achieve the vertical posture.	*May be demonstrated by:* ■ direct observation of procedure ■ peer practice ■ practical examination.

Competency statement 14.2: Specific procedure competency statements for positioning a patient in high side lying

Complete assessment against relevant fundamental competency statements (*see* Chapter 2, pp. 20, 21)	Evidence
Specific procedure competency statements for positioning a patient in high side lying	**Evidence of competency for positioning a patient in high side lying**
Demonstrate ability to: ■ teach and assess or ■ learn from assessment.	Examples of evidence of teaching, assessing and learning.
Identify reason(s) for positioning a patient in high side lying.	*May be demonstrated by:* ■ discussion with supervisor/mentor.
Identify risks, potential problems and complications of positioning a patient in high side lying and how to prevent or manage them: ■ monitor pain levels ■ monitor cardiovascular stability ■ monitor respiration and blood oxygen levels ■ monitor endurance and fatigue ■ monitor confusion and agitation ■ monitor skin integrity ■ monitor any equipment that may be affected by the position chosen, e.g. femoral catheters.	*May be demonstrated by:* ■ direct observation of appropriate monitoring of physiological responses (e.g. heart rate, respiratory rate, blood oxygen levels and pain responses) during and following the procedure ■ demonstrate or describe corrective action in the event of deterioration ■ discussion with supervisor/mentor.
Demonstrate knowledge and understanding of local and national policies, guidance and procedures in relation to positioning a patient in high side lying.	*May be demonstrated by:* ■ teaching session for peers ■ completion of workbook or educational package ■ discussion with supervisor/mentor.
Demonstrate knowledge and understanding of evidence base in relation to positioning a patient in high side lying.	*May be demonstrated by:* ■ teaching session for peers regarding the physiological consequences of changes in body posture ■ completion of workbook or educational package ■ discussion with supervisor/mentor.
Demonstrate skills that are required in relation to positioning a patient in high side lying: ■ moving and handling ■ positioning correctly with respect to the bed hinge ■ alignment of body parts to prevent soft tissue damage ■ correct use of the bed.	*May be demonstrated by:* ■ direct observation of procedure ■ practical examination ■ peer practice with critical feedback.
Prepare equipment required in relation to positioning a patient in high side lying.	*May be demonstrated by:* ■ direct observation of procedure ■ practical examination.
Demonstrate the correct procedure for positioning a patient in high side lying, including: ■ moving the patient without risk to skin integrity ■ positioning correctly with respect to the bed hinge ■ supporting the upper limbs.	*May be demonstrated by:* ■ direct observation ■ peer practice with critical feedback ■ practical examination.

Competency statement 14.3: Specific procedure competency statements for positioning a patient in side lying

Complete assessment against relevant fundamental competency statements (*see* Chapter 2, pp. 20, 21)	Evidence
Specific procedure competency statements for positioning a patient in side lying	**Evidence of competency for positioning a patient in side lying**
Demonstrate ability to: ■ teach and assess or ■ learn from assessment.	Examples of evidence of teaching, assessing and learning.
Identify reason(s) for positioning a patient in side lying including: ■ compromised venous return, e.g. pelvic/abdominal mass, pregnancy ■ global muscle weakness ■ reduced conscious levels leading to poor airway protection ■ risk of developing pressure ulcers ■ unilateral pelvic or lower limb pain ■ altered tone ■ fatigue ■ chest infection, for gravity-assisted drainage of pulmonary secretions ■ lung pathology, to optimize ventilation and perfusion matching ■ abdominal distension, e.g. ascities, bulky disease.	*May be demonstrated by:* ■ discussion with supervisor/mentor.
Identify risks, potential problems and complications of positioning a patient in side lying and how to prevent or manage them: ■ monitor pain levels ■ monitor cardiovascular stability ■ monitor respiration and blood oxygen levels ■ monitor skin integrity ■ monitor endurance and fatigue ■ monitor confusion and agitation ■ monitor any equipment which may be affected by the position chosen, e.g. femoral catheters ■ monitor level of consciousness.	*May be demonstrated by:* ■ direct observation of appropriate monitoring of physiological responses (e.g. heart rate, respiratory rate, blood oxygen levels and pain responses) during and following the procedure ■ demonstrate or describe corrective action in the event of deterioration ■ discussion with supervisor/mentor.
Demonstrate knowledge and understanding of local and national policies, guidance and procedures in relation to positioning a patient in side lying.	*May be demonstrated by:* ■ teaching session for peers ■ completion of workbook or educational package ■ discussion with supervisor/mentor.
Demonstrate knowledge and understanding of evidence base in relation to positioning a patient in side lying.	*May be demonstrated by:* ■ teaching session for peers regarding the physiological effects of positioning a patient in side lying ■ completion of workbook or educational package ■ discussion with supervisor/mentor.
Demonstrate skills that are required in relation to positioning a patient in side lying: ■ moving and handling ■ positioning correctly with respect to the bed hinge ■ alignment of body parts to prevent soft tissue damage ■ correct use of the bed.	*May be demonstrated by:* ■ direct observation of procedure ■ peer practice with critical feedback ■ practical examination.

(*Continued*)

Competency statement 14.3: (Continued)

Prepare equipment required in relation to positioning a patient in side lying.	*May be demonstrated by:* ■ direct observation of procedure ■ practical examination.
Demonstrate the correct technique for the procedure in relation to positioning a patient in side lying, including: ■ moving the patient without risk to skin integrity ■ positioning correctly with respect to the bed hinge ■ supporting the upper limbs.	*May be demonstrated by:* ■ direct observation of procedure ■ peer practice with critical feedback ■ practical examination.

Competency statement 14.4: Specific procedure competency statements for positioning a patient with raised intracranial pressure

Complete assessment against relevant fundamental competency statements (*see* Chapter 2, pp. 20, 21)	Evidence
Specific procedure competency statements for positioning a patient with raised intracranial pressure	**Evidence of competency for positioning a patient with raised intracranial pressure**
Demonstrate ability to: ■ teach and assess or ■ learn from assessment.	Examples of evidence of teaching, assessing and learning.
Identify reason(s) for positioning a patient with raised intracranial pressure.	*May be demonstrated by:* ■ discussion with supervisor/mentor ■ teaching session for peers ■ reflective text, workbook, or educational package.
Identify risks, potential problems and complications of positioning a patient with raised intracranial pressure and how to prevent or manage them: ■ monitor intracranial pressure (ICP) ■ monitor mean arterial pressure (MAP), cerebral perfusion pressure (CPP) and cardiovascular stability ■ monitor respiration and blood oxygen levels ■ monitor level of consciousness.	*May be demonstrated by:* ■ teaching session for peers ■ reflective text, workbook, or educational package ■ direct observation/appropriate monitoring of physiological responses (e.g. heart rate, blood pressure, intracranial pressure transduced from an intracranial bolt, respiratory rate, blood oxygen levels, pain responses, consciousness levels) during and following the procedure ■ demonstrate and describe corrective action in the event of deterioration ■ discussion with supervisor/mentor.
Demonstrate knowledge and understanding of local and national policies, guidance and procedures in relation to positioning a patient with raised intracranial pressure.	*May be demonstrated by:* ■ teaching session for peers ■ reflective text, workbook, or educational package ■ discussion with supervisor/mentor.
Demonstrate knowledge and understanding of evidence base in relation to positioning a patient with raised intracranial pressure, including: ■ effect of gravity and head position on cerebral venous drainage ■ effect of gravity and head position on arterial pressure ■ effect of head position on jugular venous blood flow.	*May be demonstrated by:* ■ teaching session for peers regarding the causes and adverse effects of raised intracranial pressure ■ reflective text, workbook, or educational package ■ discussion with supervisor/mentor.

Demonstrate skills that are required in relation to positioning a patient with raised intracranial pressure: ■ moving and handling ■ positioning correctly with respect to the bed hinge ■ alignment of head in relation to spine and trunk ■ correct use of the bed.	*May be demonstrated by:* ■ direct observation of procedure ■ practical examination ■ peer practice with critical feedback.
Prepare equipment required in relation to positioning a patient with raised intracranial pressure.	*May be demonstrated by:* ■ direct observation of procedure ■ practical examination.
Demonstrate the correct procedure for positioning a patient with raised intracranial pressure: ■ safe moving and handling with respect to skin integrity ■ positioning correctly with respect to the bed hinge ■ alignment of head in relation to spine and trunk ■ selection of correct head elevation angle.	*May be demonstrated by:* ■ direct observation of procedure ■ peer practice with critical feedback ■ practical examination.

Competency statement 14.5: Specific procedure competency statements for log rolling a patient with a suspected spinal injury

Complete assessment against relevant fundamental competency statements (*see* Chapter 2, pp. 20, 21)	Evidence
Specific procedure competency statements for log rolling a patient with a suspected spinal injury	**Evidence of Competency for log rolling a patient with a suspected spinal injury**
Demonstrate ability to: ■ teach and assess or ■ learn from assessment.	Examples of evidence of teaching, assessing and learning.
Identify reason(s) for log rolling a patient with a suspected spinal injury, including: ■ to physically examine the back in a person with known or suspected spinal injuries ■ to transfer to a specialized spinal board ■ pressure area care in a person with known or suspected spinal injury.	*May be demonstrated by:* ■ discussion with supervisor/mentor ■ teaching session for peers ■ reflective text, workbook, or educational package.
Identify risks, potential problems and complications of log rolling a patient with a suspected spinal injury and how to prevent or manage them: ■ monitor baseline neurology ■ monitor spinal alignment ■ monitor pain ■ monitor team log rolling team for fatigue/discomfort.	*May be demonstrated by:* ■ teaching session for peers ■ reflective text, workbook, or educational package ■ direct observation/appropriate monitoring of responses during and following the procedure and taking corrective action in the event of deterioration ■ discussion with supervisor/mentor.
Demonstrate knowledge and understanding of local and national policies, guidance and procedures in relation to log rolling a patient with a suspected spinal injury.	*May be demonstrated by:* ■ teaching session for peers ■ reflective text, workbook, or educational package ■ discussion with supervisor/mentor.

(*Continued*)

Competency statement 14.5: (Continued)

Demonstrate knowledge and understanding of evidence base in relation to: ■ spinal column anatomy ■ normal spinal alignment ■ spinal column movements ■ log rolling a patient with a suspected spinal injury.	*May be demonstrated by:* ■ teaching session for peers ■ reflective text, workbook, or educational package ■ discussion with supervisor/mentor.
Demonstrate skills that are required in relation to log rolling a patient with a suspected spinal injury: ■ moving and handling ■ effective manual cervical spine immobilization ■ effective communication ■ team leadership ■ team membership ■ assessment of baseline neurology.	*May be demonstrated by:* ■ direct observation of procedure ■ peer practice sessions ■ practical examination.
Prepare equipment required in relation to log rolling a patient with a suspected spinal injury.	*May be demonstrated by:* ■ direct observation of procedure ■ practical examination.
Demonstrate the correct technique for the procedure in relation to log rolling a patient with a suspected spinal injury: ■ safe moving and handling with respect to skin integrity and pressure area care ■ maintenance of spinal alignment throughout procedure ■ effective manual cervical spine immobilization technique ■ provision of clear commands that have been previously clarified ■ teamwork.	*May be demonstrated by:* ■ direct observation of procedure ■ peer practice sessions with critical feedback ■ practical examination.

Competency statement 14.6: Specific procedure competency statements for positioning a patient for a chest X-ray

Complete assessment against relevant fundamental competency statements (*see* Chapter 2, pp. 20, 21)	Evidence
Specific procedure competency statements for positioning a patient for a chest X-ray	**Evidence of competency for positioning a patient for a chest X-ray**
Demonstrate ability to: ■ teach and assess or ■ learn from assessment.	Examples of evidence of teaching, assessing and learning.
Identify reason(s) for positioning a patient for a chest X-ray.	*May be demonstrated by:* ■ discussion with supervisor/mentor.
Identify risks, potential problems and complications of positioning a patient for a chest X-ray and how to prevent or manage them, including: ■ monitor pain levels ■ monitor cardiovascular stability ■ monitor respiration and blood oxygen levels ■ monitor any equipment that may be affected by the position chosen, e.g. airways and venous access devices.	*May be demonstrated by:* ■ teaching session for peers ■ reflective text, workbook, or educational package ■ direct observation of appropriate monitoring of physiological responses (e.g. heart rate, blood pressure, blood oxygen levels and pain responses) during and following the procedure ■ taking corrective action in the event of deterioration or problem ■ discussion with supervisor/mentor.

Demonstrate knowledge and understanding of local and national policies, guidance and procedures in relation to positioning a patient for a chest X-ray.	*May be demonstrated by:* ■ teaching session for peers ■ discussion with supervisor/mentor.
Demonstrate knowledge and understanding of evidence base in relation to positioning a patient for a chest X-ray.	*May be demonstrated by:* ■ teaching session for peers regarding skeletal anatomy of the lungs, rib cage and upper limb and the interpretation of the portable chest X-ray ■ discussion with supervisor/mentor.
Demonstrate skills that are required in relation to positioning a patient for a chest X-ray: ■ safe moving and handling ■ positioning correctly with respect to the bed hinge ■ supporting the upper limbs ■ controlling the bed.	*May be demonstrated by:* ■ direct observation of procedure ■ peer practice with critical feedback ■ practical examination.
Prepare equipment required in relation to positioning a patient for a chest X-ray.	*May be demonstrated by:* ■ direct observation of procedure ■ practical examination.
Demonstrate the correct technique for the procedure in relation to positioning a patient for a chest X-ray, including: ■ moving the patient without risk to skin integrity ■ positioning correctly with respect to the bed hinge ■ elevating the bed to achieve an erect position ■ positioning the image plate safely ■ protracting the shoulders and supporting the upper limbs.	*May be demonstrated by:* ■ direct observation of procedure ■ peer practice with critical feedback ■ practical examination.

Competency statement 14.7: Specific procedure competency statements for completing a hoist transfer

Complete assessment against relevant fundamental competency statements (*see* Chapter 2, pp. 20, 21)	Evidence
Specific procedure competency statements for completing a hoist transfer	**Evidence of competency for completing a hoist transfer**
Demonstrate ability to: ■ teach and assess or ■ learn from assessment.	Examples of evidence of teaching, assessing and learning.
Identify reason(s) for completing a hoist transfer, including: ■ risk assessment indicates that hoist transfer to chair may be required ■ physiological stability established for commencing mobilization identified ■ benefits of sitting upright in a chair identified ■ rehabilitation plan indicating goals of sitting in a chair identified.	*May be demonstrated by:* ■ discussion with supervisor/mentor.

(Continued)

Competency statement 14.7: *(Continued)*

Identify risks, potential problems and complications of completing a hoist transfer and how to prevent or manage them: ■ monitor pain levels ■ monitor cardiovascular stability ■ monitor respiration and blood oxygen levels ■ monitor skin integrity ■ monitor endurance and fatigue ■ monitor confusion and agitation ■ monitor any equipment that may be affected by the procedure.	*May be demonstrated by:* ■ direct observation of appropriate monitoring of physiological responses (e.g. heart rate, respiratory rate, blood oxygen levels and pain responses) during and following the procedure ■ demonstrate or describe corrective action in the event of deterioration ■ discussion with supervisor/mentor.
Demonstrate knowledge and understanding of local and national policies, guidance and procedures in relation to positioning completing a hoist transfer.	*May be demonstrated by:* ■ teaching session for peers ■ completion of workbook or educational package ■ discussion with supervisor/mentor.
Demonstrate knowledge and understanding of evidence base in relation to completing a hoist transfer: ■ manufacturer's instructions for use and care of hoist equipment ■ physiological effects of upright sitting ■ rationale for early mobilization of the critically ill patient ■ reasons for use of hoist transfer.	*May be demonstrated by:* ■ teaching session for peers regarding the physiological effects of upright sitting and early mobilization of the critically ill patient ■ completion of workbook or educational package ■ discussion with supervisor/mentor.
Demonstrate skills that are required in relation to completing a hoist transfer: ■ equipment identification, safety checks and operational mechanisms ■ moving and handling a patient in bed ■ positioning the sling correctly ■ connecting the hoist and sling safely ■ protection of body parts to prevent soft tissue damage ■ management of lines, equipment and monitoring.	*May be demonstrated by:* ■ direct observation of procedure ■ peer practice with critical feedback ■ practical examination.
Prepare equipment required in relation to completing a hoist transfer.	*May be demonstrated by:* ■ direct observation of procedure ■ practical examination.
Demonstrate the correct technique for the procedure in relation to completing a hoist transfer: ■ moving the patient without risk to skin integrity ■ positioning sling correctly ■ operating hoist correctly ■ supporting and protecting the upper limbs.	*May be demonstrated by:* ■ direct observation of procedure ■ peer practice with critical feedback ■ practical examination.

466

References and further reading

Berek K, Margreiter J, Willeit J et al. (1996) Polyneuropathies in critically ill patients: a perspective evaluation. *Intensive Care Medicine* 22: 849–855.

Black CJ, Kuper M and Bellingan GJ (2007) The feasibility and impact of a multi-disciplinary team approach to weaning patients from prolonged mechanical ventilation. *Intensive Care Medicine* 33(S2): 112.

Blair E and Hickam JB (1955) The effect of change in body position on lung volume and intrapulmonary gas mixing in normal subjects. *Journal of Clinical Investigations* 34(3): 383–389.

Bloomfield SA (1997) Changes in musculoskeletal structure and function with prolonged bed rest. *Medicine and Science in Sports and Exercise* 29(2): 197–206.

Borg GA (1982) Psychophysical bases of perceived exertion. *Medicine and Science in Sports and Exercise* 1982;14:377–381.

Brower RG (2009) Consequences of bed rest. *Critical Care Medicine* 37(suppl): S422–S428.

Cecins NM, Jenkins SC, Pengelly J and Ryan G (1999) The ACBT – to tip or not to tip. *Respiratory Medicine* 93(9): 660–665.

Chang AT, Boots R, Hodges PW and Paratz J (2004) Standing with assistance of a tilt table in intensive care: a survey of Australian physiotherapy practice. *Australian Journal of Physiotherapy* 50(1): 51–55.

Chiang LL, Wang L, Wu C et al. (2006) Effects of physical training on functional status in patients with prolonged mechanical ventilation. *Physical Therapy* 86(9): 1271–1281.

Christie RJ (2008) Therapeutic positioning of the multiply-injured trauma patient in ICU. *British Journal of Nursing* 17(10): 638–642.

Convertino V, Hung J, Goldwater D and DeBusk RF (1982) Cardiovascular responses to exercise in middle-aged men after 10 days of bedrest. *Circulation* 65(1): 134–140.

Coombes A, Costa M, Trouillet J et al. (2003) Morbidity, mortality and quality-of-life outcome of patients requiring greater than or equal to 14 days of mechanical ventilation. *Critical Care Medicine* 31(5): 1373–1381.

Dean E (1985) Effect of position on pulmonary function. *Physical Therapy* 65(5): 613–618.

De Jonghe B, Cook D, Sharshar T et al (1998) Acquired neuromuscular disorders in critically ill patients: a systematic review. *Intensive Care Medicine* 24: 1242–1250.

De Jonghe B, Sharshar T, Lefaucheur F et al. (2002) Pareses acquired in the intensive care unit: a prospective multicenter study. *Journal of the American Medical Association* 288(22): 2859–2867.

Department of Health (2005) *Quality Critical Care*. London: DH.

Drakulovic MB, Torres A, Bauer TT et al. (1999) Supine body position as a risk factor for nosocomial pneumonia in mechanically ventilated patients: a randomized controlled trial. *Lancet* 354(9193): 1851–1858.

Eddleston JM, White P and Guthrie E (2000) Survival, morbidity and quality of life after discharge from intensive care. *Critical Care Medicine* 28: 2293–2299.

Fan J-Y (2004) Effect of backrest position on intracranial pressure and cerebral perfusion pressure in individuals with brain injury: a systematic review. *Journal of Neuroscience Nursing* 36(5): 278–288.

Feldman Z, Kanter MJ, Robertson CS et al. (1992) Effect of head elevation on intracranial pressure, cerebral perfusion pressure and cerebral blood flow in head-injured patients. *Journal of Neurosurgery* 76(2): 207–211.

Garnacho-Montero J, Amaya-Villar R, Garcia-Garmendia J et al (2005) Effects of critical illness polyneuropathy on the withdrawal from mechanical ventilation and the length of stay in septic patients. *Critical Care Medicine* 33: 349–354.

Gayan-Ramirez G, Testelmans D, Maes K et al. (2005) Intermittent spontaneous breathing protects the rat diaphragm from mechanical ventilation effects. *Critical Care Medicine* 33(12): 2804–2809.

General Medical Council (2013) *Good Medical Practice*. London: GMC. http://www.gmc-uk.org/gmp2013 [accessed 25 March 2013].

Gerovasili V, Stefanidis K, Vitzilaios K et al (2009) Electrical muscle stimulation preserves the muscle mass of critically ill patients: a randomized study. *Critical Care* 13(5): R161.

Grap MJ, Munro CL, Bryant S and Ashtiani B (2003) Predictors of backrest elevation in critical care. *Intensive and Critical care Nursing* 19(2): 68–74.

Griffiths H and Gallimore D (2005) Positioning critically ill patients in hospital. *Nursing Standard* 19(42): 56–64.

Griffiths RD and Hall JB (2010) Intensive care unit-acquired weakness. *Critical Care Medicine* 38(3): 779–787.

Griffiths RD and Jones C (2007) Seven lessons from 20 years of follow up of intensive care unit surviors. *Current Opinion in Critical Care* 13: 508–513.

Griffiths RD, Palmer TEA, Helliwell T et al. (1995) Effect of passive stretching on the wasting of muscle in the critically ill. *Nutrition* 11: 428–432.

Grundy D and Swain A (2002) *ABC of Spinal Cord Injury* (4e). London: MBJ Books.

Harrison P (2007) Moving and handling patients with actual or suspected spinal cord injuries. Spinal Cord Injury Centres of the United Kingdom and Ireland, The Spinal Injuries Academy and the Multidisciplinary Association of Spinal Cord Injury Profes-

sionals supported by an educational grant from Huntleigh Healthcare. www.arjo.com/admin/files/20100302122309.pdf.

Hawkins S, Stone K and Plummer L (1999) An holistic approach to turning adults. *Nursing Standard* 6(14): 51–56.

Health and Safety Executive, Manual Handling (1992) *Manual Handling Operations Regulations 1992 (as amended): guidance on the regulations L23*. London: HSE Books.

Health and Care Professions Council (2012) *Standard of Conduct, Performance and Ethics*. London: HCPC. http://www.hcpc-uk.org/assets/documents/10003B6EStandardsofconduct,performanceandethics.pdf [accessed January 2013].

Helliwell TR, Wilkinson A, Griffiths RD et al. (1998) Muscle fibre atrophy in critically ill patients is associated with the loss of myosin filaments and the presence of lysosomal enzymes and ubiquitin. *Neuropathology and Applied Neurobiology* 24:507–517.

Hermans G, De Jonghe B, Bruyninckx F and Van den Berge G (2008) Clinical review: critical illness polyneuropathy and myopathy. *Critical Care* 12(6): 238.

Herridge MS, Cheung AM, Tansey CM et al. (2003) One-year outcomes in survivors of the acute respiratory distress syndrome. *New England Journal of Medicine* 348: 683–693.

Hespel P, Op't EB, Van Leemputte M et al. (2001) Oral creatine supplementation facilitates the rehabilitation of disuse atrophy and alters the expression of muscle myogenic factors in humans. *Journal of Physiology* 536: 625–633.

Hopkins RO, Weaver LK, Collingridge D et al. (2005) Two year cognitive, emotional and quality-of-life outcomes in acute respiratory distress syndrome. *American Journal of Respiratory and Critical Care Medicine* 171(4): 340–347.

Hubmayr RD (2002) Statement of the 4th international consensus conference in critical care on ICU-acquired pneumonia. *Intensive Care Medicine* 28(11): 1521–1536.

Jenkins SC, Soutar SA and Moxham J (1988) The effects of posture on lung volumes in normal subjects and in patients pre and post coronary artery surgery. *Physiotherapy* 74(10): 492–496.

Jones AYM and Dean E (2004) Body position change and its effect on haemodynamic and metabolic status. *Heart and Lung* 33(5): 281–290.

Jones C and Griffiths RD (2000) Identifying post intensive care patients who may need physical rehabilitation. *Clinical Intensive Care* 11(1): 43–46.

Jones C, Griffiths RD, Macmillan RR and Palmer TEA (1994) Psychological problems occurring after intensive care. *British Journal of Intensive Care* 4(2): 46–53.

Jones C, Skirrow P, Griffiths RD et al. (2003) Rehabilitation after critical illness: a randomised, controlled trial. *Critical Care Medicine* 31(10): 2456–2461.

Jones C, Backman C, Capuzzo M et al. (2007) Precipitants of post traumatic stress disorder following intensive care: a hypothesis generating study of diversity in care. *Intensive Care Medicine* 33: 978–985.

Jones C, Bäckman C, Capuzzo M et al. (2009) ICU diaries reduce posttraumatic stress disorder after critical illness: a randomised, controlled trial. *Intensive Care Medicine* 35(Suppl 1): S115 abstract.

Kashihara H, Haruna Y, Suzuki Y et al. (1994) Effects of mild supine exercise during 20 days bed rest on maximal oxygen uptake rate in young humans. *Acta Physiologica Scandanavica* 616: 19–26.

Kim MJ, Hwang HG and Song HH (2002) A randomised controlled trial on the effects of body positions on lung function with acute respiratory failure patients. *International Journal of Nursing Studies* 39(5): 549–555.

Krapp K (2002) Body positioning in X-ray studies. In: Encyclopedia of Nursing & Allied Health. Andover: Gale Cengage. http://

www.enotes.com/nursing-encyclopedia/body-positioning-x-ray-studies [accessed 14 September 2010].

Kress JP, Pohlman AS, O'Connor MF and Hall JB (2000) Daily interruptions of sedative infusions in critically ill patients undergoing mechanical ventilation. *New England Journal of Medicine* **342**: 1471–1477.

Leijten FS, De Weerd AW, Poortvliet DC et al. (1996) Critical illness polyneuropathy in multiple organ dusfunctionsyndrome and weaning from the ventilator. *Intensive Care Medicine* **22b**: 856–861.

Levine S, Nguyen T, Taylor N et al. (2008) Rapid disuse atrophy of diaphragm fibres in mechanically ventilated humans. *New England Journal of Medicine* **358**: 1327–1335.

Martin UJ (2002) Whole-body rehabilitation in long-term ventilation. *Respiratory Care Clinics of North America* **8**(4): 593–609.

McWilliams DJ and Pantelides KP (2008) Does physiotherapy led early mobilisation affect length of stay on ICU. *ACPRC Journal* **40**: 5–11.

McWilliams DJ, Atkinson JFD, Conway DH et al. (2009) The impact and feasibility of a physiotherapy led, exercise based rehabilitation programme for intensive care survivors. *Physiotherapy Theory and Practice* **25**(8): 566–571.

McWilliams DJ, Westlake EV and Griffiths RD (2011) Weakness on the intensive care unit : current therapies. *British Journal of Intensive Care* **21**(2): 55–60.

Mental Capacity Act (2005) http://www.legislation.gov.uk/ukpga/2005/9/pdfs/ukpga_20050009_en.pdf [accessed 9 February 2012].

Morris PE, Goad A, Thompson C et al. (2008) Early intensive care unit mobility therapy in the treatment of acute respiratory failure. *Critical Care Medicine* **36**: 2238–2243.

National Institute for Health and Clinical Excellence (2009) *Rehabilitation After Critical Illness*. NICE clinical guidelines 83. London: NICE. www.nice.org.uk/CG83

Navajas D, Farre R, Rotger MM et al. (1988) Effect of body posture on respiratory impedance. *Journal of Applied Physiology* **64**(1): 194–199.

Navarrete-Navarro P, Ruiz-Bailén M, Rivera-Fernández R et al. (2000) Acute respiratory distress syndrome in trauma patients: ICU mortality and prediction factors. *Intensive Care Medicine* **26**(11): 1624–1629.

Nursing and Midwifery Council (2008) *The Code: standards of conduct, performance and ethics for nurses and midwives*. London: NMC. http://www.nmc-uk.org/Documents/Standards/The-code-A4-20100406.pdf [accessed 15 February 2012].

Op De Coul AAW, Verheul GAM, Leyten ACM et al. (1991) Critical illness polyneuromyopathy after artificial respiration. *Clinical Neurology and Neurosurgery* **91**(1): 27–33.

Pryor J and Webber BA (2002) Physiotherapy techniques. In: Pryor JA and Prasad SA (eds) *Physiotherapy for Respiratory and Cardiac Problems: adults and paediatrics*. London: Churchill Livingstone.

Ross J, Dean E and Abboud RT (1992) The effect of postural drainage positioning on ventilation homogeneity in healthy subjects. *Physical Therapy* **72**(11): 794–799.

Salford Royal Hospitals NHS Trust (2007) *Standards/guidelines for formal assessment, treatment and management of patients in minimally conscious/vegetative states*. Salford: Salford Royal Hospitals Foundation Trust.

Sasaki H, Hida W and Takishima T (1977) Influence of body position on dynamic compliance in young subjects. *Journal of Applied Physiology* **42**(5): 706–710.

Schweickert W, Pohlman M, Pohlman A et al. (2009) Early physical and occupational therapy in mechanically ventilated, critically ill patients: a randomised controlled trial. *Lancet* **373**: 1874–1882.

Siebens H, Anonow H, Edwards E et al. (2000) A randomised controlled trial of exercise to improve outcomes of acute hospi-

talisation in older adults. *Journal of the American Geriatrics Society* **48**(12): 1545–1552.

Staudinger T, Bojic A, Holzinger U et al. (2010) Continuous lateral rotation therapy to prevent ventilator-associated pneumonia. *Critical Care Medicine* **38**(2): 486–490.

Stewart M (1992) Chest radiography. In: Ellis ER and Alison JA (eds) *Key Issues in Cardiopulmonary Physiotherapy*, pp. 56–79. Oxford: Butterworth-Heinemann.

Stiller K (2000) Physiotherapy in intensive care: towards an evidenced-based practice. *Chest* **118**(6): 1801–1813.

Sullivan J (2000) Positioning of patients with severe traumatic brain injury: research-based practice. *Journal of Neuroscience Nursing* **32**(4): 204–209.

Talmore D, Sarge T, O'Donnell CR et al. (2006) Esophageal and transpulmonary pressures in acute respiratory failure. *Critical Care Medicine* **34**: 1389–1394.

Thomas AJ, Wright K and Mill LM (2009) The incidence of physiotherapy and rehabilitation activities within a general intensive care unit. *ACPRC Journal* **41**: 9–15.

Turner LM (1989) Cervical spine immobilization with axial traction. A practice to be discouraged. *Journal of Emergency Medicine* **7**: 385–386.

Van Pelt DC, Milbrandt EB, Qin L et al. (2007) Informal caregiver burden among survivors of prolonged mechanical ventilation. *American Journal of Respiratory and Critical Care Medicine* **175**: 167–173.

Veldhuizen JW, Verstappen FT, Vroeme JP et al. (1993) Functional and morphological adaptations following four weeks of knee immobilization. *International Journal of Sports Medicine* **14**: 283–287.

Vollman KM (2004) The right position at the right time: mobility makes a difference. *Intensive and Critical Care Nursing* **20**(4): 179–182.

Wagenmakers AJM (2001) Muscle function in critically ill patients. *Clinical Nutrition* **20**(5): 451–454.

Weissman C and Kemper M (1993) Stressing the critically ill patient: the cardiopulmonary and metabolic responses to an acute increase in oxygen consumption. *Journal of Critical Care* **8**(2): 100–108.

Williams A and Coyne SM (1993) Effects of neck position on intracranial pressure. *American Journal of Critical Care* **2**(1): 68–71.

Winkelman C (2000) Effect of backrest position on intracranial and cerebral perfusion pressures in traumatically brain-injured adults. *American Journal of Critical Care* **9**(6): 373–380.

Wong WP (1999) Use of body positioning in the mechanically ventilated patient with acute respiratory failure: application of Sackett's rules of evidence. *Physiotherapy Theory and Practice* **15**(1): 25–41.

Woodrow P (2000) Will nursing of ICU patients in semi-recumbent positions reduce rates of nosocomial infection? *Nursing in Critical Care* **5**(4): 174–178.

Zafiropoulos B, Alison JA and McCarren B (2004) Physiological responses to the early mobilisation of the intubated, ventilated abdominal surgery patient. *Australian Journal of Physiotherapy* **50**: 95–100.

Zanotti E, Felicetti G, Maini M et al. (2003) Peripheral muscle strength training in bed-bound patients with COPD receiving mechanical ventilation: effects of electrical stimulation. *Chest* **124**: 292–296.

Zerwekh JE, Ruml LA, Gottschalk F and Pak CY (1998) The effects of twelve weeks of bed rest on bone histology, biochemical markers of bone turnover, and calcium homeostasis in eleven normal subjects. *Journal of Bone and Mineral Research* **13**(10): 1594–1601.

Chapter 15

Transfer of the critically ill patient

Andrew Baker[1] and Simon M. Whiteley[2]

[1]St James's University Hospital, Leeds, UK
[2]Leeds Teaching Hospitals NHS Trust, Leeds, UK

Critical Care Manual of Clinical Procedures and Competencies, First Edition.
Edited by Jane Mallett, John W. Albarran, and Annette Richardson.
© 2013 John Wiley & Sons, Ltd. Published 2013 by John Wiley & Sons, Ltd.

Definitions

Primary transfer: Movement of patient from initial scene of injury or illness to a receiving hospital. This is the responsibility of the emergency ambulance services and is outside the scope of this chapter.

Secondary transfer: Movement of patient from one hospital facility to another. This may be **intrahospital** (between areas or departments within a single site) or **interhospital** (between sites or hospitals).

The primary focus of this chapter is on interhospital transfer and the potential problems associated with the various modes of transport. The principles, however, apply equally to intrahospital transfer and the same degree of planning and the same standards of care should be applied to critically ill patients transferred between areas in their base hospital.

Aims

The aim of any critical care transfer is to facilitate the safe transfer of the patient, avoiding any clinical deterioration, while also minimizing risk of injury to the patient, staff and, where appropriate, other road users or members of the public. The patient should normally receive at least the same standard of treatment and care during transfer that they would have received in the referring critical care unit.

Indications

Intrahospital

Critically ill patients may be moved between departments in the same hospital for a number of reasons. Typical indications include:

- escalation of level of care (e.g. movement from ward level or emergency department to critical care unit)
- from critical care unit to operating theatre (e.g. for surgical procedure/intervention)
- from critical care unit to radiology/angiography (e.g. for investigation or treatment)
- de-escalation of critical care (e.g. from level 3 to a level 2 care facility).

Interhospital

Critically ill patients are generally moved between hospitals to enable access to care not available in the referring unit. Typical indications include:

- requirement for specialist treatment or investigations not available at referring hospital (e.g. neurosurgery/cardiac surgery/vascular radiology)
- lack of critical care bed capacity in referring hospital
- repatriation to referring hospital after specialist treatment (e.g. to allow convalescence nearer to home).

It is important to distinguish between indication and degree of clinical urgency in relation to interhospital transfers. In the past, the term 'non-clinical transfer' was often used when the indication for transfer was lack of capacity. The implication was often that these transfers were clinically less urgent. Clearly, however, a transfer due to lack of capacity may still be clinically urgent and the term non-clinical is therefore best avoided (Intensive Care Society 2011).

Background

In 1997 it was estimated that more than 11 000 critically ill patients were transferred annually between hospitals in the UK each year (Mackenzie et al. 1997). Current figures are difficult to obtain because of the lack of any central recording system; however, the increased centralization of specialist services would suggest that large numbers of critically ill patients continue to require transfer between hospitals.

Evidence suggests that the transfer of critically ill patients is often poorly performed and that critical incidents are common. Concerns over the safety and organization of the transfer process has resulted in a number of organizations publishing specific guidelines on the transfer of critically ill patients (American College of Emergency Physicians 2009; Association of Anaesthetists of Great Britain and Northern Ireland 2009; Intensive Care Society 2011).

This chapter will discuss some of the recent evidence relating to transfers and discuss the factors that should be considered before embarking on a critical care transfer. Advice relating to the transfer of patients by air (rotary or fixed-wing aircraft) is included; however, aero-medical transport is a specialist area and should not be undertaken by practitioners without specific training in this area.

Physiological effects of transfer

Critically ill patients typically have limited physiological reserve and as such have limited ability to withstand the physiological stresses associated with transfer. Those accompanying a patient during transfer must therefore understand the physiology of critical illness and the potential physiological insults that can arise.

Cardiovascular system

Patients who are critically ill are frequently haemodynamically unstable. They are prone to:

- fluid shifts (systemic inflammatory response syndrome/capillary leak)
- hypotension
- myocardial ischaemia (increased myocardial oxygen demand/impaired myocardial perfusion)
- myocardial conduction defects
- dysrhythmias.

These patients are particularly susceptible to the physical effects of changes in momentum, and acceleration and deceleration forces during transfer.

Effect of movement/gravitational forces

Gravitational forces (g-forces) are experienced by passengers in all forms of transport and most people will be familiar with the effects of acceleration and deceleration in a moving vehicle. The importance of these forces in the critically ill is in their effect on intravascular fluid shifts and the potential for haemodynamic disturbance.

Depending on the mode of transport and position of the patient, these forces may act in any direction, but the effects can be most easily understood by considering the horizontal and vertical components (Figure 15.1a).

During transport in a standard road ambulance the patient is supine and normally lying facing away from the direction of travel (head toward the front of the vehicle). The patient will therefore be subjected primarily to horizontal g-forces acting along the longitudinal axis. Acceleration will tend to force blood away from the head, towards the

feet and extremities, resulting in reduced venous return, reduced cardiac output and hypotension (Figure 15.1b). Deceleration will have the opposite effect, forcing blood towards the head, leading to increased venous return, increased cerebral blood volume and potentially increased intracranial pressure (Martin 2006).

Patients transferred by air will be subject to both horizontal and vertical axis g-forces. This effect is most marked during take-off in a fixed-wing aircraft, where the combined effects of acceleration and change in posture lead to exaggerated fluid shifts and greater haemodynamic disturbance (Figure 15.1c).

In addition to the gross haemodynamic disturbances described above, acceleration and deceleration forces can result in the movement of fluid from the intravascular to interstitial compartments. In effect, fluid is forced out of the intravascular space and into the tissues. These fluid shifts may be significant in the critically ill patient with, for example, systemic inflammatory response syndrome and capillary leak. This can result in intravascular volume depletion and hypotension, with interstitial fluid accumulation, for example in the peripheral tissues (tissue oedema) and lungs (pulmonary oedema) (Martin 2006).

It is important therefore that critically ill patients are stabilized before transfer to reduce the haemodynamic consequences of movement. Consideration should be given to the use of invasive monitoring (invasive arterial pressure and or central venous pressure monitoring) if not already in situ. Hypovolaemia should be corrected and blood pressure supported with vasopressors if appropriate. Dysrhythmias should be corrected and or rate controlled (Intensive Care Society 2011).

Respiratory system

The physical movement of patients with respiratory failure can precipitate or exacerbate bronchospasm, particularly in those patients with reactive airways (for example in asthma or chronic obstructive pulmonary disease). Gravitational forces (discussed above) cause changes to distribution of blood within the lung, potentially forcing blood away from well-ventilated areas to less well-ventilated areas, resulting in ventilation/perfusion (V/Q) mismatch, which in turn leads to increased hypoxia (*see also* Chapter 5). During transfer by air the effect of altitude can have profound effects on the respiratory system.

The effects of altitude: potential for hypoxia

Transfer by air subjects critically ill patients to the effects of altitude and in particular to the effects of reduced atmospheric pressure. The extent to which the atmospheric pressure inside an aircraft is reduced during flight will depend on the type of aircraft, the altitude of the flight and whether or not the cabin is pressurized. Rotary-wing aircraft (helicopters) and small fixed-wing aircraft do not have pressurized

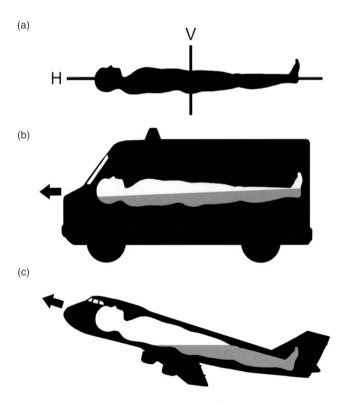

(a)

(b)

(c)

Figure 15.1 Representation of the effects of gravitational force on a patient during transfer. (a) Forces potentially acting in horizontal (H) and vertical (V) directions. (b) Effect of horizontal forces during acceleration in a land ambulance. (c) Effect of combined horizontal and vertical forces during take off in a fixed wing aircraft.

cabins. The atmospheric pressure therefore falls in direct proportion to the altitude gained (*see* Table 15.1).

In larger commercial fixed-wing aircraft/air ambulances the cabins will be pressurized during flight to maintain a cabin pressure equivalent to between 3000 and 10 000 feet, depending on the type of aircraft (Bersten and Soni 2009).

The concentration of oxygen (fractional inspired oxygen FiO_2) in the atmosphere remains relatively constant with altitude; however, as the altitude increases, and the atmospheric pressure reduces, the partial pressure of oxygen falls. This is demonstrated in Table 15.1.

Table 15.1 Effect of altitude on partial pressure of inspired oxygen

Altitude (feet) above sea level	Atmospheric pressure (kPa)	Fractional inspired oxygen (FiO$_2$)	Partial pressure inspired oxygen (kPa)
30 000	30.1	0.21	6.3
25 000	37.6	0.21	7.9
20 000	46.6	0.21	9.8
15 000	57.2	0.21	12.0
10 000	69.7	0.21	14.6
5000	84.3	0.21	17.7
Sea level	101	0.21	21.0

This fall in partial pressure of inspired oxygen leads to a corresponding fall in alveolar oxygen. This can be calculated using the alveolar air equation:

$$PAO_2 = F_iO_2 \, (P_B - P_{H_2O}) - (PaCO_2/R)$$

Where: PAO_2 = partial pressure of alveolar oxygen; FiO_2 = fractional inspired oxygen; P_B = atmospheric pressure; P_{H_2O} = water vapour pressure (6.3 kPa at 37 degrees Celsius); $PaCO_2$ = partial pressure of carbon dioxide (5.5 kPa); R = respiratory quotient (ratio of CO_2 production to O_2 consumption) typically 0.8.

Thus at 5000 feet (typical pressurized cabin) alveolar oxygen is:

$$PAO_2 = 0.21(84.3 - 6.3) - (5.7/0.8)$$
$$PAO_2 = 9.5 \text{ kPa.}$$

Allowing for a *normal* alveolar–arterial oxygen gradient of approximately 1 kPa, the arterial oxygen pressure (PaO_2) would be reduced to approximately 8.5 kPa.

The relationship between arterial PaO_2 and oxygen saturation (SaO_2) is described by the oxygen haemoglobin dissociation curve (Figure 15.2) (*see also* Chapter 5). The sigmoid shape of the curve reflects that this reduction in arterial PaO_2 will have only a minimal effect on oxygen saturation, which will be reduced to approximately 90–92%.

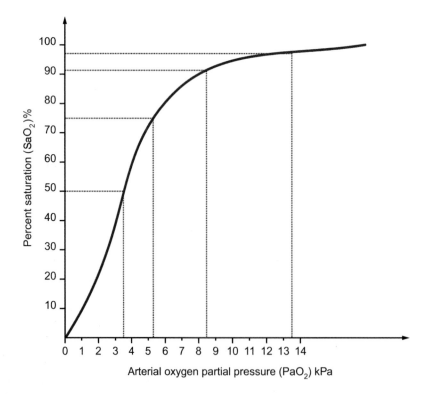

Figure 15.2 Oxygen haemoglobin dissociation curve demonstrating effect of travel in pressurized cabin at 5000 ft in a healthy individual (PaO$_2$ of 8.5 kPa and oxygen saturation of 90–92%). Further reductions in PaO$_2$ resulting from increased alveolar–arterial oxygen difference will result in steep falls in oxygen saturation.

In critically ill patients, however, with increased alveolar–arterial oxygen gradient (e.g. due to pneumonia/adult respiratory distress syndrome) the fall in arterial PaO_2 will be greater, and this in turn will lead to a greater fall in oxygen saturation with the potential for significant hypoxia.

In spontaneously breathing patients, hypoxia leads to hyperventilation (increased respiratory rate and minute volume). The resulting respiratory alkalosis increases the affinity of haemoglobin for oxygen (producing a left shift in the oxygen dissociation curve) – aiding the binding of oxygen to haemoglobin in the lungs but potentially reducing oxygen release to the tissues. Acidosis secondary to tissue hypoxia, however, has the opposite effect (producing a right shift in the oxygen dissociation curve) – aiding the off load of oxygen to the tissues (Lumb 2010).

A further potential effect of altitude-induced hypoxia is to increase hypoxic pulmonary vasoconstriction (HPV) in the lung. This physiological response to low levels of inspired oxygen effectively causes narrowing of the blood vessels in the lungs and therefore increases the resistance to the flow of blood through the lungs. This increase in right ventricular afterload could potentially result in, or exacerbate, right heart failure.

All critically ill patients should therefore receive additional inspired oxygen during air transport to reduce the potential for hypoxia. Those at risk of respiratory fatigue and/or respiratory failure should be intubated and ventilated prior to transfer.

The effects of altitude: expansion of air spaces

Boyle's law dictates that as barometric pressure decreases the volume of a gas will expand. (Boyle's law: pressure x volume = constant.) Thus as altitude increases, any gas trapped within body cavities will expand, resulting, for example, in distension of the gastrointestinal tract and enlargement of pneumothoraces. Critically ill patients transferred by air should therefore have a nasogastric tube placed (on free drainage) and any pre-existing pneumothoraces should be drained. Air trapped in fixed cavities, for example the inner ear, sinuses and skull, will also expand, leading to increased pressure within the cavity. This can lead to pain and sickness (nausea), and in the case of intracranial air to raised intracranial pressure. The presence of intracranial air is therefore a relative contraindication to air transportation (Bersten and Soni 2009).

Physiological stress response

A number of factors can contribute to an increased physiological stress response during transfer. These include haemodynamic disturbances (e.g. caused by movement and gravitational forces described above), pain and anxiety experienced by the patient, and the effects of noise and vibration (Martin 2006).

There are two main elements to the physiological stress response: neural and endocrine. Increased neural sympathetic activity leads to increased heart rate, increased myocardial contractility and increased vasoconstriction. The endocrine response includes release of adrenal corticotrophin hormone (ACTH). This in turn leads to release of catecholamines (e.g. adrenaline) from the adrenal medulla, which again increases heart rate, myocardial contractility and vasoconstriction. The resulting increase in myocardial oxygen demand may lead to myocardial ischaemia in patients with reduced/limited myocardial perfusion.

Activation of the renin-angiotensin-aldosterone system leads to further vasoconstriction (angiotensin) and salt and water retention (aldosterone), which may result in impaired ventricular function, heart failure and impaired renal function. Corticosteroid release may contribute to hypertension, fluid retention and metabolic disturbance, including hyperglycaemia.

Thus while the physiological stress response may be beneficial in counteracting some of the haemodynamic consequences of transferring a critically ill patient, exaggerated responses can be harmful. Adequate stabilization and optimization of the patient prior to transfer, together with adequate analgesia and sedation, can help to reduce the stress response.

Temperature control

Critically ill patients often have impaired ability to regulate their temperature and may be hypothermic or hyperthermic. The critical care environment is temperature and humidity controlled to minimize the impact of the environment on patients. When moved outside of the critical care unit patients are exposed to changes in environmental temperature and are at particular risk of hypothermia. Significant hypothermia is associated with physiological disturbances including depression of cardiovascular and respiratory function, reduced consciousness and metabolic derangements, including coagulopathy. All critically ill patients should therefore be appropriately wrapped to conserve heat during transfer and have their temperature monitored.

Evidence and current debates

Despite the large number of transfers of critically ill patients that take place there is relatively little in the way of good-quality research to guide clinical practice. Much of the available evidence is derived from single-centre audits and small case series or case reports, possibly reflecting the difficulty of carrying out high-quality randomized trials in this area.

Quality of patient transfers

The transfer of a critically ill patient, whether for investigation or treatment, is always intended to be of benefit to the patient, but transfer is frequently associated with an unacceptable level of risk. Evidence consistently demonstrates poor standards of care during transfers and a high level of critical incidents.

In one study for example, adverse events occurred in 34% of the transfers and of these 70% were considered avoidable (Ligtenberg et al. 2005). In another study, 59% of reported critical incidents resulted in some harm to the patient and 20% resulted in serious adverse outcomes (Flabouris et al. 2006). Critical incidents are not confined to interhospital transfers. In a study of intrahospital transfers from Australia, critical incidents occurred in 67.9% of cases. Of these, 26% related to failure to stabilize the patient prior to transfer, 49% related to equipment failure and 9% resulted in serious adverse consequences for the patient, including hypotension, decreased conscious level and raised intracranial pressure (Gillman et al. 2006).

Factors that may influence the quality of transfers include lack of adherence to national guidelines, lack of local policies, lack of involvement of senior medical and nursing staff, and inadequate training of junior practitioners (Easby et al. 2002). Clearly all those involved in transferring critically ill patients must be aware of prevailing policies and should have received suitable training.

Organization

In view of the demonstrably poor quality of many critical care transfers it has been recommended that all hospitals should have a designated medical consultant and senior nurse with responsibility for ensuring the quality and standards of transfers originating within their own organization (Intensive Care Society 2011). Those responsible should ensure that the following elements are in place.

- Locally agreed transfer guidelines/protocol (based on national guidelines).
- Transfer documentation to provide both a clinical record and audit.
- Portable monitoring suitable for use in the transfer environment.
- Portable ventilators and other equipment.
- Suitable transfer trolley (see below).
- Designated practitioners with responsibility for checking and maintaining all equipment.
- Competency-based training for practitioners involved in transfers.
- Governance arrangements, including audit and critical incident review.

Role of critical care networks

In the UK, managed critical care networks were established following publication of a review by the Department of Health (DH 2000). The aim was for critical care services to be planned and coordinated at both a regional and local level, with geographically related hospitals cooperating to ensure optimal use of resources and safe transfer of patients between units when necessary (*see also* Chapter 1). The

potential advantages include use of standardized protocols and equipment across networks and opportunities for staff training and audit. At the current time, there is little objective evidence for the benefit of networks.

Specialist transfer teams

The traditional approach to the transfer of critically ill patients has been for the referring hospital to stabilize the patient and then to arrange and carry out the transfer. There has been increasing interest over recent years, however, in the use of specialist transfer teams, either from the receiving hospital (retrieval team) or from a regional base (transfer team), to carry out transfers. These teams would typically consist of specialist medical and nursing personnel with experience in transferring critically ill patients and with all necessary equipment and monitoring to carry out the transfer. It has been suggested that the use of specialist transfer teams may be associated with improved quality of transfers and reduced risk for the patient. One study (Belligan et al. 2000) found that patients transferred to a single centre by a specialist retrieval team are less likely to be severely acidotic and hypotensive compared with patients transferred in a standard ambulance accompanied by a doctor from the base hospital.

While the authors did not identify reasons for this, it does suggest that the use of specialist retrieval teams may result in patients suffering less physiological disturbance during the transfer process. However, the evidence as to whether this improves patient outcomes is lacking and recent systematic reviews have highlighted this (Belway et al. 2006; McDonald 2006). It does seem reasonable to assume, however, that improved training and familiarity with the transfer process and equipment will to lead to improved outcomes and there is likely therefore to be increasing interest in the use of dedicated transfer teams in the future.

Timing of transfers

One issue that is important in relation to intrahospital transfers is the timing. Evidence suggests that the transfer of patients out of (discharge from) the intensive care during the nightshift hours is associated with increased morbidity and mortality (Goldfrad and Rowan 2000; Tobin and Santamaria 2006). Factors that contribute to this may include reduced staffing levels on wards, and the unplanned nature of out-of-hours discharges precipitated by capacity issues. Out-of-hours transfers/discharges should be avoided wherever possible.

Components of the transfer process

The transfer of any critically ill patient is a complex undertaking. The process can be broken down into number of key components:

- the decision to transfer
- communication
- assessment and stabilization prior to transfer
- selection of transport mode
- preparation for transfer
- safe transfer
- handover.

The decision to transfer

The decision to transfer a patient in order to receive a treatment or intervention that is not available in the referring unit is generally straightforward and the only issue that may arise is that of optimal timing. However, if the indication for transfer is lack of critical care capacity in the referring hospital, then one problem that sometimes arises is whether it is better to transfer an existing stable patient (to make room for a new and potentially less stable patient) or to transfer the new patient. In general, it is considered unethical to submit any patient to an intervention (in this case transfer to another unit) that is not in their best interests. Transferring one patient to make room for another cannot be considered to be in the first patient's best interests and is therefore normally considered unethical. There are occasions, however, when this may be the only pragmatic solution.

The decision to transfer a patient should be made by the medical consultant primarily responsible for the patient's care, in conjunction with any other involved specialists. The decision to accept a patient should be made by the medical consultant in the receiving critical care unit together with the medical consultant responsible for accepting care of the patient. There is little evidence about the rationale for the ultimate decision to transfer, and it is likely that there is huge variation between units and consultants in the decision-making process (Van Lieshout et al. 2008).

Communication

The key to coordination of the transfer process is effective communication between the referring hospital and the receiving unit. Little data exists to quantify the complexity or time spent coordinating a transfer, and this is likely to vary greatly depending on the patient and hospital characteristics. The process should begin with telephone communication between the referring and accepting medical consultants, although on average at least a further three calls are required to finalize transfer arrangement (Craig 2005). All communications should be documented in the patient notes and should include the reasons for transfer and any treatment or investigations undertaken.

Assessment and stabilization prior to transfer

Patients should be fully assessed and appropriately resuscitated and stabilized prior to transfer. For most critically ill patients optimal haemodynamic status (preload, cardiac output, blood pressure and perfusion) should be achieved to reduce the risks of haemodynamic disturbance and untoward events during transfer. The only exception to this rule is for patients with penetrating injury and/or major vascular injury (e.g. leaking aortic aneurysm), where the priority is for surgical intervention and more limited volume resuscitation has been shown to improve outcomes (Bickell et al. 1994).

Investigations that should be considered prior to transfer include full blood count (FBC), electrolytes, urea and creatinine (U&Es), blood glucose, arterial blood gas (ABG), electrocardiogram (ECG) and chest X-ray (CXR). The need for any additional investigations (e.g. X-rays, blood tests) should be balanced against the urgency of the transfer.

Selection of transport mode

There are a number of factors that influence the choice of transfer mode and these are summarized in Table 15.2.

Most critical care transfers take place by road. It is cheaper, easier to organize, requires fewer specialist practitioners and it is less of a physiological challenge to the patient than air transport. Travel by road is, however, reliant on the transport infrastructure of the particular region, and can be affected by road works and traffic conditions. There are circumstances therefore when air transportation may seem more appropriate, particularly where longer journeys are required. The perceived advantages must however be balanced against organizational delays and the requirement for transfer by road between hospital and aircraft at either end of the journey. The advantages and disadvantages of each mode of transport are summarized in Table 15.3.

In general, helicopters are more versatile than fixed-wing aircraft for moderate distance travel in that they do not require an airstrip, can take off and land in confined spaces, and in many cases can deliver patients directly to the receiving hospital without the need for road support. They are, however, more dependent on weather and may not be available in high winds or poor visibility. One prospective study that compared the outcomes of patients who had been transferred by either helicopter or road ambulance found that helicopter transfer did not reduce mortality, and may even be detrimental (Arfken et al. 1998). More research is clearly required in this area; however, the study does emphasize that

Table 15.2 Factors influencing choice of transport mode

Patient factors	Logistical factors	Available transport
■ Nature of Illness ■ Urgency of transfer	■ Length of journey ■ Traffic conditions ■ Road conditions ■ Weather ■ Terrain ■ Hospital facilities	■ Road ambulance ■ Helicopter ■ Fixed-wing aircraft

Table 15.3 Advantages and disadvantages of different modes of transport

	Indication	Advantages	Disadvantages
Road ambulance	Short distances, up to 50 miles	▪ Familiar ▪ Faster mobilization ▪ Less physiological disturbance ▪ Less dependent on weather conditions	▪ Slower ▪ Dependent on traffic conditions
Helicopter	Medium distances, 50–150 miles	▪ Faster speed of travel once airborne	▪ Cramped environment ▪ Limited access to patient ▪ Significant noise and vibration ▪ May need road transfers either end of journey if no helipad ▪ Dependent on weather conditions
Fixed-wing aircraft	Longer distances, over 150 miles	▪ Longer range ▪ Less cramped environment ▪ Less dependent on weather conditions	▪ Potential for greater physiological disturbance ▪ Need for road transfers to and from airport

air transfer should only be considered when it is deemed essential.

Fixed-wing aircraft may be used for long-distance transfers. Once airborne they are faster, quieter and expose the patient to less vibration stress than helicopters. However, they are much less versatile, relying on airports and requiring land ambulance transfers at either end of the journey.

As stated previously, the transfer of patients by air is a specialist area of medicine and practitioners without specific training in aeromedical transport should not undertake this type of transfer.

Preparation for transfer

Patients who require invasive ventilation must be stabilized on a portable ventilator prior to transfer. Transfer ventilators should be gas driven (i.e. not dependent on an electrical power supply). They should have both audible and visual disconnection alarms (to overcome noise) to alert staff to disconnection of the patient from the ventilator, and high-pressure alarms to alert staff to obstruction of the breathing system and to prevent barotrauma. An arterial blood gas should be obtained prior to departure to ensure adequate ventilation and oxygenation is achieved (Intensive Care Society 2011).

All patients should be monitored closely during transfer. The level of monitoring required will be determined by the patient's clinical condition but should normally be at least as good as that they were receiving in the referring unit prior to departure. The recommended minimum level of monitoring for critically ill and or ventilated patients includes:

▪ continuous ECG monitoring
▪ non-invasive blood pressure (NIBP)
▪ arterial oxygen saturation
▪ end tidal carbon dioxide ($ETCO_2$)
▪ temperature.

Although the minimum standard includes non-invasive blood pressure, NIBP readings can be unreliable in some critically ill patients (e.g. in the presence of arrhythmias such as atrial fibrillation). The readings can be affected by motion artefact, and the automatic pump used to inflate the blood pressure cuff can significantly shorten the battery life of portable monitors. For these reasons invasive arterial blood pressure monitoring is recommended for most transfers. Additional monitoring such as central venous pressure (CVP), pulmonary artery pressures (PAP), or intracranial pressure (ICP) may be required according to the patient's condition.

Monitors used for transfer should be small (in order to be portable and to fit on to the transfer trolley), robust, and have dual AC and battery power supply. They should be capable of displaying all required monitoring modalities (above) and the display should be clearly visible in a range of lighting conditions. Alarms should be both visual and auditory.

Safe transfer

The safety of the patient, accompanying personnel and other road users or members of the public is of paramount importance during transfer. There are a number of key issues in relation to safety.

Within the UK and European Economic Area, land ambulances must conform to the British and European standards, which state that:

without exception all persons and items, e.g. medical devices, equipment and objects normally carried on the ambulance, shall be maintained to prevent them becoming a projectile when subjected to a force of 10 g in the forward, rearward, transverse and vertical directions.

(Committee on European Standards, EN 1789, 2007)

Patients must therefore be transported using a suitable transfer trolley that is compliant with these standards. The patient must be strapped on to the trolley using a harness, including shoulder and crutch straps to prevent the patient becoming a projectile in the event of an accident. All equipment (including portable monitors, ventilator and syringe pumps) must be similarly secured to the trolley. Equipment should be below the level of the patient to lower the centre of gravity of the trolley and improve stability. Any equipment bags should be stowed in lockers or placed on the floor of the ambulance. No equipment should be allowed to rest on top of the patient trolley. A typical transfer trolley is shown in Figure 15.3.

Although portable electrical equipment such as monitoring and syringe pumps are capable of running on batteries when a mains electrical supply is unavailable, batteries should be used as little as possible during the transfer. Most modern ambulances are equipped with DC inverters, which can provide 240 V, 50 Hz AC supply (UK mains voltage). Electrical equipment should therefore be plugged in during transfer to conserve battery life. If a mains voltage power supply is not available, then additional batteries and equipment may be necessary, particularly for longer journeys.

Similarly, portable oxygen supplies should be conserved for movement between hospital bedside and ambulance (and vice versa), and for emergency use. Portable ventilators should be plugged into the ambulance oxygen supply during transfer. Ambulances generally carry sufficient oxygen to enable most transfers to take place safely; however, it is the responsibility of the transfer attendants to ensure that sufficient oxygen supplies are available for the journey.

Accompanying personnel must remain seated while the ambulance is moving and should wear seat belts at all times. The patient's physiological parameters and vital signs should be continuously monitored and recorded on documentation designed for the purpose. If the patient requires any care or interventions during the journey these should not be attempted in the back of a moving ambulance. The vehicle should be stopped (as soon as is practical) and then the patient appropriately attended to. When moving outside the ambulance high-visibility jackets should be worn.

The absolute priority during transfer is to ensure the safety of the patient, staff and other road users, and a major issue in this respect is speed of travel. For most appropriately resuscitated and stabilized critically ill patients high-speed journeys are unnecessary and should be avoided. Warning lights and sirens can be used to aid passage through traffic congestion and to enable a smooth journey, but should not be used unless absolutely necessary. The nature of the transfer is ultimately dictated by the clinical needs of

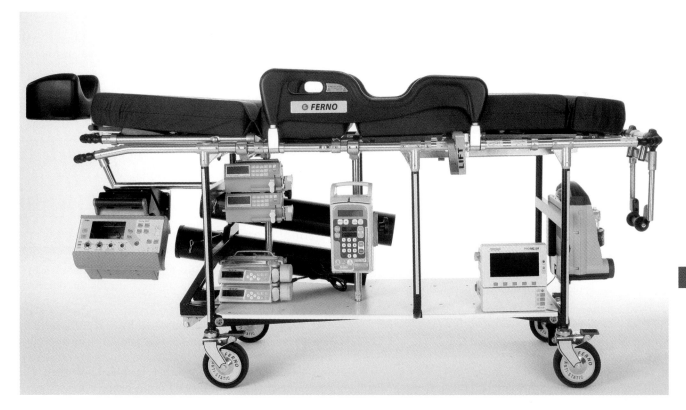

Figure 15.3 The Ferno CCT-6 p critical care transfer trolley, with secure housing for oxygen cylinders, and mountings for portable ventilator, syringe pumps, fluid pumps, monitoring and suction. Reproduced with permission from Ferno UK Ltd.

the patient and, as such, the decision to proceed at speed and/or using lights and sirens is the responsibility of the senior practitioner in attendance. Accompanying staff should therefore discuss transfer times and agree requirements with the ambulance drivers prior to departure.

Handover

Advice on the management of the patient may, where appropriate, be provided by the receiving unit prior to departure, for example when transfer is occurring to a specialist unit. The responsibility for the patient's care remains with the referring team until arrival at the receiving hospital and final handover. Handover should include a detailed history of the patient's condition, and of all treatments, care and investigations provided.

Competency statements

It is assumed that practitioners involved in the transfer of critically ill patients will have general competencies in the care of critically ill patients and in the use of the range of equipment/monitoring devices likely to be encountered during the transfer process. This will include as a minimum familiarity with the transfer trolley, and competencies in the use of the portable ventilator, portable monitoring (including invasive arterial pressure and central venous pressure monitoring), and syringe pumps.

The following competencies relate to specific steps in the transfer process and are relevant to all staff and practitioners involved.

Guidelines for transfer

Equipment

In addition to the standard items of equipment required, such as the transfer trolley, monitor and syringe pumps, etc., sufficient additional equipment, disposables and drugs should be available to enable the attendant practitioners to manage any emergency that may potentially arise during the transfer. This equipment should be stored in one place, so as to be easily accessible when required, and checked on a regular basis. Typical requirements are as follows.

Airway
- Oral/pharyngeal airways (assorted sizes)
- Laryngeal masks
- Tracheal tubes (assorted sizes)
- Intubation equipment, including laryngoscopes, Magill forceps, etc.
- Portable suction, tubing, rigid oropharyngeal suction catheter (such as a Yankauer catheter) and suction catheters
- Nasogastric tubes

Ventilation
- Self-inflating bag-valve-mask with oxygen reservoir and tubing
- Portable ventilator and tubing
- Portable oxygen supply

Circulation
- Syringes and needles (assorted sizes)
- Alcohol and chlorhexidine skin preparation
- Intravenous cannulae (assorted sizes)
- Arterial cannulae
- Central venous cannulae and insertion pack (for insertion prior to transfer)
- Syringe drivers/fluid pumps

Drugs and fluids
Including:

- Anaesthetic/sedative agents
- Muscle relaxants
- Bronchodilators
- Anti-dysrhythmic drugs
- Inotropes/vasopressors
- Emergency drugs (cardiac arrest/anaphylaxis, etc.)
- Intravenous fluids.

Portable monitoring
Including:

- Transport monitor
- Cables and sensors (ECG, blood pressure, oxygen saturation, end tidal CO_2 temperature, invasive pressures)
- Spare batteries.

Transfer trolley (CEN compliant)
Including:

- Oxygen cylinder housing
- Mounting for syringe pumps
- Mounting for portable monitoring
- Mounting for portable ventilator
- Secure harness for restraining patient.

Personal protective equipment
- Warm clothing
- High-visibility jacket (for moving outside ambulance)
- Portable telephone (plus contact details of referring/receiving unit)

The critically ill patient should normally be accompanied by two attendants during transfer. One should be an appropriately trained and experienced doctor and the other a suitably experienced nurse or other healthcare worker. The procedure guidelines at the end of the chapter provide guidance on the steps that should be undertaken to facilitate safe transfer. Some of the steps described may be role-specific but are included, recognizing that good and effective communication between all team members is vital.

Procedure guideline 15.1: Decision to transfer

Action	Rationale
1 Decision to transfer made by medical consultant in charge of critical care unit and/or consultant responsible for the patient in accordance with local/national guidelines.	To ensure appropriateness of transfer.
2 In all cases the decision must be made in the best interests of the patient and be clearly documented in the notes. In the case of patients who lack capacity it may be necessary to involve relatives or independent medical capacity advocates.	To ensure the patient's best interests are maintained (Mental Capacity Act 2005).

Procedure guideline 15.2: Communication

Action	Rationale
1 Utilize national, regional or local bed bureaux to identify potentially available bed in receiving unit.	To identify potentially available beds in target receiving units.
2 Confirm availability of bed in the receiving unit.	To ensure capacity in receiving unit.
3 Ensure that patient is appropriately referred to, and accepted by, the receiving unit.	To ensure appropriateness of transfer and that the patient's care needs can be met at receiving hospital. (Where appropriate, advice may also be received regarding the ongoing management of the patient.)
4 Where possible, explain and discuss the need for transfer and the approximate times of departure and arrival with the patient and/or the patient's relatives.	To ensure that the patient and or the patient's relatives understand the need for transfer and give their consent/assent. To ensure good communication with the patient and/or patient's relatives and to minimize anxiety and distress.
5 Ensure all notes and relevant investigations are copied and available.	To provide optimal handover of care at receiving unit.
6 Ensure that transfer documentation required to record patient's observations and treatment provided during the transfer is available.	To enable documentation of care during transfer and aid handover of care at receiving unit.
7 Arrange appropriate ambulance (air or road) using agreed priorities. Choice will depend on the distance of transfer, physiological state of the patient and the relative risks of the different modes of transport, availability and training of staff and practitioners.	To ensure appropriate type of vehicle or mode of transport available in appropriate time frame.
8 Confirm return travel arrangements for staff and equipment.	To aid smooth repatriation.
9 Telephone receiving unit prior to departure and advise estimated time of arrival.	To minimize disruption and delays at receiving unit.

Procedure guideline 15.3: Assessment and stabilization prior to transfer

Action	Rationale
Airway	
1 Assess whether patient is maintaining their own airway and has adequate cough/gag reflexes.	To determine whether the airway is adequate and/or the need for endotracheal intubation.
2 If airway is not maintained or cough/gag reflexes are inadequate, secure airway by endotracheal intubation.	To ensure adequate and safe airway during transfer and reduce the risk of aspiration of gastric contents.
3 If airway is adequate but may become compromised later, for example due to airway swelling caused by facial burns, secure airway by endotracheal intubation.	To ensure adequate and safe airway during transfer.
4 If intubated, check position of the endotracheal tube on a chest X-ray.	To confirm correct placement of the endotracheal tube.
Breathing	
5 Assess adequacy of the patient's breathing, including respiratory rate, work of breathing (use of accessory muscles, intercostal recession, paradoxical breathing), air entry breath sounds, oxygen saturations and arterial blood gas.	To identify potentially reversible problems with breathing and/or ventilation and guide to further management.
6 Obtain a chest X-ray.	To complement clinical examination above and identify any other problems.
7 Treat any potentially reversible causes of inadequate oxygenation and/or ventilation such as bronchospasm, pneumothorax/pleural effusion/pulmonary oedema.	To optimize respiratory function.
8 If oxygenation and/or ventilation remain inadequate, intubate and ventilate prior to transfer.	To ensure optimal oxygenation and or ventilation during transfer.
9 Obtain repeat arterial blood gas.	To confirm adequacy of ventilation and oxygenation prior to transfer.
10 If chest drains are in situ, check that these are functioning correctly. (NB Do not clamp chest drains during transfer. Keep underwater seal drains below the level of the patient.)	To prevent re-accumulation of pleural collections and potential deterioration during transfer.
Circulation	
11 Assess cardiovascular system, including heart rate and rhythm, preload (central venous pressure), blood pressure and perfusion.	To assess haemodynamic status and guide optimization prior to transfer.
12 If there is evidence of hypovolaemia, correct with fluids. Consider the need for central venous pressure monitoring to guide fluid replacement.	To optimize preload and reduce haemodynamic disturbances associated with transfer.
13 Control blood loss where possible. Consider transfusion of packed red cells if haemoglobin is less than 8 g/dL.	To reduce blood loss and optimize oxygen delivery.
14 Commence inotropes or vasopressors as appropriate. Consider the use of haemodynamic monitoring such as oesophageal Doppler or LiDCO to guide therapy (*see* Chapter 6).	To optimize cardiac output and blood pressure and reduce haemodynamic disturbance during transfer.

Central nervous system (CNS)

15	Assess Glasgow Coma Scale (GCS), pupillary size and reaction to light. Look for abnormal movements, including seizures, and evidence of agitation or pain (*see* Chapter 11).	To identify potential brain injury/encephalopathy/coma and patients at risk of airway compromise (due reduced conscious level).
16	Control agitation with anxiolytics and/or sedative agents.	To reduce the risk of injury during transfer.
17	Control any seizures with appropriate anticonvulsant drugs.	To reduce the risks associated with prolonged seizures and reduce the risk of injury during transfer.
18	If there is evidence of potential brain injury/encephalopathy/coma, uncontrolled seizures, or unmanageable agitation intubate and ventilate prior to transfer. (NB All patients with a GCS 8 or less must be intubated prior to transfer.)	To provide safe airway and ventilation during transfer, reduce brain metabolic rate for oxygen (effect of sedation) and reduce the risks of further (secondary) brain injury.
19	If evidence of, or potential for, raised intracranial pressure, transfer the patient with 10–15° head-up tilt and maintain mean arterial pressure above 80 mmHg, PaO_2 of 13 kPa and $PaCO_2$ of 4.5–5 kPa.	To increase venous drainage from the brain, ensure adequate cerebral perfusion pressure and optimal oxygenation and ventilation.

Gastrointestinal tract

20	In awake and unintubated patients consider the need for antiemetic prior to transfer.	To reduce the risks of motion sickness during transfer.
21	In all patients consider the requirement for a nasogastric (NG) tube prior to transfer. All intubated/ventilated patients should have a NG tube inserted and be placed on free drainage prior to transfer.	To reduce the risks of gut distension (particularly air transfers) and the risks of passive regurgitation of stomach contents and potential contamination of the airway.

Renal system

22	Consider the need for urinary catheterization. Most patients should be catheterized prior to transfer.	To improve patient comfort and to allow monitoring of urine output and fluid balance.
23	Assess patients urine output. If less than 1 mL/kg/h consider need for further fluid boluses and/or diuretics.	To maintain urine output and prevent acute kidney injury.

Temperature

24	Check core temperature.	To identify abnormalities of temperature and to provide baseline prior to transfer.
25	If the patient is pyrexial, give antipyretics and institute cooling measures.	To reduce the physiological consequences associated with high temperature.
26	If the patient is hypothermic, institute active warming if appropriate. (NB Exclusion – patients being actively cooled after cardiac arrest.)	To reduce the physiological consequences associated with low temperature.
27	Ensure the patient is appropriately wrapped and insulated prior to transfer.	To avoid development of hypothermia during transfer.

(Continued)

Procedure guideline 15.3: (*Continued*)

Biochemistry

30 Review available biochemical results to ensure that parameters are within acceptable ranges including: (a) Potassium (K^+) 3.5–5 mmol/L. (b) Blood glucose 4–10 mmol/L. (c) Blood gas. Oxygenation and ventilation adequate and acid-base balance improving. (Institute corrective therapies if not.)	To identify underlying pathology, assess results of resuscitation and to ensure the patient is safe for transfer. (a) To reduce risk of cardiac dysrhythmia precipitated by hypo- or hyperkalaemia. (b) To avoid risks associated with hypo- or hyperglycaemia. (c) To provide confirmation that effective resuscitation has been achieved. Worsening metabolic acidosis may signify a serious deterioration of the patient's underlying condition.
31 Document assessment, care and treatment provided.	To: ■ provide an accurate record of care ■ monitor the effectiveness of procedures ■ reduce the risk of duplication of treatment ■ acknowledge accountability for actions ■ facilitate communication and continuity of care. (NMC 2008; HCPC 2012; GMC 2013)

Procedure guideline 15.4: **Preparation for transfer**

Action	Rationale
1 Ensure that all transfer equipment, disposables, etc., are available, checked and correctly functioning.	To ensure safety during the transfer process.
2 Check that the patient is adequately resuscitated and stabilized (*see* Procedure guideline 15.3).	To reduce risks of haemodynamic disturbance and deterioration during transfer.
3 Check that the patient has adequate venous access for transfer. Minimum requirements two peripheral venous cannulae. Consider need for central venous access if not already in place.	To provide safe and secure access for drugs and fluid during transfer.
4 Transfer the patient to transport trolley and secure with appropriate harness.	To ensure patient safety during transfer.
5 Transfer to portable monitors if not already done. Ensure appropriate standards of monitoring in place, including as a minimum: ■ ECG ■ non-invasive blood pressure ■ oxygen saturation ■ end tidal carbon dioxide (ventilated patients) ■ temperature.	To enable monitoring of the patient's condition during the transfer.
6 Consider the need for invasive arterial blood pressure monitoring if not already in place.	To improve reliability of blood pressure monitoring during transfer.
7 Check that all transfer equipment (ventilators, monitors, syringe pumps, etc.) is appropriately secured to transport trolley and functioning correctly.	To comply with safety regulations and ensure patient and staff safety during transfer.
8 Stabilize the patient on transport ventilator if this has not already been done and check blood gases prior to departure.	To ensure effective ventilation being achieved prior to departure.

9 Check that any drugs and fluids likely to be required during the transfer are available.	To prevent adverse events associated with interruption to treatment caused by failure of drug infusions, etc. To ensure that adequate drugs and fluid are available to deal with any unexpected or adverse events.
10 Check that resuscitation equipment is available (including self-inflating bag-valve-mask for ventilating the patient).	To ensure that equipment to deal with unexpected or adverse events is available.
11 Check that the patient's clinical records including X-rays, CT scans, blood results, etc., are available (or copied) and transferred with the patient.	To enable effective handover at receiving unit.
12 Ensure transfer documentation (to be completed during transfer) is available.	To provide record of the patient's condition and care during transfer and for clinical audit purposes.
13 Ensure all staff involved in transfer (including ambulance staff) are briefed and ready to depart.	To reduce the risk of adverse events during the transfer.
14 Transfer equipment to portable oxygen and power supplies (batteries) and ensure that all equipment is functioning correctly.	To prepare for departure.
15 Ensure practitioners are appropriately dressed for climate and check availability of high-visibility jackets and any other personal safety equipment.	To ensure comfort and safety.
16 Ensure mobile telephone communication available for staff.	To enable contact with base or receiving hospital in case of unexpected difficulty.
17 Transfer patient to waiting ambulance.	To begin transfer.

Procedure guideline 15.5: Carrying out safe transfer

Action	Rationale
1 Ensure transfer trolley is safely secured in the ambulance and all equipment safely stowed.	To ensure safety of patient and staff.
2 Transfer oxygen and power supplies to ambulance and check that all equipment is functioning correctly.	To conserve portable oxygen and power supplies.
3 Check lighting, heating and humidity controls are appropriately set.	To ensure comfort and safety of staff and patient.
4 Agree urgency and required speed of travel with ambulance drivers, bearing in mind the needs of the patient and the requirement for safety.	To avoid unnecessary high-speed journeys and minimize risk to patient, staff and other road users.
5 Carry out final patient assessment and safety check before departure.	To ensure the patient's condition is stable prior to departure, minimizing the requirement for additional care and interventions once mobile.
6 Take seat in the ambulance and wear seat belt. (Ensure that monitors and vital equipment are visible.)	To reduce risk of injury to self and others and to enable safe monitoring of the patient.
7 Carry out transfer while monitoring the environment, the patient, and oxygen and power supplies.	To ensure safety of the patient during transfer and prevent or detect clinical deterioration and/or adverse events.
8 Document patient vital signs, treatments and any interventions/critical incidents.	To: ■ provide an accurate record of care ■ monitor the effectiveness of procedures ■ reduce the risk of duplication of treatment ■ acknowledge accountability for actions ■ facilitate communication and continuity of care. (NMC 2008; HCPC 2012; GMC 2013)

Procedure guideline 15.6: **Handover**

Action	Rationale
1 Transfer the patient from the ambulance to the receiving hospital unit (reverse procedures in Procedure guidelines above).	To enable completion of transfer.
2 Transfer the patient to the receiving unit bed, ventilator, monitoring and infusion pumps, and syringe pumps, etc., ensuring no interruption to vital treatments.	To safely complete transfer process.
3 Provide detailed handover of patient to the receiving hospital, including details of history investigations and treatment.	To transfer care and responsibility to the receiving unit staff and to ensure that they have all the necessary information to manage the patient.

Competency statement 15.1: **Specific procedure competency statements for decision making in relation to transfer**

Complete assessment against relevant fundamental competency statements (*see* Chapter 2, pp. 20, 21)	Evidence
Specific procedure competency statement for decision making in relation to critical are transfers	**Evidence of competency in decision making in relation to critical care transfers**
Demonstrate ability to: ■ teach and assess or ■ learn from assessment.	*May be demonstrated by:* ■ examples of evidence of teaching, assessing and learning.
Demonstrate understanding of the indications for transfer of critically ill patients, including: ■ escalation of level of care ■ specialist surgical procedure/intervention/treatment or investigation ■ de-escalation of critical care ■ repatriation.	*May be demonstrated by:* ■ discussion with supervisor/mentor ■ teaching session for peers.
Demonstrate ability to balance the risk and benefits of patient transfer, including: ■ advantages and disadvantages of different modes of transport from physiological and time perspectives.	*May be demonstrated by:* ■ discussion with supervisor/mentor ■ teaching session for peers ■ direct observation of clinical practice.
Demonstrate understanding of the ethical issues in relation to the decision making process, including: ■ acting in the patient's best interests ■ capacity to consent ■ requirements of the Mental Capacity Act.	*May be demonstrated by:* ■ discussion with supervisor/mentor ■ teaching session for peers.
Demonstrate knowledge of national, regional and local policies in relation to transfer process.	*May be demonstrated by:* ■ discussion with supervisor/mentor ■ teaching session for peers.

Competency statement 15.2: Specific procedure competency statements for communication in relation to transfer

Complete assessment against relevant fundamental competency statements (*see* Chapter 2, pp. 20, 21)	Evidence
Specific procedure competency statements for communication in relation to critical are transfers	**Evidence of competency in communication in relation to critical care transfers**
Demonstrate ability to: ■ teach and assess or ■ learn from assessment.	*May be demonstrated by:* ■ examples of evidence of teaching, assessing and learning.
Demonstrate understanding of the importance of good communication between staff in receiving and referring units in ensuring safe and effective transfer.	*May be demonstrated by:* ■ discussion with supervisor/mentor ■ teaching session for peers.
Demonstrate the ability to communicate effectively with members of the multidisciplinary team at both referring and receiving hospitals, including ability to convey essential information relating to patient's: ■ history ■ investigations ■ treatment ■ personal circumstances.	*May be demonstrated by:* ■ direct observation of clinical practice.
Demonstrate understanding of the importance of good record keeping during all stages of care as an aid to communication handover and audit.	*May be demonstrated by:* ■ discussion with supervisor/mentor ■ teaching session for peers.

Competency statement 15.3: Specific procedure competency statements for assessment and stabilization prior to transfer

Complete assessment against relevant fundamental competency statements (*see* Chapter 2, pp. 20, 21)	Evidence
Specific procedure competency statements for assessment and stabilization of critically ill patients prior to transfer	**Evidence of competency in assessment and stabilization of critically ill patients prior to transfer**
Demonstrate ability to: ■ teach and assess or ■ learn from assessment.	*May be demonstrated by:* ■ examples of evidence of teaching, assessing and learning.
Demonstrate knowledge and understanding of the pathophysiology of critical illness.	*May be demonstrated by:* ■ discussion with supervisor/mentor ■ teaching sessions for peers.
Demonstrate understanding of the importance of stabilization and optimization of the patient's condition prior to transfer, including the need for: ■ safe and secure airway ■ effective ventilation ■ haemodynamic stability ■ optimization of organ perfusion ■ adequate sedation and analgesia.	*May be demonstrated by:* ■ discussion with supervisor/mentor ■ teaching sessions for peers.
Demonstrate knowledge and skills (appropriate to role) required to asses and stabilize the patient prior to transfer, including: ■ intubation and ventilation ■ optimization of haemodynamic status ■ optimization of organ perfusion ■ provision of adequate sedation and analgesia.	*May be demonstrated by:* ■ direct observation of clinical practice.

Competency statement 15.4: Specific procedure competency statements for preparation for transfer

Complete assessment against relevant fundamental competency statements (*see* Chapter 2, pp. 20, 21)	Evidence
Specific procedure competency statements for preparation of a critically ill patient for transfer	**Evidence of competency for preparation of a critically ill patient for transfer**
Demonstrate ability to: ■ teach and assess or ■ learn from assessment.	*May be demonstrated by:* ■ examples of evidence of teaching, assessing and learning.
Demonstrate understanding of the equipment needed for transfer and ability to prepare and check equipment prior to use.	*May be demonstrated by:* ■ discussion with supervisor/mentor ■ teaching sessions for peers ■ direct observation of clinical practice.
Demonstrate knowledge and understanding of the necessary steps to ensure preparation of a critically ill patient for transfer, including minimum standards for monitoring.	*May be demonstrated by:* ■ discussion with supervisor/mentor ■ teaching sessions for peers ■ direct observation of clinical practice.
Demonstrate safe preparation of patient for transfer, including movement of patient to transfer trolley and safe approach to securing patient and equipment.	*May be demonstrated by:* ■ direct observation of clinical practice.
Demonstrate safe use of the transfer equipment, including portable ventilator, portable monitoring and syringe pumps.	*May be demonstrated by:* ■ direct observation of clinical practice.
Demonstrate understanding of the benefits of pre-transfer check lists to aid preparation.	*May be demonstrated by:* ■ discussion with supervisor/mentor ■ teaching sessions for peers.

Competency statement 15.5: Specific procedure competency statements for carrying out safe transfer

Complete assessment against relevant fundamental competency statements (*see* Chapter 2, pp. 20, 21)	Evidence
Specific procedure competency statements for carrying out safe transfer of a critically ill patient	**Evidence of competency for carrying out safe transfer of a critically ill patient**
Demonstrate ability to: ■ teach and assess or ■ learn from assessment.	*May be demonstrated by:* ■ examples of evidence of teaching, assessing and learning.
Demonstrate familiarity with the proposed mode of transport and demonstrate knowledge and understanding of the limitations/problems associated with it. (NB Practitioners without specific training in air transportation should not undertake patient transfers by air.)	*May be demonstrated by:* ■ discussion with supervisor/mentor ■ teaching sessions for peers.

Demonstrate knowledge and understanding of the physiological effects of transportation and the transport environment on the critically ill, including effects of: ■ acceleration/deceleration forces ■ noise ■ vibration ■ environmental temperature.	*May be demonstrated by:* ■ discussion with supervisor/mentor ■ teaching sessions for peers.
Demonstrate knowledge and understanding of the safety issues involved during transfer, including: ■ safe stowage of equipment ■ avoidance of excessive speed ■ appropriate use of lights and sirens to facilitate journey.	*May be demonstrated by:* ■ discussion with supervisor/mentor ■ teaching sessions for peers ■ direct observation of clinical practice.
Demonstrate knowledge and skills required to deal with problems encountered during transfer, including deterioration of the patient, and potential equipment failure.	*May be demonstrated by:* ■ discussion with supervisor/mentor ■ teaching sessions for peers ■ direct observation of clinical practice.

Competency statement 15.6: Specific procedure competency statements for handover following patient transfer

Complete assessment against relevant fundamental competency statements (*see* Chapter 2, pp. 20, 21)	Evidence
Specific procedure competency statements for handover following patient transfer	**Evidence for competency for handover following patient transfer**
Demonstrate ability to: ■ teach and assess or ■ learn from assessment.	*May be demonstrated by:* ■ examples of evidence of teaching, assessing and learning.
Demonstrate knowledge and understanding of the importance of keeping accurate records during transfer.	*May be demonstrated by:* ■ discussion with supervisor/mentor ■ teaching sessions for peers ■ direct observation of clinical practice.
Demonstrate knowledge and understanding of the importance of handover to the receiving unit in ensuring seamless care.	*May be demonstrated by:* ■ discussion with supervisor/mentor ■ teaching sessions for peers.
Demonstrate ability to provide effective handover including identifying relevant information, investigation and treatments.	*May be demonstrated by:* ■ direct observation of clinical practice.

References and further reading

Andrews PJD, Piper IR and Dearden NM (1990) Secondary insults during intrahospital transport of head-injured patients. *Lancet* 335: 327–330.

Arfken CL, Shapiro MJ, Bessey PQ and Littenberg B (1998) Effectiveness of helicopter vs ground ambulance for interfacility transport. *Journal of Trauma* 45(4): 785–790.

American College of Emergency Physicians (2009) Appropriate interhospital patient transfer. *Annals of Emergency Medicine* 54: 141.

Association of Anaesthetists of Great Britain and Ireland (2009) *AAGBI Safety Guideline: Interhospital transfer*. London: AAGBI.

Belligan G, Olivier T, Batson S and Webb A (2000) Comparison of a specialist retrieval team with current UK practice for the hospital transport of critically ill patients. *Intensive Care Medicine* 26(6): 740–744.

Belway D, Henderson W, Keenan S et al. (2006) Do ppecialist transport personnel improve hospital outcome in critically ill patients transferred to higher centres? A systematic review. *Journal of Critical Care* 21: 8–18.

Bersten AD and Soni N (eds) (2009) *Oh's Intensive Care Manual* (6e). Oxford: Butterworth-Heinemann.

Bickell WH, Wall MJ Jr, Pepe PE et al. (1994) Immediate versus delayed fluid resuscitation for hypotensive patients with penetrating torso injuries. *New England Journal of Medicine* 331(17): 1105–1109.

Committee on European Standards (2007) *Medical Vehicles and their Equipment*. EN 1789. Brussels: European Committee for Standardization.

Cook CJ and Allan C (2008) Are trainees equipped to transfer critically ill patients? *Journal of the Intensive Care Society* 9(2): 145–147.

Craig SS (2005) Challenges in arranging interhospital transfers from a small regional hospital: an observational study. *Emergency Medicine Australasia* 17(2): 124–131.

Deasy C and O'Sullivan I (2007) Transfer of patients – from the spoke to the hub. *Irish Medical Journal* 100(7): 538–539.

Department of Health (2000) *Comprehensive Critical Care. A review of adult critical care services*. London: DH.

Department of Health (2009) *Emergency Services Review*. London: DH.

Easby J, Clarke FC and Bonner S (2002) Secondary inter-hospital transfers of critically ill patients: completing the audit cycle. *British Journal of Anaesthesia* 89: 354.

European Society for Intensive Care Medicine (2011) *Patient Transportation: skills and techniques*. Brussels: The European Society for Intensive Care Medicine.

Flabouris A, Runciman WB and Levings B (2006) Incidents during out-of-hospital patient transportation. *Anaesthesia and Intensive Care* 34(2): 228–236.

General Medical Council (2013) *Good Medical Practice*. London: GMC. http://www.gmc-uk.org/gmp2013 [accessed 25 March 2013].

Gillman L, Leslie G, Williams T et al. (2006) Adverse events experienced while transferring the critically ill patient from the emergency department to the intensive care unit. *Emergency Medicine Journal* 23(11): 858–861.

Goldfrad C and Rowan K (2000) Consequences of discharges from intensive care at might. *Lancet* 355: 1138–1142.

Gray A, Bush S and Whiteley S (2004) Secondary transport of the critically ill and injured adult. *Emergency Medicine Journal* 21(3): 281–285.

Health and Care Professions Council (2012) *Standard of Conduct, Performance and Ethics*. London: HCPC. http://www.hcpc-uk.org/assets/documents/10003B6EStandardsofconduct,performanceandethics.pdf [accessed January 2013].

Intensive Care Society (2011) *Guidelines for the Transport of the Critically Ill Adult*. London: ICS. http://www.ics.ac.uk/intensive_care_professional/standards_and_guidelines/transport_of_the_critically_ill_adult_2011 [accessed 20 March 2012].

Iwashyna TJ, Christie JD, Moody J et al. (2009) The structure of Critical Care Transfer Networks. *Medical Care* 47(7): 787–793.

Ligtenberg JJ, Arnold LG, Stienstra Y et al. (2005) Quality of interhospital transport of critically ill patients: a prospective audit. *Critical Care* 9(4): R446–451.

Lumb AB (2010) *Nunn's Applied Respiratory Physiology* (7e). Edinburgh: Churchill Livingstone.

Mackenzie PA, Smith EA and Wallace PGM (1997) Transfer of adults between intensive care units in the United Kingdom: postal survey. *British Medical Journal* 314: 1455–1456.

Martin T (2006) *Aeromedical Transportation: a clinical guide*. Aldershot: Ashgate.

McDonald AC (2006) Critical care transport teams: searching for evidence of effectiveness. *Journal of Critical Care* 21(1): 17–18.

Mental Capacity Act (2005) http://www.legislation.gov.uk/ukpga/2005/9/pdfs/ukpga_20050009_en.pdf [accessed 09 February 2012].

Nursing and Midwifery Council (2008) *The Code: standards of conduct, performance and ethics for nurses and midwives*. London: NMC. http://www.nmc-uk.org/Documents/Standards/The-code-A4-20100406.pdf [accessed 15 February 2012].

Royal College of Anaesthetists (2009) *CCT in Anaesthesia, II. Competency Basic Level (Speciality Training Years 1 and 2) Training and Assessment. A manual for trainees and trainers* (2e). London: Royal College of Anaesthetists.

Spencer C, Watkinson P and McCluskey A (2005) Training and assessment of competency of trainees in the transfer of critically ill patients. *Anaesthesia* 60: 413–414.

Stevenson A, Fiddler C, Craig M and Gray A (2005) Emergency department organisation of critical care transfers in the UK. *Emergency Medicine Journal* 22(11): 795–798.

Thomson DP and Thomas SH (2003) Guidelines for air-medical dispatch. Services Committee of the National Association of EMS Physicians. *PreHospital Emergency Care* 7(2): 265–271.

Tobin AE and Santamaria JD (2006) After-hours discharges from intensive care are associated with increased mortality. *Medical Journal of Australia* 184: 334–337.

Van Lieshout EJ, De Vos R, Binnekade JM et al (2008) Decision making in interhospital transport of critically ill patients: national questionnaire survey amongst critical care physicians. *Intensive Care Medicine* 34(7): 1269–1273.

Yentis S, Hirsch N and Smith G (2009) *A-Z of Anaesthesia and Intensive Care* (4e). New York: Elsevier.

Chapter 16

Rehabilitation from critical illness

Catherine I. Plowright[1] and Christina Jones[2]

[1]Medway NHS Foundation Trust and Canterbury Christ Church University, Canterbury, Kent, UK
[2]Whiston Hospital and Institute of Ageing and Chronic Disease, University of Liverpool, Liverpool, UK

Critical Care Manual of Clinical Procedures and Competencies, First Edition.
Edited by Jane Mallett, John W. Albarran, and Annette Richardson.
© 2013 John Wiley & Sons, Ltd. Published 2013 by John Wiley & Sons, Ltd.

Definition

To rehabilitate is to restore (someone) to health or normal life by therapy after illness (Oxford English Dictionary 2010). For patients recovering from critical illness, rehabilitation includes physical, psychological and cognitive domains.

Aims and indications for rehabilitation

The aim of rehabilitation is return the patient to as close to, or better than, their normal health as possible. The latter is possible in some cases because, for example, their medication has been optimized or they have managed to stop smoking (Jones et al. 2001a). The time taken to return to a level of activity similar to that prior to critical illness depends on a number of things, such as the patient's length of stay in a critical care unit (Jones and Griffiths 2000). It is typically between 9 and 12 months after hospital discharge, or longer (National Institute for Health and Clinical Excellence 2009).

All patients admitted to a critical care unit should be assessed to ensure that any potential rehabilitation needs are recognized and an appropriate plan devised. This includes the following:

- All patients admitted to a critical care environment should have a short clinical assessment performed to determine their risk of developing physical and non-physical morbidity, for example anxiety, depression.
- All patients at risk of physical and non-physical morbidity should have a comprehensive clinical assessment performed to identify their rehabilitation needs.
- Patients identified at risk, for example showing significant muscle mass loss, should have short-term and medium-term rehabilitation goals set based on a comprehensive clinical assessment.
- Rehabilitation should be instigated as early as clinically possible, based on the assessment and any rehabilitation needs.

Background

Rehabilitation and critical care

In England and Wales, about 100 000 people are admitted to critical care units every year, and the majority of them are discharged home (Intensive Care National Audit & Research Centre – Case Mix Programme 2010). About 20% of patients admitted to critical care units die in this setting, with a hospital mortality of 28% of all admissions (Intensive Care National Audit & Research Centre – Case Mix Programme 2010). However, the perception among many healthcare professionals, patients and their families is that the recovery will be rapid and that individuals will return to the quality of life they had before they became critically ill (NICE 2009).

For patients who have been discharged from critical care, their recovery is often uncertain and they will typically experience a number of physical and non-physical problems. Patients who have had a prolonged critical illness of weeks, or in some cases months, have greater long-term difficulties (Jones et al. 2000). However, some who have spent relatively short periods of time (that is, less than 5 days) in critical care may experience substantial health problems, particularly psychological issues such as anxiety and depression (Jones et al. 2007; Granja et al. 2008; NICE 2009). Regardless of the period of time they were critically ill, some patients do have an uneventful recovery and practitioners need to remember and consider this when planning discharge (NICE 2009).

Effect of critical illness on patients' families

Many families are affected by the rehabilitation needs of patients who have been critically ill, and they may have emotional, physical and financial difficulties themselves (NICE 2009). In addition to the impact on patients and their families, there is an effect on society when patients and their relatives do not return to being fully functioning members of society (NICE 2009; Davidson et al. 2012).

Patients' and relatives' stories, outlining their individual experiences regarding critical illness, have started to appear on websites such as Healthtalkonline (www.healthtalkonline. org), ICUSteps (www.icusteps.org) and Patient Opinion (www.patientopinion.org.uk). These are valuable in assisting practitioners to develop an understanding of the impact of critical illness on patients and families.

Healthtalkonline is a web site that includes individual interviews with patients and family. The stories can be searched for particular themes, for example receiving an 'ICU diary'. ICUSteps is a support group set up by people who had been critical care patients and their family members. The aim of ICUSteps is to help those who have suffered a life-threatening injury or illness, allowing patients to come to terms with their experience and find support and reassurance in the long recovery period. An example from ICUSteps of unmet rehabilitation needs is demonstrated by 'Mandy's story', covering her husband's 3 weeks in ITU, 3 weeks on a ward and then going home.

Mandy's story

'The preceding weeks had been very stressful and seeing just how unhappy he had become, against my better judgement, I helped him with the aid of his walking frame to the car and took him home. All the way home all I could think was "What have I done?". By then though it was too late. Eventually, somehow, as he was still very weak from being immobile for so long, we made it home, upstairs and into bed where I cared for him. I feel I must have gone a bit insane myself at that time, because that is when the consequences of what I'd helped him to do really became apparent to me.

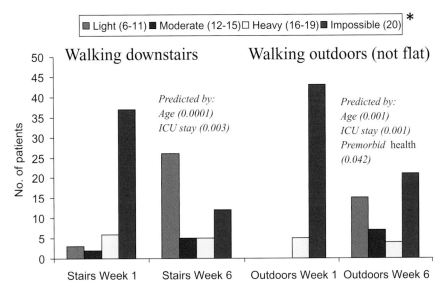

Figure 16.1 Factors related to difficulty with activities at 1 and 6 weeks post 'ICU' discharge (Jones and Griffiths 2000). *Numbers in table refer to Borg exertion scale ratings (1982) made by the patient when undertaking the specific activity at week 1 then at week 6.

I couldn't sleep, afraid that something would happen to him in my care, and he had no medication . . . I spent time on the phone to my GP surgery struggling to convince them that I needed a home visit . . . I was contacted by the physiotherapy department at the hospital . . . The community occupational therapy unit came and fitted disabled aids to the bath, toilet, etc., and taught him how to manage stairs . . . Everything he did physically was of great effort and he would spend a lot of time resting. He was still very afraid, and I couldn't really appreciate what he was feeling, but later discovered it was fear of having lost several weeks of his life and a feeling of unreality to his existence. Thankfully, in a psychological sense, his return home enabled him gradually to come to terms with his trauma.' (www.icusteps.org, accessed 13 January 2011)

Review of components of rehabilitation from critical care

Muscle loss and weakness

The need for physical rehabilitation is driven by the accelerated muscle mass loss that takes place during critical illness (Griffiths and Hall 2010). Research, using paired muscle biopsies, has shown losses of up to 3% from Type 1 muscle fibres and 4% from Type 2 (Helliwell et al. 1998). Type 1 fibres are slow to fatigue and give stamina, while Type 2 fibres are quicker to tire and allow short bursts of speed. In addition, the protein loss from muscle during multi-organ failure can reach up to 2% per day (Gamrin et al. 1997). Such losses happen very quickly but require good nutrition, particularly a good protein and vitamin intake, and the

stimulation of exercise to replace during recovery (*see also* Chapter 12).

Factors that identify patients requiring physical rehabilitation depend on the demand that the activity places on the body. For example, age and length of stay in a critical care unit are predictors of difficulty in walking downstairs and walking on uneven ground. Pre-morbid health also has a negative impact on the latter (Jones and Griffiths 2000) (Figure 16.1). In addition, loss of muscle mass results in weakness and critical illness, and motor and sensory polyneuropathy further complicate physical rehabilitation (Fletcher et al. 2003). Although mobilizing a critically ill patient with polyneuropathy is a significant challenge, longer-term recovery is possible if the patient is able to rebuild muscle bulk through rehabilitative exercise (*see* Chapter 14).

Cognitive deficits

There are a number of cognitive problems that can occur following critical illness. These can be very distressing and are often not recognized (Griffiths and Jones 2007).

Most research into cognitive function in critically ill patients has focused on those with adult respiratory distress syndrome (ARDS). At 2 years after discharge from a critical care unit, 47% of people still have cognitive impairment (Hopkins et al. 1999). Deficits in memory, decision making and attention have been shown, with the defects principally involving executive function. This controls and manages other cognitive processes and is responsible for planning, cognitive flexibility, abstract thinking, rule acquisition, initiating appropriate action, suppressing inappropriate actions and selecting relevant sensory information. Defects in executive function have also been demonstrated in critical care patients at 3 (Jones et al. 2006), 6 (Jackson et al. 2003) and 9 months after discharge from a critical care unit (Sukantarat et al. 2005). Therefore, patients who have experienced a critical illness may demonstrate a dysexecutive syndrome (poor executive function), which may vary in severity and result in problems with memory, problem solving and making social decisions (Griffiths and Jones 2007).

Absent-mindedness has also been reported in post-recovery critical care patients (Griffiths and Jones 2007). This can manifest as an increased incidence of slips of action, i.e. forgetting part of an action, such as putting the kettle on without putting water in it. This becomes very irritating to the patient and makes them feel out of control.

The patient's partner or a close family member may in some cases compensate for the patient's cognitive deficits. This may be demonstrated by family members remembering hospital appointments for patients and managing financial affairs, for example. This may be a cause of stress among relatives and they should be given information so that they understand what is happening to the patient (Griffiths and Jones 2007).

Psychological problems precipitated by the patient's experiences of critical illness include a wide range of diagnoses from anxiety, depression, post-traumatic stress disorder (PTSD), agoraphobia, panic attacks and hospital phobia (Jones and Griffiths 2005). Such psychological problems can affect ongoing rehabilitation and care, especially when patients become panic stricken, for example when coming to the hospital for appointments. Approximately 10% of patients who have received critical care may develop new-onset PTSD. This is often triggered by frightening delusional memories, such as nightmares, hallucinations and paranoid delusions from when they were critically ill (Jones et al. 2001a; Granja et al. 2005; Jones et al. 2007). Such memories are usually described by patients as being very vivid and realistic. Where these are their only memories of their illness it can be very difficult for patients to separate reality from delusion. Patients with the full diagnosis of PTSD and where no help is offered may become socially isolated and alienated from others. In addition, they may not return to their normal life as a means of allowing them to cope with their symptoms. Alcohol and drug abuse can occur in this patient group in an effort to self-medicate to control their symptoms (Jones and Griffiths 2007).

Rehabilitation

Rehabilitation following critical illness aims to optimize the patient's physical, emotional, cognitive and social recovery by implementing patient-centred strategies that reflect the individual's needs. This requires a practitioner to coordinate the process to ensure that aspects of the patient's rehabilitation needs are not missed. National guidelines (NICE 2009) highlight that rehabilitation should:

- address both physical and non-physical problems
- start as soon as the patient is admitted to critical care

- include ongoing assessment of rehabilitation needs throughout the patient's hospital stay and at discharge home.

The guidelines suggest the use of two well-validated screening tools for assessing anxiety, depression and symptoms of PTSD. These are the Hospital Anxiety and Depression Scale (HADS; Zigmond and Snaith 1983) and the Post Traumatic Syndrome 14 Question Inventory (PTSS-14; Twigg et al. 2008), both of which can be completed by the patient. Although these screening tools are very short and easy to score in a clinical setting, the HADS is only available to purchase by those individuals or organizations with the relevant qualifications and/or training and experience. The relevant score obtained indicates whether there is a potential need for referral for specialist psychological therapy.

Rehabilitation interventions

There is evidence of efficacy of specific rehabilitation interventions in critical care units and following discharge, including that of early rehabilitation while the patient is still critically ill. This can result in, for example, an increase in distance walked in 6 minutes, isometric quadriceps force and patients' subjective wellbeing at hospital discharge (Burtin et al. 2009). Simply mobilizing patients early during their stay in the critical care unit reduces their length of stay in critical care and reduces hospital stay (Morris et al. 2008). In addition, self-directed exercises, psychological advice and information about the after-effects of critical illness (in the form of an 'ICU Recovery Manual Rehabilitation Programme' [Jones et al. 2003]), have been shown to improve physical function-related quality of life at 6 months. This programme also produced some reduction in depression at 2 months post critical care discharge (Jones et al. 2003). The 'ICU Recovery Manual Rehabilitation Programme' has been devised to guide the patient through the first 6 weeks of their recovery and is used from about one week after discharge from a critical care unit. This guidance enables the patient to take control of their recovery by devising their own individual exercise programme to regain their strength. A cohort of the patients in the Jones et al. (2003) study also recorded their smoking habits and this showed an increased rate of smoking cessation among the intervention patients at both 2 and 6 months (Jones et al. 2001b).

Research has also indicated that other types of programme may lead to some improvements in patients' rehabilitation. The 'Programme of Enhanced Physiotherapy and Structured Exercise' (PEPSE) comprises of a 2-hour outpatient class combined with two sessions at the patient's home. The outpatient class is based on circuit training, with the patient moving from one exercise station to the next, targeting different muscle groups. A small, non-randomized study of eight patients showed an increase in the distance the patient walked in 6 minutes and a reduction in anxiety and depression (McWilliams et al. 2009).

Diaries

Diaries have been shown to be meaningful for patients and their families (Robson 2008; Storli et al. 2008). Two studies have highlighted the use of diaries as a basis for systematic follow-up where patients seek to understand their memories (Bäckman and Walther 2001; Storli and Lind 2009). Egerod and Christensen (2009) identified that diaries showed the presence of nurses and were a source of comfort, encouragement and a method of installing hope in patients. The use of diaries and hospital records have been compared and it was shown that the diary provided a more comprehensive story that could help the patient to construct or reconstruct their critical illness narrative (Egerod and Christensen 2010).

Since the 1980s, diaries written by practitioners and family members have been used by nursing staff in critical care. The use of diaries is expanding in many countries where they are utilized as a method to assist patients come to terms with their critical illness experience (Storli et al. 2008). They are used in approximately half the critical care units in Norway (Gjengedal et al. 2010); around a third of Danish critical care units (Egerod et al. 2007); 75% of Swedish critical care units (Åkerman et al. 2010); and increasingly in the UK, Italy and Portugal (Jones et al. 2010).

The efficacy of providing patients with an ICU diary to aid psychological recovery after discharge has been tested in two randomized, controlled trials (RCT). The diary documented the day-to-day details of the patient's stay and were written by their family and practitioners. A small RCT (n = 36) investigating the incidence of anxiety and depression after critical illness measured with HADS demonstrated a reduction for those patients receiving a diary (Knowles and Tarrier 2009). A larger trial with 352 patients (who had stayed in critical care units) completing the 3-month follow-up assessment reviewed the impact of diaries on new-onset PTSD. These diaries additionally included photographs.

Patients were randomized to an intervention group, who received their diary at one month post critical care discharge (by which time they had left hospital), while the control group were given their diary at 3 months following discharge. There was a reduced incidence of new-onset PTSD in the intervention group of 5%, compared with 13.1% for the controls (p = 0.03) (Jones et al. 2010). The effect was most noticable in the intervention group, who were showing the highest levels of symptoms of PTSD prior to receiving the diary.

Counselling

Currently in the UK, the provision of specialist counselling services for patients who have undergone a prolonged period of critical care is confined to a few centres. In the UK, the National Institute of Clinical Excellence (NICE 2004a, 2004b, 2006) has produced a number of treatment guidelines for anxiety, depression and PTSD. All the guidelines have at their core:

1 the need for assessment in high-risk groups
2 appropriate and timely referral
3 a 'watch and wait' approach for those patients with low symptom levels
4 advice that psychoactive medication should only be used if patients do not engage in psychotherapy.

For patients undergoing counselling common themes are:

- trying to make sense of what happened in the critical care unit
- coming to terms with physical changes (which in some cases may be permanent)
- coping with distressing flashbacks or nightmares (Barnett 2006; Jones et al. 2008).

The flashback and nightmares experienced by some patients are associated with a diagnosis of PTSD. Forms of psychotherapy for the treatment of PTSD that have been supported by NICE (2006) include eye movement desensitization and reprocessing (EMDR) and cognitive behavioural therapy (CBT). EMDR was developed to resolve symptoms resulting from disturbing and unresolved life experiences. It uses a structured approach to address past, present and future aspects of disturbing memories (Shapiro 2002). CBT can involve: examining beliefs that might be unhelpful or unrealistic; gradually encouraging patients to face activities that may have been avoided; and enabling them to try out new ways of reacting to situations (Olatunji et al. 2010). Clinical experience with counselling patients who had stayed in a critical care unit (Jones et al. 2008) supports the use of EMDR. EMDR alone or in combination with CBT results in most patients becoming non-symptomatic or the PTDS becoming subclinical (Jones et al. 2008). The patients themselves report that they feel significantly better and able to return to their normal life.

Summary

Individualized rehabilitation strategies should be considered during and after discharge from critical care in order to improve patient outcomes. Application of appropriate interventions may:

- reduce the length of stay in critical care
- reduce the length of hospital stay after discharge from critical care
- minimize hospital readmission rates (Morris et al. 2008)
- decrease pressure on primary care resources.

Furthermore, tailored rehabilitation programmes may help patients return to their previous level of activities sooner, which will result in substantial benefits for recovering patients and their families (Jones et al. 2003).

Procedure guideline 16.1: Rehabilitation during and following critical illness

Action	Rationale
1 Where possible, explain and discuss the procedure with the patient. If the patient lacks the capacity to make decisions the practitioner must act in the patient's best interests.	To ensure that the patient understands the procedure and gives their valid consent. To ensure the patient's best interests are maintained (Mental Capacity Act 2005).
2 Ensure the rehabilitation needs of all patients admitted to critical care units are assessed: (a) during critical care (b) prior to discharge from the critical care unit (c) during ward-based care (d) 2–3 months following discharge from critical care.	To enable the physical and non-physical needs of the patient to be identified as soon as possible (NICE 2009).
3 For (a), (b), (c) undertake short clinical assessment to identify patients requiring physical rehabilitation. This should include the following factors: ■ unable to get out of bed independently ■ anticipated long duration of critical care stay ■ obvious significant physical or neurological injury ■ lack of cognitive functioning to continue exercise independently ■ unable to self-ventilate on 35% oxygen or less ■ presence of pre-morbid respiratory or mobility problems ■ unable to mobilize independently over short distances.	To identify physical rehabilitation needs of the patient as soon as possible (NICE 2009).
4 For (a), (b), (c) undertake short clinical assessment to identify patients requiring psychological rehabilitation. This should include the following factors: ■ recurrent nightmares – particularly where patients report trying to stay awake to avoid nightmares ■ intrusive memories of traumatic events that have occurred prior to admission (for example road traffic accidents) or during their critical care stay (for example delusional experiences) ■ new and recurrent anxiety or panic attacks ■ expressing the wish not to talk about their illness or changing the subject quickly off the topic.	To identify psychological needs of the patient as soon as possible (NICE 2009).
5 For (a) and (b) complete an 'ICU diary' for all patients staying more than 72 hours on a critical care unit.	To address information needs and reduce the risk of new onset PTSD (Jones et al. 2010).
6 For (b), (c) or (d) go through the ICU diary with the patient when they report feeling ready to listen to the story and look at the photographs.	To address information needs and reduce the risk of new onset PTSD (Jones et al. 2010).
7 For (d) undertake a clinical assessment of any remaining physical rehabilitation needs, including: ■ If patient appears to be recovering at a slower rate than anticipated ■ If the patient has developed unanticipated physical problems not previously anticipated.	To identify physical problems that may need further rehabilitation (NICE 2009).
8 For (d) apply appropriate screening tools for assessing psychological needs: ■ for anxiety and depression administer the Hospital Anxiety and Depression Scale (HADS) ■ or symptoms of PTSD administer the Post Traumatic Syndrome 14 Question Inventory (PTSS-14).	To identify psychological problems that may need further rehabilitation (NICE 2009).

9 Document any assessment and care provided.

To:
- provide an accurate record
- monitor effectiveness of procedure
- reduce the risk of duplication of treatment
- provide a point of reference or comparison in the event of later questions
- acknowledge accountability for actions
- facilitate communication and continuity of care.

(NMC 2008; HCPC 2012; GMC 2013)

Competency statement 16.1: Specific procedure competency statements for rehabilitation of critically ill patients

Complete assessment against relevant fundamental competency statements (*see* Chapter 2, pp. 20, 21)	Evidence
Specific procedure competency statements for rehabilitation of critically ill patients	**Evidence of competency for rehabilitation of critically ill patients**
Demonstrate ability to: - teach and assess or - ability to learn from assessment.	Examples of evidence of teaching, assessing and learning.
Explain the meaning of 'critical care rehabilitation' (NICE 2009), including: - rehabilitation is the process of physical and psychological recovery, helping people cope with the physical, psychological and emotional effects associated with critical illness and with being a patient in critical care - rehabilitation can help patients get physically and psychologically stronger through the use of gentle exercise programmes, advice and support.	*May be demonstrated by:* - discussion with supervisor/mentor - teaching session.
Identify reasons why rehabilitation of critically ill patients is essential, including: - to return the patient to as close to their normal health state prior to the critical illness experience - to reduce the length of stay in critical care - to reduce hospital stay after discharge from critical care - to minimize hospital readmission rates - to reduce the use of primary care resources.	*May be demonstrated by:* - discussion with supervisor/mentor - teaching session for peers - completion of a reflective text/essay.
Explain functional assessment (NICE 2009) and what it should include: - an assessment to examine the patient's daily functional ability - physical dimensions, non-physical dimensions.	*May be demonstrated by:* - discussion with supervisor/mentor - teaching session for peers - completion of a reflective text/essay.
Identify the times when assessment of the rehabilitation needs should be conducted, including: - during the patient's critical care stay and as early as clinically possible - before discharge from critical care - during ward-based care - before discharge to home or community care - 2–3 months after discharge from critical care.	*May be demonstrated by:* - discussion with supervisor/mentor - teaching session for peers - completion of a reflective text/essay.

(*Continued*)

Competency statement 16.1: (Continued)

Explain and list the differences between physical and non-physical morbidity. For example: ■ physical weakness may include inability/partial ability to sit, rise to standing, or to walk, fatigue, pain, breathlessness, swallowing difficulties, incontinence, inability/partial ability to self-care (NICE 2009) ■ non-physical problems may include nightmares, flashbacks, memory loss, low self esteem, relationship difficulties.	*May be demonstrated by:* ■ discussion with supervisor/mentor ■ teaching session for peers ■ completion of a reflective text/essay.

Identify and discuss examples that may indicate that the patient is at risk of developing physical and non-physical morbidity (NICE 2009), including:
■ physical:
  ○ unable to get out of bed independently
  ○ unable to self-ventilate on 35% oxygen or less
  ○ lack of independent mobility over short distances
■ non-physical:
  ○ recurrent nightmares
  ○ new and recurring panic or anxiety attacks
  ○ intrusive memories of traumatic events.
	May be demonstrated by:
	■ discussion with supervisor/mentor
	■ teaching session for peers
	■ completion of a reflective text/essay.

Discuss the effectiveness of a variety of screening and assessment tools available to assist in rehabilitation of patients following a critical illness. For example: ■ Hospital Anxiety and Depression Scale (HADS) ■ Post Traumatic Syndrome 14 Question Inventory (PTSS-14) ■ Rivermead Mobility Index ■ CAM-ICU.	*May be demonstrated by:* ■ discussion with supervisor/mentor ■ teaching session for peers ■ completion of a reflective text/essay.
Identify the variety of tools available to assist in rehabilitation of patients following a critical illness: ■ 'ICU Recovery Manual Rehabilitation Programme' ■ Programme of Enhanced Physiotherapy and Structured Exercise (PEPSE).	*May be demonstrated by:* ■ discussion with supervisor/mentor ■ teaching session for peers ■ implementation into practice.
Identify the advantages and disadvantages of using patient diaries in a critical care environment: ■ source of comfort and encouragement ■ a method of installing hope to patients ■ provides a story to help the patient construct or reconstruct their critical illness ■ assist patients come to terms with their critical illness ■ reduce incidence of PTSD.	*May be demonstrated by:* ■ discussion with supervisor/mentor ■ teaching session for peers ■ implementation into practice.
Identify and discuss the common themes that patients having counseling following critical illness experience and the therapies that can be used: ■ trying to make sense of what happened in CCU ■ coming to terms with physical changes ■ eye movement desensitization and reprocessing therapy ■ cognitive behavioural therapy.	*May be demonstrated by:* ■ discussion with supervisor/mentor ■ teaching session for peers.

References

Åkerman E, Granberg-Axéll A, Ersson A et al. (2010) Use and practice of the patient diaries in Swedish intensive care units: a national survey. *Nursing in Critical Care* 15(1): 26–33.

Bäckman C and Walther SM (2001) The photo-diary and follow-up appointmenet on ICU: Giving back time to patients and relatives. In: Ridley S (ed.) *Critical Care Focus 12 – The Psychological Challenges of Intensive Care*, pp. 39–49. Oxford: Blackwell Publishing.

Barnett L (2006) Intensive care: an existential perspective. *Therapy Today* 17(5): 10–15.

Borg GA (1982) Psychophysical basis of perceived exertion. *Medical Science Sports Exercise* 14: 377–381.

Burtin C, Clerckx B, Robbeets C et al. (2009) Early exercise in critically ill patients enhances short-term functional recovery. *Critical Care Medicine* 37(9): 2499–2505.

Davidson J, Jones C and Bienvenu OJ (2012) Family response to critical illness: postintensive care syndrome – family. *Critical Care Medicine* 40(2). DOI 10.1097/CCM.0b013e318236ebf9.

Egerod I and Christensen D (2009) Analysis of patient diaries in Danish ICUs: a narrative approach. *Intensive and Critical Care Nursing* 25(5): 268–277.

Egerod I and Christensen D (2010) A comparative study of ICU patients' diaries vs hospital charts. *Qualitative Health Research* 22(10): 1446–1456.

Egerod I, Schwartz-Nielson KH, Hansen GM and Lærkner E (2007) The extent and application of patient diaries in Danish ICUs in 2006. *Nursing in Critical Care* 12(3): 159–167.

Fletcher SN, Kennedy DD, Ghosh IR et al. (2003) Persistent neuromuscular and neurophysiologic abnormalities in long-term survivors of prolonged critical illness. *Critical Care Medicine* 31: 1012–1016.

Gamrin L, Andersson K, Hultman E et al. (1997) Longitudinal changes of biochemical parameters in muscle during critical illness. *Metabolism* 46: 756–762.

General Medical Council (2013) *Good Medical Practice*. London: GMC. http://www.gmc-uk.org/gmp2013 [accessed 25 March 2013].

Gjengedal E, Storli SL, Norlemann Holme A and Eskerud RS (2010) An act of caring – patient diaries in Norwegian intensive care units. *Nursing in Critical Care* 15(4): 176–184.

Granja C, Lopes A, Moreira S et al. (2005) Patients' recollections of experiences in the intensive care unit may affect their quality of life. *Critical Care* 9: R96–R109.

Granja C, Gomes E, Amaro A, Ribeiro O et al., the JMIP Study Group (2008) Understanding posttraumatic stress disorder-related symptoms after critical care: the early illness amnesia hypothesis. *Critical Care Medicine* 36(10): 2901–2909.

Griffiths RD and Jones C (2007) Delirium, cognitive dysfunction and posttraumatic stress disorder. *Current Opinion in Anaesthesiology* 20: 124–129.

Griffiths RD and Hall J (2010) Intensive care unit-acquired weakness. *Critical Care Medicine* 38 (3): 779–787.

Health and Care Professions Council (2012) *Standard of Conduct, Performance and Ethics*. London: HCPC. http://www.hcpc-uk.org/assets/documents/10003B6EStandardsofconduct,performanceandethics.pdf [accessed January 2013].

Helliwell TR, Wilkinson A, Griffiths RD et al. (1998) Muscle fibre atrophy in critically ill patients is associated with the loss of myosin filaments and the presence of lysosomal enzymes and ubiquitin. *Neuropathology and Applied Neurobiology* 24: 507–517.

Hopkins RO, Weaver LK, Pope D et al (1999) Neurophysiological sequelae and impaired health status in survivors of severe acute respiratory distress syndrome. *American Journal of Respiratory and Critical Care Medicine* 160: 50–56.

Intensive Care National Audit & Research Centre – Case Mix Programme 2010. https://www.icnarc.org [accessed 19 January 2011].

Jackson JC, Hart RP, Gordon SM et al. (2003) Six month neuropsychological outcome from medical intensive care unit patients. *Critical Care Medicine* 31(4): 1226–1234.

Jones C and Griffiths RD (2000) Identifying post intensive care patients who may need physical rehabilitation. *Clinical Intensive Care* 11(1): 35–38.

Jones C and Griffiths RD (2005) Psychological Stress in adult ICU patients and relatives. In: Ridley S (ed.) *Critical Care Focus 12 – The Psychological Challenges of Intensive Care*, pp. 39–49. Oxford: Blackwell Publishing.

Jones C and Griffiths RD (2007) Patient and caregiver counselling after the intensive care unit: what are the needs and how should they be met? *Current Opinion in Critical Care* 13: 503–507.

Jones C, Griffiths RD, Humphris GH and Skirrow PM (2001a) Memory, delusions, and the development of acute posttraumatic stress disorder-related symptoms after intensive care. *Critical Care Medicine* 29(3): 573–580.

Jones C, Griffiths RD, Skirrow P and Humphris GH (2001b) Smoking cessation through comprehensive critical care. *Intensive Care Medicine* 27: 1547–1549.

Jones C, Skirrow P, Griffiths RD et al. (2003) Rehabilitation after critical illness: a randomized, controlled trial. *Critical Care Medicine* 31: 2456–2461.

Jones C, Griffiths RD, Slater T et al. (2006) Significant cognitive dysfunction in non-delirious patients identified during and persisting following critical illness. *Intensive Care Medicine* 32(6): 923–926.

Jones C, Bäckman C, Capuzzo M et al. (2007) Precipitants of posttraumatic stress disorder following intensive care: a hypothesis generating study of diversity in care. *Intensive Care Medicine* 33(6): 978–985.

Jones C, Hall S and Jackson S (2008) Benchmarking a nurse-led ICU counselling initiative. *Nursing Times* 104(38): 32–34.

Jones C, Bäckman C, Capuzzo M et al. and RACHEL group (2010) Intensive care diaries reduce new onset PTSD following critical illness: a randomised, controlled trial. *Critical Care* 14: R168.

Knowles RE and Tarrier N (2009) Evaluation of the effect of prospective patient diaries on emotional well-being in intensive care unit survivors: a randomised control trial. *Critical Care Medicine* 37: 184–191.

McWilliams DJ, Atkinson D and Carter A (2009) Feasibility and impact of a structured, exercise-based rehabilitation programme for intensive care survivors. *Physiotherapy Theory in Practice* 25(8): 566–571.

Mental Capacity Act (2005) http://www.legislation.gov.uk/ukpga/2005/9/pdfs/ukpga_20050009_en.pdf [accessed 9 February 2012].

Morris PE, Goad A and Thompson C (2008) Early intensive care unit mobility therapy in the treatment of acute respiratory failure. *Critical Care Medicine* 36: 2238–2243.

National Institute of Clinical Excellence (2004a) *Anxiety: management of anxiety (panic disorder, with or without agoraphobia, and generalised anxiety disorder) in adults in primary, secondary and community care*. London: NICE. www.nice.org.uk/pdf/CG022NICEguideline.pdf [accessed 25 January 2011].

National Institute of Clinical Excellence. (2004b) *Depression: management of depression in primary and secondary care – NICE guidance*. London: NICE. www.nice.org.uk/CG023NICEguideline.pdf [accessed 25 January 2011].

National Institute of Clinical Excellence (2006) *Post-traumatic Stress Disorder – the management of PTSD in adults and children in primary and secondary care*. London: NICE. www.nice.org.uk/ CG026NICEguideline.pdf [accessed 25 January 2011].

National Institute of Clinical Excellence (2009) *Rehabilitation After Critical Illness*. London: NICE. http://guidance.nice.org.uk/ CG83 [accessed 17 November 2010].

Nursing and Midwifery Council (2008) *The Code: standards of conduct, performance and ethics for nurses and midwives*. London: NMC. http://www.nmc-uk.org/Documents/Standards/ The-code-A4-20100406.pdf [accessed 15 February 2012].

Olatunji BO, Cisler JM and Deacon BJ (2010) Efficacy of cognitive behavioral therapy for anxiety disorders: a review of meta-analytic findings. *Psychiatric Clinics of North America* 33(3): 557–577.

Oxford English Dictionary (2010) Oxford: Oxford University Press.

Robson W (2008) An evaluation of patient diaries in intensive care. *Connect. The World of Critical Care Nursing*. 6(2): 34–37.

Shapiro F (2002) *EMDR as an Integrative Psychotherapy Approach: experts of diverse orientations explore the paradigm prism*. Washington, DC: American Psychological Association.

Storli S and Lind R (2009) The meaning of follow-up in intensive care: patients' perspective. *Scandinavian Journal of Caring Sciences* 23(1): 45–56.

Storli S, Lindseth A and Asplund K (2008) A journey in quest of meaning: A hermeneutic – phenomenological study on living with memories from intensive care. *Nursing in Critical Care* 13(2): 86–89.

Sukantarat KT, Burgess PW, Williamson RCN and Brett SJ (2005) Prolonged cognitive dysfunction in survivors of critical illness. *Anaesthesia* 60: 847–853.

Twigg E, Humphris GH, Jones C et al. (2008) Use of a screening questionnaire for post-traumatic stress disorder (PTSD) on a sample of UK ICU patients. *Acta Anaesthesiologica Scandinavia* 52: 202–208.

Zigmond AS and Snaith RP (1983) The Hospital Anxiety and Depression Scale. *Acta Psychiatrica Scandinavica* 67: 361–370.

Useful websites

Healthtalkonline: http://www.healthtalkonline.org
ICUSteps: http://www.icusteps.org
Patient Opinion: http://www.patientopinion.org.uk

Chapter 17

Withdrawal of treatment and end of life care for the critically ill patient

The Royal Marsden NHS Foundation Trust, London, UK

Critical Care Manual of Clinical Procedures and Competencies, First Edition.
Edited by Jane Mallett, John W. Albarran, and Annette Richardson.
© 2013 John Wiley & Sons, Ltd. Published 2013 by John Wiley & Sons, Ltd.

Definition

End of life is a state of progressive decline, which is irreversible. It is often used to describe the last few hours or days of a person's life or can refer to those whose terminal condition is incurable.

End-of-life care can be defined as:

care that helps all those with advanced, progressive, incurable illness to live as well as possible until they die. It enables the supportive and palliative care needs of both patient and family to be identified and met throughout the last phase of life and into bereavement. It includes management of pain and other symptoms and provision of psychological, social, spiritual and practical support.

(National Audit Office 2008: 6)

Aims and indications

End of life care (EOLC) is sometimes used synonymously with palliative care; however, there are differences between the two. EOLC pertains to the last phases of life, whereas palliative care predominantly relates to symptom relief (which may be provided at times other than the end of life). However, symptom relief can also be given at the end of life, so palliative care can encompass EOLC (see the definition of palliative care by the World Health Organization [Sepúlveda et al. 2002]; *see* Box 17.1).

Box 17.1 Palliative care

Facets of palliative care provision*

- Provides relief from pain and other distressing symptoms
- Affirms life and regards dying as a normal process
- Intends neither to hasten nor postpone death
- Integrates the psychological and spiritual aspects of patient care
- Offers a support system to help patients live as actively as possible until death
- Offers a support system to help the family cope during the patient's illness and in their own bereavement
- Uses a team approach to address the needs of patients and their families, including bereavement counselling, if indicated
- Will enhance quality of life, and may also positively influence the course of illness
- Is applicable early in the course of illness, in conjunction with other therapies that are intended to prolong life, such as chemotherapy or radiation therapy, and includes those investigations needed to better understand and manage distressing clinical complications

(Sepúlveda et al. 2002, reproduced with permission from Elsevier)

*NB While the definition represents facets of care provision, the defining characteristic of palliative care is the management of symptoms.

Background

As patients receiving critical care can deteriorate (sometimes rapidly and suddenly) to the point of dying, the focus for this chapter is EOLC. This will include the processes leading up to end of life, the care involved around decision making, withdrawal of care, care of the dying and care after death within the context of critical care practice.

Competence and skill in planning for end of life (EOL), in administering EOLC, and providing patients and their families with support, demands professional expertise. In addition, EOLC requires practitioners to have a detailed understanding of normal and abnormal pathophysiological changes that develop during this phase. Recognizing symptoms associated with the dying patient and knowledge of the effects that many therapeutic interventions used with patients receiving critical care will enable practitioners to identify changes in clinical condition and prevent some of the undesirable side effects caused. Therefore, an appreciation of clinical changes experienced by individuals at the end of life, an understanding of ventilation, effects of hypoxia and inotropes (*see* Chapters 5 and 7), and brainstem function (*see* Chapter 11), is necessary, along with some understanding of opioid and sedation and symptom-management pharmacology (*see* Chapter 10).

Recent data indicate that 16.1% of patients die in critical care. In the UK (Intensive Care National Audit Centre [ICNARC] 2012) this represents a sixth of all admissions to these environments. While there have been several UK initiatives to try and improve EOLC, few have specifically referred to, or focused on, critical care, despite the substantial number of critical care deaths. The National Gold Standard Framework (2011) was an NHS initiative that aimed to improve care for those nearing death across the acute and community sector. Toolkits have also been developed (discussed on p. 502), to provide some guidance around identifying, assessing, planning and finding support in end of life (National Gold Standard Framework 2011). Similarly, the *End of Life Care Strategy* (Department of Health 2008) and the *National End-of-Life Care Programme* (DH, 2009) were introduced to meet the wide disparities in EOLC in service provision (National Clinical Institute for Excellence 2004). Recently, difficulties encountered in critical care have been summarized as:

staff inevitably focus on trying to ensure that the person survives. The availability of intensive care and organ support may make it harder to accept that the person is dying. In this context it is important that staff are aware of the person's preferences . . . Wherever possible, relatives and carers should be involved in discussions about whether or not to intensify, or to withdraw, life-sustaining treatment and, if the person lacks capacity, then decisions must be made in their best interests and the family must be consulted as part of the process. In this context, death may occur rapidly and it is essential that families are involved in order to gain their acceptance and understanding.

(DH 2008: 65)

Despite this, the focus of strategic documents is on patients requiring care in the community setting or patients with chronic conditions. Little guidance is available for patients not expected to survive in critical care units, except that they should be transferred to another area (DH 1996: 16; NB this document is currently being revised). However, this is not always possible for a variety of reasons (see below). Nevertheless, some of the broad EOLC principles apply to acute care.

Pre-EOLC considerations: at the beginning

Patients will need EOLC in critical care for one of two reasons.

1   Patients who are expected to survive but who deteriorate and die in critical care (unexpected death). This may include patients who rapidly deteriorate despite active measures to sustain life.
2   Patients for whom the chances of critical care survival are unknown, or low at presentation, and who continue to deteriorate (expected death).

In either of these situations, a decision to forego life-sustaining treatment (DFLST) or withdrawal to precipitate dying may be required.

In the case of unexpected dying, withdrawal of active treatment may occur. This refers to treatment that has been initiated and is then stopped or gradually reduced. That is, the withdrawal of all active treatment other than comfort measures. This does not include 'placing an upper limit on treatment (withholding treatment) and does not include changing the aims of treatment (for example, the decision to leave a patient ventilator dependent rather than to wean them from the ventilator' (Wunsch et al. 2005: 824). In the case of patients who are not expected to survive, a decision needs to be made as to whether to withdraw or withhold treatment. Withholding treatment refers to treatment that is purposefully not initiated (or there is a limitation placed on existing treatment). That is, decisions are made to cease, place limitations on, or de-escalate critical care treatment or therapy. Each of the trajectories will guide and influence decisions to initiate EOLC.

Assessment by critical care teams, critical care outreach teams (CCOT), or medical emergency teams (METs) where they exist, are vital at this pre-EOL stage (Jones et al. 2007; Calzavacca et al. 2010; Pattison et al. 2010). These teams can be influential and might decide whether patients:

■   are for 'active' treatment (i.e. all options for treatment should be considered and no limitation placed on treatment options)
■   should be admitted to critical care
■   should have treatment withheld

■   should have a 'limitation of care' order (e.g. for a certain maximum level of treatment such as not for ventilation), or a Do Not Attempt Resuscitation order
■   should not be admitted to a critical care unit due to their clinical condition and where survival outcome is poor. In such circumstances critical care teams might choose to care for these patients in a ward environment.

However, decision making may not be straightforward as the situation can be complex. For example, deciding to treat, or even palliate, a patient with advanced disease who is in respiratory distress with non-invasive ventilation might mean a critical care admission is inevitable, even though the patient could die in critical care. There are many ethical and resource implications to be considered in admitting patients to critical care, or continuing critical care treatment in patients for whom it would be futile (i.e. it would confer no benefit on survival or quality of life). In the context of clinical situations, medical futility has been defined as a treatment which:

■   does not need to be provided, as it is questionable (i.e. unreasonable to initiate, implausible and unlikely to work)
■   is non-beneficial.

Therefore, having reviewed all available patient data, the intervention would not improve the individual's recovery nor chances of survival (Barnato et al. 2005; Mason and Laurie 2006).

While many critical care treatments can prolong life, in some instances they may be delaying the dying process. Recognizing this distinction and when to act accordingly is vital for the patient and family. Following consensus discussions with family and clinical team 'Do Not Attempt Cardiopulmonary Resuscitation' (DNACPR) orders might be implemented and communicated to all staff to ensure life-saving interventions are not undertaken (BMA, UK Resuscitation Council and RCN 2007). Good planning at this stage, even before admission to critical care, means it is more likely that patients will not receive unnecessary interventions and will receive timely EOLC that reflects their expressed needs, and that this managed in a sensitive and compassionate manner.

Prognosis

A patient's prognosis plays an important part in determining whether to actively treat, or withdraw or withhold treatment and initiate EOLC. Prognostic models and indices are useful in deciding the most appropriate route for the patient (Seymour 2001). However, they are not completely reliable or wholly accurate. Indeed, models and indices such as Simplified Acute Physiology Score (SAPS) (Le Gall et al. 1984), Acute Physiological and Chronic Health Evaluation

(APACHE II and III) (Knaus et al. 1985), Mortality Prediction Model (MPM) (Teres et al. 1987), Sequential Organ Failure Assessment (SOFA) (Vincent et al. 1998) are poor prognosticators in certain chronic conditions (such as cancer) (Soares et al. 2004).

In addition, combining prognoses for different pathologies or illnesses increases clinical uncertainty about the expected course of the patient's outcome (Pattison et al., in press). Clinical judgement, however, when compared with prognostic models is found to be better (Scholz et al. 2004; Rocker et al. 2004; Copeland-Fields et al. 2001). Notably, nurses' estimation of mortality was more pessimistic than doctors' predictions of a patient's survival (Rocker et al. 2004; Festic et al. 2012). Doctors were found to be more accurate predictors of outcome. Critical care nurses' pessimism could have implications for their involvement in decision making, and doctors' confidence in nurses' contributions (discussed below). Practitioners have to respond to how patients' conditions might change from an expected trajectory and plan care around this. Such changes can cause difficulties for the multiprofessional team who are trying to plan treatment and care in a very dynamic, rapid-changing situation. More complex trajectories inevitably create difficulties around decisions because there are more opportunities for uncertainty related to whether patients are likely or not to die. Practitioners have to address these issues before EOLC planning can be considered. The corollary of dealing with clinical uncertainty means that there will be uncertainty in deciding to withdraw or withhold treatment and initiate EOLC.

In summary:

- prognostication is important for deciding whether patient management should be curative and resuscitation driven, or whether it should adopt a palliative model of care
- prognostication is difficult because of the complexities relating to multiple pathologies and varying responses to treatment and care
- prognostic models are of limited use, especially in specific circumstances
- practitioners' judgement *might* turn out to be better than prognostic models in predicting outcome.

Post prognosis: EOLC in critical care environments

Tools that facilitate best care at EOL

A number of tools have been developed to facilitate good EOLC. The advent of integrated care pathway tools such as the Liverpool Care Pathway for Intensive Care Units (LCP-ICU) (Marie Curie Palliative Care Institute 2007), based on the Liverpool Care Pathway (LCP) (Ellershaw and Ward 2003) have helped practitioners to address EOLC in critical care settings. The LCP-ICU does not prescribe *how* to

provide care or withdraw treatments, rather it highlights the medical interventions that should be considered for withdrawal and provides prompts for communication, spiritual and psychological care. Evidence concerning pathways for care of dying patients is scant at present (Hardy et al. 2007; Veerbeek et al. 2008; Chan and Webster 2010), although a large national study is currently under way to assess the impact of the LCP-ICU on quality of care (Ellershaw et al. 2010). The National Gold Standards Framework and the National End of Life Care Programme also provide guidance for service planning in the form of a toolkit (DH 2009; National Gold Standards Framework 2011). The latter also offers guidance on how to implement preferred priorities for care. However, the focus of these tools is on advanced care planning, and guidance specific to critical care is minimal. Therefore, they have limitations in their use with the critically ill patient.

Consensus guidelines for end of life in critical care have been developed (Truog et al. 2008), and although these are US-based, many of the core concepts transcend international boundaries. The guidelines cover principles of family communication, processes of withdrawing treatment, ethical principles of killing and letting die, and after-death psychological care.

Tools that measure the quality and delivery of care include:

- the Toolkit of Instruments to Measure End of Life Care (TIME). This provides measures of quality at the end of life from varying perspectives (www.chcr.brown.edu/pcoc/toolkit.htm)
- the NHS-based End of Life Care Quality Assessment tool, part of the National End of Life Care Intelligence Network, measures quality at an organizational level. (http://www.elcqua.nhs.uk).

These toolkits have some relevance for critical care practice and provide resources, educational and training packages in one place for practitioners.

Tools that measure quality of dying such as the Quality of Death and Dying (QODD) (Curtis et al. 2002) have been validated in critical care and widely accepted in these environments (Hales et al. 2010). A newer initiative IPAL-ICU, Improving Palliative Care in the ICU, was launched in 2010 for worldwide use and to try to illustrate how generic EOL tools can be applied to critical care (*see* http://www.capc.org/ipal-icu). There are also many tools specific to critical care.

Guidance for EOLC

The British Medical Association (BMA) (2007) has produced guidance around decision making and withdrawal practices, and more recently the General Medical Council (GMC 2010) published new documentation on decision making for patients at the end of life. The aims of these publications are to ensure high-quality treatment and care at EOL (BMA 2007; GMC 2010). The role of nurses in terms of EOLC has been delineated in *The Nursing Contribution to the Provision of Comprehensive Critical Care for Adults* (DH 2001):

> Nursing supports the patient and their family in making the transition towards the restoration of health, and when it is accepted that survival is not possible, nursing supports the patient and family through the process of dying and the early stages of bereavement.
>
> (DH 2001: 5)

These policies and guidelines offer structure around providing information for patients and families in EOL situations. Beyond this, nurses and allied health professionals also have a role in inputting into EOL decision making and in planning for withdrawal and EOLC (see below).

Assessment of need for 'Do Not Attempt Cardiopulmonary Resuscitation' orders

In the situation where the prognostic outlook is poor and irreversible, 'Do Not Attempt Cardiopulmonary Resuscitation' (DNACPR) orders have to be considered and are often difficult to undertake. In addressing a DNACPR order in a timely manner, practitioners are trying to ensure patients are not unnecessarily resuscitated at EOL. A joint statement from the British Medical Association, Resuscitation Council and Royal College of Nursing (2007) indicates that the responsibility for the decision of DNACPR order should not rest solely with the senior medical consultant-in-charge.

Assessment should focus on ensuring that, where possible, patient and family wishes are taken into account (although, legally, they do not necessarily have to be adhered to [BMA, UK Resuscitation Council and RCN 2007]), and that decisions are planned and individualized to the individual's expressed preferences. Decisions around DNACPR do not have to be discussed with patients and families (but there must be a full written record and transparency in all decisions), but this is good practice (GMC 2010). Rare situations where DNACPR is not discussed might include:

> When a clinical decision is made that CPR should not be attempted, because it will not be successful, and the patient has not expressed a wish to discuss CPR, it is not necessary or appropriate to initiate discussion with the patient to explore their wishes regarding CPR.
>
> (BMA, UK Resuscitation Council and RCN 2007: 9)

There are four main situations where it is deemed inappropriate to attempt resuscitation (BMA, UK Resuscitation Council and RCN 2007).

1 Where cardiopulmonary resuscitation (CPR) is unlikely to succeed (i.e. breathing and heart would not restart).

2 Where the burden of CPR, or of surviving, outweighs benefits to the patient. However, in this situation the patient's views should be sought. Burden here refers to the physical, emotional and psychological consequences of undergoing resuscitation. For example, potential for brain damage in prolonged hypoxia, fractured ribs during chest compression and possible related pneumothoraces, as well as quality of life considerations for the outcome of CPR).

3 Where a patient who is capable of making a decision has consistently stated or recorded that they do not wish to be resuscitated. Patients' previously stated wishes should be taken into account.

4 Where there is an Advanced Directive (RCP 2009) that states the patient does not wish to be resuscitated (BMA, UK Resuscitation Council and RCN 2007).

Some hospitals now provide information leaflets for patients outlining consequences of resuscitation and DNACPR so that individuals and families are aware of the possible outcomes. The UK Resuscitation Council provides an example of a patient leaflet about CPR (Resuscitation Council 2008) that is important, as patients' decisions are informed by such knowledge. DNACPR decisions should not override clinical judgement (BMA, UK Resuscitation Council and RCN 2007). It is important to note that having a DNACPR order in situ does not necessarily mean the patient is not for active treatment.

Process for obtaining a DNACPR order

The principles and process for obtaining a DNACPR order echo that of breaking bad news (see below). One study showed that only 14% of patients wished to discuss DNACPR if they became critically ill, although 90% wished to discuss this during their hospital stay (Gorton et al. 2008). This highlights that timing for discussion needs to be carefully considered. The legal requirements are that decisions made are clearly documented and that practitioners act in the patient's best interest (BMA, UK Resuscitation Council and RCN 2007). Since the introduction of the Mental Capacity Act and Court of Protection in 2007, where there is discrepancy or dispute over 'best interest' or capacity to make decisions, an application to the Court can be made for judgement (Mental Capacity Act 2005; BMA, UK Resuscitation Council and RCN 2007). In the UK, the DNACPR form must be signed and completed by the senior practitioner (or designated deputy), which is usually a consultant physician, but in rare circumstances it can be a nurse (for example in the hospice setting where the nurse may be the most senior clinician). Entries must be dated and any discussion must be documented. Changes in a patient's condition might necessitate a review of the DNACPR order (for example consideration of a reversal of an order in the event of patient recovery). Regular review of the patient's condition and the DNACPR decision should occur.

Assessment of need for discussion of withdrawal of treatment

Incidence of withdrawal and withholding treatment

Once prognosis and DNACPR have been considered, withdrawal or withholding treatment is usually the next step (although DNACPR can occur concurrently with withdrawal as part of care planning when patients' conditions are reviewed).

Withdrawal of treatment in the UK occurs with approximately 9.9% of all admissions (and around 60% of all patients who die in critical care) (Wunsch et al. 2005). This figure does not include withholding treatment or withholding cardiopulmonary resuscitation (CPR). Withdrawal of active treatment will quickly precipitate death in critical care. The average time to death following withdrawal is 2–4 hours (Wunsch et al. 2005). Therefore, withdrawal must be appropriate and timely and this forms part of EOLC planning.

Legal and ethical issues

There are many ethical and legal aspects linked with withdrawal or withholding decisions (often referred to as 'decisions to forego life-sustaining treatment' or DFLSTs). There may be reluctance by practitioners to consider DFLSTs, which might mean that decisions are delayed or not made. As a result of those 'non-decisions', the potential window for timely EOLC can be lost (Pattison et al., in press). Despite some professional guidance for withdrawal of treatment (BMA 2007; GMC 2010), and admission and discharge (DH 1996), the processes leading to decisions to withhold or withdraw treatment and subsequent provision of care at the end of life can be fraught with problems and perceived risks. For example, perceived risks of litigation and difficulties concerning perceptions of 'killing' (an act) and 'letting die' (an omission) complicate the issues (Shaw 2007; Truog et al. 2008).

Case law in 1993 (*Airedale National Health Service Trust v Bland* [1993] AC 789) and in 2002 (*Re B [Adult: Refusal of Medical Treatment]* [2002] 2 AER 449) clarified practice in the UK in relation to turning off ventilation (and thus precipitate death) for patients reliant on artificial mechanical ventilation for survival. It was ruled that survival should not be at all costs (such as quality of life). This action was perceived as an 'omission', rather than an 'act', because it was deemed cessation of ongoing treatment. This has set the precedent for current practice in the UK around withdrawal. The ethical concept of non-maleficence (doing no harm) is particularly implicated in decisions to forego life-sustaining treatments (DFLSTs). Beauchamp and Childress (2005)

emphasize need for frameworks specifically for such decisions. Moral rules supported by the principle of non-maleficence include:

- do not kill
- do not cause pain or suffering.

(Beauchamp and Childress 2005: 117)

There is an ongoing ethical debate about whether withdrawal is more consequential than withholding treatment (Beauchamp and Childress 2005; Gedge et al. 2007). Both withdrawal and withholding treatment will result in patient death. This is because the underlying physiological processes (that is the patient is deteriorating or not improving despite critical care treatments) related to dying cause patients to die, not the act of withdrawing or withholding (Winter and Cohen 1999). As an act, rather than an omission, withdrawal of treatment can lead to a causality-temporality association where practitioners might consider that their actions caused the death to happen. (For example, did my action of stopping inotropes at that point lead to the patient's death or would it have happened anyway?) Practitioners may also have fears and feelings of killing patients. This might explain a subsequent reticence to undertake DFLSTs and to initiate timely EOLC.

The administration of bolus opiates and benzodiazepines can cause concern for practitioners who might be concerned they are hastening a patient's death. There is evidence to suggest that increasing opiates and benzodiazepines and, after withdrawal, to enhance patients' comfort, has no effect on time to death; however, they may decrease consciousness (Chan et al. 2004; Truog et al. 2008; Puntillo et al. 2010a). Practitioners need to decide what approach is most appropriate in each case.

Avoiding prolongation of dying and decisions about transfer

Practitioners must consider whether making decisions to initiate or continue with treatment prolongs what would have been an inevitable critical care death in a futile situation. Forming prognoses is part of decision-making processes and often highly influential in determining futility (Tonelli 2007). With unclear prognosis and where there are ethical complexities (for example families demanding treatment where practitioners do not feel it is appropriate), it is more likely that decisions are delayed and for futility to remain undetermined. Futility may be because of advanced disease, irreversible condition (e.g. trauma), impending death (independent of ventilation), or other existing pathophysiologies. Modern medicine can now prolong life, even when death is imminent, which raises questions about quality of life considerations (Truog et al. 2008). Prolonging life is often inextricably linked with prolonging dying, which can go against principles of beneficence and non-maleficence upon which practitioners codes of conduct are founded (Bradshaw 1999; Beauchamp and Childress 2005). Therefore, practitioners should avoid any practices that prolong inevitable and imminent death (such as delaying decisions).

Decisions relating to withdrawing and withholding treatment near the end of a patient's life are contextualized by critical care and technology in critical care. Whether technology is always appropriately used in critical care is debatable (Locsin 1998; Cook et al. 1999; Seymour 2001). Perceptions can differ between professions, with one study outlining how significantly more nurses believed that withdrawal decisions were unnecessarily delayed compared with doctors (Jensen et al. 2011). Continuing with technology and delaying withdrawal of treatment might be used after the point of futility (i.e. the point at which it is recognized that dying is inevitable and imminent) to allow families, next of kins and friends (referred to collectively in this chapter as families) time to adjust to the hopelessness of a situation. However, this could be contentious as a patient's dying trajectory might be extended for the benefit of families, so this has to be carefully considered. Indeed, it might be regarded as unethical to rush families and make DFLSTs so patients can be transferred from critical care to receive EOLC on the ward. Transferring patients (DH 1996) does not acknowledge impracticalities of imminently dying patients and preparation for discharge (e.g. with extubation of endotracheal breathing tubes or disconnection from ventilators), which could precipitate immediate death. These situations compounds difficult decisions about transferring patients out of critical care at EOL (Campbell et al. 1999; Cook et al. 2003; O'Mahony et al. 2003; Marr and Weismann 2004; Pattison 2006a; Chotirmall et al. 2010). Some patients cannot be transferred because they still require ventilation and will, therefore, require care in critical care (DH 1996; Wunsch et al. 2005). The consideration of potential situations around transfer such as these, form part of EOLC planning in critical care.

Care around withdrawal: care in the last days and hours

Diagnosing dying

This forms an important part of the discussion around withdrawal of treatment and is clearly linked with prognosis. Recognizing dying is an important skill that comes with experience (see Table 17.1). The level of organ failure and physical recognition of dying can contribute to prognosis debates (also referred to as prognostication), which in turn contributes to diagnosing dying. Withdrawal of treatment can precede diagnosis and recognition of dying. Patients sometimes are visibly dying only after or at withdrawal.

However, when patients are receiving critical care it is more difficult to recognize dying because the usual cues may

Table 17.1 Stages, signs and symptoms of dying in ICU patients

Stage of dying	Signs
Early stage	Can include: ■ loss of appetite ■ inability to take oral medication ■ general weakness (the patient is bedbound) ■ increasing sleepiness or delirium (Furst and Doyle 2005)
Mid-stage	Can include: ■ loss of swallowing function ■ increasing obtundation (decrease in mental alertness and pain sensations)
Late-stage	Can include: ■ Cheyne-Stokes respiration ■ agonal breathing ■ skin mottling ■ loss of consciousness Of particular use in diagnosing dying in patients receiving critical care are: ■ hypotension refractory to inotropic support ■ cardiac failure refractory to support (or other irreversible organ failure) ■ irreversible delirium and in certain diagnoses: ■ advanced cachexia (loss of body mass that cannot be reversed nutritionally) (Furst and Doyle 2005; Towers 2010)

not be present or obvious, or the signs may be due to other reasons. For example:

■ changes in breathing are not obvious if the patient is mechanically ventilated, for example if the patient would have agonal breaths (shallow, slow, irregular breaths of 3–4/min), or Cheyne–Stokes breathing (similarly, increasingly shallower breaths with periods of apnoea)

■ skin changes that can occur when a person is dying (such as grey pallor and mottling) can be present, but may be due to other factors. For instance, certain drugs cause skin flushing (cardiac drugs, such as glyceryl trinitrate), or peripheral shutdown and mottling (inotropes, such as high doses of noradrenaline).

Monitoring offers an additional aid in recognizing dying patients who may be heavily sedated and ventilated. Changes in blood pressure and cardiac rhythm changes can indicate dying. However, families can fixate on monitors, which can make care of dying patients more difficult, therefore nurses must assess the appropriateness of continuing monitoring. Where the patient has been made DNACPR and is dying, if monitoring is not stopped then alarms must be silenced (in case alarms go off when patient is asystolic, for instance).

Consultation and communication of decision to withdraw treatment with patient, next of kin and significant others

Multidisciplinary teams are expected to reach difficult decisions, in consultation with family members, about when to allow a patient to die in a dignified manner (BMA, UK Resuscitation Council and RCN 2007).

Complexity may arise when the patient is being managed by two clinical teams (for example the referring team and the critical care team) as this may hamper decision making and prospects for the dying patient's care (Cassell et al. 2003). Introduction of palliative care teams into critical care multidisciplinary team meetings can have a positive and helpful effect on decision making (Nelson et al. 2010; Scheunemann et al. 2011). Likewise, in ethically difficult cases, using clinical ethics committees, ethicists or lay people (such as chaplains) can be beneficial in reducing interprofessional conflict (Truog et al. 2008). Best practice is that patients and families, where possible and appropriate, are consulted (BMA 2007). Planning for meetings is very important, and toolkits might help in this respect (Gay et al. 2009; Nelson et al. 2009).

Patients

In a critical care setting, patients are only rarely able to contribute to consultations concerning withdrawal or withholding treatment or care at the end of their lives because they are frequently unable to communicate or heavily sedated. In these situations, families are often consulted to gain a perspective on patient's preferences for care.

In the UK, since the advent of the Mental Capacity Act in 2005 (which came into force in 2007), independent mental capacity advocates (IMCAs) have been introduced who can offer a neutral perspective in the case of incapacitated patients with no family available and where there is disagreement with practitioners' positions. Cases can also be referred to the Court of Protection for review. This new legislation supersedes the principle of 'best interest', and means practitioners can no longer act unilaterally in situations of disagreement where there is no family and the patient is incapacitated. The Court of Protection now assumes the responsibility for determining incapacitated patients' 'best interests' (The Stationery Office, 2007).

Specifically, the Court of Protection has the powers to:

- decide whether a person has capacity to make a particular decision for themselves
- make declarations, decisions, or orders on financial or welfare matters affecting people who lack capacity to make such decisions

- appoint deputies to make decisions for people lacking capacity to make those decisions
- decide whether a Lasting Power of Attorney (LPA) or Enduring Power of Attorney (EPA) is valid
- remove deputies or attorneys who fail to carry out their duties
- hear cases concerning objections to register an LPA or EPA and make decisions about whether or not an LPA or EPA is valid (The Stationery Office 2007).

Where patients *are* able to contribute to decisions their views should ideally be taken into account. However, where patients seek further treatment in situations where there would be no benefit to continuing, this has to be handled carefully and sensitively by the critical care practitioner and the team caring for the patient. Meeting patient requests for treatment (such as a trial on non-invasive ventilation, or continuation of antibiotics) might be considered acceptable by the healthcare team if that action ameliorates the dying patient's psychological needs. The perceived benefit might, therefore, be classified as psychological, as there will be no physiological benefits. However, this could result in significant resource or ethical issues (i.e. it may do considerable harm).

Patients may have also made advanced decisions about critical care treatment. Valid and applicable advance decisions to refuse treatment have the same legal status as decisions made by people with capacity at the time of treatment (The Stationery Office, 2007). In this situation practitioners must be aware that patients may have refused treatment in advance.

Families/Next of kin/Significant others

Family, next of kin and significant others' perspectives can present difficulties for teams because their opinions may not always reflect what patients would have wanted. Some studies have demonstrated that families tend towards over-aggressive (wanting treatment in the face of futility and reluctance to withdraw) care approaches and equally, other work has reported that patients expected more aggressive management (Danis et al. 1998; Tilden et al. 1995; Swigart et al. 1996; Lynn et al. 1997; Sulmasy et al. 2002). Family contribution has legitimacy if the patient's preferences or values are known to the healthcare team (Truog et al. 2008). In the absence of patients' voice, these perspectives can be used as a proxy. Furthermore, the tension between treating patients and caring for families is complex for critical care teams who often have to provide psychological support to families when patients are at EOL (Pattison et al., in press).

Practitioners and the clinical team have to support patients and families at this stage of critical illness, to death and beyond, as the policy document (DH 2001) outlines. Managing conflict, which is often present during end of life decision making in critical care (Abbott et al. 2001; Azoulay et al. 2009) is part of this process and often falls to nurses, who are continually present with families and patients, and who might even act as mediators (Pattison et al., in press). Sensitive discussion is key.

Nurses and allied health professionals

Nurses' disenfranchisement and dissatisfaction with decision making in critical care at the EOL has been noted in several studies (Baggs and Schmitt 1995; Jezuit 2000; Kirchhoff and Beckstrand 2000; Kirchhoff et al. 2000; Melia 2001; Ferrand et al. 2003; Keenan et al. 2003; Robichaux and Clark 2006; Latour et al. 2009) and their influence on doctors found to be limited (SUPPORT Principle Investigators 1995; Jezuit 2000; Abbott et al. 2001; Melia 2001; Puntillo et al. 2001; Ahrens et al. 2003; Keenan et al. 2003; Carlet et al. 2004). In a recent European study, nurses felt they were routinely involved in DFLSTs only 60% of the time (Latour et al. 2009).

This raises important questions for nurses who have to provide care at the end of a patient's life.

- Why are some nurses not involved in DFLSTs?
- Where nurses are involved in DFLSTs, to which specific aspects do they contribute?

Nurses, and potentially by extension, allied health professionals, may choose not to get involved for four main reasons.

- There are emotional ramifications of engagement, particularly as they are with families and patients by the bedside for up to 12 hours a day. Nurses might have to invest emotionally in determining EOLC plans. This might increase the risk of their burnout (Meltzer and Huckabay 2004; Piers et al. 2011).
- Poor educational preparation may leave nurses and allied health professionals lacking in confidence to contribute to professional debates about DFLSTs.
- Lack of experience and knowledge among nurses and therapists may impact on the quality of care patients and families receive, and their subsequent involvement in DFLSTS (Baggs and Schmitt 1995; Latour et al. 2009; Pattison et al., in press). This is likely to hold for allied health professionals too.
- Conflict between nurses, allied health professionals and doctors (as well as managing conflict between families or patients and teams) is also a significant issue for contribution and involvement (Cassell et al. 2003; Ferrand et al. 2003; Frick et al. 2003; Keenan et al. 2003; Pattison 2006b; Hamric and Blackhall 2007; Azoulay et al. 2009; Piers et al. 2010).

Once decisions have been made to initiate EOLC, there is scope for nurses' roles to increase in relation to planning EOLC and how decisions to withdraw treatment might affect EOLC (Long-Sutehall et al. 2011; Coombs et al. 2012).

Communication and breaking bad news: supporting the family

Individualized communication, advanced care planning and identification of patient's needs in the last days of life are key to improving EOL provision (Addicott and Ashton 2010). Communication strategies, such as written information for families, have been shown to reduce the intensity of critical care treatment provided by practitioners. That is fewer resources were used because clinicians were more likely to initiate EOLC (Lautrette et al. 2007; Scheunemann et al. 2011). Communication difficulties have been identified by families and patients as a significant barrier to good EOLC in critical care (SUPPORT Principal Investigators 1995; Counsell and Guin 2002; Kirchhoff et al. 2002). Evidence suggests that families need accurate and timely information from professionals, and preferably from consultant doctors (Popejoy et al. 2009; Wåhlin et al. 2009). Keeping lines of communication open and honesty enhance trust between practitioners, which in turn enhances EOLC (Seymour 2001). For families, helpful practitioner behaviours have centred on minimizing conflict (Abbott et al. 2001; Cassell et al. 2003), and having family conferences (Glavan et al. 2008).

An important part of family communication in EOL centres on breaking bad news, because critically ill patients are rarely able to contribute at this stage. The SPIKES (Setting, Perception, Invitation, Knowledge, Emotions, Strategy and Summary) (Baile et al. 2000) approach to breaking bad news has been widely adopted in areas such as cancer, but is applicable to settings such as critical care. This involves six steps.

1 Setting up the interview (rehearsing what will be discussed, arranging for privacy, involving significant others, connecting with patient, minimizing interruptions).
2 Assessing patient's Perception (or family's).
3 Obtaining an Invitation to give information (and assess how much information families would like).
4 Giving Knowledge and information to the patient and/or family (warning patients you have bad news to give, then give the bad news, using non-technical language, avoiding bluntness unless requested).
5 Addressing patient's and family's Emotions with empathic responses. Empathic response is outlined as: watching for emotion; identifying it (clarify with patient/family and asking what they are thinking/feeling); identifying reason for emotion (it may *not* be related to bad news); and finally, giving a connecting or validating response (letting the patient or family know you empathize – an empathic affirmation).

507

6 Providing a Strategy (e.g. for managing EOLC) and summary.

Nelson et al.'s (2009) concept of preparing for family meetings includes creating a family meeting planner, a family meeting guide and a documentation template. Having timely family meetings for those close to death, or with poor prognosis, is emphasized and is good practice (Nelson et al. 2009, 2010; Arnold et al. 2010). As part of the IPAL-ICU resources, Arnold et al. (2010) outlined five fundamental principles for communicating EOL issues in critical care. These communication principles can be used by all practitioners (families often use nurses and therapists after meetings to clarify issues) and are summarized in Procedure guideline 17.1.

Cultural issues

Cultural issues, a group's values and worldview (Breslin 1993), can encompass age, ethnicity, religion and socioeconomic situations. The most recent UK census reported 7.9% of the population coming from ethnic groups (Office for National Statistics 2003). Ethnicity and cultural needs have to be considered at EOL. Cultural practices at the end of a patient's life in critical care can be considered in the following main areas: communication; decision making; attitudes regarding life support, do not resuscitate orders, advance directives (ADs); and withdrawal issues (Searight and Gafford 2005; Doolen and York 2007). Carey and Cosgrove (2006) also highlight the disastrous effects of misunderstanding and failing to engage with different cultural groups in relation to care at the end of life. Assessment of cultural issues that affect communication is an important part of planning care for dying patients (Kagawa-Singer and Blackhall 2001). Strategies might be needed to help deal with these issues, such as understanding the need to communicate only with the senior member of family. Truth-telling, common in Western societies, might be considered overtly blunt, rude and disrespectful in other cultures (Surbone 2006). Linguistic sensitivity should be displayed, as language can easily be misinterpreted, especially if English is not the first language. This might also have ramifications for decision making about care at the end of a patient's life within the family unit.

Withdrawal and withholding treatment practices vary with religious cultures, such as sects of Sunni and Shiite Islam that do not believe treatment should be withdrawn once instigated (although it can be acceptable to withhold) (Clarfield et al. 2003; Ankeny et al. 2005). This is also true of sects of orthodox Judaism (Clarfield et al. 2003; Ankeny et al. 2005). However, individuals might hold different beliefs to those of their religion. Spiritual beliefs might also differ (Speck et al. 2004). Practitioners should enquire whether there are any cultural needs that should be met, or that they need to be aware of. Where patients cannot contribute to these discussions, families should be consulted.

Review of practical components of withdrawal of treatment and end of life care

Once futility has been determined and teams have decided to withdraw or withhold treatment, the next stage is planning EOLC. This encompasses withdrawal and timing of withdrawal of treatment, because death will occur very soon afterwards in most cases of withdrawal (Wunsch et al. 2005). The ultimate goal of EOLC in critical care is to ensure a 'good death' for patients (discussed below) and withdrawal can be an important part of achieving this. This guidance is not meant to be prescriptive, because that does not allow for individualized care, but to offer guidance in each area of withdrawal.

When to withdraw

Decisions to withdraw treatment will cause distress, and families and patients should be informed that the moment of death cannot be predicted by practitioners. In some situations it might be appropriate to wait an hour or two for a family member to arrive before initiating withdrawal of treatment, and nurses are often able to make these decisions autonomously around timing of withdrawal (and if withdrawal has been agreed by consultant-in-charge). Where possible, it is preferable to offer to care for patients in a single room for privacy and a quieter environment.

How and when to withdraw treatment

It can sometimes be more difficult to withdraw long-standing critical care support (rather than recently instituted interventions) because it can be seen as more consequential and part of someone's 'normal' life or treatment. Staged approaches to withdrawing treatment do occur, but equally attention should be paid to avoid prolonging dying (Harper and Chapman 2010; MacIver and Ross 2010). Procedure guideline 17.2 outlines specific areas of treatment that should be considered around withdrawal.

Extubation

Withdrawal of treatment might involve extubation and, as such, is included as an option in the Liverpool Care Pathway ICU (LCP-ICU). This means that the patient will no longer be mechanically ventilated and it may be possible to transfer them to the ward (if that is viewed as appropriate). However, a proportion of patients will still require ventilation and will therefore require EOLC and die in critical care (DH 1996; Wunsch et al. 2005; Pattison 2006a).

'Terminal weaning' or extubation of dying ventilated patients is considered ethically contentious (Faber-Langendoen et al. 1996; Tasota and Hoffman 1996; Way et al. 2002; Cook et al. 2003; Fartoukh et al. 2005; Campbell 2007) because there is a risk of airway obstruction, which may precipitate immediate death. The presence of post-laryngeal oedema and copious secretions (and, hence, obstruction) is a risk post extubation (François et al. 2007). Where there is a significant risk of airway obstruction or pulmonary haemorrhage (where 'blood aerosol' may be an infection risk) extubation is contraindicated.

If a patient is receiving muscle relaxant (neuromuscular blockade/paralysing agent) medication to aid ventilation compliance, extubation should not be considered until the medication would have worn off (Pace 1996). Since the medication effectively paralyses the respiratory muscles, once extubated the patient would not be able to breathe unsupported and could die as a result of an 'act' not 'omission' (an important ethical, moral and legal distinction). However, this can be difficult to address, as neuromuscular blockade agents typically have a long half-life and in patients with renal and liver failure delayed clearance might mean an unacceptable length of time before ventilation withdrawal (Truog et al. 2008). In this situation, extubation would not be appropriate. In addition, the process of weaning someone off a ventilator purely to be extubated might, in fact, prolong dying or cause distress compared with extubation without weaning, and study findings have differed on this (Campbell et al. 1999; Faber-Langendoen and Lanken 2000). Nevertheless, extubation is indicated in some cases, such as situations where patients have suffered extensive, irreversible neurological deficits and are likely to be unaware (Fartoukh et al. 2005; MacIver and Ross 2010).

Withdrawing ventilator-supported respiration, the most frequently withdrawn treatment in critical care (Pace 1996; Prendergast and Luce 1997; Cook et al. 2003), commonly involves turning off ventilators or reducing the levels of oxygen to that consistent with room air. Procedure guideline 17.4 outlines specific aspects of extubation care.

Care of the dying patient during extubation

Procedure guideline 17.3 outlines some further practicalities to be considered around extubation that should be associated with end of life care practices.

Further EOLC considerations in the last days and hours

Procedure guideline 17.4 outlines further EOLC considerations for practitioners, beyond withdrawal. These cover dignity, pain, anxiety, comfort, wound and elimination care, psychological care, delirium and patient aesthetics (appearance and associated wellbeing).

Sudden or unexpected dying

Sudden death, by definition, cannot be planned for. However, compassionate care after death might help bereaved families and critical care teams to deal with aspects of this situation better. Where patients suddenly deteriorate, as opposed to

gradually decline, planning is more of a challenge, as EOLC has to be initiated very quickly. Withdrawal of treatment when the patient's condition is declining rapidly often precipitates a very quick death, so where it has been decided withdrawal is appropriate, families (and patients) will need substantial psychological support. Family liaison, pastoral care teams, social workers and spiritual advisers are important people to help with family advice and offer support. Bereavement services are very important in sudden death (Wright 1996).

Brainstem function measurement and death

There is currently a code of practice for brainstem function measurement and the diagnosis of brainstem death (DH 1998). There is no statutory legal definition for death in the UK, although 'irreversible loss of the capacity for consciousness, combined with irreversible loss of the capacity to breathe' (DH 1998: 7) is the most commonly used definition. Since there is no legal framework for, or statutory definition of, death, brainstem death is diagnosed using consensus practice and is regarded as equating to patient death. Brainstem death is the:

> irreversible loss of the capacity for consciousness, combined with irreversible loss of the capacity to breathe. The irreversible cessation of brainstem function (brain stem death) whether induced by intracranial events or the result of extra-cranial phenomena, such as hypoxia, will produce this clinical state and therefore brain stem death equates with the death of the individual.
> (DH 1998: 7)

There should be no doubt when verifying death that the patient's condition is due to irremediable brain damage and caused by *known* aetiology (DH 1998). Measurement of brainstem death therefore requires assessment of underlying aetiology and certain conditions to be excluded, particularly when patients are deeply unconscious, such as:

- hypothermic coma
- depressant drug-induced coma
- potentially reversible causes (e.g. hypernatraemia, diabetes insipidus coma).

There should also be delay in testing after hypoxic brain injury to ensure this is not reversible.

Cessation of spontaneous breathing also needs further investigation to rule out reversible causes, including:

- persistence of sedation
- suppression of breathing by opioids or neuromuscular blockade drugs

Box 17.2 Brainstem function measurements and care following brainstem death

Indictors of brainstem death:

- Fixed pupils, no corneal reflex – when brushed with tissue no blink reflex. (Take care not to damage cornea)
- Absent vestibulo-ocular reflex – following injection of 50 mL iced water injected into each ear over one minute (tympanic membrane should be visible and head flexed at 30°)
- No motor responses from cranial nerve stimulation – to painful stimuli
- No gag reflex – to spatula placed on the back of the tongue
- No gag reflex response – to suction catheter stimulation
- No ventilator response – when disconnected from ventilator for 10 minutes and the partial pressure of carbon dioxide ($PaCO_2$) has reached 6.65 kPa (the threshold for respiratory stimulation). Hypoxia should be avoided by administration of 6 L/min of oxygen during test via nasal cannulae (or administration of 5% oxygen where available, with 100% oxygen for 10 minutes pre-test and then 5% during test for 5 minutes). NB With chronic respiratory disease expert help may be required due to higher hypercapnic drive (these patients will normally exist with a high $PaCO_2$ and therefore it could be more difficult to determine brain death)

(DH 1998)

- baclofen (used to treat spasticity and in multiple sclerosis, and sometimes in alcoholism), which has been seen to mimic brain death in baclofen overdose-induced coma (Ostermann et al. 2000; Bell et al. 2004)
- lidocaine overdose or thiopental overdose (central nervous system depressant used in anaesthesia).

Box 17.2 outlines the brainstem function measurements and care following brainstem death.

The brainstem function measurements can be used from 2 months of age (DH 1998). The test should be repeated by independent medical practitioners with at least 5 years' experience. Timing of the repeat is subject to discretion (DH 1998) and there is no consensus as to minimum time between tests. If patients are being considered for organ donation, transcranial Dopplers (measures the blood flow through the brain's blood vessels) or occasionally cerebral angiography (provides images of the blood vessels in and around the brain) may be appropriate as confirmatory tests. This is particularly necessary where there is disagreement or where one of the aforementioned reversible causes is present (Bell et al. 2004).

Brainstem death

Patients can be classified as brain dead once neuromuscular blockade has stopped, tests have been carried out and brain-stem death has been verified (DH 1998). Death is pronounced on verification by a second practitioner, but time of death is taken from the first practitioner's pronunciation of brainstem death.

Brainstem death can be distressing and difficult for families to comprehend, especially as patients still might appear 'alive'. This is because there may be complex-spontaneous motor movements and, therefore, ongoing limb and trunk movements (spinal reflexes) and a heartbeat (although these will cease within days usually even with continued ventilation) (DH 1998). False-positive triggering of the ventilator may also occur in patients who are brain dead (Wijdicks et al. 2010). These patients, however, have no capacity for consciousness.

Critical care teams have to be very sensitive in how support machines are turned off and how much time families might need to adjust to the situation. However, this needs tempering against the fact that patients are dead and delay might compromise potential organs for donation (Bell et al. 2004; Shemie 2010). Organ donation is frequently considered in these cases (discussed below). To ensure organs are perfused and functioning when they are removed might mean that artificial ventilation support (and sometimes cardiac bypass or inotropes) may need to be continued until brainstem tests have been carried out. In some situations (such as heart transplantation) it is better to donate from a patient whose heart is still beating. At this point transplantation teams would be involved and advise on care after death (see www.uktransplant.org.uk).

After-death care

Last offices, or preparing the body of a patient who has died, is a large topic in itself. In view of this, only the specific considerations for after-death care in critical care is considered here (see Pattison 2008a, 2008b; Hills and Albarran 2010; Dougherty and Lister 2011 for further details). It should be noted that there may be social, cultural or religious considerations that might impact on how last offices are undertaken (see Neuberger 1999; Speck 2003; Dougherty and Lister 2011).

Communicating procedures around death

Practitioners have to use their judgement and discuss with families whether they wish to view the patient before or after last offices. The opportunity should also be offered, as appropriate, for families to be involved in hygiene and last office care following death. This is important culturally, as well as emotionally, for some families. Families should be briefly informed of processes to be undertaken, but it is usually unnecessary to provide exact details, because this in itself can be distressing. Where there are specific cultural or religious requirements to be undertaken the family might even guide last offices. For patients who have died and need repatriating to another country, individual hospital policy guidelines and individual country requirements (via the relevant High Commission) should be referred to. It might be appropriate to inform other patients around the bed space that the patient has died (liaise with senior staff in event of uncertainty with how to deal with this situation).

Helping the family to understand procedures after death will often fall on nurses as they are frequently those who first meet with families after patients have died. The website www.direct.gov.uk has a checklist, 'What to do after a death', which can help families. Where the family verbalizes that they feel the death was unnatural or even that it was interfered with, professionals have a responsibility to explore these feelings carefully (and be aware of legislation). Their legal entitlement to a post-mortem should be clarified.

Preparing the body of the patient who has died

Last offices is an important act in the rite of passage in moving the person who has died into the world of the dead (Van Gennep 1972), and people from all cultures recognize rituals and procedures after death (Dougherty and Lister 2011). Before undertaking last offices, it must be ascertained (with the person verifying the death) whether the patient's case is to be referred to the coroner (DH 2008). Indications for referrals are given in Procedure guideline 17.5.

Infection risk

Where patients have died and there is high risk of infection (for example with HIV or hepatitis B), precautions need to be taken for the safety of those coming into contact with the body (such as family, practitioners, porters and mortuary technicians). In addition, some infections can be transmitted through expiration after death, particularly when rolling patients (for example tuberculosis). In the case of highly infectious patients (e.g. including those who have diseases that are notifiable), 'packing' (the filling of orifices with cotton wool, gauze, or padding) should be considered (Dougherty and Lister 2011; Pattison 2008a) to prevent fluid leakage. In certain cases (i.e. typhus, severe acute respiratory syndrome, yellow fever, anthrax, plague, rabies and smallpox), viewing should not be permitted given the high risk of transmission after death (Health and Safety Advisory Committee 2003). Patients' bodies with an infection risk should be labelled as such on the forms accompanying the body. There should also be nationally recognized hazard labels on the body bag and on the patient. Linen and waste should be treated as infected.

A brief summary of procedures after death is outlined in Procedure guideline 17.5. In-depth guidance is available from Dougherty and Lister (2011) on this.

Considerations before showing families the deceased patient (either before or after last offices)

The following actions should be carried out to assist the family following the patient's death.

- Prepare the family for what they might see (for example inform them if the patient still has an endotracheal or tracheal tube, etc.).
- Invite the family into the bed space or room, which has been cleared of unnecessary equipment.
- Accompany the family but respect the need for privacy should the family require it. The family might want a religious or spiritual leader to accompany them and this should be facilitated wherever possible.
- Anticipate questions.
- Offer to contact other relatives on behalf of the family, as appropriate.
- Advise about local (and national) bereavement support services that can be accessed.
- Offer the family the opportunity to discuss care (at that time or in the future). This might need to be a booked appointment with senior practitioner-in-charge.
- Provide family with a point of contact with the hospital.

Families' time with patient in unit after the patient's death

How long a patient should remain in the ward (where there can be a relatively elevated temperature) is contentious (there could potentially be early onset of rigor mortis), and the senior practitioner will have to exercise discretion about when to send the patient to the mortuary (Dougherty and Lister 2011). Professional judgement should be exercised according to each family's circumstances (for example there could be a short delay in family arriving) and to the situation on the ward (side rooms may be easier for the family and other patients). Generally, 1–2 hours would be considered the upper limits for a patient to remain in the critical care unit after last offices have been carried out. However, families may wish to view the patient in the chapel of rest or mortuary after the patient's body has been transferred. The patient should be laid out in a presentable state before the family sees them. Problems can arise because critical care patients can leak a substantial amount of bodily fluids from orifices, wounds and puncture sites after death which might result in skin excoriation, maceration, degradation and slippage (where the skin sloughs off the body) (Pattison 2008a). Again, local and unit policies and guidelines can vary on this. Auditing practices of this area of care is important to assess whether care provision and standards are being met (Hills and Albarran 2009).

Bereavement care

The bereaved family may find it difficult to comprehend the death of their family member and it can take great sensitivity and skill to support them at this time. Explaining all procedures as fully as appropriate can help understanding of the practices at the end of life. Culture, gender and other factors can affect grief; families may experience shock, despair, denial, anger, aggression, or become helpless, silent, or withdrawn (Pattison 2008b; Hills and Albarran 2010). Being aware of possible reactions enhances sensitivity, especially where reactions differ from cultural norms (Pattison 2008b). Offering bereavement care services may be useful to families during the difficult period immediately after death and in the future. The local services are listed below and additionally there are national bereavement services such as the charity CRUSE (www.cruse.org.uk). There may be extreme distress, which is a difficult situation to handle, and other family members are likely to be of most benefit to a distressed family at this point (Pattison 2008a). The LCP-ICU asks for patients' GPs to be notified of death (Marie Curie Palliative Care Institute 2007) and family members may also wish for their own GP to be contacted for additional support (for example help accessing local bereavement or counselling services). Practitioners need to maintain a high degree of sensitivity when outlining the paperwork and processes because families frequently have to attend the hospital in order to collect the documentation for registering the death. The 'What to do after a death' checklist (available online at www.direct.gov.uk) can help families.

Bereavement care also extends to psychological care of staff working in critical care. Burnout and moral distress (the distress associated with a situation where the ethically appropriate course of action is known but cannot be taken [Elpern et al. 2005) are noted among critical care nurses and doctors in several studies (Meltzer and Huckabay 2004; Embriaco et al. 2007; Poncet et al. 2007). This phenomenon has not been researched in allied health professionals but is likely to also be an issue. Compassion fatigue may occur (also described as secondary traumatic stress disorder) and is associated with the stress of helping, or wanting to help, another undergoing trauma or stress (Sabo 2006). Where psychological support services exist for staff these can be useful, as can unit support such as staff outings and support groups (Intensive Care Society 1998). This may be particularly important following difficult critical care deaths. Structured, externally facilitated, debrief sessions might be appropriate in ethically complex cases that unsettle teams. Critical incident stress debriefing, such as after a traumatic unit death, where an event (and associated feelings and actions) is discussed in depth, can be useful (Hanna and Romana 2007). Managers and senior practitioners need to be sensitive to the burden of caring for EOL patients and think carefully about staffing allocation. Staff support needs to be viewed as an integral part of unit management, especially in an area where a sixth of all patients cared for die (ICNARC 2009). Practitioners should be encouraged to engage with EOLC, and where they do, they might have a better experience themselves (Pattison 2011).

Competencies

Delivering individualized EOL care requires sensitivity, empathy and compassion. These behaviours together with regular information giving should underpin all care interventions to meet the needs of the patient and family. Competency tools in EOLC have been developed for nurses (St Christopher's Hospice 2009) and practitioners (National Health Service 2009a).

Sayers and DeVries (2008) describe 'being sensitive' as comprising two core features:

- 'being aware' physically, emotionally and professionally
- 'responding and reacting to the needs of others' in a manner that encompasses a multitude of attitudes and moral behaviours.

Empathy can be defined as the ability to sense another's world as it were your own (Rogers 1957). Achieving measures for assessing competency for empathy has been described as difficult (Yu and Kirk 2008). This may be because empathy has been conceptualized in different ways including:

- a human trait
- a professional state
- a communication process
- caring
- a special relationship.

The key elements of empathy include moral, emotive, cognitive and behavioural domains (Kunyk and Olson 2001; Yu and Kirk 2008). The specific procedure competency statements for end of life care (EOLC) outlines some of the fundamental interpersonal skills needed in EOLC.

Compassion, underpinning NHS values is responding with 'humanity and kindness to each person's pain, distress, anxiety or need. We search for the things we can do, however small, to give comfort and relieve suffering' (NHS 2009b: 12. It is about the inclination to share others' feelings and to show concern for patients' comfort and wellbeing Zhang et al. (2001).

Further information can be found at: www.endoflifecare. nhs.uk (NHS 2009a). The Competency statement 17.1 (*see also* Procedure guideline 17.1) outlines some key points that demonstrate how to give empathetic, sensitive, compassionate responses to families.

Conclusion

End of life care encompasses many issues of ethics, communication considerations and clinical care. Practitioners working in the arena of critical care have important roles in decision making, EOLC planning, and subsequent care before and after death. This is a specialist area where a good death in critical care, even an unexpected death, is possible with careful planning and forethought.

Procedure guideline 17.1: Communication strategies at end of life (based on Arnold et al. 2010 in IPAL-ICU)

Procedure

Action	Rationale
1 Ask-tell-ask. Ask the family to describe their current understanding: '*What is the most important thing you would like to talk about today?*' Asking also means seeking permission to discuss patients' condition. Next, give the family clinical information about the patient in clear language, remembering to chunk information (giving two to three take-home messages). Finally, ask them how much they understood and if they need clarification.	To help frame the family's understanding, negotiate the agenda and determine concerns. Chunking information can help the family digest complex information at difficult times (Arnold et al. 2010). Assessing understanding will minimize opportunities for confusion.
2. Ask for more information if required to understand the situation: 'Tell me more.' Invite the family to explain where they are in the conversation and consider three levels of conversation. ■ *What is happening?* Try to understand how the family feel about the information given. ■ *How do the family feel about this?* Try and ascertain the emotions the family feel related to the conversation (they might seek validation from professional for their emotion). ■ *What does this mean for the family?* Address what that new information means to the family and their identity. Practitioners might ask: '*Could you say something about how you are feeling about what we've discussed?*'	Empathy and validating emotions can help the family process information. These lines of questions open up communication about how they are feeling about the conversation (Arnold et al. 2010).
3 Use reflections rather than questions to learn more. Paraphrase what has been said, with (complex) or without (simple) adding an interpretation of meaning.	To facilitate or demonstrate empathy. Reflective statements can help with empathy and also allow the family to retain control of conversation. Reflections also use tonal inflections to statement rather than questions to elicit greater, deeper responses (Arnold et al. 2010). Adding interpretation of meaning must be done cautiously in case there is misinterpretation by professionals.
4 Use skills for responding to emotion. Attend appropriately to emotional reactions. Allow time for reactions and ensure the family is not pressurized into making or contributing to decisions. This might include providing an accepting response (a response that makes family not feel judged and that validates their feelings and the importance of their contribution). This might include a statement such as: '*It sounds like you are worried that (patient) would not have wanted this treatment. Some people in this situation would be angry about this.*'	To facilitate empathy and trust. Receiving bad or emotional news can make it harder to hear cognitive information and to make decisions. The family can feel pressurized into decisions and have been shown to be less satisfied with care if this occurs (Keenan et al. 2000; Heyland et al. 2003). Empathically responding can help with trust, and for families to feel heard and appreciated (Arnold et al. 2010).
5 Assess the family members' informational, decision-making and coping style. Assess how people have coped in similar situations before, e.g. 'Have you had anything like this ever happen before?' and asking how people explicitly coped. Provide appropriate levels of information.	To appropriately react to the individual's different responses. Appropriate adaptation of responses can help emphasize the value placed on the individual involved in decision making or receiving bad news. For example, some people will seek information to help them manage and others might use emotion-focused approaches and avoid information, distance themselves and engage in denial of their situation (Arnold et al. 2010).

(Continued)

6 Document care.	To:
	■ provide an accurate record
	■ monitor effectiveness of procedure
	■ provide a point of reference or comparison in the event of later questions
	■ acknowledge accountability for actions
	■ facilitate communication and continuity of care.
	(NMC 2008; HCPC 2012; GMC 2013)

Procedure guideline 17.2: Considerations concerning withdrawal of treatment

Procedure

Action	Rationale
Antibiotics	
1 Antibiotics, therapeutic or prophylactic, should be in most cases stopped. Rarely, it might be appropriate to continue (where it is part of symptom management and the sequelae of stopping would be worse than continuing).	Antibiotics do not need to be continued if it has been decided to initiate EOLC and where they will not aid in controlling symptoms. Treating infection might prolong end of life (Stiel et al. 2011). Fever can be treated with comfort measures such as paracetamol.
Blood products	
2 Generally, blood product administration is stopped.	At EOL there is an important resource issue around whether EOL patients should receive blood products in order to improve their EOL experience (McGrath and Leahy 2009), or whether bleeding should be controlled in other ways (e.g. topical and intravenous tranexamic acid, vitamin K administration, packing, pressure bandages, haemostatic droooings). Dark towels might also be necessary to reduce the appearance of blood. In certain haematological diseases, however, patients may have relied on blood products to keep bleeding under control in their disease. In these instances it may be appropriate to continue to administer blood products. Therefore, decisions need to be made on a case-by-case basis.
Nutrition, hydration and nasogastric tubes	
3 Consider whether or not to withdraw nutrition and hydration support.	Continuing nutrition and hydration could prolong dying. Withdrawing nutrition and hydration has been historically ethically contentious (the precedent was with the Airedale NHS Trust v. Bland case). However, withdrawal of this is now common practice in EOL in critical care (Harper and Chapman 2010).
4 Feeding tubes should be removed unless they are an aid to managing symptoms.	Where nasogastric or orogastric tubes provide symptomatic relief (e.g. in case of abdominal obstruction, vomiting [Harper and Chapman 2010], or gross abdominal distension) they should be left in situ.
Inotropic drugs	
5 Inotropes can be stopped (again this can lead to immediate death, so timing is imperative so that everyone is prepared for that possibility).	These drugs should not be gradually reduced unless for a good reason (as gradually reducing the dose can, ultimately, prolong dying). Abrupt discontinuation does not result in discomfort (Truog et al. 2008).
Implanted cardiac defibrillators	
6 Where possible, implanted cardiac defibrillators should be deactivated. There are additional considerations for patients with implanted cardiac defibrillators that extend to care after death.	Deactivation will prevent the implanted cardiac defibrillator delivering an electric shock to the patient if they develop cardiac arrest with a shockable rhythm (Dimond 2004; Kobza and Erne 2007; Pattison 2008a).

7 Pressure support (the support patients require when mechanically ventilated) and positive end expiratory pressure (PEEP) should be reduced. Some intensivists favour also reducing oxygen levels to 21% (room air) and then allowing the patient to die (Rocker 2010).	Reducing the amount of pressure support and PEEP (ensuring there is no potential respiratory distress during reduction) is more likely to result in less respiratory distress overall. The dying process can be reduced if the oxygen is decreased to 21% but it should be ensured that this action does not lead to 'air hunger'.
8 Ensure patients are well sedated and have adequate analgesia.	To enhance comfort.
9 Suction should be limited to only where necessary (where copious secretions could cause distress); regular suction is inappropriate.	Suction could precipitate coughing and discomfort. Regular suction is not needed because only symptomatic relief is being given (not prevention of infection).
10 Ventilation via a T-piece is often used prior to extubation (El-Khatib and Bou-Khalil 2008), and also has a place in end of life (Way et al. 2002). 'T-piecing', as it is referred to, involves maintaining the endotracheal or tracheal tube airway in situ and administering of oxygen (usually around 21%, but not necessarily) with no additional ventilatory support (so patients are on less support which might be desirable for them or their family).	This can results in less respiratory effort. However, this only occurs in patients who do not have a lot of secretions, as secretions can increase endotracheal resistance, which mean patients have to make more effort to breath (El-Khatib and Bou-Khalil 2008).
11 Intravenous fluids, total parenteral nutrition and gastric feeds should all stop in preparation for withdrawing ventilation (Kompanje et al. 2008).	Reducing fluids and feeds will minimize secretions (Kompanje et al. 2008).
12 Tools such as the Respiratory Distress Observation Scale should be considered in patients unable to communicate (Campbell et al. 2010).	Assessment tools such as the Respiratory Distress Observation Scale are validated for use with, and can help practitioners assess distress in, patients unable to communicate (Campbell et al. 2010). This is because dyspnoea can be an issue in both ventilated and non-ventilated patients. Specific underlying causes are important to consider (such as chronic obstructive pulmonary disease) and for which steroids can be very helpful in symptomatic relief (Arai et al. 2010). Limiting fluids also ensures patients do not develop fluid overload, which compromises breathing. Bronchodilators will dilate airways in patients struggling to breathe and might help relieve discomfort.
13 Techniques for managing breathlessness during withdrawal of ventilatory support in EOL should be used with patients who are aware and anxious. This includes using relaxation techniques such as guided imagery, relaxation tapes and/or music. Techniques for managing air hunger include using fans, opening windows and using moist, cool flannels/towels to cheeks or forehead (Puntillo et al. 2010a).	It is important to minimize as much as possible any distress caused by breathlessness. Cool cloths to the face increase airflow to trigeminal nerve dermatomes in the cheeks and can be soothing (Puntillo et al. 2010a).
14 Document care provided.	To: ■ provide an accurate record ■ monitor effectiveness of procedure ■ reduce the risk of duplication of treatment ■ provide a point of reference or comparison in the event of later questions ■ acknowledge accountability for actions ■ facilitate communication and continuity of care. (NMC 2008; HCPC 2012; GMC 2013)

Procedure guideline 17.3: Extubation care at end of life

Procedure

Action	Rationale
1 Where possible, explain and discuss the procedure with the patient. If the patient lacks the capacity to make decisions the practitioner must act in the patient's best interests.	To ensure that the patient understands the procedure and gives their valid consent. To ensure the patient's best interests are maintained (Mental Capacity Act 2005).
2 Review analgesia. Ensure any analgesia required has taken effect (Bakker et al. 2008; Kompanje et al. 2008; Rocker 2010).	To ensure the patient remains comfortable and has adequate analgesia. Analgesia reduces the risk of the patient being in pain and reduces the risk of dyspnoea (Bakker et al. 2008; Kompanje et al. 2008).
3 Review sedation and neuromuscular blockade medications with team.	To ensure respiratory muscles can be used and the patient can breathe spontaneously.
4 Prepare linen or drapes before extubation.	To cover the patient's chest so their body does not get sprayed with secretions or blood.
5 Use universal infection prevention and control precautions and wear goggles.	To reduce the risk of infection. Extubation can lead to coughing and cause a fine spray (aerosol) to be expelled around the patient – and thus spread of infection and blood- and droplet-borne viruses.
6 Warn the family and patient about the potential for obstruction or stridor. Consider administering methylprednisolone prior to extubation (François et al. 2007; Kompanje et al. 2008).	To try to reduce the family and patient's distress. Stridor can be noisy and distressing for those witnessing (or experiencing it) and is common in obstruction. Warning families might reduce anxiety associated with this procedure. Methylpredisolone has been suggested in the management of extubation stridor at EOL. Steroids might reduce inflammation of upper airways and thus reduce stridor (François et al. 2007; Kompanje et al. 2008).
7 Ensure the patient is not dependent on high levels of PEEP pressure support and FiO$_2$ before extubation (Rocker 2010).	Extubation in a situation of a high level of respiratory support might cause respiratory distress (acute breathlessness or 'air hunger') on extubation (Puntillo et al. 2010a; Rocker 2010). Although staged withdrawal is not best practice as it can prolong dying (Harper and Chapman 2010), planning for extubation might also sometimes include withdrawing ventilation support in phases to ensure patients are not extubated straight from a high level of support (Rocker 2010).
8 Document care provided.	To: ■ provide an accurate record ■ monitor effectiveness of procedure ■ reduce the risk of duplication of treatment ■ provide a point of reference or comparison in the event of later questions ■ acknowledge accountability for actions ■ facilitate communication and continuity of care. (NMC 2008; HCPC 2012; GMC 2013)

Procedure guideline 17.4: Considerations for end of life care for patients in critical care units

Procedure

Action	Rationale
1 Where appropriate, and where possible, explain and discuss the procedure with the patient. If the patient lacks the capacity to make decisions the practitioner must act in the patient's best interests.	To ensure that the patient understands the procedure and gives their valid consent. To ensure the patient's best interests are maintained (Mental Capacity Act 2005).

Dignity

2 Ensure the family holds an enduring memory of their loved one's death as a calm and dignified event (despite any previous suffering and also even though death is in a highly technological and busy environment). Compassionate care is essential.	Dignified death is a premise of good EOLC (Levy et al. 2005; DH, 2008). Practitioners have a professional duty to maintain dignity in all of their care (NMC 2008; HCPC 2012; GMC 2013). Despite the emphasis on a 'good death', dignity is not always upheld (National Audit Office 2008). However, critical care nurses' endeavour to provide dignified EOLC has been noted (Fridh et al. 2009). Being in receipt of compassion characterizes a good patient experience and reduces anxiety (Schantz 2007; Firth-Cozens and Cornwell 2009).

Pain

3 Assess patient's pain (*see also* Chapter 10). Consider the use of pain scales in assessment of pain in ventilated patients and patients with reduced consciousness. Use non-verbal cues such as grimacing, sweating, dyspnoea, raised heart rate and/or blood pressure. Consider involving the family to interpret patient's level of pain.	Pain scales such as the Pain Behaviour Scale (Payen et al. 2001) and the Critical Care Pain Observation Tool (Gélinas et al. 2006) are validated for use in patients receiving ventilation. In unconscious patients, pain management is more challenging as levels of pain are very difficult to assess. One study showed that more than 50% of seriously ill hospitalized patients had pain (Nelson et al. 2001). Puntillo et al's (2010b) study of ventilated patients at high risk of dying showed that pain was distressing (although tiredness, thirst and shortness of breath were worse). Pain can exacerbate breathlessness. Unconscious patients are unable to contribute to pain assessment and therefore non-verbal cues have to be used instead. Grimacing, sweating, dyspnoea, raised heart rate and/or blood pressure can all indicate pain in critical care patients unable to communicate (Puntillo et al. 2010a). Families might be familiar with the patient's pain, through proximity with the patient, and can contribute to pain assessment.
4 Consider allowing a temporary increase in consciousness and, therefore, possibly an increased level of pain or discomfort, if patients wish to contribute to EOL decisions (Truog et al. 2008). The ethics of this should be considered at length (Batchelor et al. 2003; Tonelli 2005).	3. There might occasionally be times when it is acceptable to reduce analgesia and sedation in order for patients to be mentally capable of contributing to EOL decision making (Truog et al. 2008). However, practitioners have to be certain that any potential patient distress from reducing analgesia and sedation is outweighed by their wishes and ability to contribute to discussions about treatments. There is debate over the issue of arousing patients purely to contribute to decisions (Batchelor et al. 2003; Tonelli 2005).

(Continued)

Procedure guideline 17.4: (*Continued*)

5 Maintain adequate sedation and analgesia. Use guidance such as the Liverpool Care Pathway and local protocols for pain management. Long-acting opiates such as morphine or diamorphine are often drugs of choice.	The long action of these opiates lessens the risk of breakthrough pain. Although where patients are on fentanil and their dying trajectory is predicted to be very rapid – it might be appropriate to continue with administering fentanil preparations. NB Alfentanil would rarely be used due to its short half-life, except in circumstances where renal clearance was an issue for EOL symptoms – such as increased morphine-related myoclonic jerks, respiratory depression (DH, Renal NSF Team and Marie Curie Palliative Care Institute 2008).
6 Administer prescribed analgesics. Most opioids are given via intravenous (IV) drug administration at EOL in critical care, particularly if patients are already on IV analgesia. Palliative care teams can be consulted for advice if there is doubt over route of administration and drug efficacy.	Changing route of administration to that usually used in palliative care (i.e. to sub-cutaneous [Ellershaw and Ward 2003]) might temporarily affect opioid uptake and result in inconsistent drug delivery. Palliative care teams are able to provide advice in this area and will consider any analgesia that they think will alleviate the patient's pain.
7 Achieve a therapeutic dose.	Patients might have a high tolerance for analgesia, based on their medical history and previous analgesic use (for example whether they are a frequent opioid user, or were previously receiving high levels of analgesia in ITU, or have a history of IV drug abuse). It is important to achieve a therapeutic dose and not to under-dose. Evidence suggests that high-dose opioids do not significantly depress respiration (Estfan et al. 2007; Bakker et al. 2008). The patient's underlying history of analgesia is an important consideration (Puntillo et al. 2010a).

Comfort

8 Ensure the patient's comfort is maintained. Ensure patients have regular eye, mouth care and hygiene care. Saliva substitutes and ice chips can help relieve symptoms of thirst (*see* Chapter 12 for guidance on this). Involve the palliative care team to ensure all aspects of comfort have been considered (Nelson and Danis 2001; Spuhler 2010).	Regular eye and mouth care enhance patient comfort (Marie Curie Palliative Care Institute 2007; Spuhler 2010). Thirst can worsen near the end of life, particularly if hydration has been stopped. Thirst was the most distressing and intense symptom for ventilated patients at high risk of dying (Puntillo *et al.* 2010b). Hygiene care (bed baths, washes, using wipes) might help where patients have pruritis, equally it might exacerbate any pruritis so a judgement has to be made as to what will cause patients less distress.

Anxiety

9 Use sensitive language and offer reassurance about presence is important for both patient and their family. Consider using a leaflet to help families deal with EOL situations and bereavement (Lautrette et al. 2007).	Anxiety may be an issue for the patient and also their family (Pochard et al. 2001; Puntillo et al. 2010b), some of whom might even have post-traumatic stress disorder (PTSD) (Azoulay et al. 2005; McAdam et al. 2010).

Psychological care/Distress

10 Observe for patients who will be awake during withdrawal of treatment and care and minimize their distress. This might involve providing sedation or analgesia.	Psychological distress in patients who are aware of their situation at the end of their life is not uncommon (Gao et al. 2010), and psychological support might even be helpful for some of these patients (Crunkilton and Rubins 2009).
11 Encourage the family to be present to help calm the patient's distress.	Families can provide a reassuring presence.

12 Assess and address patients' and families' spiritual and religious needs wherever possible.	End of life can provoke spiritual and religious questioning and spirituality and religiosity is often of intense importance to families and patients at the end of life. Having spiritual and religious awareness and wellness, might enhance emotional health (Candy et al. 2012).

Delirium/Confusion

13 Ensure the environment is soothing. For example, provide appropriate lighting and avoid unnecessary stimuli or obtrusive noise. Where appropriate, include the familiar presence of family or staff (Pattison 2005; Truog et al. 2008).	Delirium may be caused or compounded by a range of critical care interventions or illnesses such as pain, hypoxia and dyspnoea.
14 Manage terminal agitation and delirium with prescribed sedation. This may be better managed with haloperidol rather than usual sedating agents (Marie Curie Palliative Care Institute 2007; Truog et al. 2008).	To ameliorate the symptoms of terminal agitation and delirium which may be distressing for patients and can be distressing for relatives. Haloperidol is the drug of choice in ICU related delirium (NICE 2010), and can be used in EOL situations (Marie Curie Palliative Care Institute 2007; Truog et al. 2008).

Wound care and pressure relief

15 Assess appropriateness of dressing wound (e.g. trauma, burns, or surgical wounds) dressings. Reinforcing existing dressings might be more appropriate if there is strikethrough or leakage.	A judgement should be made as to whether it is appropriate to redress a wound because it might cause additional pain or discomfort to the patient to undergo a wound change or dressing.
16 An assessment should be made regarding the appropriateness of pressure relief care.	This is because it might be more beneficial to not disturb a patient (who might be in pain) for pressure relief positioning when the patient will soon or imminently die.

Elimination care and hygiene

17 Maintain suitable appearance and hygiene needs. The need to change bedding frequently for hot, clammy patients should be balanced against overly disturbing patients.	The benefit of moving and changing the patient needs to be balanced against the possibility of pain, etc. For example, replacing stoma dressings can cause discomfort. However, in elimination care this has to be balanced again patients' hygiene needs towards the end of their life. Opioid use can cause constipation and this may need to be managed with appropriate medication (aperients) or interventions (enema) but again this needs to be balanced against overall comfort.
18 Manage patient's elimination. An assessment should be made concerning the risk of developing constipation when opioids are used and of developing diarrhoea, for example when laxatives are utilized.	It is important to manage (as best as possible) the patient's elimination in order to promote comfort. Depending on the situation it may be appropriate to administer aperients or laxatives. It is likely that a catheter is already in situ to facilitate fluid balance measurement. If not, a decision should be made as to whether the presence of a urinary catheter is beneficial overall.

Aesthetics and personalizing care

19 Provide personalizing care, such as apply the patient's favourite body moisturizer or perfume. Play music, use the patient's own clothes and pillows or bedding.	Personalizing care can help preserve what Seymour (2001) terms 'personhood'. Ensuring the aesthetics of care are attended to, such as brushing hair how patients would have liked, shaving (as appropriate) and other personalized care, creates a more pleasing environment for the patient and their family. It might also be appropriate and helps to create a sense of the person beyond the patient and this has to be balanced against unnecessarily disturbing patients.

519

(Continued)

Procedure guideline 17.4: (*Continued*)

Environment and documentation

20 Consider (as outlined earlier) the appropriateness of monitoring, equipment and documentation.	Fixation on monitoring of patients' vital signs can make care of dying patients more difficult, therefore nurses must assess the appropriateness of continuing monitoring. Try to remove as much equipment from the bed space as possible to enhance the environment. Documentation of procedures, discussions and nursing or medical care should continue, but observations should not be recorded hourly, at the most 4-hourly, or less. If the patient is on an EOLC pathway (such as the LCP-ICU) this should be completed.
21 Consider displaying 'Get to know me' posters (see Massachussetts General hospital and IPAL-ICU websites in references) by patients' bedsides.	Learning about the patient can also help with helping staff to view the patient as a person, and thus enhance personhood.
22 Document care provided.	To: ■ provide an accurate record ■ monitor effectiveness of procedure ■ reduce the risk of duplication of treatment ■ provide a point of reference or comparison in the event of later questions ■ acknowledge accountability for actions ■ facilitate communication and continuity of care. (NMC 2008; HCPC 2012; GMC 2013)

Procedure guideline 17.5: Summary of procedures after death

Procedure

Action	Rationale
Preparing the patient for the mortuary	
1 After washing the patient, all deceased critical care patients should be placed in a zipped, waterproof plastic body bag. Absorbent sheets or incontinence pads can be placed either side of the patient's head.	There is a risk of leakage from gastrointestinal losses as there can be movement of secretions and fluid into the GI tract (and subsequently out of the mouth) (Pattison 2008a).
2 Consider leaving intact recent surgical dressings for wounds. Reinforcement of the dressing should be sufficient (Dougherty and Lister 2011; Pattison 2008a).	Wounds could leak, for example large amputation wounds (Dougherty and Lister 2011; Pattison 2008a).
3 Apply petroleum jelly to lips and perioral area.	Petroleum jelly may prevent skin excoriation or corrosion if stomach contents aspirate (Dougherty and Lister 2011; Pattison 2008a).
4 Suction oropharynx if previously intubated or if the patient had a tracheostomy.	Even if the patient is not obviously leaking from the oral cavity, secretions may accumulate in the oropharynx in previously intubated and trachestomy patients (Pattison 2008a).

Verifying death (before any after-death care)

5 Verification should be documented in the clinical notes. Verification of death is carried out by a medical doctor in critical care.

Verification of death can be complex in critical care (as exemplified in the case of brainstem death).

6 Inform next of kin and family, as appropriate, of processes to be undertaken. Offer the opportunity, as appropriate, for families to be involved.

Informing families (detail usually unnecessary) and offering them the opportunity to assist might help them feel involved and to understand what needs to be done.

7 Ask the nurse-in-charge to inform relevant part of organization of death, or leave a message and follow up first thing in the morning if 'out of hours'.

To prevent unnecessary delays for families and processing of death certification.

8 Ascertain if there are any religious or cultural implications for care of the patient who has died. (For extensive guidance on specific religious/cultural practices when caring for the patient who has died, please see Dougherty and Lister 2011.)

For instance, it is considered offensive to raise the notion of post-mortem (PM) with Hindu families, unless it is what is referred to as a 'legal PM' (i.e. required by law, rather than requested by a medical practitioner) (Speck 2003). Cultural sensitivity is important in all care (Leininger 1988), and sensitivities might be heightened at EOL.

Coroner referral and post-mortem

9 Practitioners need to determine if the patient is a candidate for review of death via the coroner. If the death was sudden and unexpected, but the coroner is satisfied that the death was due to natural causes, no inquest is required (HMSO 2004). (See www.dh.gov.uk and www.hta.gov.uk for more information regarding when to refer to the coroner or when post-mortems are indicated.)

Deaths that are referred to the coroner include:
- those notifiable specific cases where the coroner must be informed (for example deaths within 24 hours of an operation, patients with mesothelioma, or deaths following occupational health treatment)
- a death that is sudden and unexpected
- where a person has been ill but the doctor confirming the death is not certain why it happened at that particular time
- those where death has been the result of an accident or unusual circumstances.

Preparation of the patient's body may be different according to reason for referral. Tubes, appliances and dressings will need to stay in place until discussed with the coroner.

10 By law a coroner can order a post-mortem examination to be undertaken (DH 2003). If the patient is likely to require a post-mortem (which may not be a coroner's [or 'legal'] PM, but a PM requested by the consultant-in-charge, or even family, to answer a specific query over the cause of death) it is wise to prepare the family for what this might entail.

Preparing the family might help allay anxiety or fear around the procedure. The Department of Health (2003) has written guidance for families regarding this.

Organ donation

11 It is important to contact local or regional transplantation teams (*see* www.uktransplant.org.uk for local numbers if these are unavailable on your unit).

Local transplant teams can offer specialist advice. Tissues and organs that can be transplanted include: heart (including valves), lungs, kidneys, pancreas, liver, small bowel. Other tissues transplanted include: corneas, brain, skin, tracheae, bone. Faces and hands have more recently been transplanted (but this is not yet common practice).

(Continued)

Procedure guideline 17.5: *(Continued)*

12 The wishes of the deceased donor should take precedence in all cases. However, if patients did not have the capacity to consent before they died (and had not made their wishes known) they can still donate.	The patient's wishes are paramount in this instance.
13 Check the organ donor register. Registration as an organ donor (on the NHS Organ Donor Register) is deemed consent for organ donation. It can be difficult for teams to manage situations where families object to organ donation but the Human Tissue Authority (2004, Human Tissue Act, section 15 of Code 2) provides clinical guidance for dealing with such situations. It is stated that families do not have the legal right to veto or overrule the deceased patient's wishes. If wishes are unknown then professionals need to help facilitate a decision with sensitive discussion with the family (Pattison 2010). Once a decision has been made, it must be respected (HTA 2009).	Regulations published by the Department of Health deem adults who did not have capacity (i.e. were unconscious before death) able to donate tissue if certain approvals have been met by the Human Tissue Authority (HTA). Clinical teams, the HTA and any family members should be jointly involved in the decision about the appropriateness of donation. An independent assessor may be required. Children can donate their organs after death but have to have expressed a previous wish that they wanted to donate their organs (and be competent to do so). Parents and legal guardians can donate their child's organs where the child's wishes are unknown (UK Transplant 2009). Donation is a difficult decision and it is unacceptable to attempt to change decisions at this sensitive time (HTA 2009).
14 Document care provided.	To: ■ provide an accurate record ■ monitor effectiveness of procedure ■ reduce the risk of duplication of treatment ■ provide a point of reference or comparison in the event of later questions ■ acknowledge accountability for actions, and ■ facilitate communication and continuity of care. (NMC 2008; HCPC 2012; GMC 2013)

Competency statement 17.1: Specific procedure competency statements for end of life care

Complete assessment against relevant fundamental competency statements (see Chapter 2, pp. 20, 21)	Evidence
Specific procedure competency statements for end of life care	**Evidence of competency for end of life care**
Demonstrate ability to: ■ teach and assess or ■ learn from assessment.	Examples of evidence of teaching, assessing and learning.
Identify reason(s) for providing EOLC in critical care, including: ■ dying a 'good death' ■ what to consider at withdrawal/withholding stage in preparation for EOLC ■ understand implications of communication styles.	*May be demonstrated by:* ■ discussion with supervisor/mentor of correct procedure and issues relating to a 'good death' ■ communicating in a timely and appropriate manner any changes or concerns regarding EOLC with the multidisciplinary team ■ observation in practice.

Identify risks, potential problems and complications for EOLC:
- withholding and/or withdrawing treatment
- infection risk from the patient's body
- unexpected or sudden death
- cultural differences in caring for a patient's body
- need for coroner referral/post-mortem.

May be demonstrated by:
- discussion with supervisor/mentor
- observation in practice
- communicating in a timely and appropriate manner any changes or concerns regarding EOLC with the multidisciplinary team.

Demonstrate knowledge and understanding of local and national policies, guidance, and procedures in relation to EOLC:
- withdrawal and withholding treatment
- do not attempt cardiopulmonary resuscitation
- brainstem death diagnosis guidance
- last offices and after-death care.

May be demonstrated by:
- discussion with supervisor/mentor of relevant manufacturer, local and national guidelines and policies.

Demonstrate knowledge and understanding of evidence base in relation to EOLC:
- research into patient and family perceptions of 'good death'
- evidence for brainstem death
- care at EOL in relation to stages of dying.

May be demonstrated by:
- direct observation and discussion with supervisor/mentor.

Demonstrate skills that are required in relation to EOLC:
- interpersonal skills (communication)
- sensitivity
- empathy
- compassion
- knowledge and application of withdrawal practices.

May be demonstrated by:
- direct observation and discussion with supervisor/mentor of skills required at EOLC.

Prepare equipment required in relation to last offices:
- hygiene
- pads/gauze
- body bag, etc.

May be demonstrated by:
- direct observation and discussion with supervisor/mentor of correct procedure for last offices.

Demonstrate the correct technique for the procedure in relation to last offices:
- preparing the patient's body according to culture and whether there is a need for coroner referral/post-mortem
- minimize infection risk
- withholding or withdrawing treatment
- supporting the family.

May be demonstrated by:
- direct observation and discussion with supervisor/mentor of correct procedure for last offices.

References and further reading

Abbott KH, Sago JG, Breen CM et al. (2001) Families looking back: one year after discussion of withdrawal or withholding of life-sustaining support. *Critical Care Medicine* **29**(1): 197–200.

Addicott R and Ashton R (eds) (2010) *Delivering better care at end of life: the next steps report* from the Sir Roger Bannister Health Summit, Leeds Castle, 19–20 November 2009. London: Kings Fund. http://www.institute.nhs.uk/nhs_alert/nhs_institute_alerts_archive/Improvement_archive.html [accessed 19 May 2010].

Ahrens T, Yancey V and Kollef M (2003) Improving family communications at the end of life: implications for length of stay in the intensive care unit and resource use. *Amercian Journal of Critical Care* **12**: 317–324.

Airedale NHS Trust v. Bland [1993] 1 All ER 821 HL.

Ankeny RA, Clifford R, Jordens CFC et al. (2005) Religious perspectives on withdrawal of treatment from patients with multiple organ failure. *Medical Journal of Australia* **183** (11/12): 616–621.

Arai S, McAdam J and Puntillo K (2010) Dyspnoea. In: Rocker GM, Azoulay E, Puntillo K and Nelson J (eds) *End of Life Care in the ICU: from advanced disease to bereavement*, pp. 66–67. Oxford: Oxford University Press.

Arnold R, Nelson J, Prendergast T et al. (2010) Educational modules for the critical care communication (C3) course – a communication skills training program for intensive care fellows. http://www.capc.org/palliative-care-professional-development/Training/c3-module-ipal-icu.pdf [accessed 11 February 2011].

Azoulay E, Pochard F, Kentish-Barnes N et al.; FAMIREA Study Group (2005) Risk of post-traumatic stress symptoms in family members of intensive care unit patients. *American Journal of Respiratory and Critical Care Medicine* **171**(9): 987–994.

Azoulay E, Timsit JF, Sprung CL et al. and the Conflictus Study Investigators and for the Ethics Section of the European Society of Intensive Care Medicine (2009) Prevalence and factors of intensive care unit conflicts: the conflicus study. *American Journal of Respiratory and Critical Care Medicine* **180**(9): 853–860.

Baggs JG and Schmitt MH (1995) Intensive care decisions about level of aggressiveness of care. *Research in Nursing and Health* **18**:(4) 345–355.

Baile WF, Buckman R, Lenzi R et al. (2000) SPIKES – a six-step protocol for delivering bad news: application to the patient with cancer. *The Oncologist* 5: 302–311.

Bakker J, Jansen TC, Lima A and Kompanje EJO (2008) Why opioids and sedatives may prolong life rather than hasten death after ventilator withdrawal in critically ill patients. *American Journal of Hospice & Palliative Care* 25(2): 152–154.

Barnato AE, Labor RE, Freeborne NE et al. (2005) Qualitative analysis of Medicare claims in the last 3 years of life: a pilot study. *Journal of the American Geriatric Society* 53(1): 66–73.

Batchelor A, Jenal L, Kapadia F et al. (2003) Ethics roundtable debate: should a sedated dying patient be wakened to say goodbye to family? *Critical Care* 7: 335–338 (DOI 10.1186/cc2329).

Beauchamp TL and Childress JF (2005) *Principles of Biomedical Ethics* (5e). London: Oxford University Press.

Bell MDD, Moss E and Murphy PG (2004) Brainstem death testing in the UK – time for reappraisal? *British Journal of Anaesthesia* **92**(5): 633–640.

Bradshaw A (1999) The virtue of nursing: the covenant of care. *Journal of Medical Ethics* 25(6): 477–481.

Breslin R (1993) *Understanding Culture's Influence on Behavior*. New York, NY: Harcourt Brace.

British Medical Association (BMA) (2007) *Withholding and Withdrawing Life-Prolonging Medical Treatment: guidance for medical decision-making* (3e). London: BMA.

British Medical Association, UK Resuscitation Council and Royal College of Nursing (2007) *Decisions Relating to Cardiopulmonary Resuscitation. A joint statement from the British Medical Association, the Resuscitation Council (UK) and the Royal College of Nursing*. London: BMA.

Calzavacca P, Licari E, Tee A et al. (2010) The impact of Rapid Response System on delayed emergency team activation patient characteristics and outcomes – a follow-up study. *Resuscitation* 81(1): 31–35.

Campbell ML (2007) How to withdraw mechanical ventilation: a systematic review of the literature. *AACN Advance in Critical Care* 18(4): 397–403.

Campbell ML, Bizek KS and Thill M (1999) Patient responses during rapid terminal weaning from mechanical ventilation: a prospective study. *Critical Care Medicine* 27: 73–77.

Campbell ML, Templin T and Walch J (2010) A Respiratory Distress Observation Scale for patients unable to self-report dyspnea. *Journal of Palliative Medicine* 13(3): 285–290.

Candy B, Jones L, Varagunam M et al. (2012) Spiritual and religious interventions for well-being of adults in the terminal phase of disease. *Cochrane Database Systematic Review* May 16; 5: CD007544.

Carey SM and Cosgrove JF (2006) Cultural issues surrounding end-of-life care. *Current Anaesthesia and Critical Care* 17(5): 263–270.

Carlet J, Thijs LG, Antonelli M et al. (2004) Challenges in end-of-life care in the ICU: statement of the 5th International Consensus Conference in Critical Care, Brussels, Belgium, April 2003. *Intensive Care Medicine* 30: 770–784.

Cassell J, Buchman TG, Streat S and Stewart RM (2003) Surgeons, intensivists, and the covenant of care: administrative models and values affecting care at the end of life – updated. *Critical Care Medicine* 31(5): 1551–1559.

Chan JD, Treece PD, Engelberg RA et al. (2004) Narcotic and benzodiazepine use after withdrawal of life support: association with time to death? *Chest* 126(1): 286–293.

Chan R and Webster J (2010) End-of-life care pathways for improving outcomes in caring for the dying. *Cochrane Database of Systematic Reviews*; Issue 1, Art No: CD008006. DOI: 10.1002/14651858.CD008006.pub2.

Chotirmall SH, Flynn MG, Donegan CF et al. (2010) Extubation versus tracheostomy in withdrawal of treatment – ethical, clinical, and legal perspectives. *Journal of Critical Care* 25(2): 360. E1–8. doi: 10.1016/j.jcrc.2009.08.007. Epub 21 Oct 2009.

Clarfield, AM; Gordon, M; Markwell, H; Alibhai, SMH (2003) Ethical issues in end-of-life geriatric care: the approach of three monotheistic religions – Judaism, Catholicism, and Islam. *Journal of American Geriatric Society* 51: 1149–1154.

Cook DJ, Giacomini M, Johnson N and Willms D (1999) Life support in the intensive care unit: a qualitative investigation of technological purposes. *Canadian Medical Association Journal* **161**(9): 1109–1113.

Cook D, Rocker G, Marshall J and Sjokvist P (2003) Withdrawal of mechanical ventilation in anticipation of death in the intensive care unit. *New England Journal of Medicine* 349(12): 1123–1132.

Coombs MA, Addington-Hall J and Long-Sutehall T (2012) Challenges in transition from intervention to end of life care in intensive care: a qualitative study. *International Journal of Nursing Studies* 49(5): 519–527.

Copeland-Fields L, Griffin T, Jenkins T et al. (2001) Comparison of outcome predictions made by physicians, by nurses, and by using the Mortality Prediction Model. *American Journal of Critical Care* 10: 313–319.

Counsell C and Guin P (2002) Exploring family needs during withdrawal of life support in critically ill patients. *Critical Care Nursing Clinics of North America* 14: 187–191.

Crunkilton DD and Rubins VD (2009) Psychological distress in end-of-life care: a review of issues in assessment and treatment. *Journal of Social Work in End-of-Life & Palliative Care* 5(1/2): 75–93.

Curtis JR, Patrick DL, Engelberg RA et al. (2002) A measure of the quality of dying and death. Initial validation using after-death interviews with family members. *Journal of Pain and Symptom Management* 24(1): 17–31.

Danis M, Patrick DL, Southerland LI and Green ML (1998) Patients' and families' preferences for medical intensive care. *Journal of the American Medical Association* 260(6): 797–802.

Department of Health (1996) *Guidelines on Admission to and Discharge from Intensive Care and High Dependency Units*. London: NHS Executive.

Department of Health (DH) (1998) *A Code of Practice for the Diagnosis of Brain Stem Death*. London: DH.

Department of Health (2001) *The Nursing Contribution to the Provision of Comprehensive Critical Care: the review of adult critical care services*. London: NHS Executive.

Department of Health (2003) *Families and Post Mortems: a code of practice*. London: DH.

Department of Health (2008) *End of Life Care Strategy – promoting high quality care for all adults at the end of life*. London: DH. http://www.dh.gov.uk/en/Publicationsandstatistics/Publications/PublicationsPolicyAndGuidance/DH_086277 [accessed 10 January 2011].

Department of Health (2009) *National End of Life Care Programme*. http://webarchive.nationalarchives.gov.uk/+/www.dh.gov.uk/en/Healthcare/IntegratedCare/Endoflifecare/DH_086083. Last modified 12.4.2009 [accessed 3 January 2011].

Dimond B (2004) Health and safety considerations following the death of a patient. *British Journal of Nursing* 13(11): 673–676.

Doolen J and York N (2007) Cultural differences with end-of-life care in the critical care unit. *Dimensions of Critical Care Nursing* **26**(5): 194–198.

Dougherty L and Lister S (eds) (2011) *Royal Marsden Manual of Clinical Procedures* (8e). Oxford: Blackwell.

Dying Matters (2011) http://www.dyingmatters.org/site/about-us [accessed 3 March 2011].

El-Khatib MF and Bou-Khalil P (2008) Clinical review: liberation from mechanical ventilation. *Critical Care* **12**: 221.

Ellershaw J, Haycox AR and Perkins L (2010) *The Impact of the Liverpool Care Pathway on Care at the End of Life*. NIHR Service delivery and organisation programme. http://www.sdo.nihr.ac.uk/projdetails.php?ref=08-1813-256 [accessed 3 March 2011].

Ellershaw J and Ward C (2003) Care of the dying patient: the last hours or days of life. *British Medical Journal* **326**: 30–34.

Elpern EH, Covert B and Kleinpell R (2005) Moral distress of staff nurses in a medical intensive care unit. *American Journal of Critical Care* **14**(6): 523–530.

Embriaco N, Papazian L, Kentish-Barnes N et al. (2007) Burnout syndrome among critical care healthcare workers. *Current Opinion in Critical Care* **13**(5): 482–488.

Estfan B, Mahmoud F, Shaheen P et al. (2007) Respiratory function during parenteral opioid titration for cancer pain. *Palliative Medicine* **21**(2): 81–86.

Faber-Langendoen K and Lanken PN (2000) Dying patients in the intensive care unit: forgoing treatment, maintaining care. *Annals of Internal Medicine* **133**(11): 886–893.

Faber-Langendoen K, Spomer A and Ingbar D (1996) A prospective study of withdrawing mechanical ventilation from dying patients. *American Journal of Respiratory and Critical Care Medicine* **153**: A365.

Fartoukh M, Brun-Buisson C and Lemaire F (2005) Terminal extubation in 5 end-of-life patients in intensive care units. *Presse Med* **34**(7): 495–501. English translation available at http://www.em-consulte.com/article/158963 [accessed 30 September 2010].

Ferrand E, Lemaire F, Regnier B et al. (2003) Discrepancies between perceptions by physicians and nursing staff of intensive care unit end-of-life decisions. *American Journal of Respiratory and Critical Care Medicine* **167**(10): 1310–1315.

Festic E, Wilson ME, Gajic O et al. (2012) Perspectives of physicians and nurses regarding end-of-life care in the intensive care unit. *Journal of Intensive Care Medicine* **27**(1): 45–54.

Firth-Cozens J and Cornwell J (2009) *The Point of Care: enabling compassionate care in acute hospital settings*. London The Kings Fund.

François B, Bellissant E, Gissot V et al.; Association des Réanimateurs du Centre-Ouest (ARCO) (2007) 12-h pretreatment with methylprednisolone versus placebo for prevention of postextubation laryngeal oedema: a randomised double-blind trial. *Lancet* **369**(9567): 1083–1089.

Frick S, Uehlinger DE and Zuercher Zenklusen RM (2003) Medical futility: predicting outcome of intensive care unit patients by nurses and doctors – a prospective comparative study. *Critical Care Medicine* **31**: 456–461.

Fridh I, Forsberg A and Bergbom I (2009) Doing one's utmost: nurses' descriptions of caring for dying patients in an intensive care environment. *Intensive and Critical Care Nursing* **25**(5): 233–241.

Furst CJ and Doyle D (2005) The terminal phase. In: Doyle D, Hanks G, Cherny N and Calman K (eds) *Oxford Textbook of Palliative Medicine* (3e), pp. 1117–1133. Oxford: Oxford University Press.

Gao W, Bennett MI, Stark D et al. (2010) Psychological distress in cancer from survivorship to end of life care: prevalence, associ-ated factors and clinical implications. *European Journal of Cancer* **46**(11): 2036–2044.

Gay EB, Pronovost PJ, Bassett RD and Nelson JE (2009) The intensive care unit family meeting: making it happen. *Journal of Critical Care* **24**(4): 629.e1–12.

Gedge E, Giacomini M and Cook D (2007) Withholding and withdrawing life support in critical care settings: ethical issues concerning consent. *Journal of Medical Ethics* **33**: 215–218.

Gélinas C, Fillion L, Puntillo KA et al. (2006) Validation of the critical-care pain observation tool in adult patients. *American Journal of Critical Care* **15**(4): 420–427.

General Medical Council (2010) *Treatment and Care Towards the End of Life: good practice in decision making*. London: GMC. http://www.gmc-uk.org/guidance/ethical_guidance/end_of_life_care.asp [accessed March 2012].

General Medical Council (2013) *Good Medical Practice*. London: GMC. http://www.gmc-uk.org/gmp2013 [accessed 25 March 2013].

Glavan BJ, Engelberg RA, Downey L and Curtis JR (2008) Using the medical record to evaluate quality end-of-life care in the intensive care unit. *Critical Care Medicine* **36**(4): 1138–1146.

Gorton AJ, Jayanthi NV, Lepping P and Scriven MW (2008) Patients' attitudes towards 'do not attempt resuscitation' status. *Journal of Medical Ethics* **34**(8): 624–626.

Hales S, Zimmermann C and Rodin G (2010) Review: the quality of dying and death: a systematic review of measures. *Palliative Medicine* **24**(2): 127–144.

Hamric AB and Blackhall LJ (2007) Nurse-physician perspectives on the care of dying patients in intensive care units: collaboration, moral distress, and ethical climate. *Critical Care Medicine* **35**: 422–429.

Hanna DR and Romana M (2007) Debriefing after a crisis. *Nursing Management* **38**(8): 38–42, 44–55, 47.

Hardy JR, Haberecht J, Maresco-Pennisi D and Yates P (2007) Australian Best Care of the Dying Network, Queensland. Audit of the care of the dying in a network of hospitals and institutions in Queensland. *Internal Medicine Journal* **37**(5): 315–319.

Harper J and Chapman L (2010) The Liverpool Care Pathway for patients dying in intensive care in the UK. In: Rocker GM, Azoulay E, Puntillo K and Nelson J (eds) *End of Life Care in the ICU: from advanced disease to bereavement*, pp. 278–281. Oxford: Oxford University Press.

Health and Safety Advisory Committee (HSAC) (2003) *Safe Working and the Prevention of Infection in the Mortuary and Post-Mortem Room*. London: HSAC/HSE.

Health and Care Professions Council (2012) *Standard of Conduct, Performance and Ethics*. London: HCPC. http://www.hcpc-uk.org/assets/documents/10003B6EStandardsofconduct,performanceandethics.pdf [accessed January 2013].

Heyland DK, Cook DJ, Rocker GM et al. (2003) Decision-making in the ICU: perspectives of the substitute decision-maker. *Intensive Care Medicine* **29**(1): 75–82.

Hills M and Albarran J (2009) Last offices care and service for the newly bereaved: an audit of practice. *Nursing Times* **105**(23): 14–16.

Hills M and Albarran JW (2010) After death 1: caring for bereaved relatives and being aware of cultural differences. *Nursing Times* **106**(27): 19–20.

HMSO (2004) *Reforming the Coroner and Death Certification Service. A Position Paper*. London: HMSO.

Human Tissue Act (2004) http://www.hta.gov.uk/legislationpolicies andcodesofpractice/legislation.cfm [accessed 8 September 2010].

Human Tissue Authority (2009) http://www.hta.gov.uk/legislation policiesandcodesofpractice/codesofpractice/code3post-mortem.

cfm?FaArea1=customwidgets.content_view_1&cit_id=693&cit_parent_cit_id=680 [accessed 8 September 2010].

Human Tissue Authority (2009) *Code of practice 2: Donation of solid organs for transplantation*. London: Department of Health. http://www.hta.gov.uk/legislationpoliciesandcodesofpractice/codesofpractice/code2donationoforgans.cfm?faArea1=customwidgets.content_view_1&cit_id=669 [accessed 10 September 2010].

Intensive Care National Audit Centre [ICNARC] (2009) Summary statistics case-mix programme 2007–8. https://www.icnarc.org/documents/summary%20statistics.pdf [accessed 12 April 2012].

Intensive Care National Audit Centre [ICNARC] (2012) Summary statistics case-mix programme 2010–11. https://www.icnarc.org/documents/Case%20Mix%20Programme%20(CMP)%20Summary%20Statistics%202010-11.pdf [accessed 25 June 2012].

Intensive Care Society (1998) *Guidelines for Bereavement Care in Intensive Care Units*. London: ICS. http://www.ics.ac.uk/intensive_care_professional/standards_and_guidelines/bereavement_care_in_the_icu [accessed 3 March 2011].

Jensen HI, Ammentorp J, Erlandsen M and Ording H (2011) Withholding or withdrawing therapy in intensive care units: an analysis of collaboration among healthcare professionals. *Intensive Care Medicine* 37(10): 1696–2705.

Jezuit DL (2000) Suffering of critical care nurses with end-of-life decisions. *Medsurg Nursing* 9(3): 145–152.

Jones DA, McIntyre T, Baldwin I et al. (2007) The medical emergency team and end-of-life care: a pilot study. *Critical Care Resuscitation* 9(2): 151–156.

Kagawa-Singer M and Blackhall LJ (2001) Negotiating cross-cultural issues at the end of life: 'you got to go where he lives'. *Journal of the American Medical Association* 286: 2993–3001.

Keenan SP, Mawdsley C, Plotkin D et al. (2000) Withdrawal of life support: how the family feels, and why. *Journal of Palliative Care* 16. 10–44.

Keenan SP, Mawdsley C, Plotkin D and Sibbald WJ (2003) Critical Care Research Network. Interhospital variability in satisfaction with withdrawal of life support: room for improvement? *Critical Care Medicine* 31(2): 626–631.

Kirchhoff KT and Beckstrand RL (2000) Critical care nurses' perceptions of obstacles and helpful behaviours in providing end-of-life care to dying patients. *American Journal of Critical Care* 9(2): 96–105.

Kirchhoff KT, Spuhler V, Walker L et al. (2000) Intensive care nurses' experiences with end-of-life care. *American Journal of Critical Care* 9(1): 36–42.

Kirchhoff KT, Walker L, Hutton A et al. (2002) The vortex: families' experiences with death in the intensive care unit. *American Journal of Critical Care* 11(3): 200–209.

Knaus WA, Draper EA, Wagner DP and Zimmerman JE (1985) Prognosis in acute organ-system failure. *Annals of Surgery* 202: 685–693.

Kobza R and Erne P (2007) End-of-life decisions in ICD patients with malignant tumors. *Pacing and Clinical Electrophysiology* 30(7): 845–849.

Kompanje EJO, van der Hoven B and Bakker J (2008) Anticipation of distress after discontinuation of mechanical ventilation in the ICU at the end of life. *Intensive Care Medicine* 34(9): 1593–1599.

Kunyk D and Olson K (2001) Clarification of conceptualizations of empathy. *Journal of Advanced Nursing* 35(3): 317–325.

Latour JM, Fulbrook P and Albarran JW (2009) EfCCNa survey: European intensive care nurses' attitudes and beliefs towards end-of-life care. *Nursing in Critical Care* 14(3): 110–121.

Lautrette A, Darmon M, Megarbane B et al. (2007) Communication strategy and brochure for relatives of patients dying in the ICU. *New England Journal of Medicine* 356(5): 469–478.

Le Gall JR, Loirat P, Alperovitch A et al. (1984) A simplified acute physiology score for ICU patients. *Critical Care Medicine* 12(11): 975–977.

Leininger M (1988) *Caring: an essential human need*. Detroit: Wayne State University Press.

Levy CR, Ely EW, Payne K et al. (2005) Quality of dying and death in two medical ICUs: perceptions of family and clinicians. *Chest* 127(5): 1775–1783.

Locsin RC (1998) Technologic competence as caring in critical care nursing. *Holistic Nursing Practice* 12(4): 50–56.

Long-Sutehall T, Willis H, Palmer R et al. (2011) Negotiated dying: a grounded theory of how nurses shape withdrawal of treatment in hospital critical care units. *International Journal of Nursing Studies* 48(12): 1466–1474.

Lynn J, Teno JM, Phillips RS et al. (1997) Perceptions by family members of the dying experience of older and seriously ill patients. *Annals of Internal Medicine* 126(2): 97–106.

MacIver J and Ross HJ (2010) Withdrawal of ventricular assist device support. In: Rocker GM, Azoulay E, Puntillo K and Nelson J (eds) *End of Life Care in the ICU: From advanced disease to bereavement*, pp. 258–261. Oxford: Oxford University Press.

Marie Curie Palliative Care Institute (2007) Liverpool Care Pathway – Intensive Care Unit. http://www.liv.ac.uk/mcpcil/liverpool-care-pathway/pdfs/LCP-ICU-version11.pdf [accessed 3 February 2011].

DH, Renal NSF Team and Marie Curie Palliative Care Institute (2008) Guidelines for LCP prescribing in advanced chronic kidney disease. http://www.renal.org/pages/media/Guidelines/National%20LCP%20Renal%20Symptom%20Control%20Guidelines%20%2805.06.08%29%20%28printable%20pdf%29.pdf [accessed 3 March 2011].

Marr L and Weismann DE (2004) Withdrawal of ventilatory support from the dying adult patient. *Journal of Supportive Oncology* 2(3): 283–288.

Mason K and Laurie G (2006) *Mason and McCall Smith's Law and Medical Ethics* (8e). Oxford: Oxford University Press.

McAdam J, Arai S and Puntillo K (2010) Anxiety. In: In: Rocker GM, Azoulay E, Puntillo K and Nelson J (eds) *End of Life Care in the ICU: From advanced disease to bereavement*, pp. 68–73. Oxford: Oxford University Press.

McGrath P and Leahy M (2009) Catastrophic bleeds during end-of-life care in haematology: controversies from Australian research. *Supportive Care in Cancer* 17(5): 527–537.

Melia KM (2001) Ethical issues and the importance of consensus for the intensive care team. *Social Science and Medicine* 53: 707–719.

Meltzer LS and Huckabay LM (2004) Critical care nurses' perceptions of futile care and its effect on burnout. *American Journal of Critical Care* 13: 202–208.

Mental Capacity Act (2005) http://www.legislation.gov.uk/ukpga/2005/9/pdfs/ukpga_20050009_en.pdf [accessed 9 February 2012 at].

National Audit Office (NAO) (2008) *End of Life Care*. London: The Stationery Office.

National Gold Standard Framework (2011) The Gold Standards Framework. http://www.goldstandardsframework.nhs.uk/The GSFToolkit [accessed 2 February 2011.

National Health Service (NHS) (2009a) *Common Core Competences and Principles for Health and Social Care Workers Working with Adults at the End of Life*. Leicester: NHS. http://www.endoflifecareforadults.nhs.uk/publications/core competencesguide

National Health Service (NHS) (2009b) *The NHS Constitution: the NHS belongs to us all*. London: NHS.

National Institute for Clinical Excellence (NICE) (2004) *Improving Supportive and Palliative Care for Adults with Cancer*. London: NICE.

National Institute for Health and Clinical Excellence (NICE) (2010) *Clinical Guideline 103: Delirium: diagnosis, prevention and management*. London: NICE. http://www.nice.org.uk/CG103 [accessed March 2012].

Nelson J and Danis M (2001) End-of-life care in the intensive care unit: where are we now? *Critical Care Medicine* 29(2; suppl): 2.

Nelson JE, Meier DE, Oei EJ et al. (2001) Self-reported symptom experience of critically ill cancer patients receiving intensive care. *Critical Care Medicine* 29: 277–282.

Nelson JE, Walker AS, Luhrs CA et al. (2009) Family meetings made simpler: a toolkit for the intensive care unit. *Journal of Critical Care* 24(4): 626.e7–14.

Nelson JE, Bassett R, Boss RD et al. for the Improve Palliative Care in the Intensive Care Unit Project (2010) Models for structuring a clinical initiative to enhance palliative care in the intensive care unit: a report from the IPAL-ICU Project (Improving Palliative Care in the ICU). *Critical Care Medicine* 38: 1765–1772.

Neuberger J (1999) *Dying Well: a guide to enabling a good death*. Cheshire: Hochland and Hochland.

Nursing and Midwifery Council (NMC) (2008) *The Code of Conduct*. London: NMC.

Office for National Statistics (2003) *Population Size*. http://www.statistics.gov.uk/cci/nugget.asp?id=273 [accessed 2 September 2010].

O'Mahony S, McHugh M, Zallman L and Selwyn P (2003) Ventilator withdrawal: procedures and outcomes. Report of a collaboration between a critical care division and a palliative care service. *Journal of Pain and Symptom Management* 26(4): 954–961.

Ostermann ME, Young B, Sibbald WJ and Nicolle MW (2000) Coma mimicking brain death following baclofen overdose. *Intensive Care Medicine* 26(8): 1144–1146.

Pace NA (1996) Withholding and withdrawing medical treatment. In: Pace NA and McLean SAM (eds) *Ethics and the Law in the Intensive Care Unit*, pp. 47–67. Oxford: Oxford University Press.

Pattison N (2005) Psychological implications of admission to critical care. *British Journal of Nursing* 14(13): 708–714.

Pattison NA (2006a) A critical discourse analysis of provision of end-of-life care in key UK critical care documents. *Nursing in Critical Care* 11(4): 198–208.

Pattison N (2006b) Integration of palliative care and critical care at end of life. In: Woodward S (ed.) *Neuroscience Nursing*, Chapter 13. London: MA Healthcare.

Pattison N (2008a) Care of patients who have died. *Nursing Standard* 22(28): 42–48.

Pattison N (2008b) Caring for patients after death. *Nursing Standard* 22(51): 48–56.

Pattison N (2010) Organ donation. In: Woodhouse J and Baldwin M (eds) *Key Concepts in Palliative Care*. London: Sage.

Pattison N (2011) End-of-life care: an emphasis on care. *Nursing in Critical Care* 16(3): 113–115.

Pattison N, Carr S, Turnock C and Dolan S (2013) Viewing in slow motion': patients', families', nurses' and doctors' perspectives on end-of-life care in critical care. *Journal of Clinical Nursing* (in press).

Pattison N, Ashley S, Farquhar-Smith P et al. (2010) Thirty-day mortality in critical care outreach patients with cancer: an investigative study of predictive factors related to outreach referral episodes. *Resuscitation* 81(12): 1670–1675.

Payen JF, Bru O, Bosson JL et al. (2001) Assessing pain in critically ill sedated patients by using a behavioral pain scale. *Critical Care Medicine* 29: 2258–2263.

Piers R, Azoulay E, Ricou B, DeKeyser F et al. (2010) Preliminary results from the APPROPRICUS study (APPROPRIATENESS OF CARE IN THE ICU). European Society Intensive Care Medicine Conference. Barcelona. October 2010.

Piers RD, Van den Eynde M, Steeman E et al. (2011) End-of-life care of the geriatric patient and nurses' moral distress. *Journal of the American Medical Directors Association* 13(1): 80.e7–13.

Pochard F, Azoulay E, Chevret S and Zittoun R (2001) Symptoms of anxiety and depression in family members of intensive care unit patients: ethical hypothesis regarding decision-making capacity. *Critical Care Medicine* 29: 1893–1897.

Poncet MC, Toullic P, Papazian L et al. (2007) Burnout syndrome in critical care nursing staff. *American Journal of Respiratory and Critical Care Medicine* 175: 698–704.

Popejoy LL, Brandt LC, Beck M and Antal L (2009) Intensive care unit nurse perceptions of caring for the dying: every voice matters. *Journal of Hospice & Palliative Nursing* 11(3): 179–186.

Prendergast TJ and Luce JM (1997) Increasing incidences of withholding and withdrawal of life support from the critically ill. *American Journal of Respiratory and Critical Care Medicine* 155: 15–20.

Puntillo KA, Benner P, Drought T et al. (2001) End-of-life issues in intensive care units: a national random survey of nurses' knowledge and beliefs. *American Journal of Critical Care* 10(4:) 216–229.

Puntillo K, Arai S and McAdam J (2010a) Pain. In: Rocker GM, Azoulay E, Puntillo K and Nelson J (eds) *End of Life Care in the ICU: from advanced disease to bereavement*, pp. 60–63. Oxford: Oxford University Press.

Puntillo KA, Arai S, Cohen NH et al. (2010b) Symptoms experienced by intensive care unit patients at high risk of dying. *Critical Care Medicine* 38(11): 2155–2160.

Resuscitation Council (2008) *Decisions about Cardiopulmonary Resuscitation. Model patient information leaflet*. London: Resuscitation Council. http://www.resus.org.uk/pages/deccprmd.htm [accessed 30 September 2010].

Robichaux CM and Clark AP (2006) Practice of expert critical care nurses in situations of prognostic conflict at the end of life. *American Journal of Critical Care* 15: 480–491.

Rocker G (2010) ICU care during life support withdrawal. A personal view from Canada. In: Rocker GM, Azoulay E, Puntillo K and Nelson J (eds) *End of Life Care in the ICU: from advanced disease to bereavement*, pp. 252–257. Oxford: Oxford University Press.

Rocker GM, Heyland DK, Cook DJ et al. (2004) Most critically ill patients are perceived to die in comfort during withdrawal of life support: a Canadian multicentre study. *Canadian Journal of Anaesthesia* 51(6): 623–630.

Rogers C (1957) The necessary and sufficient conditions of therapeutic personality change. *Journal of Consulting Psychology* 21(2): 95–103.

Royal College of Physicians (2009) *Advance Care Planning. National Guidelines*. London: RCP. http://bookshop.rcplondon.ac.uk/contents/pub267-e5ba7065-2385-49c9-a68e-f64527c15f2a.pdf [accessed March 2012].

Sabo B (2006) Compassion fatigue and nursing work: can we accurately capture the consequences of caring work? *International Journal of Nursing Practice* 12: 136–142.

Sayers KL and de Vries K (2008) Concept development of 'being sensitive in nursing. *Nursing Ethics* 15(3): 289–303.

Schantz ML (2007) Compassion: a concept analysis. *Nursing Forum* 42(2): 48–55.

Scheunemann LP, McDevitt M, Carson SS and Hanson LC (2011) Randomized, controlled trials of interventions to improve communication in intensive care: a systematic review. *Chest* 139(3): 543–554.

527

Scholz N, Bäsler K and Saur P et al. (2004) Outcome prediction in critical care: physicians' prognoses vs. scoring systems. *European Journal of Anaesthesiology* 21(8): 606–611.

Searight HR and Gafford J (2005) Cultural diversity at the end of life: issues and guidelines for family physicians. *American Family Physician* 71: 515–522.

Sepúlveda C, Marlin A, Yoshida T and Ullrich A (2002) Palliative care: the World Health Organization's global perspective. *Journal of Pain and Symptom Management* 24(2): 91–96.

Seymour JE (2001) *Critical Moments – death and dying in intensive care*. Buckingham: Open University Press.

Shaw D (2007) The body as unwarranted life support: a new perspective on euthanasia. *Journal of Medical Ethics* 33(9): 519–521.

Shemie SD (2010) Organ and tissue donation in the ICU. IIn: Rocker GM, Azoulay E, Puntillo K and Nelson J (eds) *End of Life Care in the ICU: from advanced disease to bereavement*, pp. 341–346. Oxford: Oxford University Press.

Skrobik Y (2010) Delirium in the critically ill patient at the end of life: issues and management. In: Rocker GM, Azoulay E, Puntillo K and Nelson J (eds) *End of Life Care in the ICU: from advanced disease to bereavement*, pp. 74–77. Oxford: Oxford University Press.

Soares M, Fontes F, Dantas J et al. (2004) Performance of six severity-of-illness scores in cancer patients requiring admission to the intensive care unit: a prospective observational study. *Critical Care* 8(4): R194–R203.

Speck P (2003) Spiritual/religious issues in care of the dying. In: Ellershaw J and Wilkinson S (eds) *Care of the Dying: a pathway to excellence*, pp. 90–105. Oxford: Oxford University Press.

Speck P, Higginson I and Addington-Hall J (2004) Spiritual needs in health care. *British Medical Journal* 329(7458): 123–124.

Spuhler V (2010) The Role of teams in palliative ICU care. In: Rocker GM, Azoulay E, Puntillo K and Nelson J (eds) *End of Life Care in the ICU: from advanced disease to bereavement*, pp. 156–160. Oxford: Oxford University Press.

St Christopher's Hospice (2009) End-of-life care competencies for nurses and health and social are staff working in the community, care homes and hospitals *End of Life Care* 3(3).

Stiel S, Krumm N, Pestinger M et al. (2011) Antibiotics in palliative medicine-results from a prospective epidemiological investigation from the HOPE survey. *Support Care Cancer* 28 Jan [Epub ahead of print].

Sulmasy DP, McIlvane JM, Pasley PM and Rahn M (2002) A scale for measuring patient perceptions of the quality of end-of-life care and satisfaction with treatment: the reliability and validity of QUEST. *Journal of Pain and Symptom Management* 23(6): 458–470.

SUPPORT Principal Investigators (1995) A controlled trial to improve care for seriously ill hospitalized patients: The Study to Understand Prognoses and Preferences for Outcomes and Risks of Treatments (SUPPORT). *Journal of the American Medical Association* 274(20): 1591–1598.

Surbone A (2006) Cultural aspects of communication in cancer care. *Recent Results in Cancer Research* 168: 91–104.

Swigart V, Lidz C, Butterworth V and Arnold R (1996) Letting go: family willingness to forgo life support. *Heart and Lung* 25(6): 483–494.

Tasota FJ and Hoffman LA (1996) Terminal weaning from mechanical ventilation: planning and process. *Critical Care Nursing Quarterly* 19(3): 36–51.

Teres D, Lemeshow S, Avrunin JS and Pastides H (1987) Validation of the mortality prediction model for ICU patients. *Critical Care Medicine* 15(3): 208–213.

The Stationery Office (2007) *Mental Capacity Act: Code of Practice* London: The Stationery Office.

Tilden VP, Tolle S, Garland M and Nelson CA (1995) Decisions about life-sustaining treatment: impact of physicians' behaviours on the family. *Archives of Internal Medicine* 155(6): 633–638.

Tonelli MR (2005) Waking the dying: must we always attempt to involve critically ill patients in end-of-life decisions? *Chest* 127(2): 637–642.

Tonelli MR (2007) What medical futility means to clinicians. *HEC Forum* 19(1): 83–93.

Towers A (2010) Diagnosing dying. In: Rocker GM, Azoulay E, Puntillo K and Nelson J (eds) *End of Life Care in the ICU: from advanced disease to bereavement*, pp. 2–3. Oxford: Oxford University Press.

Truog RD, Campbell ML, Curtis JR et al. and the American Academy of Critical Care Medicine (2008) Recommendations for end-of-life care in the intensive care unit: a consensus statement by the American College [corrected] of Critical Care Medicine. *Critical Care Medicine* 36(3): 953–963.

UK Transplant (2009) *How to Become a Donor*. www.uktransplant. org.uk [accessed 1 September 2010].

Van Gennep A (1972) *The Rites of Passage*. Chicago: Chicago University Press.

Veerbeek L, van Zuylen L, Swart SJ et al. (2008) The effect of the Liverpool Care Pathway for the dying: a multi-centre study. *Palliative Medicine* 22(2): 145–151.

Vincent JL, de Mendonça A, Cantraine F et al. (1998) Use of the SOFA score to assess the incidence of organ dysfunction/failure in intensive care units: results of a multicenter, prospective study. Working group on 'sepsis-related problems' of the European Society of Intensive Care Medicine. *Critical Care Medicine* 26(11): 1793–1800.

Wåhlin I, Ek A-C and Idvall E (2009) Empowerment in intensive care: patient experiences compared to next of kin and staff beliefs. *Intensive and Critical Care Nursing* 25(6): 332–340.

Way J, Back AL and Curtis JR (2002) Clinical review: withdrawing life support and resolution of conflict with families. *British Medical Journal* 325: 1342–1345.

Weaver K, Morse J and Mitcham C (2008) Ethical sensitivity in professional practice: concept analysis. *Journal of Advanced Nursing* 62(5): 607–618.

What to do after a death checklist. http://www.direct.gov.uk/prod_consum_dg/groups/dg_digitalassets/@dg/@en/documents/digitalasset/dg_170740.pdf [accessed 2 September 2010].

Wijdicks EF, Varelas PN, Gronseth GS, Greer DM; American Academy of Neurology (2010) Evidence-based guideline update: determining brain death in adults: report of the Quality Standards Subcommittee of the American Academy of Neurology. *Neurology* 74(23): 1911–1918.

Winter B and Cohen S (1999) ABC of intensive care. Withdrawal of treatment. *British Medical Journal* 319: 306–308.

Wright B (1996) *Sudden Death – a research base for practice* (2e). Edinburgh: Churchill Livingstone.

Wunsch H, Harrison DA, Harvey S and Rowan K (2005) End-of-life decisions: a cohort study of the withdrawal of all active treatment in intensive care units in the United Kingdom. *Intensive Care Medicine* 31: 823–831.

Yu J and Kirk M (2008) Measurement of empathy in nursing research: systematic review. *Journal of Advanced Nursing* 64(5): 440–454.

Zhang Z, Luk W, Arthur D and Wong T (2001) Nursing competencies: personal characteristics contributing to effective nursing performance. *Journal of Advanced Nursing* 33(4): 467–474.

Useful websites

www.bma.org.uk
www.chcr.brown.edu/pcoc/toolkit.htm
www.citizensadvice.org.uk
www.cruse.org.uk
www.direct.gov.uk
www.endoflifecare.nhs.uk
www.gmc.org.uk
www.hsac.gov.uk
www.hta.org.uk
www.resus.org.uk
www.tneel.uic.edu/tneel.asp
www.uktransplant.org.uk

For religious aspects:
Buddhist Hospice Trust: www.buddhisthospice.org.uk
Hindu Council UK: www.hinducounciluk.org
Hospital Chaplaincies Council: www.nhs-chaplaincy-spiritualcare.org.uk
Jainism: www.jainism.org
Jehovah's Witnesses: www.watchtower.org
National Spiritual Assembly of the Bahais of the United Kingdom: www.bahai.org.uk
Rastafarianism: www.rastafarian.net
Zoroastrian Trust Funds of Europe: www.ztfe.com
www.bbc.co.uk/religion/religions/judaism
www.bbc.co.uk/religion/religions/sikhism
www.bbc.co.uk/religion/religions/zoroastrian

Chapter 18

Cardiopulmonary resuscitation

Jackie S. Younker[1] and Jasmeet Soar[2]

[1]*University of the West of England, Bristol, UK*
[2]*Southmead Hospital, Bristol, UK*

Critical Care Manual of Clinical Procedures and Competencies, First Edition.
Edited by Jane Mallett, John W. Albarran, and Annette Richardson.
© 2013 John Wiley & Sons, Ltd. Published 2013 by John Wiley & Sons, Ltd.

Definition

Cardiac arrest is when the heart stops beating – when caused by heart disease this is referred to as a primary cardiac arrest. Cardiac arrest rapidly leads to loss of consciousness and respiratory arrest – this is called cardiorespiratory arrest. The terms cardiac arrest and cardiorespiratory arrest are often used interchangeably. Respiratory arrest is when the breathing stops; when this occurs first, without cardiac arrest it is called a primary respiratory arrest. If a primary respiratory arrest is not treated rapidly, cardiac arrest will rapidly follow.

Cardiopulmonary resuscitation (CPR) is the term used to describe the clinical interventions used to restart the heart after cardiac arrest and support life.

The complexity of interventions used during CPR can be further divided into basic and advanced life support level interventions.

Aims and indications

The aim of CPR basic and advanced life support is to restore life to those who suffer a cardiac arrest. Indications for commencing CPR include:

- cardiac arrest
- respiratory arrest
- cardiorespiratory arrest.

The commonest cause of a primary cardiac arrest is ischaemic heart disease, and the presenting cardiac arrest rhythm is ventricular fibrillation (VF) or pulseless ventricular tachycardia (VT). Ventricular fibrillation and pulseless VT are termed 'shockable rhythms', as they can be treated with defibrillation – an electric shock to the heart. Cardiac arrest occurring after airway, breathing and circulation problems more commonly presents with an initial rhythm of asystole (no cardiac electrical activity) or pulseless electrical activity (PEA). In PEA cardiac arrest, the electrocardiogram (ECG) shows a rhythm that is normally compatible with a cardiac output. Asystole and PEA are 'non-shockable rhythms' (Nolan 2011). Most in-hospital cardiac arrests, including those that occur in critical care units, have a non-shockable rhythm most commonly caused by hypoxaemia or hypovolaemia (Meaney et al. 2010; Kutsogiannis et al. 2011).

Background

Anatomy and physiology

Cardiac arrest occurs due to a failing respiratory, cardiovascular, or neurological system, that is ABCDE (Airway, Breathing, Circulation, Disability, Exposure) problems (see also Chapter 3). Coronary artery disease is the commonest cause of primary cardiac arrest with a shockable rhythm. Hypoxaemia (low oxygen levels in the blood) and/or hypovolaemia (a decrease in circulating volume) are the com-

monest causes of cardiac arrest with a non-shockable rhythm.

Heart and coronary vessels

The heart has four muscular chambers (two atria and two ventricles) that pump blood. Like all muscles the heart needs oxygen and nutrition to work effectively; it therefore needs its own blood supply – the coronary circulation. The left ventricle pumps oxygenated blood into the aorta through the aortic valve; the aorta is a large artery that branches and supplies oxygenated blood to the body. Two arterial branches come off the aorta just above the aortic valve and supply blood to the heart – the right and left coronary arteries. The right coronary artery predominantly supplies blood to the right side of the heart. The left coronary artery divides into two, into the left anterior descending artery and the circumflex artery (Tortora and Derrickson 2011) (see Chapter 6, Figure 6.1, and Figure 18.1).

Coronary artery disease occurs when there is a build up of cholesterol on the inner wall of the artery (a coronary plaque). Plaques can rupture (fissuring), causing:

- bleeding into the plaque blocking the lumen of the artery
- constriction of the arterial smooth muscle (vasospasm) causing further narrowing
- blood clot formation (thrombus) on the surface of the plaque.

The extent and location of coronary artery occlusion and resultant reduction in blood flow and oxygen supply to the heart muscle determines whether the patient develops angina, or an acute coronary syndrome (unstable angina, non-ST elevation myocardial infarction, ST-segment myocardial infarction). Arrhythmias (see also Chapter 6), including VF/VT, can occur due to:

- conduction problems in areas of heart muscle that become ischaemic. This can be due to a poor coronary artery blood flow or infarction due to no coronary artery blood flow
- reperfusion (reperfusion-injury; see below) when a coronary artery occlusion is treated by unblocking an artery with percutaneous coronary intervention [PCI] or thrombolysis.

Oxygen delivery

Hypoxaemia can cause cardiac arrest even when there is an adequate coronary blood supply. Oxygen constitutes 21% of the air we breathe and is inspired into the lungs through the upper airway (mouth, nose, pharynx) and into the lungs via the trachea. Oxygen then passes into the lung alveoli where gas exchange takes place – oxygen diffuses into the small blood vessels (capillaries) that surround the alveoli. In the blood, oxygen binds to haemoglobin that is carried in red blood cells. Venous blood (low oxygen levels) is pumped

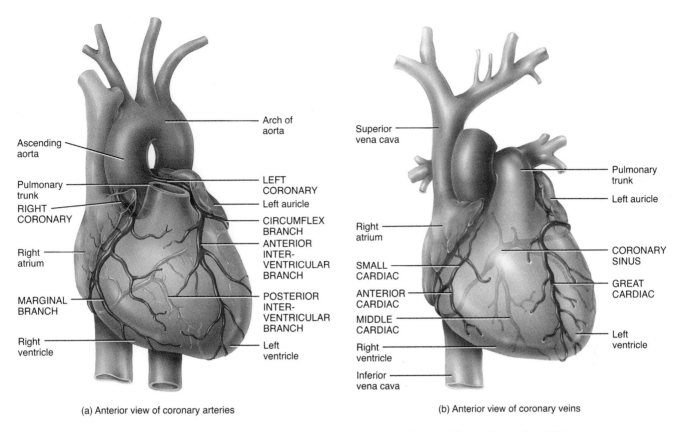

(a) Anterior view of coronary arteries

(b) Anterior view of coronary veins

Figure 18.1   The coronary circulation (from Tortora and Derrickson 2011, reproduced with permission from Wiley).

into the lungs by the right ventricle, through the pulmonary valve via the pulmonary artery. Blood oxygenated in the alveoli returns to the left side of the heart, via the pulmonary vein into the left atrium. It then passes through the left atrioventricular (mitral) valve into the left ventricle. The left ventricle in turn pumps the oxygenated blood to the body and tissues via the aorta (Tortora and Derrickson 2011) (*see also* Chapter 6).

The cells of the body require oxygen and glucose to generate energy to allow them to function (*see also* Chapters 3 and 5). This energy comes in the form of adenosine-5'-triphosphate (ATP) that is generated in mitochondria, which are found inside cells. Lack of ATP caused by lack of oxygen will therefore cause cells to fail and, with prolonged ischaemia, die. Failure in this oxygen delivery pathway will therefore lead to hypoxaemia, cell failure and cardiac arrest. Successful resuscitation and restoration of a spontaneous circulation (ROSC) and oxygenation to the cells after a period of ischaemia is termed reperfusion. Paradoxically, reperfusion itself increases the rate of cell failure and death (Collard and Gelman 2001; De Groot and Rauen 2007). This process is called ischaemia-reperfusion injury, and brain cells are particularly vulnerable to this (Nolan et al. 2008). Many of the interventions carried out on the critical care unit after initial successful resuscitation aim to prevent or limit ischaemia-reperfusion injury and further cell death and organ failure.

Cardiopulmonary resuscitation and coronary perfusion pressure

When cardiac arrest occurs, the heart stops pumping blood and blood tends to pool in the veins and right side of the heart (Frenneaux 2003). Chest compressions restore blood flow by direct compression of the heart and by increasing the pressure in the chest (intrathoracic pressure). Chest compressions generate a cardiac output and coronary blood flow. Studies show that the pressure in the coronary arteries (coronary perfusion pressure = CPP) determines successful ROSC (Paradis et al. 1990). Coronary perfusion pressure is the difference in pressure between the aorta and the left ventricle at the end of diastole. Pauses in chest compression cause CPP to rapidly fall in a matter of seconds (Frenneaux 2003). Furthermore, an excessive ventilation rate during CPR also causes a decrease in CPP. To maintain a good CPP, current CPR guidelines therefore emphasize the importance of high-quality chest compressions (see below), with minimal interruption and slow ventilation rates (Nolan et al. 2010b).

Incidence and causes of cardiac arrest

The incidence of in-hospital cardiac arrest ranges from 1 to 5 per thousand admissions (Nolan 2011). Fewer than 20% of patients who have an in-hospital cardiac arrest survive to leave hospital (Meaney et al. 2010). Patients who have a sudden monitored VF/VT cardiac arrest have the best chance of survival. This usually occurs in patients who are being treated for a myocardial infarction on a coronary care unit – this type of arrest accounts for only small proportion of in-hospital arrests. Most in-hospital cardiac arrest patients have a cardiac arrest that follows a period of deterioration that is often not recognized or treated adequately (Smith 2010). These patients tend to have a 'non-shockable' cardiac arrest rhythm and tend to have a poor outcome. In this group, prevention of cardiac arrest is the key intervention (NICE 2007).

The Chain of Survival describes the interventions that contribute to survival after a cardiac arrest (Figure 18.2) – all four links in the chain must be strong (Nolan et al. 2006). They are:

- early recognition and call for help – to prevent cardiac arrest
- early cardiopulmonary resuscitation (CPR) – to gain time to allow other interventions
- early defibrillation – to restart the heart
- post-resuscitation care – to restore quality of life.

Cardiac arrest rapidly leads to death if not treated immediately. The current standard of care for patients having an in hospital cardiac arrest (Gabbott et al. 2005) is:

- cardiorespiratory arrest must be recognized immediately
- help should be summoned using a standard telephone number (2222 in the UK) (NPSA 2004)
- cardiopulmonary resuscitation (CPR) must be started immediately
- defibrillation, if indicated, is attempted as soon as possible (within 3 minutes).

Evidence for guidelines

The scientific evidence for resuscitation is reviewed and published every 5 years by the International Liaison Committee on Resuscitation (ILCOR) (Nolan et al. 2010a). Resuscitation guidelines for clinical practice are based on the ILCOR consensus on science and treatment recommendations. This international process has ensured that the treatment of cardiac arrest is similar worldwide. The guidelines used in the UK are produced by the Resuscitation Council (UK), most recently in 2010 (Resuscitation Council (UK) 2010). In turn, these UK guidelines are based on the European Resuscitation Council 2010 Guidelines (Nolan et al. 2010b). To ensure guidelines and their implementation actually result in improvements in patient care and outcomes, national audits of in- and out-of-hospital cardiac arrest have been established (Grasner et al. 2011). In the UK, the National Cardiac Arrest Audit (NCAA; http://www.resus.org.uk/pages/ncaa.htm) enables hospitals to collect cardiac arrest data in a standardized manner, audit local outcomes and benchmark against other hospitals. This should help identify areas for improvement in patient care both at a local and national level.

In-hospital resuscitation

The actions after in-hospital cardiac arrest depend on the following.

1 The patient's location (clinical or non-clinical area; monitored or unmonitored patients).
2 The skills of the staff who respond to the cardiac arrest.
3 The number of responders.
4 The equipment available

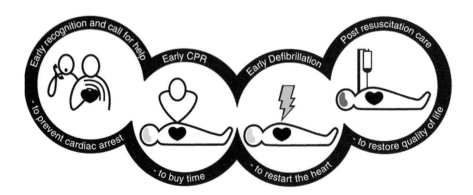

Figure 18.2   The chain of survival (from Nolan et al. 2006, reproduced with permission from Elsevier).

5   The hospital system for response to cardiac arrest and medical emergencies (for example, medical emergency team [MET], cardiac arrest team).

(Deakin et al. 2010a)

Location

Patients who have monitored cardiac arrests are usually diagnosed rapidly and have the best chance of survival (Meaney et al. 2010). Unmonitored ward patients often have a period of deterioration followed by an unwitnessed cardiac arrest – survival in these patients is poor. Hospitals should have a system in place to identify the deteriorating patient based on vital sign measurements and an early warning score (Smith 2010) (*see* Chapter 3). Patients who are identified as being at high risk of cardiac arrest should be cared for in a monitored area with facilities for immediate resuscitation. Arrests can also occur in non-clinical areas (e.g. car parks, corridors). Depending on the location of the cardiac arrest, and access to the patient, it may be appropriate to call for an ambulance in addition to the hospital resuscitation team.

Skills of the staff who respond to the cardiac arrest

The division between basic life support and advanced life support is arbitrary; in practice, the resuscitation process is a continuum. Basic and advanced life support include common skills. Irrespective of level of training, all practitioners should be able to recognize cardiac arrest, call for help and start CPR (Gabbott et al. 2005) – practitioners in critical care areas should have more advanced skills than those who are not involved regularly in resuscitation. Staff should use those resuscitation skills they have been trained to do.

Basic life support (BLS) in clinical settings should include chest compressions and ventilation with the use of airway adjuncts (e.g. oropharyngeal airway, pocket mask or bag-mask with or without oxygen). BLS training should ideally include training in the use of an automated external defibrillator (AED). An AED enables staff who are not competent in rhythm recognition skills to treat VF/pulseless VT cardiac arrest. Immediate Life Support (ILS) and Advanced Life Support (ALS) refer specifically to the Resuscitation Council (UK) training courses (Perkins and Lockey 2002; Soar et al. 2003). Both these courses include basic as well as 'advanced' resuscitation skills. ILS is aimed at clinical staff who rarely attend cardiac arrests but may need to start CPR while awaiting the arrival of a resuscitation team. ILS training as part of a hospital-wide improvement plan has been shown to decrease the number of cardiac arrests and increase initial survival and survival to discharge if cardiac arrest occurs (Spearpoint et al. 2009). Advanced Life Support (ALS) is aimed at doctors and senior nurses working in acute areas who may be resuscitation team leaders and members. Resuscitation skills and knowledge decay within a year after training so regular (e.g. at least annual) refreshers are needed to maintain skills, especially for those who rarely use the skills in clinical practice (Yang et al. 2012).

Non-technical skills are important to ensure cardiac arrest patients receive the best possible care (Flin et al. 2010). These consist of situational awareness, decision making and team working, including team leadership and task management. Communication tools such as SBAR (**S**ituation, **B**ackground, **A**ssessment, **R**ecommendation; *see also* Chapter 3) or RSVP (**R**eason, **S**tory, **V**ital signs, **P**lan) ensure rapid effective communication and handovers (Nolan 2011).

Number of responders

The first priority of the person attending a cardiac arrest patient is to ensure that help is on its way. Usually other practitioners are nearby, enabling several actions to be undertaken simultaneously. Survival rates from in-hospital cardiac arrest tends to be lower at nights and weekends – this may reflect the fact that fewer staff are available, failure to detect cardiac arrest early, or that more experienced staff are not available (Peberdy et al. 2008). Higher nursing staff-to-patient ratios are also associated with a lower incidence of ward cardiac arrest and deaths (Aiken et al. 2002; Needleman et al. 2002; Tourangeau et al. 2006).

Equipment and medicines available

The equipment used for CPR (including defibrillators) and the layout of equipment and medicines should be standardized throughout a hospital and checked on a regular basis (ideally daily) to ensure it is ready for use (Dyson and Smith 2002; Gabbott et al. 2005) (list of equipment in Procedure guideline 18.1).

Resuscitation team

Traditionally, cardiac arrest teams are only called once cardiac arrest occurs. Many hospitals now have teams that are called as part of an early warning or rapid response system (e.g. MET) before cardiac arrest occurs (Deakin et al. 2010a). Recognizing deteriorating patients at risk of cardiac arrest will enable some cardiac arrests to be prevented. This will also identify patients for whom CPR is unlikely to be beneficial, and those who do not wish to have CPR. In these cases a Do Not Attempt CPR (DNACPR) decision may be appropriate (*see also* Chapter 17).

Resuscitation team members should meet for introductions and plan roles at the beginning of each shift. They should also have a debriefing after resuscitation events. This should be based on what they actually did during the arrest, as research suggests this helps to improve performance at subsequent arrests (Edelson et al. 2008).

Initial management of the 'collapsed' patient

The initial management of a collapsed patient is summarized by the Resuscitation Council (UK) in-hospital resuscitation algorithm (Figure 18.3).

Personal safety

The first priority after a patient collapses is to ensure personal safety. In practice, the risks to those performing CPR are extremely small (Soar et al. 2010). Musculoskeletal injuries can occur when moving patients and guidance for safe handling during resuscitation is available (Resuscitation Council (UK) 2009). There are very few isolated reports of disease transmission to rescuers. Personal protective equipment (e.g. gloves, aprons, masks, eye protection) should be used according to local infection control policies, especially when the patient is known to have an infection with a high

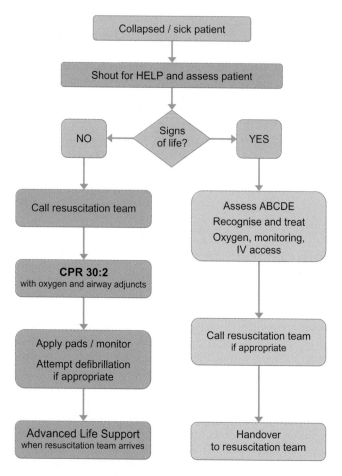

Figure 18.3 In-hospital resuscitation algorithm. ABCDE – airway, breathing, circulation, disability, exposure; CPR – cardiopulmonary resuscitation; IV – intravenous. (Reproduced with the kind permission of the Resuscitation Council [UK].)

risk of transmission or harm to the rescuer (e.g. human immunodeficiency virus [HIV], tuberculosis) (Soar et al. 2010).

Recognizing cardiac arrest and calling for help

When a patient collapses, or is apparently unconscious, the first member of staff attending should first shout for help to ensure help is coming and then assess the patient by gently shaking the shoulders and asking loudly, 'Are you all right?'. If the patient is responsive, they are not in cardiac arrest, but may still be at risk of deterioration. An ABCDE approach can be used to identify and treat conditions, and start monitoring while awaiting help (*see* Chapter 3). Oxygen therapy should be adjusted according to the patient's oxygen saturation measured with a pulse-oximeter. Both too little oxygen and low blood oxygen levels (hypoxaemia) and too much oxygen leading to high blood oxygen levels (hyperoxaemia) can be potentially harmful to patients. Emergency oxygen guidance from the British Thoracic Society therefore recommends adjusting inspired oxygen to target oxygen saturations (O'Driscoll et al. 2008):

- age less than 70 years – target oxygen saturation 94–98%
- age over 70 years – target oxygen saturation 92–98%
- chronic obstructive airways disease – target oxygen saturation 88–92%.

In practice, this means starting high-flow oxygen with a non-rebreathing mask to correct any hypoxaemia as part of the ABCDE approach, and then adjusting the flows or changing to another oxygen mask system as soon as pulse oximetry monitoring is available.

If the patient is unresponsive on 'shaking and shouting', the patient should be turned on their back and the airway opened using a head tilt and chin lift (Figure 18.4). If there is a suspected cervical spine injury, a jaw thrust can be used to minimize any neck movements – the priority is an open airway and adequate ventilation, so small amounts of head tilt may still be required. Efforts to protect the cervical spine must not prevent oxygenation and ventilation (Resuscitation Council (UK) 2010).

Once the airway is open, breathing is assessed by looking for chest movement, listening for breath sounds and by feeling for air on the rescuer's cheek.

Occasional gasps, slow, laboured and noisy breaths ('agonal breathing') occur in about half of cardiac arrests and can last for several minutes – this is a sign of cardiac arrest and should not be mistaken for a sign of life (Bobrow et al. 2008). Once CPR starts, agonal breathing will often continue as brain perfusion improves. The presence of gasping during CPR does not indicate ROSC, but does indicate that CPR is more likely to be successful and therefore resuscitation efforts should be continued (Bobrow et al. 2008).

Pulse checks alone are an unreliable method of diagnosing cardiac arrest (Ruppert et al. 1999). Mistaking that there is

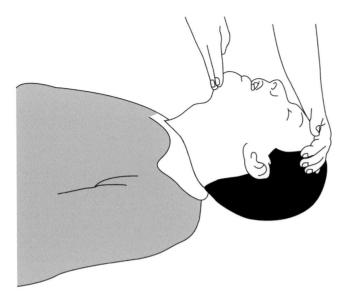

Figure 18.4 Head tilt/chin lift manoeuvre (from Dougherty and Lister 2011, reproduced with permission from Wiley).

a pulse when one is absent will result in no CPR starting and an adverse effect on survival, whereas starting CPR in a patient with a difficult-to-feel pulse is unlikely to be harmful (White et al. 2010). Assessment of the presence of a carotid pulse should therefore be done simultaneously with the breathing check only by those skilled in clinical assessment and resuscitation. The whole assessment process including breathing and pulse checks should take less than 10 seconds – delays in starting CPR worsen the chances of survival (Resuscitation Council (UK) 2010).

In monitored patients in critical care areas, a rapid clinical assessment of the patient is essential as well as the information provided by the monitors. In addition to changes in patient signs, monitoring may show:

- changes in the monitored ECG to a cardiac arrest rhythm
- a decrease in the continuously monitored invasive blood pressure
- a decrease in end-tidal carbon dioxide.

They will all help diagnose cardiac arrest (Heradstveit et al. 2012).

If the patient is unconscious, unresponsive and not breathing normally, one person starts CPR while a colleague gets help and equipment. The priority is to ensure that help and resuscitation equipment and medicines are coming, so the lone rescuer should get help before starting CPR. In the UK, the National Patient Safety Agency has recommended that all hospitals use the same number (2222) to summon a resuscitation team (NPSA 2004). A single national number decreases uncertainty and delays when contacting the switchboard to summon the resuscitation team and improves patient safety. This is important especially for agency staff and staff on rotations between hospitals.

Some critical care units and similar settings often manage cardiac arrests 'in-house' using the expertise already present among the unit's staff, and do not call the resuscitation team. All staff need to know the system for getting help in their unit.

Starting CPR

Cardiopulmonary resuscitation is started by giving 30 chest compressions followed by two ventilations. The advanced life support algorithm provides a standardized approach to cardiac arrest management (Figure 18.5).

Starting CPR with chest compressions does not require any special equipment and prevents any delays in starting CPR caused by delays in starting ventilations. Chest compressions during in-hospital CPR are often too slow and too shallow, with frequent interruptions (Abella et al. 2005). Interruptions to chest compression during a cardiac arrest increase the 'no-flow time' (where blood does not circulate as no compressions take place) and this has been shown to result in worse survival (Christenson et al. 2009).

High-quality chest compressions

The correct hand position for chest compression is the middle of the lower half of the sternum and the recommended depth of compression is at least 5–6 cm and the rate is 100–20 compressions per minute (that is, about two compressions per second) (Nolan et al. 2010b).

An in-hospital cardiac arrest study showed that chest compressions deeper than 5 cm were associated with improved defibrillation success and ROSC (Edelson et al. 2006). The chest should be allowed to completely recoil at the end of each compression, as leaning (not allowing full recoil of the chest at the end of a chest compression) on the chest is associated with decreased coronary perfusion pressure (Niles et al. 2011). Prompt and/or feedback devices that provide real-time guidance to rescuers can be used to increase chest compression quality, but have not been shown to improve patient survival (Yeung et al. 2009; Hostler et al. 2011).

Studies show that the quality of chest compression performance decays in terms of depth and rate after about 2 minutes, often before the rescuer complains of fatigue (Sugerman et al. 2009). It is therefore important that the person providing chest compressions should change at about every 2 minutes, or earlier if they are unable to give high-quality chest compressions. This change should be done with minimal interruption to compressions.

Mechanical chest compression devices (e.g. AutoPulse, LUCAS) are available, but no studies have shown that they improve survival compared to high-quality standard chest compressions. These devices may have a role in situations where the rescuer's access to the patient's chest is difficult, such as during coronary angiography in the cardiac catheter laboratory, or during patient transport.

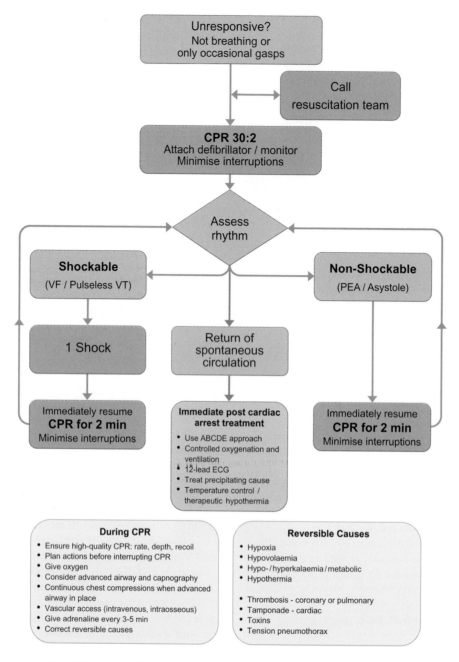

Figure 18.5 Adult advanced life support algorithm (reproduced with the kind permission of the Resuscitation Council [UK]).

Airway and ventilation

The choice of airway and ventilation technique used during CPR depends on the experience and skills of the rescuer (Nolan and Soar 2008). No specific method of airway management during CPR has so far been shown to be superior in high-quality studies (Deakin et al. 2010a). A pocket mask or self-inflating bag-mask (for example an Ambu bag) with a two-person technique, with an oropharyngeal ('Guedel')

airway, are the commonest techniques for initially providing ventilations during CPR (*see* Chapter 5, Figure 5.5, and Figure 18.6). Mouth-to-mouth ventilations are rarely used in clinical settings as airway equipment is usually rapidly available, there are often clinical reasons to avoid contact with the patient and CPR is started with compressions first.

Two quick breaths (inspiratory time one second) with a volume to cause a visible chest rise should be given every 30 compressions. This provides adequate ventilation, minimizes

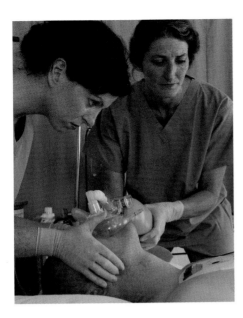

Figure 18.6 Two-person technique for bag-mask ventilation (reproduced with the kind permission of the Resuscitation Council [UK]).

interruption to compressions and minimizes the risks of gastric insufflation. Inflating the stomach during CPR makes subsequent ventilation more difficult. Oxygen should be added as soon as available. High-flow oxygen (10–15 L/min) with a bag-mask and reservoir will provide an 85% inspired oxygen.

The use of supraglottic airway devices (e.g. laryngeal mask airway, i-gel) is becoming more common during CPR (Nolan and Soar 2008). These can allow more effective ventilation than a bag-mask, are much easier to insert than a tracheal tube and, importantly, can be inserted without interrupting chest compressions. Research shows effective laryngeal mask airway and i-gel use during cardiac arrest by nursing staff who had received a relatively small amount of training (Baskett 1994; Larkin et al. 2012). The use of these devices also appears to be associated with a lower incidence of regurgitation and aspiration of gastric contents compared with bag-mask use (Stone et al. 1998).

Tracheal intubation should only be attempted by those who are trained, competent and experienced in this skill (*see also* Chapter 5). Several studies suggest that a large number of tracheal intubations (80 to 150) need to be performed to achieve a 90–95% success rate (Konrad et al. 1998; Bernhard et al. 2012). The two main problems with tracheal intubation use during CPR are unrecognized oesophageal intubation and prolonged interruption to chest compressions to enable intubation (Wang et al. 2009). Both these problems are more common with inexperienced intubators. Waveform capnography to detect exhaled carbon dioxide should be used for confirming tracheal tube placement during CPR and subsequent monitoring (Cook et al. 2011) (*see* Chapter 5). During CPR the end-tidal carbon dioxide is usually low and improves with high-quality chest compressions. If ROSC occurs during chest compressions, the end-tidal carbon dioxide will rise further (Heradstveit et al. 2012).

Chest compressions can be given continuously without interruptions for ventilations once the trachea is intubated. Compressions should then be given at 100–120/min and ventilations at 10/min. In patients with a tracheal tube, a self-inflating bag, 'Waters circuit' with supplemental oxygen, or a mechanical ventilator, can be used for ventilation. Pressure limit settings on a mechanical ventilator can, however, result in inadequate tidal volumes during chest compressions. Effective oxygenation and ventilation can be maintained during CPR with a tidal volume of approximately 500 mL given over an inspiratory time of one second. This tidal volume will cause a visible chest rise (Baskett et al. 1996).

Defibrillation

Early defibrillation is the key intervention for VF/ VT cardiac arrest as the likelihood of defibrillation being successful declines rapidly with time. If there is no CPR, every minute delay in attempted defibrillation increases mortality by about 10% (Deakin et al. 2010b). Performing chest compressions while awaiting the arrival of a defibrillator halves the risk of death over each passing minute. Delays in attempting defibrillation are common after a VF/VT cardiac arrest on a general ward or outpatient department (Chan et al. 2008). Automated external defibrillators (AEDs) that advise whether a shock is needed have a role in areas where practitioners lack skills in rhythm recognition and there may be delays in the resuscitation team arriving. The use of AEDs in clinical areas where manual defibrillation is rapidly available may be detrimental, as rhythm analysis by the AED can lead to increased interruptions in chest compressions and only a small proportion of in-hospital arrests have a shockable rhythm (Chan et al. 2010; Gibbison and Soar 2011).

Prolonged interruptions in chest compressions for a defibrillation adversely affect shock success. Every 5-second increase in the duration of the pre-shock pause (the interval between stopping chest compressions and delivering a shock) almost halves the chance of successful defibrillation (Edelson et al. 2006). To minimize interruptions in chest compressions, current guidelines for manual defibrillation recommend the following.

1 A brief pause in chest compressions for rhythm analysis and confirming a shockable rhythm.
2 Then continuing chest compressions while the defibrillator is charged.
3 Once defibrillator is charged, chest compressions are paused and the shock delivered. No one should touch the patient during the delivery of the shock.
4 Chest compressions are immediately resumed after shock delivery.

To achieve this safely, actions should be planned before stopping chest compressions. Defibrillator charging during compressions was shown to be safe in a single-centre US study (Edelson et al. 2010). Indeed, risks to rescuers during defibrillation are much less than perceived, but it remains essential that no one touches the patient during shock delivery (Hoke et al. 2009; Petley et al. 2011).

There is a small risk of fire in an oxygen-enriched atmosphere by sparking from poorly applied defibrillator paddles. This risk is much smaller if self-adhesive pads are used. To further minimize the risk of fire during defibrillation:

- remove any oxygen mask or nasal cannulae to at least 1 m away from the patient's chest
- leave a ventilation bag (e.g. self-inflating bag) connected to the tracheal tube or supraglottic airway device, or disconnect the ventilation bag and remove it at least 1 m from the patient's chest
- if the patient is connected to a ventilator, leave the ventilator tubing (breathing circuit) connected to the tracheal tube. If the ventilator tubing is disconnected, ensure that it is kept at least 1 m from the patient or, better still, switch the ventilator off and use a ventilation bag; modern ventilators generate massive oxygen flows when disconnected.

If VF/VT occurs during cardiac catheterization, or in the early in-hospital post-operative period following cardiac surgery (when chest compressions can disrupt vascular sutures), attempt up to three shocks before starting chest compressions. In terms of the ALS algorithm these three 'stacked' defibrillation attempts would count as the first shock.

Drugs and vascular access

Drugs have a secondary role for the treatment of cardiac arrest as there is very limited evidence as to whether they improve patient survival (Olasveengen 2012). Adrenaline is used during CPR because its vasopressor effects result in greater coronary and brain perfusion during CPR. Studies suggest that its use during CPR increases the chances of ROSC (Olasveengen et al. 2009; Jacobs et al. 2011). There are no studies that show improved long-term survival, and some even suggest harm (Callaway 2012). Amiodarone (an anti-arrhythmic) is given if three defibrillation attempts for VF have been unsuccessful. In these circumstances, amiodarone increases the chances of successful defibrillation and appears to be more effective than lidocaine (Kudenchuk 1999; Kudenchuk et al. 1999). Similar to adrenaline, there is no evidence that amiodarone improves long-term survival. Drugs should be given intravenously (IV). Drugs need to reach the heart and circulation to act during CPR. Even with IV administration, this can take several minutes to occur during CPR. The use of a flush (e.g. 20 mL 0.9% sodium chloride bolus) of fluid infusion can improve the time taken for drugs given into a peripheral vein to reach the heart during CPR. If IV access cannot be rapidly established, the intra-osseous (IO) route should be used. Intra-osseous drug administration during CPR can be as effective as peripheral IV administration (Weiser et al. 2012). The tracheal route is no longer recommended for giving drugs during CPR, as large drug doses in a large volume of diluent are needed, and absorption of drugs by this route is unreliable during CPR (Deakin et al. 2010a) (see Problem solving table 18.1).

Problem solving table 18.1: In-hospital resuscitation

Problem	Possible causes	Preventative measures	Suggested action
Equipment/medicines not working, or unavailable, or expired	■ No checks ■ Not replaced after use ■ No formal checking procedures ■ User errors ■ Batteries run out	■ Daily equipment check using a checklist ■ Restocking and checking after every use ■ Train practitioners to use equipment ■ Ensure chargers/spare batteries available	■ Responsible person identified for daily checks ■ Audit of checking procedures, equipment availability ■ Training of practitioners
Delays in getting help	■ Delayed call to team ■ Team sent to wrong location ■ Pager system failure ■ Team or individuals busy elsewhere	■ Daily radiopager test calls ■ Use early warning scoring systems	■ Emergency simulation drills in situ with debriefing to test systems and train practitioners

Failure to follow current guidelines, communication problems during resuscitation	■ Poor team working and communication	■ Improved training in human factors and team members meet and plan each day	■ Daily resuscitation team meeting at beginning of shift to discuss roles and responsibilities
Inappropriate resuscitation attempted in dying patient	■ Decision regarding CPR not made beforehand or DNACPR decision not adequately communicated to carers	■ Decisions regarding CPR considered as part of end of life care. Effective communication of DNACPR decisions	■ Action plan based on audit of DNACPR decision making and whether national guidance and local policies followed

Identifying reversible causes

Once CPR has been established, potentially reversible causes should be ruled out using the '4 Hs and 4 Ts' approach (see Figure 18.5). In addition to the history, clinical assessment and blood sampling for blood gas analysis, the ultrasound (e.g. echocardiography) assessment can be used to help identify reversible causes of cardiac arrest, including pericardial effusion (tamponade), tension pneumothorax and pulmonary embolism (Breitkreutz et al. 2010). The scan should be performed with only brief (less than 10 s) interruptions in chest compressions and requires specialist training (Price et al. 2010). The recognition and treatment of reversible causes is summarized in Table 18.1.

Post-cardiac arrest care

The quality of care immediately after initial successful resuscitation determines survival (Nolan and Soar 2010). After successful resuscitation, patients often develop a systemic inflammatory response, especially after a prolonged resuscitation. The post-cardiac arrest syndrome consists of:

1 post-cardiac arrest brain injury
2 post-cardiac arrest myocardial dysfunction
3 systemic ischaemia/reperfusion response
4 disease process that caused cardiac arrest.

Intensive care treatments after cardiac arrest are essential to ensure survival with a good neurological outcome. An ABCDE approach is used to manage the patient (Deakin et al. 2010a). Those who remain comatose after resuscitation, require sedation, tracheal intubation, ventilatory support and 'ICU' treatments. Currently, only a third of patients admitted to a critical care facility after cardiac arrest survive to hospital discharge, and about 80% of these survivors have good neurological function (Nolan et al. 2007). Critical care patients who die after an out-of-hospital cardiac arrest most commonly die because they have an irreversible brain injury caused by prolonged hypoxaemia. Those admitted after an in-hospital cardiac arrest tend to die from multiple organ failure, often related to the condition that caused the cardiac arrest in the first place (Laver et al. 2004). The critical care interventions required to improve survival are summarized in the Table 18.2 (Nolan et al. 2008).

Diagnosing death

If CPR fails to restore a circulation and a decision is made to stop CPR, death must be diagnosed and confirmed according to the code of practice of the Academy of Medical Royal Colleges (AoMRC 2008) (see also Chapter 17). This includes observing cardiac and respiratory arrest for a minimum of 5 minutes (AoMRC 2008). Immediately after CPR has stopped, there can be a transient cardiac output or gasping. This is important, as there have been cases where families have been informed of their relative's death before formal procedures to confirm death have taken place. Families have then been taken to their relative who is still breathing and showing signs of life (NPSA 2012).

Table 18.1 Recognition and treatment of reversible causes

Reversible cause	Recognition	Treatment during CPR
Hypoxia	All cardiac arrest patients become hypoxic if not treated rapidly	Ensure lungs are ventilated with supplemental oxygen during CPR
Hypovolaemia	Look for evidence of bleeding (e.g. trauma) or fluid losses	Stop bleeding and/or fluid losses and give IV/IO fluids and blood products
Hypothermia	<ul><li>History of cold exposure</li><li>Measure temperature</li></ul>	Provide external warming (radiant heater, warming blankets) or internal warming (warm fluids, bladder irrigation, cardiopulmonary bypass) May need prolonged resuscitation
Hypo-hyperkalaemic/ metabolic	Review:<ul><li>history</li><li>any available blood results</li><li>past medical history (e.g. for diabetes)</li><li>check blood during CPR (e.g. for blood gas, electrolytes and blood glucose)</li></ul>	Correct any abnormality, for example: – IV glucose for hypoglycaemia – IV potassium for hypokalaemia – IV calcium, insulin/glucose for hyperkalaemia
Thrombosis – coronary or pulmonary	<ul><li>History of chest pain for coronary thrombosis</li><li>Recent surgery and/or immobility for pulmonary embolism</li></ul>	Consider thrombolysis during CPR
Tamponade	<ul><li>Small complexes on ECG</li><li>Echocardiography shows fluid collection around heart</li></ul>	Conduct pericardiocentesis (drainage of fluid from around the heart)
Toxins	<ul><li>History of drug ingestion/reaction.</li><li>Clinical signs, e.g. pinpoint pupils after opioid</li></ul>	Give specific antidote, for example:<ul><li>naloxone for opioid</li><li>lipid for local anaesthetics</li></ul>
Tension pneumothorax	<ul><li>Decreased air entry</li><li>Hyper-resonance to percussion on affected side of chest</li><li>Conduct ultrasound assessment</li></ul>	Decompress tension in chest with a needle in second intercostal space mid-clavicular line, or with a thoracostomy (finger-size hole in chest wall) in fifth intercostal space, mid-clavicular line

IV – intravenous, IO – intra-osseous.

Table 18.2 Post-cardiac arrest care interventions

	Intervention	Comment
Post-cardiac arrest brain injury	Control oxygenation	Aim for oxygen saturations of 94–98%. Avoid hyperoxaemia as too much oxygen may increase neuronal cell death
	Control of blood glucose	Aim for blood glucose 4–10 mmol/L using insulin and feeding protocol. Both hypo- and hyperglycaemia worsen outcome (Finfer et al. 2009; *see also* Chapter 8)
	Control of seizures	Seizures increase mortality. In a sedated, ventilated patient who has received muscle relaxants, EEG monitoring is needed to recognize seizure activity. Treat with benzodiazepines, phenytoin, sodium valproate, propofol, or a barbiturate. If myoclonus, treat with clonazepam
	Targeted temperature management ('therapeutic hypothermia')	Hypothermia is neuroprotective. Cool patients to 32–34°C and maintain for 24 h and rewarm at 0.25 °C/hour. Avoid hyperthermia Cooling decreases damage to neurones caused by ischaemia-reperfusion injury. Patients should be rewarmed slowly to avoid overwarming and hyperthermia
Post-cardiac arrest myocardial dysfunction	Fluid resuscitation Inotropic support	This can be guided by blood pressure, heart rate, urine output, and rate of plasma lactate clearance and central venous oxygen saturations. After cardiac arrest 'myocardial stunning' (reversible myocardial dysfunction) is common and usually resolves after 48–72 h
	Mechanical circulatory support	An intra-aortic balloon pump or extra-corporeal support ('ECMO') may be indicated in those with severe cardiogenic shock
Ischaemia-reperfusion injury	Critical care supportive therapies	No specific additional therapies. Cooling may prevent ischaemia-reperfusion injury. Apply usual critical care bundles
Disease process that caused cardiac arrest	Coronary reperfusion after myocardial infarction	Percutaneous coronary intervention (PCI; *see also* Chapter 6) should be considered in all those with a primary cardiac arrest, especially if 12-lead ECG shows myocardial infarction

Procedure guideline 18.1: **Resuscitation**

Equipment

These lists are based on guidance from the Resuscitation Council (UK) (reproduced with the kind permission of the Resuscitation Council [UK]). Please check website for latest guidance.

Airway and breathing

- Pocket mask with oxygen port
- Oxygen mask with reservoir
- Self-inflating bag with reservoir
- Clear face masks, size 3, 4, 5
- Oropharyngeal airways, sizes 2, 3, 4
- Nasopharyngeal airways, sizes 6, 7

  with appropriate syringes, lubrication and ties/tapes/scissors
- Oxygen cylinder (with key if necessary)
- Oxygen tubing
- Magill forceps (a specific type of angled forceps)
- Stethoscope
- Tracheal tubes, cuffed sizes 6, 7, 8
- Tracheal tube introducer (stylet)

- Portable suction (battery or manual) with rigid oropharyngeal suction catheter (such as a Yankauer catheter) and soft suction catheters
- Supraglottic airway device, e.g. laryngeal mask airways (LMA) (sizes 4, 5), or i-gel (sizes 3, 4), ProSeal LMAs (sizes 4, 5), or LMA Supreme (sizes 4, 5)
- Bougie
- Laryngoscope (handles, blades [standard and long], batteries) and spare
- Syringes, lubrication and ties/tapes/scissors for tracheal tube
- Waveform capnography – with appropriate tubing and connector (battery-operated)

Circulation

- Defibrillator
  - manual and or automated external defibrillator
  - pacing facility if needed
- Adhesive defibrillator pads
- Razor
- ECG electrodes
- Intravenous cannulae (selection of sizes) and 2% chlorhexidine/alcohol wipes, tourniquets and dressings
- Adhesive tape

- Intravenous infusion set
- 0.9% sodium chloride (1000 mL)
- Selection of needles and syringes, e.g. 2.5, 5, 10 20 mL
- Intra-osseous access device
- Central venous access – 'Seldinger' kit (specific type of device that uses a guide wire for insertion; *see also* Chapter 6)
- Ultrasound/echocardiography

Other items

- Clock/timer
- Gloves, aprons, eye protection
- Urinary catheter

- Nasogastric tube
- Sharps container and waste bag

Large scissors

- 2% chlorhexidine/alcohol wipes
- Blood sample tubes
- IV extension set, three-way taps and bungs
- Pressure bags for infusion
- Blood gas syringe

- Blood glucose monitor with appropriate strips
- Drug labels
- Manual handling equipment
- Forms for recording events and audit
- Access to algorithms, emergency drug doses

First-line cardiac arrest medicines for IV/IO use

- Adrenaline 1 mg (=10 mL 1:10000) pre-filled syringe × 3
- Amiodarone 300 mg prefilled syringe × 1

Medicines for peri-arrest use

- Adenosine, 6 mg × 10
- Atropine, 1 mg × 3
- Adrenaline, 1 mg (=10 mL 1:10000) × 10
- Amiodarone, 300 mg × 1
- Calcium chloride, 10 mL 10% × 1
- Chlorphenamine, 10 mg × 2
- Hydrocortisone, 100 mg × 2
- Glucose, 500 mL 10% or 500 mL 20% or 50 mL 50%

- Intralipid, 20% 1000 mL
- Lidocaine, 100 g × 1
- Magnesium sulphate, 2 g (= 8 mmol) × 1
- Midazolam 10 mg × 1
- Naloxone, 400 micrograms × 5
- Potassium chloride, 40 mmol × 1
- Sodium bicarbonate, 8.4%, 50 mL × 1

(Continued)

Procedure guideline 18.1: (Continued)

Procedure

Action	Rationale
1 **Ensure personal safety.** Check that the patient's surroundings are safe.	To ensure personal safety and that of resuscitation team members. This is the first priority during any resuscitation attempt.
2 Put gloves on as soon as possible. Consider other personal protective equipment if the patient has a known infection. Be careful with patients exposed to poisons or corrosive substances.	To reduce the risk of infection, poisoning, or harm from corrosive substances. The risk of infection is much lower than perceived. There are isolated reports of infections such as tuberculosis (TB) and severe acute respiratory distress syndrome (SARS). Transmission of HIV during CPR has never been reported. Poisons such as hydrogen cyanide or hydrogen sulphide can be potentially dangerous so it is best to avoid mouth-to-mouth ventilation and exhaled air. Corrosive chemicals are easily absorbed through the skin and respiratory tract and contact should be avoided.
3 Use safe manual handling when moving patients.	To avoid injury to the patient and practitioners involved in moving the patient.
4 **Check the patient for a response.** Shout for help first if you see a patient collapse or find a patient apparently unconscious. Assess if they are responsive (shake and shout). Gently shake their shoulders and ask loudly: 'Are you all right?'	A patient who is responsive will not need CPR, but will require urgent medical assessment. If other practitioners are nearby it will be possible to undertake actions simultaneously.

If the patient responds

Action	Rationale
5(A) Call for help according to local protocols. This may be a resuscitation team or medical emergency team. Assess the patient using the Airway-Breathing-Circulation-Disability-Exposure (ABCDE) approach.	Urgent medical attention is required for a patient who collapses, but is able to respond to 'shake and shout'. Using the ABCDE approach will provide a systematic method of patient assessment. Problems can be dealt with as they arise during the assessment.
6(A) Assess if the patient lacks the capacity to make decisions. The practitioner must act in the patient's best interests, or according to the patient's wishes if known.	To ensure that the patient understands the procedure and gives their valid consent. To ensure the patient's best interests are maintained (Mental Capacity Act 2005).
7(A) Give the patient oxygen. Titrate oxygen therapy according to the pulse oximetry. Attach monitoring and record observations (pulse oximetry, ECG and blood pressure).	To manage patients with serious illness requiring supplemental oxygen if hypoxaemic. The British Thoracic Society recommends adjusting inspired oxygen to target oxygen saturations (O'Driscoll et al. 2008): ■ age less than 70 years – target oxygen saturation 94–98% ■ age over 70 years – target oxygen saturation 92–98% ■ chronic obstructive airways disease – target oxygen saturation 88–92%. Use appropriate oxygen delivery technique to achieve target, e.g. nasal cannulae at 2–6 L/min (preferably), simple face mask at 5–10 L/min, or face mask with reservoir mask at 10–15 L/min.
8(A) Gain intravenous access.	To ensure that a route is available for any medications that are required.

9(A)	Prepare for handover using a structured technique.	To provide a structured and thorough handover. It is recommended to use SBAR (Situation, Background, Assessment, Recommendation) or RSVP (Reason, Story, Vital signs, Plan).

If the patient is unresponsive

5(B)	Begin the sequence of resuscitation based on your training and experience in assessment of breathing and circulation in sick patients.	Survival is adversely affected if there are delays in diagnosis of cardiac arrest and starting CPR. This must be avoided.
6(B)	Shout for help (if not done already).	To obtain assistance and so colleagues can call the resuscitation team.
7(B)	Position the patient on their back. Open the airway using head tilt and chin lift Look in the mouth. Remove any visible debris with forceps or suction.	To assess for any obstruction to the upper respiratory tract and obtain a clear airway.
7(C,i)	Maintain an open airway and look, listen and feel to determine if the patient is breathing normally. This should take less than 10 s. That is: ■ look for chest movement, any other movement or signs of life ■ listen at the patient's mouth for breath sounds ■ feel for air on your cheek.	To rapidly diagnose cardiac arrest and avoid delay in commencing CPR if necessary. Evidence shows that even trained healthcare staff cannot assess the pulse sufficiently reliably to confirm cardiac arrest.
7(D,i)	If the patient does not have signs of life (based on lack of purposeful movement, normal breathing, coughing), start CPR until more help arrives or the patient shows signs of life.	To commence CPR as soon as possible. Agonal breathing (occasional gasps, slow, laboured, or noisy breathing) is common in the early stages of cardiac arrest and is a sign of cardiac arrest and should not be confused as a sign of life. Agonal breathing can also occur during chest compressions as cerebral perfusion improves, but is not indicative of a return of spontaneous circulation.
7(C,ii)	If competent in the assessment of sick patients, check for breathing and assess the carotid pulse at the same time. The whole assessment should take less than 10 s.	Absence of a carotid pulse provides further evidence to support diagnosis of cardiac arrest and commence CPR.
7(D,ii)	If the patient has no signs of life, no pulse, or if there is any doubt, start CPR immediately.	Starting CPR on a very sick patient with a low cardiac output is unlikely to be harmful and may be beneficial.
8(B)	Assess the patient to confirm cardiac arrest even if the patient is monitored in a critical care area.	A rapid clinical assessment of the patient is essential to confirm cardiac arrest. Patient monitors will provide useful information and alerts but do not make the diagnosis.
9(B)	If there is a risk of cervical spine injury, establish a clear upper airway by using jaw thrust or chin lift in combination with manual in-line stabilization (MILS) of the head and neck by an assistant (if enough personnel are available).	To reduce the risk of worsening any existing cervical spine injury. The jaw thrust is required if there is a risk of cervical spine injury. However, establishing a patent airway, oxygenation and ventilation takes priority over concerns about a potential cervical spine injury. If life-threatening airway obstruction persists despite effective application of jaw thrust or chin lift, add head tilt a small amount at a time until the airway is open.
10(A)	*If there is a pulse or other signs of life:* ■ call for urgent medical assessment ■ assess the patient using the ABCDE approach ■ give oxygen ■ attach monitoring ■ gain intravenous access.	To ensure the patient has appropriate review and treatment as soon as possible. The patient is at high risk of further deterioration and cardiac arrest and needs continued observation until the team arrives. Follow the actions and rationale from action 5a.

(Continued)

Procedure guideline 18.1: (Continued)

10(B) *If there is no pulse or signs of life:*

- continue CPR following the resuscitation guidance provided by Resuscitation Council (UK) and ask a colleague to call the resuscitation team.
- if alone, leave the patient to get help and equipment.
- bring the resuscitation equipment and a defibrillator to the patient.

To use an evidence-based technique to resuscitate the patient. To avoid interruptions to CPR and reduce 'no-flow time'.

To ensure expert resuscitation practitioners and equipment are on coming before starting CPR. Chest compressions and ventilations alone buy time, but alone are unlikely to be effective for successful resuscitation.

Resuscitation technique

Chest compressions

(a) Quickly place the heel of one hand in the centre of the chest with the other hand on top. The hands should be in the middle of the lower half of the sternum.

(a) To ensure the hands are in the correct position for chest compressions.

(b) Give 30 chest compressions followed by 2 ventilations. Provide chest compressions at a depth of 5–6 cm and a rate of 100–120 compressions/min.

(b) To ensure high-quality chest compressions.

(c) Allow the chest to recoil completely after each compression. Take about the same amount for compression and relaxation of chest wall and minimize interruptions to chest compression (hands-off time).

(c) To avoid a reduction in coronary perfusion pressure caused by incomplete recoil of chest at end of each chest compression. To reduce 'no-flow time'.

(d) A feedback device and/or prompt may be used if available.

(d) To help ensure high-quality chest compressions. A palpable carotid or femoral pulse is not reliable for assessing effective arterial flow.

(e) The person doing chest compressions should change every 2 minutes when possible.

(e) The person doing chest compressions will get tired and may not be able to maintain high-quality chest compressions. The change in the person doing compressions should be done with minimal interruption (Resuscitation Council UK 2010).

Airway and ventilation

(f) Use whatever equipment is immediately available for airway and ventilation.
A pocket mask may be used with an oral airway and should be readily available.
Use a supraglottic airway device (e.g. laryngeal mask airway [LMA]) and self-inflating bag or bag mask if competent and according to local policy.

(f) The patient may require an airway adjunct to maintain an open airway and ensure adequate ventilations. Tracheal intubation is only recommended if someone who is trained, competent and experienced is available. Otherwise simple airway manoeuvres, airway adjuncts and a bag mask should be used.

(g) Give breaths with an inspiratory time of about one second and enough volume to produce a visible chest rise. Avoid rapid or forceful breaths.

(g) Rapid forceful breaths can inflate the stomach as well as the lungs. This increases the chances of regurgitating gastric contents and lung injury due to aspiration of gastric contents.

(h) Add supplemental oxygen as soon as possible.

(h) To correct hypoxaemia by giving a high inspired oxygen concentration.

(i) If competent, intubate the patient's trachea. Intubation should be performed with minimal interruption in chest compression. Monitor end-tidal carbon dioxide with waveform capnography.

(i) Tracheal intubation enables continuous chest compressions (see below). Prolonged interruptions in chest compressions worsen chances of survival. Waveform capnography should be routinely available for confirming tracheal tube placement (in the presence of a cardiac output and during CPR) and subsequent monitoring of an intubated patient. Waveform capnography can also be used to monitor the quality of CPR (Resuscitation Council UK 2010).

(j) Once the patient's trachea is intubated, continue chest compressions uninterrupted (except for defibrillation or pulse checks) at a rate of 100–120/min and ventilate the lungs at approximately 10 breaths/min (e.g. do not stop chest compressions for ventilation).

(k) Consider mouth-to-mouth ventilation if airway and ventilation equipment are not available. If there are clinical reasons to avoid mouth-to-mouth contact, continue chest compressions until help or airway equipment arrives.

When the defibrillator is available

(l) Apply self-adhesive defibrillation electrode pads to the patient and analyse the cardiac rhythm. Electrode pads should be applied while chest compressions are ongoing.

(m) For automated external defibrillation (AED) users, switch on the machine and follow the audiovisual prompts.

(n) For manual defibrillation, deliver a shock while minimizing the interruption to chest compressions.

(o) Assess the heart rhythm during a brief pause in chest compressions. If the rhythm is 'shockable' (ventricular fibrillation/pulseless ventricular tachycardia), charge the defibrillator and restart chest compressions.

(p) When the defibrillator is charged and everyone except for the person doing chest compressions is clear, pause the chest compressions, rapidly ensure everyone is clear of the patient and then deliver the shock.

(q) Restart chest compressions immediately after the shock is delivered.
Continue resuscitation until the resuscitation team arrives, or the patient shows signs of life, or until the next rhythm assessment after 2 minutes.

(r) Use a watch or clock to time cycles of about 2 minutes.

11(A) *If the patient is not breathing and has a pulse (respiratory arrest)*
Ventilate the patient's lungs (see 10(B)(g), 10(B)(h), 10(B)(i) airway and ventilation).
Check for a pulse every 10 breaths (about every minute).

(j) To reduce the 'no flow' time and improve chances of successful resuscitation.

(k) To minimize risks to resuscitator. In most clinical areas equipment for ventilation should be immediately available. Starting chest compressions while awaiting airway equipment should not result in a significant delay.

(l) To enable rapid assessment of heart rhythm. Use of adhesive electrode pads as opposed to defibrillation paddles enables chest compressions to continue while the pads are applied.

(m) AEDs allow those who are not confident in rhythm recognition to use a defibrillator by following the audiovisual prompts. The AED will advise a shock if the patient has a shockable rhythm.

(n) Manual defibrillators allow brief pauses for rhythm assessment and shock delivery. They can also be charged during chest compressions. Minimizing interruptions in chest compressions ('no-flow time' or 'hands-off time') improves survival.

(o) The length of the pre-shock pause, the interval between stopping chest compressions and delivering a shock, is inversely proportional to the chance of successful defibrillation. Every 5-second increase in the duration of the pre-shock pause almost halves the chance of successful defibrillation, therefore it is critical to minimize the pause (Edelson et al. 2006).

(p) To minimize the 'no-flow time' while ensuring the safety of resuscitation practitioners.

(q) To minimize 'no-flow time'. Successful defibrillation is not always apparent immediately after shock delivery. Chest compressions should therefore resume for 2 minutes, unless the patient shows signs of life such as regaining consciousness and purposeful movement.

(r) To help plan any interruption to CPR before completing the cycle (Resuscitation Council UK 2010).

All patients in respiratory arrest will develop cardiac arrest if the respiratory arrest is not treated rapidly and effectively (Meaney et al. 2010).

(Continued)

Procedure guideline 18.1: *(Continued)*

11(B) *If the patient has a monitored and witnessed cardiac arrest on cardiac surgery critical care unit or cardiac catheter laboratory* Confirm cardiac arrest and shout for help. If the initial rhythm is VF/VT, give up to three quick, successive shocks. Start chest compressions immediately after the third shock and continue for 2 minutes.	To treat quickly patients who have a monitored and witnessed cardiac arrest in the catheter laboratory or early after cardiac surgery. Consider this three-shock strategy for an initial, witnessed VF/VT cardiac arrest if the patient is already connected to a manual defibrillator.
12 Document care and result.	To: ■ provide an accurate record ■ monitor effectiveness of procedure ■ reduce the risk of duplication of treatment ■ provide a point of reference or comparison in the event of later questions ■ acknowledge accountability for actions ■ facilitate communication and continuity of care. (NMC 2008; HCPC 2012; GMC 2013)

Data from Resuscitation Council (UK) 2010.

Competency statement 18.1: Specific procedure competency statements for recognition of cardiac arrest and starting CPR

(These standards are based on those used by the Resuscitation Council [UK])

Complete assessment against relevant fundamental competency statements (*see* Chapter 2, pp. 20, 21)

Specific procedure competency statements for recognition of cardiac arrest and starting CPR	Evidence of competency for recognition of cardiac arrest and starting CPR
Demonstrate ability to: ■ teach and assess or ■ learn from assessment.	Examples of evidence of teaching, assessing and learning.
Check responsiveness, open airway, look listen and feel for breathing to identify cardiac arrest and call for help.	On manikin – recognizes cardiac arrest, uses pulse check if trained to do so, calls for help. Discussion – understands that agonal breathing is a sign of cardiac arrest.
Starts high-quality CPR.	On manikin – provides CPR with correct hand position, depth, rate, duty cycle and recoil of compressions, 30:2 ratio. Avoids unnecessary interruptions in chest compression.

Competency statement 18.2: Specific procedure competency statements for defibrillation – AED

Complete assessment against relevant fundamental competency statements (*see* Chapter 2, pp. 20, 21)	Evidence
Specific procedure competency statements for defibrillation – AED	**Evidence of competency for defibrillation – AED**
Demonstrate ability to: ■ teach and assess or ■ learn from assessment.	Examples of evidence of teaching, assessing and learning.
Demonstrates safe and effective use of an automated external defibrillator.	On manikin – switches on AED and correctly follows AED audiovisual prompts. Correct pad placement and safe shock delivery.

Competency statement 18.3: Specific procedure competency statements for defibrillation – manual

Complete assessment against relevant fundamental competency statements (*see* Chapter 2, pp. 20, 21)	Evidence
Specific procedure competency statements for defibrillation – manual	**Evidence of competency for defibrillation – manual**
Demonstrate ability to: ■ teach and assess or ■ learn from assessment.	Examples of evidence of teaching, assessing and learning.
Before defibrillation – identifies skill levels and allocates tasks accordingly.	On manikin – identifies shockable rhythm and prepares team; explains sequence team will follow to minimize interruptions to chest compression; allocates roles.
Demonstrates safe shock delivery with minimal interruption to chest compression.	On manikin – pads applied, rhythm check, team stands clear except person doing chest compressions, defibrillator charged, compressions stop, shock delivery, resume CPR.

Competency statement 18.4: Specific procedure competency statements for airway assessment and ventilation

Complete assessment against relevant fundamental competency statements (see Chapter 2, pp. 20, 21)	Evidence
Specific procedure competency statements for airway assessment and ventilation	**Evidence of competency for airway assessment and ventilation**
Demonstrate ability to: ■ teach and assess or ■ learn from assessment.	Examples of evidence of teaching, assessing and learning.
Open the airway using head tilt/chin lift and jaw thrust manoeuvre, establishing patency. Demonstrates use of suction.	On manikin – airway is cleared and opened.
Demonstrate correct sizing and insertion of oropharyngeal and nasopharyngeal airway.	On manikin – open airway with use of adjuncts.
Demonstrate effective ventilation using a self-inflating bag-mask with supplemental oxygen.	On-manikin – ensure visible chest rise on ventilation at correct rate.
Demonstrates the use of a supraglottic airway, e.g. laryngeal mask airway.	On manikin – correct insertion procedure and visible chest rise on ventilation.
Can prepare equipment and assist during rapid sequence induction and tracheal intubation.	On manikin – prepares equipment, including waveform capnography, demonstrates assistance during tracheal intubation.

References

Abella BS, Alvarado JP, Myklebust H et al. (2005) Quality of cardiopulmonary resuscitation during in-hospital cardiac arrest. *Journal of the American Medical Association* **293**: 305–310.

Aiken LH, Clarke SP, Sloane DM et al. (2002) Hospital nurse staffing and patient mortality, nurse burnout, and job dissatisfaction. *Journal of the American Medical Association* **288**: 1987–1993.

Academy of Medical Royal Colleges (2008) *A Code of Practice for the Diagnosis and Confirmation of Death*. London: Academy of Medical Royal Colleges. http://www.aomrc.org.uk/publications/reports-a-guidance/doc_details/42-a-code-of-practice-for-the-diagnosis-and-confirmation-of-death.html

Baskett PJ (1994) The use of the laryngeal mask airway by nurses during cardiopulmonary resuscitation: results of a multicentre trial. *Anaesthesia* **49**: 3–7.

Baskett P, Nolan J and Parr M (1996) Tidal volumes which are perceived to be adequate for resuscitation. *Resuscitation* **31**(3): 231–234.

Bernhard M, Mohr S, Weigand MA et al. (2012) Developing the skill of endotracheal intubation: implication for emergency medicine. *Acta Anaesthesiologica Scandinavica* **56**: 164–71.

Bobrow BJ, Zuercher M, Ewy GA et al. (2008) Gasping during cardiac arrest in humans is frequent and associated with improved survival. *Circulation* **118**: 2550–2554.

Breitkreutz R, Price S, Steiger HV et al. (2010) Focused echocardiographic evaluation in life support and peri-resuscitation of emergency patients: a prospective trial. *Resuscitation* **81**: 1527–1533.

Callaway CW (2012) Questioning the use of epinephrine to treat cardiac arrest. *Journal of the American Medical Association* **307**: 1198–1200.

Chan PS, Krumholz HM, Nichol G and Nallamothu BK (2008) Delayed time to defibrillation after in-hospital cardiac arrest. *New England Journal of Medicine* **358**: 9–17.

Chan PS, Krumholz HM, Spertus JA et al. (2010) Automated external defibrillators and survival after in-hospital cardiac arrest. *Journal of the American Medical Association* **304**: 2129–2136.

Christenson J, Andrusiek D, Everson-Stewart S et al. (2009) Chest compression fraction determines survival in patients with out-of-hospital ventricular fibrillation. *Circulation* **120**: 1241–1247.

Cook TM, Woodall N, Harper J and Benger J (2011) Major complications of airway management in the UK: results of the Fourth National Audit Project of the Royal College of Anaesthetists and the Difficult Airway Society. Part 2: intensive care and emergency departments. *British Journal of Anaesthesia* **106b**: 632–642.

Collard CD and Gelman S (2001) Pathophysiology, clinical manifestations and prevention of ischemia-reperfusion injury. *Anesthesiology* **94**: 1133–1138.

Deakin CD, Nolan JP, Soar J et al. (2010a) European Resuscitation Council Guidelines for Resuscitation 2010 Section 4. Adult advanced life support. *Resuscitation* **81**: 1305–1352.

Deakin CD, Nolan JP, Sunde K and Koster RW (2010b) European Resuscitation Council Guidelines for Resuscitation 2010 Section 3. Electrical therapies: automated external defibrillators, defibrillation, cardioversion and pacing. *Resuscitation* **81**: 1293–1304.

De Groot H and Rauen U (2007) Ischemia-reperfusion injury: process in pathogenetic networks: a review. *Transplant Proceedings* **39**: 481–484.

Dougherty L and Lister S (eds) (2011) *The Royal Marsden Hospital Manual of Clinical Nursing Procedures* (8e). Oxford: Wiley-Blackwell.

Dyson E and Smith GB (2002) Common faults in resuscitation equipment – guidelines for checking equipment and drugs used in adult cardiopulmonary resuscitation. *Resuscitation* 55: 137–149.

Edelson DP, Abella BS, Kramer-Johansen J et al. (2006) Effects of compression depth and pre-shock pauses predict defibrillation failure during cardiac arrest. *Resuscitation* 71: 137–145.

Edelson DP, Litzinger B, Arora V et al. (2008) Improving in-hospital cardiac arrest process and outcomes with performance debriefing. *Archives of Internal Medicine* 168: 1063–1069.

Edelson DP, Robertson-Dick BJ, Yuen TC et al. (2010) Safety and efficacy of defibrillator charging during ongoing chest compressions: a multi-center study. *Resuscitation* 81: 1521–1526.

Finfer S, Chittock DR, Su SY et al. (NICE-SUGAR Study Investigators) (2009) Intensive versus conventional glucose control in critically ill patients. *New England Journal of Medicine* 360(13): 1283–1297.

Flin R, Patey R, Glavin R and Maran N (2010) Anaesthetists' non-technical skills. *British Journal of Anaesthiology* 105: 38–44.

Frenneaux M (2003) Cardiopulmonary resuscitation; some physiological considerations. *Resuscitation* 58: 259–265.

Gabbott D, Smith G, Mitchell S et al. (2005) Cardiopulmonary resuscitation standards for clinical practice and training in the UK. *Resuscitation* 64: 13–19.

General Medical Council (2013) *Good Medical Practice*. London: GMC. http://www.gmc-uk.org/gmp2013 [accessed 25 March 2013].

Gibbison B and Soar J (2011) Automated external defibrillator use for in-hospital cardiac arrest is not associated with improved survival. *Evidence Based Medicine* 16: 95–6.

Grasner JT, Herlitz J, Koster RW et al. (2011) Quality management in resuscitation–towards a European cardiac arrest registry (EuReCa). *Resuscitation* 82: 989–994.

Health and Care Professions Council (2012) *Standard of Conduct, Performance and Ethics*. London: HCPC. http://www.hcpc-uk.org/assets/documents/10003B6EStandardsofconduct,performance andethics.pdf [accessed January 2013].

Heradstveit BE, Sunde K, Sunde GA et al. (2012) Factors complicating interpretation of capnography during advanced life support in cardiac arrest – a clinical retrospective study in 575 patients. *Resuscitation* 83(7): 813–818.

Hoke RS, Heinroth K, Trappe HJ and Werdan K (2009) Is external defibrillation an electric threat for bystanders? *Resuscitation* 80: 395–401.

Hostler D, Everson-Stewart S, Rea TD et al. (2011) Effect of real-time feedback during cardiopulmonary resuscitation outside hospital: prospective, cluster-randomised trial. *British Medical Journal* 342: d512.

Jacobs IG, Finn JC, Jelinek GA et al. (2011) Effect of adrenaline on survival in out-of-hospital cardiac arrest: A randomised double-blind placebo-controlled trial. *Resuscitation* 82: 1138–1143.

Konrad C, Schupfer G, Wietlisbach M and Gerber H (1998) Learning manual skills in anesthesiology: Is there a recommended number of cases for anesthetic procedures? *Anesthesia and Analgesia* 86: 635–639.

Kudenchuk PJ (1999) Intravenous antiarrhythmic drug therapy in the resuscitation from refractory ventricular arrhythmias. *American Journal of Cardiology* 84: 52R–55R.

Kudenchuk PJ, Cobb LA, Copass MK et al. (1999) Amiodarone for resuscitation after out-of-hospital cardiac arrest due to ventricular fibrillation. *New England Journal of Medicine* 341: 871–878.

Kutsogiannis DJ, Bagshaw SM, Laing B and Brindley PG (2011) Predictors of survival after cardiac or respiratory arrest in critical care units. *Canadian Medical Association Journal* 183(14): 1589–1595.

Larkin C, King B, D'agapeyeff A and Gabbott D (2012) iGel supraglottic airway use during hospital cardiopulmonary resuscitation. *Resuscitation* 83(6): e141.

Laver S, Farrow C, Turner D and Nolan J (2004) Mode of death after admission to an intensive care unit following cardiac arrest. *Intensive Care Medicine* 30(11): 2126–2128.

Meaney PA, Nadkarni VM, Kern KB et al. (2010) Rhythms and outcomes of adult in-hospital cardiac arrest. *Critical Care Medicine* 38: 101-1-8.

Mental Capacity Act (2005) http://www.legislation.gov.uk/ukpga/2005/9/pdfs/ukpga_20050009_en.pdf [accessed 9 February 2012].

National Institute for Health and Clinical Excellence (2007) *NICE clinical guideline 50. Acutely Ill Patients in Hospital: recognition of and response to acute illness in adults in hospital*. London: NICE.

National Patient Safety Agency (2004) *NPSA Patient Safety Alert 02. Establishing a standard crash call telephone number in hospitals*. London: NPSA.

National Patient Safety Agency (2012) *National Patient Safety Agency National Reporting and Learning Service Signal – diagnosis of death after cessation of cardiopulmonary resuscitation*. London: NPSA.

Needleman J, Buerhaus P, Mattke S et al. (2002) Nurse-staffing levels and the quality of care in hospitals. *New England Journal of Medicine* 346: 1715–1722.

Niles DE, Sutton RM, Nadkarni VM et al. (2011) Prevalence and hemodynamic effects of leaning during CPR. *Resuscitation* 82(Suppl 2): S23–26.

Nolan J (2011) *Advanced Life Support*. London: Resuscitation Council (UK).

Nolan JP and Soar J (2008) Airway techniques and ventilation strategies. *Current Opinion in Critical Care* 14: 279–286.

Nolan JP and Soar J (2010) Postresuscitation care: entering a new era. *Current Opinion in Critical Care* 16: 216–222.

Nolan J, Soar J and Eikeland H (2006) The chain of survival. *Resuscitation* 71: 270–271.

Nolan JP, Laver SR, Welch CA et al. (2007) Outcome following admission to UK intensive care units after cardiac arrest: a secondary analysis of the ICNARC Case Mix Programme Database. *Anaesthesia* 62: 1207–1216.

Nolan JP, Neumar RW, Adrie C et al. (2008) Post-cardiac arrest syndrome: epidemiology, pathophysiology, treatment, and prognosis. A Scientific Statement from the International Liaison Committee on Resuscitation; the American Heart Association Emergency Cardiovascular Care Committee; the Council on Cardiovascular Surgery and Anesthesia; the Council on Cardiopulmonary, Perioperative, and Critical Care; the Council on Clinical Cardiology; the Council on Stroke. *Resuscitation* 79: 350–379.

Nolan JP, Hazinski MF, Billi JE et al. (2010a) Part 1: Executive summary: 2010 International Consensus on Cardiopulmonary Resuscitation and Emergency Cardiovascular Care Science With Treatment Recommendations. *Resuscitation* 81(Suppl 1): e1–25.

Nolan JP, Soar J, Zideman DA et al. (2010b) European Resuscitation Council Guidelines for Resuscitation 2010 Section 1. Executive summary. *Resuscitation* 81: 1219–1276.

Nursing and Midwifery Council (2008) *The Code: standards of conduct, performance and ethics for nurses and midwives*. London: NMC. http://www.nmc-uk.org/Documents/Standards/The-code-A4-20100406.pdf [accessed 15 February 2012].

O'Driscoll BR, Howard LS and Davison AG (2008) BTS guideline for emergency oxygen use in adult patients. *Thorax* 63(Suppl 6): vi1–68.

Olasveengen TM (2012) Can drugs ever improve outcome after cardiac arrest? *Resuscitation* 83(6): 663–664.

Olasveengen TM, Sunde K, Brunborg C et al. (2009) Intravenous drug administration during out-of-hospital cardiac arrest: a randomized trial. *Journal of the American Medical Association* 302: 2222–2229.

Paradis NA, Martin GB, Rivers EP et al. (1990) Coronary perfusion pressure and the return of spontaneous circulation in human cardiopulmonary resuscitation. *Journal of the American Medical Association* 263(8): 1106–1113.

Peberdy MA, Ornato JP, Larkin GL et al. (2008) Survival from in-hospital cardiac arrest during nights and weekends. *Journal of the American Medical Association* 299: 785–792.

Perkins G and Lockey A (2002) The advanced life support provider course. *British Medical Journal* 325: S81.

Petley GW, Cotton AM and Deakin CD (2011) Hands-on defibrillation: theoretical and practical aspects of patient and rescuer safety. *Resuscitation* 83(5): 551–556.

Price S, Ilper H, Uddin S et al. (2010) Peri-resuscitation echocardiography: training the novice practitioner. *Resuscitation* 81: 1534–1539.

Resuscitation Council (UK) (2009) *Guidance for Safer Handling During Resuscitation in Healthcare Settings*. London: Resuscitation Council (UK).

Resuscitation Council (UK) (2010) *Resuscitation Guidelines 2010*. London: Resuscitation Council (UK).

Ruppert M, Reith MW, Widmann JH et al. (1999) Checking for breathing: evaluation of the diagnostic capability of emergency medical services personnel, physicians, medical students, and medical laypersons. *Annals of Emergency Medicine* 34: 720–729.

Smith GB (2010) In-hospital cardiac arrest: is it time for an in-hospital 'chain of prevention'? *Resuscitation* 81: 1209–1211.

Soar J, Mancini ME, Bhanji F et al. (2010) Part 12: Education, implementation, and teams: 2010 International Consensus on Cardiopulmonary Resuscitation and Emergency Cardiovascular Care Science with Treatment Recommendations. *Resuscitation* 81(Suppl 1): e288–330.

Soar J, Perkins GD, Harris S et al. (2003) The immediate life support course. *Resuscitation* 57: 21–26.

Spearpoint KG, Gruber PC and Brett SJ (2009) Impact of the Immediate Life Support course on the incidence and outcome of in-hospital cardiac arrest calls: an observational study over 6 years. *Resuscitation* 80: 638–643.

Stone BJ, Chantler PJ and Baskett PJ (1998) The incidence of regurgitation during cardiopulmonary resuscitation: a comparison between the bag valve mask and laryngeal mask airway. *Resuscitation* 38: 3–6.

Sugerman NT, Edelson DP, Leary M et al. (2009) Rescuer fatigue during actual in-hospital cardiopulmonary resuscitation with audiovisual feedback: a prospective multicenter study. *Resuscitation* 80: 981–984.

Tortora GJ and Derrickson B (2011) *Principles of Anatomy and Physiology* (13e). New Jersey: John Wiley and Sons.

Tourangeau AE, Cranley LA and Jeffs L (2006) Impact of nursing on hospital patient mortality: a focused review and related policy implications. *Quality and Safety in Health Care* 15: 4–8.

Wang HE, Simeone SJ, Weaver MD and Callaway CW (2009) Interruptions in cardiopulmonary resuscitation from paramedic endotracheal intubation. *Annals of Emergency Medicine* 54: 645–652 e1.

Weiser G, Hoffmann Y, Galbraith R and Shavit I (2012) Current advances in intraosseous infusion – a systematic review. *Resuscitation* 83: 20–26.

White L, Rogers J, Bloomingdale M et al. (2010) Dispatcher-assisted cardiopulmonary resuscitation: risks for patients not in cardiac arrest. *Circulation* 121: 91–97.

Yang CW, Yen ZS, McGowan JE et al. (2012) A systematic review of retention of adult advanced life support knowledge and skills in healthcare providers. *Resuscitation* 83(9): 1055–1060.

Yeung J, Meeks R, Edelson D et al. (2009) The use of CPR feedback/prompt devices during training and CPR performance: a systematic review. *Resuscitation* 80: 743–751.

Useful websites

European Resuscitation Council: www.erc.edu
International Liaison Committee on Resuscitation (ILCOR): www.ilcor.org
Resuscitation Council UK: www.resus.org.uk

Index

Critical Care Manual of Clinical Procedures and Competencies, First Edition.
Edited by Jane Mallett, John W. Albarran, and Annette Richardson.
© 2013 John Wiley & Sons, Ltd. Published 2013 by John Wiley & Sons, Ltd.